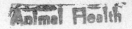

THE MYCOPLASMAS

VOLUME II

THE MYCOPLASMAS

EDITORS

M. F. Barile

Mycoplasma Branch
Bureau of Biologics
Food and Drug Administration
Bethesda, Maryland

S. Razin

Biomembrane Research Laboratory
Department of Clinical Microbiology
The Hebrew University–Hadassah Medical School
Jerusalem, Israel

J. G. Tully

Mycoplasma Section
Laboratory of Infectious Diseases
National Institute of Allergy and Infectious Diseases
National Institutes of Health
Bethesda, Maryland

R. F. Whitcomb

Plant Protection Institute
Federal Research, Science and Education Administration
U.S. Department of Agriculture
Beltsville, Maryland

THE MYCOPLASMAS

VOLUME II

Human and Animal Mycoplasmas

Edited by

J. G. TULLY

Mycoplasma Section
Laboratory of Infectious Diseases
National Institute of Allergy and Infectious Diseases
National Institutes of Health
Bethesda, Maryland

and

R. F. WHITCOMB

Plant Protection Institute
Federal Research, Science and Education Administration
U.S. Department of Agriculture
Beltsville, Maryland

ACADEMIC PRESS New York San Francisco London 1979
A Subsidiary of Harcourt Brace Jovanovich, Publishers

ACADEMIC PRESS, INC.
111 Fifth Avenue, New York, New York 10003

United Kingdom Edition published by
ACADEMIC PRESS, INC. (LONDON) LTD.
24/28 Oval Road, London NW1 7DX

Library of Congress Cataloging in Publication Data
Main entry under title:

The Mycoplasmas.

  Includes bibliographies.
  CONTENTS: v. 1. Cell biology. v. 2. Host parasite
interrelationships.
  1. Mycoplasmacales. 2. Mycoplasma diseases.
I. Barile, Michael Frederick, (Date)   [DNLM:
1. Mycoplasma.   QW143 M9973]
QR352.M89   589.9   78–20895
ISBN 0–12–078402–5

PRINTED IN THE UNITED STATES OF AMERICA

79 80 81 82   9 8 7 6 5 4 3 2 1

CONTENTS

Contents vii

IV. Classification   220
V.   Identification   223
VI. Canine and Feline Mycoplasma Flora   224
VII. Host–Parasite Interaction   229
     References   233

8 / MURINE AND OTHER SMALL-ANIMAL MYCOPLASMAS
Gail H. Cassell and Auriol Hill

I.   Introduction   235
II. Murine Mycoplasmas   236
III. Mycoplasmas of Other Small Animals   261
IV. Detection and Control: Remaining Problems and Future Outlook   264
     References   268

9 / *Mycoplasma pneumoniae* INFECTIONS OF MAN
Wallace A. Clyde, Jr.

I.   Introduction   275
II. Epidemiology   279
III. Disease Characteristics   281
IV. Diagnosis   289
V.   Therapy   296
VI. Prevention   298
     References   302

10 / MYCOPLASMAS IN HUMAN GENITOURINARY INFECTIONS
David Taylor-Robinson and William M. McCormack

I.   Mycoplasmas in the Human Genitourinary Tract   308
II.   Collection and Handling of Specimens for the Isolation of Genital
      Mycoplasmas   310
III. Methods Used for the Laboratory Diagnosis of Genital Mycoplasmal
      Infection   312
IV.   Epidemiology   315
V.   Role of Genital Mycoplasmas in Diseases of Men   321
VI.   Role of Genital Mycoplasmas in Diseases of Women   331
VII. Role of Genital Mycoplasmas in Disorders of the Urinary Tract   339
VIII. Role of Genital Mycoplasmas in Disorders of Reproduction   342
IX.   Conclusions   357
      References   357

11 / MYCOPLASMAS AS ARTHRITOGENIC AGENTS
Barry C. Cole and John R. Ward

I.   Introduction   367
II. Mycoplasma-Induced Arthritis in Animals   368

LIST OF CONTRIBUTORS

Numbers in parentheses indicate the pages on which the authors' contributions begin.

Michael F. Barile (425), Mycoplasma Branch, Division of Bacterial Products, Bureau of Biologics, Food and Drug Administration, Bethesda, Maryland 20014

Gail H. Cassell (235), Department of Microbiology, University of Alabama in Birmingham, Birmingham, Alabama 35294

Wallace A. Clyde, Jr. (275), Departments of Pediatrics and Microbiology and Immunology, University of North Carolina School of Medicine, Chapel Hill, North Carolina 27514

Barry C. Cole (191, 367), Division of Arthritis, Departments of Medicine and Microbiology, University of Utah College of Medicine, Salt Lake City, Utah 84132

Albert M. Collier (475), Department of Pediatrics and Frank Porter Graham Child Development Center, University of North Carolina School of Medicine, Chapel Hill, North Carolina 27514

G. S. Cottew (103), C.S.I.R.O. Division of Animal Health, Animal Health Research Laboratory, Parkville, Melbourne, Victoria 3052, Australia

Gerald W. Fernald (399), Department of Pediatrics, University of North Carolina School of Medicine, Chapel Hill, North Carolina 27514

R. N. Gourlay (49), Agricultural Research Council, Institute for Research on Animal Diseases, Compton, Newbury, Berkshire RG16 ONN, England

Auriol Hill (235), Medical Research Council, Laboratory Animals Centre, Woodmansterne Road, Carshalton, Surrey SM5 4EF, England

C. J. Howard (49), Agricultural Research Council, Institute for Research on Animal Diseases, Compton, Newbury, Berkshire RG16 ONN, England

F. T. W. Jordan (1), Subdepartment of Avian Medicine, University of Liverpool Veterinary Field Station, Leahurst, Neston, Wirral L64 7TE, England

Ruth M. Lemcke (177), Agricultural Research Council, Institute for Research on Animal Diseases, Compton, Newbury, Berkshire RG16 ONN, England

William M. McCormack [1] (307), Channing Laboratory, Harvard Medical School, Boston, Massachusetts

Søren Rosendal [2] (217), FAO/WHO Collaborating Center for Animal Mycoplasmas, Institute of Medical Microbiology, University of Aarhus, Aarhus C, DK 8000, Denmark

Norman L. Somerson (191), Department of Medical Microbiology, Ohio State University College of Medicine, Columbus, Ohio 43210

David Taylor-Robinson (307), Division of Communicable Diseases, MRC Clinical Research Centre, Watford Road, Harrow, Middlesex, England

John R. Ward (367), Department of Medicine, University of Utah College of Medicine, Salt Lake City, Utah 84132

P. Whittlestone (133), University of Cambridge, Department of Clinical Veterinary Medicine, Cambridge CB3 OES, England

[1] Present address: State Laboratory Institute, 305 South Street, Jamaica Plain, Massachusetts 02130.

[2] Present address: Department of Veterinary Microbiology and Immunology, Ontario Veterinary College, University of Guelph, Guelph, Ontario N1G2W1, Canada.

FOREWORD

Mycoplasmas are of consuming interest to biologists as intellectual puzzles for a variety of good reasons: they are the smallest known free-living creatures; their surfaces offer relatively clean models for the study of biological membranes; their viruses represent yet-open ground for students of phage; and their taxonomy and wide distribution in nature, in both animals and plants, are still complicated matters for those concerned with systematics and evolution.

They are, in addition, a problem for medicine. It is hard to imagine a class of microorganisms displaying so many instances of disease in so many species of animals—and now plants—with so few evidences of pathogenicity for man. Apart from primary atypical pneumonia, certain infections of the genitourinary system, and scattered reports of secondary invasion of the blood, the mycoplasmas appear to have stayed away from the human host. But the evidence for this is, of course, entirely negative: they are not cultivable from the tissues where they have, at various times, been suspected of being involved. Although there are striking analogies between the pathology of veterinary infections and human disease (rheumatoid arthritis and polyarteritis, for example), there is no immunologic evidence for infection by strains other than *M. pneumoniae* and the ureaplasmas.

It must be remembered, however, that it took something over 20 years of work by competent microbiology and virology laboratories before the Eaton agent was recognized as a mycoplasma, and the existence of plant pathogens has only recently come to light. The possibility still exists that other species of mycoplasma, still undetected, are subtly at work as disease agents in human beings, where they may be waiting to be found when the methods for isolating and growing such peculiar microorganisms are improved by more fundamental research into their nature.

Meanwhile, even if they turn out to be relatively nonpathogenic for humans, the mycoplasmas offer excellent models for the study of mechanisms of tissue damage in infection, perhaps containing answers to fundamental questions about the types of injury caused by unrelated, more conventional microbial agents. These models, readily available in experimental mycoplasma infections of laboratory animals (including, notably, poultry), permit study of the ways in which spectacularly widespread chronic granulomatous lesions, polyarteritis, arthritis, endocarditis, encephalitis, autoimmune reactions, pneumonia, and upper respiratory tract disease can be subjected to detailed study by experimental pathologists. The exotoxins of certain mycoplasmas and the toxicity demonstrable in suspensions of whole mycoplasma provide potentially informative models in themselves.

In particular, the exuberant infiltrations of infected tissues by lymphocytes, plasma cells, and macrophages, the multiplicity of autoimmune serological reactions, the vascular lesions resembling those of hypersensitivity, and the evidences, here and there, of cross-reactivity between mycoplasma antigens and those of the infected host all suggest the usefulness of these agents as models for research on the pathogenesis of human diseases believed to be based on autoimmunity, whether or not mycoplasmas are actually implicated in such diseases.

An enormous amount of work has been done on mycoplasma pathogenicity in animals, much of it summarized in the chapters of this volume, and a great deal more remains to be carried out. The sheer spadework of sorting out the pathogens from commensals and possible symbionts, and devising the cultural and immunologic techniques needed for specific identification, has required great effort on the part of many different laboratories, most of them committed to veterinary pathology. Much of the groundwork has thus been laid out in something like order, and one hopes that greater numbers of investigators primarily concerned with the mechanisms of human disease will now recognize the abundance of scientific opportunities and turn their attention to this rich field.

Lewis Thomas
Memorial Sloan-Kettering Cancer Center

PREFACE

"The Mycoplasmas," a comprehensive three-volume series, encompasses the various facets of mycoplasmology, emphasizing outstanding developments made in the field during the past decade. The pronounced information explosion in mycoplasmology was prompted primarily by the discovery of insect and plant mycoplasmas and mycoplasma viruses in the early 1970s, which attracted many new workers from different disciplines. During this period significant progress in the field of animal and human mycoplasmas was also made, providing important new insights into the nature of host–parasite relationships and into the mechanisms by which mycoplasmas infect and cause disease in man and animals.

Mycoplasmas are the smallest and simplest self-replicating microorganisms, and their use as models for the study of general biological problems has contributed considerably to our understanding of cell biology, particularly in the field of biological membranes. Volume I deals with the cell biology of the mycoplasmas, largely concentrating on problems regarding their classification, phylogenetics, and relatedness to wall-covered bacteria; their unique molecular biology, energy metabolism, transport mechanisms, antigenic structure, and membrane biochemistry. The characterization, ultrastructure, and molecular biology of the mycoplasma viruses, as well as the special properties of several groups of mycoplasmas, are also included.

Volume II is concerned with host–parasite relationships of mycoplasmas in man and animals. In part, emphasis is placed on recent developments in the study of classical mycoplasmal diseases of animals, such as cattle, sheep, goats, swine and chickens. On the other hand, new information on the host range of mycoplasmas made it necessary to describe the mycoplasma flora of hosts not previously known to harbor mycoplasmas (for example, equines) or to document the increasing number of new mycoplasmas found in some other animal hosts (as observed in canines, felines, and nonhuman primates). This volume also offered the opportunity to record current knowledge about mycoplasmal diseases of man, including those involving the respiratory and genitourinary tracts. Humoral and cellular immune responses to mycoplasmas, which are assuming an ever-increasing significance in our understanding of the pathogenesis of human and animal mycoplasmal diseases, are covered in detail. The volume closes with reviews on mycoplasmas as arthritogenic agents and the interaction of mycoplasmas with cell and organ cultures.

Volume III represents the first serious attempt not only to present an extensive and critical review of the rapidly expanding field of plant and insect mycoplasmas but to integrate these important new subdisciplines into the total field of mycoplasmology. Many of the contributions involve current information on an entirely new group of helical mycoplasmas (spiroplasmas), stressing their part in plant and insect diseases. Tick-borne spiroplasmas and their possible role in vertebrate disease are also discussed here. Additional coverage in this volume updates our knowledge of other suspected mycoplasmal plant diseases, as well as vector transmission of mycoplasmas and spiroplasmas, and discusses the chemotherapy of mycoplasmal plant diseases.

Thus, this three-volume series provides a standard reference work for every mycoplasmologist and a current exhaustive treatment of recent advances in mycoplasmology for other interested microbiologists, cellular and molecular biologists, membrane biochemists, clinicians, veterinarians, plant pathologists, and entomologists.

M. F. Barile
S. Razin
J. G. Tully
R. F. Whitcomb

1 / AVIAN MYCOPLASMAS

F. T. W. Jordan

I. INTRODUCTION

Organisms which would almost certainly now be regarded as avian mycoplasmas were first recovered by Nelson (1935) from fowl coryza. He described them as coccobacilliform bodies. In a series of experiments he

THE MYCOPLASMAS, VOL. II
Copyright © 1979 by Academic Press, Inc.
All rights of reproduction in any form reserved.
ISBN 0-12-078401-7

demonstrated the association of these organisms with disease of the upper respiratory tract in the chicken, either alone (Nelson, 1936a,b) or together with *Haemophilus gallinarum* (Nelson, 1938). He grew the organisms in chick embryos, cell culture (Nelson, 1936c,d), and cell-free medium (Nelson, 1939).

Further isolations of what were probably mycoplasmas were made by Delaplane and Stuart (1943) from chronic respiratory disease (CRD) of chickens and infectious sinusitis of turkeys. They considered the organism to be a virus. Van Herick and Eaton (1945) isolated a pleuro-pneumonia-like organism (PPLO) from chick embryos, and de Blieck (1948) recognized coryza in chickens due to coccobacilliform bodies. Markham and Wong (1952) showed that the agents associated with CRD and infectious sinusitis of turkeys could both be propagated in Edward's PPLO broth and suggested that both agents resembled PPLOs. Chu (1954) pointed out some of the difficulties of correlating disease and infection with these organisms. He indicated the probability of several different types varying in pathogenicity and reemphasized the importance of synergism with other pathogens.

The first published evidence for the existence of antigenically different strains of avian mycoplasmas was that of Adler *et al.* (1957) and Adler and Yamamoto (1957). Immunological and other differences among strains were demonstrated, and classification was attempted by various workers, including Adler *et al.* (1958), Yamamoto and Adler (1958a,b), Edward and Kanarek (1960), Kleckner (1960), Moore *et al.* (1960), Kelton and Van Roekel (1963), Roberts (1964), Yoder and Hofstad (1964), Dierks *et al.* (1967), Sabry (1968), and Barber (1969), culminating in the classification of Fabricant (1969). Procedures for classification have advanced in recent years, and the subject has received considerable stimulus from the Board of the WHO/FAO Programme on Comparative Mycoplasmology; the present position is indicated in Section II.

Avian mycoplasmas have been studied mainly in association with domestic poultry, and most of the recognized avian species have been isolated from these hosts. Their distribution seems to be worldwide. However, *Mycoplasma gallisepticum* has been isolated from pheasant (Osborn and Pomeroy, 1958), chuka partridge, *Alectoris graeca* (Wichmann, 1957; Yoder and Hofstad, 1964), peacock, *Pavo cristatus* (Wills, 1955), and bobwhite quail, *Colinus virginianus* (Madden *et al.*, 1967); *M. gallinarum* from a blackheaded gull, *Larus ridibundus* (Amin, 1977); *M. synoviae* from a guinea fowl, *Numida meleagridis* (Pascucci *et al.*, 1976); and *M. anatis* from a teal, *Anas crecca,* and a scaup, *Aythya marila*, from zoological gardens (Amin, 1977) and from several birds from aviaries (Amin, 1977). Serotype L has been recovered only from pigeons, and many untyped mycoplasmas have been recovered from poultry, wild birds, and birds from zoological gardens (Amin, 1977) and from pigeons (Gerlach, 1977; Shimizu *et al.*, 1978). Shimizu (1978) also isolated serotype D from many Galliformes and *M. gallinarum* from varieties of avian species.

There are also reports of some species of avian mycoplasmas being recovered from mammals (Taylor-Robinson and Dinter, 1968; Ernø *et al.*, 1973; R. H. Leach, 1977 personal communication).

In domestic poultry several species of mycoplasmas are of considerable economic importance because of their association with disease and reduced production, but in other avian species the significance of mycoplasma infection in disease is yet to be determined.

II. CLASSIFICATION

Mycoplasmas isolated from avian species are classified according to the criteria laid down by the ICSB Subcommittee on the Taxonomy of Mycoplasmatales (Subcommittee, 1972, 1978).

Currently there are 11 recognized avian species or serotypes of the genus *Mycoplasma*; three *Acholeplasma* species have been isolated from birds, and there are reports of recovery of ureaplasmas from chickens. The preponderance of isolates of typed and untyped organisms seem to be in the genus *Mycoplasma*.

Some details of the recognized species and serotypes are given below, although it is appreciated that taxonomically the serotype designation is outdated for organisms which possess a species name.

1. *Mycoplasma gallisepticum* (Edward and Kanarek, 1960). Serotype A (Kleckner, 1960); type strain PG31 (Edward and Freundt, 1973) was derived from strain X95 of Markham (Yoder and Hofstad, 1964), who recovered it from the respiratory tract of a chicken; it is probable that the coccobacilliform bodies of Nelson (1936b), de Blieck (1948), and Chu (1954) fall into this category; serotype S6 (Adler *et al.*, 1958; Zander, 1961) and serotype A (Kleckner, 1960; Yoder and Hofstad, 1964; and Dierks *et al.*, 1967) are strains of *M. gallisepticum*. This organism is associated with disease in chickens and turkeys. The species ferments glucose and does not hydrolyze arginine.

2. *Mycoplasma gallinarum* (Freundt, 1955). Serotype B (Kleckner, 1960); type strain PG16 (Edward and Freundt, 1956) was derived from strain "fowl" of Chu from the trachea of a chicken; B serotypes (Kleckner, 1960; Yoder and Hofstad, 1964; Dierks *et al.*, 1967) are strains of this species. The species seems to be generally apathogenic for the chicken and turkey, but its exact properties in this respect require further study.

Kleven *et al.* (1978) showed a synergistic effect with avian infectious bronchitis virus in causing air sacculitis in the chicken. It does not ferment glucose but it hydrolyzes arginine.

3. Serotype C (Adler *et al.*, 1958). Type strain CKK (adopted by the Board of the WHO/FAO Programme on Comparative Mycoplasmology, 1974) was originally isolated by Fabricant from the trachea of a chicken (Barber, 1969). Little is known of the pathogenicity of this serotype. It ferments glucose and does not hydrolyze arginine.

4. Serotype D (Kleckner, 1960). Type strain DD (adopted by the Board of the WHO/FAO Programme on Comparative Mycoplasmology, 1974) was originally isolated by Fabricant from the trachea of a chicken (Barber, 1969). Little is known of the pathogenicity of this serotype. It ferments glucose and does not hydrolyze arginine.

5. *Mycoplasma iners* (Edward and Kanarek, 1960). Serotype E (Kleckner, 1960); type strain PG30 (Edward and Kanarek, 1960) was derived from an isolate from the respiratory tract of a chicken (Barber and Fabricant, 1971). It seems to be nonpathogenic for the chicken and turkey. It does not ferment glucose but hydrolyzes arginine.

6. Serotype F (Kleckner, 1960). Type strain WR1 (adopted by the Board of the WHO/FAO Programme on Comparative Mycoplasmology, 1974) was originally isolated by Roberts (1963) from air sac lesions in adult turkeys. It causes air sacculitis in turkeys but not chickens following air sac inoculation (Roberts, 1963), but its role as a primary pathogen is doubtful (Wise *et al.*, 1970). It ferments glucose and does not hydrolyze arginine.

7. *Mycoplasma meleagridis* (Yamamoto *et al.*, 1965). Serotype H (Kleckner, 1960); type strain 17529 (Yamamoto and Bigland, 1964) was isolated from the infraorbital sinus of a turkey. The organism is pathogenic for turkeys but not chickens. It does not ferment glucose; it hydrolyzes arginine and shows phosphatase activity.

8. Serotype I [Yoder and Hofstad (1964), although they had previously (Yoder and Hofstad, 1962) designated it strain Iowa]. Type strain 695 (Yoder and Hofstad, 1962) was derived from air sac lesions of pipped turkey embryos. This serotype comprises the strains I, J, K, N, Q, and R of Dierks *et al.* (1967). Although they are all antigenically sufficiently similar to be included in this serotype, there are quantitative differences in antigenic components. The species kills turkey and chicken embryos and causes mild air sac lesions in turkeys and exudative lesions in the hock and foot pad of chicks following inoculation at these sites (Yoder and Hofstad, 1962). It ferments glucose and hydrolyzes arginine.

9. Serotype L (Yoder and Hofstad, 1964). Type strain 694 (adopted by the Board of the WHO/FAO Programme on Comparative Mycoplasmol-

ogy, 1974) was originally isolated from pigeon turbinates (Yoder and Hofstad, 1964). The pathogenicity of this strain has not been determined; it has only been recovered from pigeons under natural conditions. It does not ferment glucose; it hydrolyzes arginine and shows phosphatase activity.

10. *Mycoplasma synoviae* (Olson *et al.*, 1963). Serotype S (Dierks *et al.*, 1967); type strain WVU 1853 (Olson *et al.*, 1964), which was originally isolated from the purulent exudate from the hock joint of a broiler-type chicken, was referred to as "culture 8" (Olson *et al.*, 1957). The organism is pathogenic for the chicken and turkey. It has a specific requirement for nicotinamide adenine dinucleotide (NAD) in artificial culture; it ferments glucose and does not hydrolyze arginine.

11. *Mycoplasma anatis* (Roberts, 1964). The type strain is 1340 (adopted by the Board of the WHO/FAO Programme on Comparative Mycoplasmology, 1974). The organism causes lesions in ducks (Roberts, 1964; Amin and Jordan, 1978a), but its significance is still to be determined. It ferments glucose, does not hydrolyze arginine, and shows phosphatase activity.

12. *Acholeplasma laidlawii* (Freundt, 1955). Type strain PG8 (Edward and Freundt, 1973) was originally isolated from sewage (Laidlaw and Elford, 1936). It has been recovered from the infraorbital sinus of a chicken with coryza (Adler *et al.*, 1961; Adler and Shifrine, 1964; *Mycoplasma laidlawii* var. *inocuum*), and also from air sacculitis of goslings (Stipkovits *et al.*, 1975). It is of doubtful pathogenicity for chickens but kills goose embryos (Kisary *et al.*, 1976).

13. *Acholeplasma axanthum* (Tully and Razin, 1970). Type strain S743 (Tully and Razin, 1970) was recovered from murine tissue culture cell lines (Friend *et al.*, 1966). It has also been recovered from goose embryos (Stipkovits *et al.*, 1975). It is pathogenic for goose and chicken embryos and, together with a parvovirus, causes lesions in goslings (Kisary *et al.*, 1976).

14. *Acholeplasma equifetale* (Kirchhoff, 1974). Recently this organism was isolated from the trachea and cloaca of a broiler-type chicken (Amin, 1977) and identified (Bradbury, 1978).

15. *Mycoplasma columbinum* and *Mycoplasma columborale*. (Shimizu *et al.*, 1978). Recently these two species have been isolated from pigeons in Japan.

III. ISOLATION AND IDENTIFICATION

The isolation of avian mycoplasmas from field material is influenced by several factors (Table I) which can be classified into two main groups: (1)

those associated with the organs and tissues of the host, and (2) those concerned with the provision of growth requirements.

Recovery in many cases is perhaps more likely early in infection before the organisms have declined in number or have been eliminated from the host, or before the tissues have been invaded by other organisms. However, an increase in mycoplasma number, and thus ease of isolation, sometimes follows concomitant infection with certain pathogens such as the virus of avian infectious bronchitis or Newcastle disease (Corstvet and Sadler, 1966a; Jordan and Kulasegaram, 1968). That the reverse sometimes occurs has been shown by Amin (1977). The influence of multiple mycoplasma infection of a tissue on the isolation of one particular species has not been critically studied, although it is possible that mycoplasmas present in greater number and/or which grow more rapidly under the conditions provided might suppress the other(s).

Antimycoplasma substances, whether they be drugs in the tissue, antisera, or inhibitors released from tissues after death, may influence the recovery of these organisms (Tully and Rask-Nielsen, 1967; Kaklamanis *et al.*, 1969, 1971; Mårdh and Taylor-Robinson, 1973; Barile, 1974; Rashid and Jordan, 1978).

Various complex media have been used for the recovery of mycoplasmas from field material (Fabricant, 1969; Frey *et al.*, 1973; Barile, 1974; Whittlestone, 1974; Power and Jordan, 1976a). They all seem to support growth of the common avian pathogens. NAD is necessary for the

TABLE 1. **Factors Influencing the Isolation of Mycoplasma from Avian Field Material**

Those associated with the organs and tissues of the host:
  Duration of infection (number of viable organisms)
  Intercurrent infection with viruses, bacteria, molds, and multiple mycoplasmas
  Antimycoplasma substances—drugs, antisera, and tissue inhibitors
  Choice and quantity of tissue and/or exudate
  Transfer and treatment of tissue—swab, inoculum, homogenate, scrapings and washings
Those concerned with the provision of growth requirements:
  Artificial media
    Components (for growth; indicator of growth; inhibitors of contaminants)
    Form (agar, semisolid agar, overlay, broth)
    pH
    Temperature
    Humidity
    Gaseous environment
    Restreaking
  Embryonated eggs
  Organ culture
  Cell culture
  Complex adaptive techniques

isolation of *M. synoviae*. Agar, semisolid agar, broth, and overlay have all been advocated (Timms, 1967; Olson, 1978; Yamamoto, 1978; Yoder, 1978; Barile, 1974; Whittlestone, 1974), and it is common practice to inoculate more than one type of medium when attempting recovery from the field. A pH of 7.5 or more is usually used, except for ureaplasmas (Stipkovits, 1976; Koshimizu and Magaribuchi, 1977). A temperature of 36° or 37°C is usual, and additional carbon dioxide for the incubation of plates is recommended by Fabricant (1969) and Barile (1974). This had not been found necessary by Amin and Jordan (1978b) in the isolation of a wide variety of mycoplasmas from avian field material. Barile (1974) also advised "restreaking" for the growth of more fastidious organisms.

Chick embryo inoculation has been shown to be a sensitive method for the recovery of certain avian mycoplasmas (Fabricant, 1958, 1969). However, it may not be satisfactory for all strains and species of the organism, since Ghazikhanian and Yamamoto (1974b) showed that it did not support the growth of one laboratory-adapted strain of *M. meleagridis*. Organ culture and cell culture may be helpful in the recovery of fastidious mycoplasmas, but they should be from stock known to be mycoplasma-free, and their evaluation has yet to be undertaken. This applies also to the complex adaptive techniques advocated by Whittlestone (1974).

The recognition of an isolate from field material is based on the morphology of the colonies on agar medium and by serological methods such as their examination by immunofluorescence and/or by growth inhibition. Identification of an isolate by immunofluorescence can be rapidly performed using the method of Rosendal and Black (1972) or of Bradbury *et al.* (1976). These methods have the merit of readily detecting mixed cultures. Recently the agar gel precipitation test was advocated for the identification of an isolate (Aycardi *et al.*, 1971; Sahu and Olson, 1976a,b; Nonomura and Yoder, 1977).

The identification of a new isolate subsequent to cloning follows the procedure outlined by the ICSB subcommittee (Subcommittee, 1972, 1979) and includes biochemical and serological tests.

IV. MYCOPLASMAS IN DOMESTIC POULTRY

A. Species of Poultry and Species of Mycoplasmas

It is probable that mycoplasma infections of domestic chickens, turkeys, ducks, and geese existed prior to the isolation of coccobacillary bodies from a chronic respiratory disease of chickens by Nelson (1935).

However, intensive management and the increasing use of live vaccines, which have become a feature of poultry production over the last 25–30 years, have exacerbated and prolonged diseases of the respiratory tract and increased the transmission of mycoplasmas. Concomitant with this has been the rapid development of diagnostic techniques for recognizing the presence of mycoplasma infections, both by isolation of the organism and by serology. Thus their incidence is apparent wherever poultry are kept.

The mycoplasmas isolated from domestic poultry include those described in Section II, except for serotype L which seems to be confined to the pigeon, and in addition several untyped strains. Reference has also been made to pathogenicity which is considered in greater detail in Section V.

B. Disease in Domestic Poultry Caused by Mycoplasma Pathogens

In this section, the term "pathogen" is reserved for organisms which cause disease in chicks, poults, ducklings, and goslings and in older birds, but does not include those that cause only embryo mortality or lesions following inoculation of embryonated eggs.

The organisms isolated from poultry may be classified pathogenically into three groups: (1) those known to be pathogenic, (2) some for which circumstantial evidence suggests a pathogenic role but for which there is at present insufficient confirmation, and (3) others which appear to be nonpathogenic.

Those known to be pathogenic are *M. gallisepticum* and *M. synoviae* for the chicken and turkey, *M. meleagridis* for the turkey, and *A. axanthum* for the goose. However, the virulence of strains within at least the first three species varies considerably.

Those which may be pathogenic under certain circumstances include *M. gallinarum* for the chicken, *M. anatis* for the duck, *A. laidlawii* for the goose and duck, and a ureaplasma isolated from chickens and turkeys.

The remaining serotypes and untyped mycoplasmas are either nonpathogenic or insufficient information is available about them to place them in either of the other groups.

It is proposed to consider the diseases in poultry caused by the above-named pathogens. For each organism in turn the following aspects of disease are outlined: epidemiology, clinical disease, lesions, pathogenesis, diagnosis, and control.

1. *Mycoplasma gallisepticum* Infection of Chickens and Turkeys

The most common manifestation of this infection is disease of the respiratory tract; in chickens and turkeys it is tracheitis and air sacculitis, and in turkeys sinusitis and air sacculitis.

Disease probably associated with this organism was first described by Dodd (1905) in turkeys. The infection is worldwide, but it is probably of economic importance mainly when stock are kept under intensive systems of management. Synergism between mycoplasma and other avian pathogens is also important in this respect. For the chicken these include the viruses of Newcastle disease or infectious bronchitis either as natural infections or as live vaccines. They also include avian pathogenic strains of *Escherichia coli*, while for the turkey they include certain strains of *E. coli* and influenza A virus. Turkeys, however, are more susceptible to *M. gallisepticum*, and the organism alone causes disease in them more frequently than in chickens. Multiple infections with *M. gallisepticum* and other mycoplasma species occur, but their significance in disease production is not known.

Mortality in poultry is relatively rare, and economic loss is caused by reduced production of layers, broiler chickens, and turkeys, downgrading of carcasses and suboptimal hatchability, and suboptimal grading of chicks and poults.

a. Epidemiology. The main features of epidemiological importance associated with the causal organism are (1) the existence of one antigenic type; (2) variation in virulence (Fabricant and Levine, 1963; Nutor, 1969; Truscott *et al.*, 1974; Power and Jordan, 1976a) and tropism; the latter is seen in the proclivity of the S6 strain for the brain of the turkey (Yamamoto and Adler, 1958a), for the chicken and turkey (Varley and Jordan, 1978b,c), and for arterial walls (Clyde and Thomas, 1973a); and of the A514 strain for the hock and foot joints of turkey poults (Varley and Jordan, 1978c) and an undesignated strain for the trachea of turkeys (Rhoades *et al.*, 1965); (3) survival of the organism away from the host for only a few days under conditions likely to be reflected in the field (Beard and Anderson, 1967; Chandiramani *et al.*, 1966; Wright *et al.*, 1968; Yoder, 1978; Polak-Vogelzang, 1977); (4) susceptibility of the organism to various drugs, but drug-resistant strains occur (Fahey, 1957; Domermuth, 1958, 1960; Kiser *et al.*, 1961; Yoder *et al.*, 1961; Newnham and Chu, 1965; Griffin, 1969; Truscott *et al.*, 1974; Kuniyasu *et al.*, 1974; Meroz *et al.*, 1976); it also readily succumbs to common disinfectants; (5) persistence of infection in the chicken and turkey, which may extend up to 18 months or longer.

The more important epidemiological features concerning the host seem to be genetic constitution, age, immune status, intercurrent infection with other microorganisms, and also debilitating factors. For instance, although the organism has been recovered from several avian species apart from the chicken and turkey, it is only in these two species that it has been shown to be pathogenic. Although the influence of age on resistance to disease has not been adequately examined, resistance apparently increases with age, particularly in the chicken.

Protection of the respiratory system resulting from a previous infection or vaccination has been reviewed by Jordan (1975b). Although some degree of immunity can be attained, it seems to be vulnerable to a superimposed infection of the bird with such viruses as Newcastle disease virus (NDV) and infectious bronchitis virus. However, it is not known what would result if the birds were also protected against these viruses. Fabricant and Levine (1963) demonstrated the elimination of egg transmission of *M. gallisepticum* following infection of young birds with a virulent organism. Later, Fabricant (1977) showed that it was possible to reduce a fall in egg production in laying birds caused by the mycoplasma by vaccination of 9- to 12-week-old pullets with an autogenous organism via the drinking water. Exacerbation or amelioration of disease by *M. gallisepticum* may occur in the course of one or more intercurrent infections. In many instances of exacerbation it seems to be the consequence of a synergistic rather than an additive mechanism, and organisms which on their own may be only mildly pathogenic can cause severe disease in multiple infections. The sequence of infection with the pathogens involved and the period between infections may determine the outcome of the interaction. Brief reviews involving multiple infections have been produced by Bankowski (1961) and by Fabricant (1969) and Jordan (1972, 1975a). References to the organisms concerned include, for the chicken, NDV (Corstvet and Sadler, 1966a,b; Sato, 1970; Sato *et al.*, 1970), infectious bronchitis virus (Calnek and Levine, 1957; Adler *et al.*, 1962; Fabricant, 1969; Varley and Jordan, 1978a), infectious laryngotracheitis virus (Bezrukava, 1965), influenza A virus (Ranck *et al.*, 1970), avian adenovirus (Berry, 1969; Aghakhan *et al.*, 1976), reovirus (Fahey and Crawley, 1954; Subramanyan and Pomeroy, 1960; Simmonds and Lukert, 1972); *H. gallinarum* (Nelson, 1938; Adler and Yamamoto, 1956; Kato, 1965), *E. coli* (Gross, 1956, 1958, 1961; Fabricant, 1969; see also Thornton, 1971, who was unable to confirm this), and molds (Matuka *et al.*, 1968).

It is of interest that under certain circumstances *M. gallisepticum* may have an inhibitory effect on intercurrent pathogens. For instance, infection with *M. gallisepticum* of chick embryo tracheal organ culture

(Nonomura, 1973) or chickens themselves (Nonomura and Sato, 1975) reduces or inhibits the replication of a mild strain of NDV given subsequently. It had little effect, however, on more virulent virus. There is a suggestion from the observations of Katzen *et al.* (1969) that *M. gallisepticum* infection might have an ameliorative influence on Marek's disease. It has been shown also that infection of a chicken tracheal organ culture with *M. gallinarum* protected against *M. gallisepticum* (Taylor-Robinson and Cherry, 1972) and that a previous infection of chickens with *M. synoviae* reduces the severity of disease and the antibody titer produced by later infection with *M. gallisepticum* (Bradbury, 1975). In the turkey less intensive study has been made of mixed infection, but synergism has been reported with *E. coli* (Gross, 1956) and influenza A virus (Ranck *et al.*, 1970).

Certain debilitating factors are known to exacerbate disease with *M. gallisepticum,* including trauma such as scarification of the trachea (Corstvet and Sadler, 1966a), excess ammonia (Sato *et al.*, 1973), and social stress (Gross and Siegel, 1965; Gross and Colmano, 1969, 1971).

The spread of *M. gallisepticum* (Yoder, 1978) occurs almost entirely by direct means, through the egg or by infected airborne droplets from the respiratory system of carriers or clinically affected stock. The relatively short survival time of the organism away from the host greatly reduces fomite transmission, although it can occur. An unusual example of the latter is live infectious laryngotracheitis vaccine contaminated with *M. gallisepticum* (Benton *et al.*, 1967). Evidence of egg-borne transmission in the chicken has been provided by Van Roekel *et al.* (1952), Cover and Waller (1954), Fahey and Crawley (1954), Fabricant and Levine (1963), Yoder and Hofstad (1965), and Yoder (1969), and in the turkey by Jerstad *et al.* (1949), Hofstad (1957), and Osborn and Pomeroy (1958). Furthermore, *M. gallisepticum* has been isolated from the oviduct of the female and semen of the male by Yoder and Hofstad (1964). The proportion of infected eggs laid by a flock varies considerably and may be intermittent. Airborne or contact transmission has been described by Fahey and Crawley (1955), and both egg transmission and airborne spread may be influenced by intercurrent infections which stimulate multiplication of the mycoplasma. The rapidity of spread of disease within a flock is also probably influenced by these factors and intensive management, but it is variable, sometimes quite slow and at other times rapid. Spread from flock to flock on the same farm but in different pens when there is no direct contact is often slow or may not occur at all.

b. Clinical disease. Under experimental conditions the incubation period may vary between 1 and 3 weeks (Delaplane and Stuart, 1943; Van Roekel *et al.*, 1952; Hofstad, 1952). However, signs may not appear following infection and in some cases do not appear until precipitated by intercurrent infection (Calnek and Levine, 1957) or other debilitating factors, and this may be true of most natural infections in the chicken.

The most common clinical signs of the natural condition are associated with disease of the respiratory tract and include coryza, coughing, sneezing, and rales. Coryza is generally more severe in turkeys than in chickens, and is characterized by swelling of one or both infraorbital sinuses, hence the name "sinusitis." It may be so severe as to close the eyelids completely. Nasal exudate is often more profuse in the turkey, and the wing feathers are often soiled where the birds have attempted to wipe away the discharge. In both the chicken and turkey mild conjunctivitis with a frothy exudate in the eye may be the only sign of coryza, or it may be the prodromal indication of more severe disease. When the air sacs alone are affected, there are no specific clinical signs. Other specific clinical signs are generally relatively rare and include ataxia of turkeys that is associated with brain lesions, and lameness associated with lesions and swelling of the hock in chickens. An unusual condition observed by Power and Jordan (1976b) was unilateral enlargement of the eyeball of chickens 3–4 weeks of age following experimental infection of 18-day-old embryos with the A514 strain of *M. gallisepticum*. The condition occurred in a small proportion of chicks, and the organism could be recovered from the anterior segment of affected eyes but not from normal ones.

Nonspecific signs include lowered egg production and growth rate, but intercurrent infection also influences these signs (Blake, 1962; McMartin and Wilson, 1968).

In uncomplicated infection the disease may be inapparent or very mild and may last no longer than a few weeks, but signs and lesions are exacerbated and the course of disease prolonged, sometimes for several months, when multiple infections or debilitating factors play a significant part.

c. Lesions. Gross lesions are seen most commonly in the respiratory tract, much less frequently in the oviduct, and rarely in the hocks, and have only been reported from experimental infection in the brain and eye.

Gross lesions of the respiratory tract may be so mild as to be imperceptible or consist only of excess mucus or catarrhal exudate in the nares, sinuses, trachea, and lungs, and edema of the air sac walls. Caseous exudate may appear later, particularly in the air sacs and attached to the air sac walls. Mucus causes dilatation of the infraorbital sinuses and, especially in turkeys, it may become tenacious and later caseous. In disease exacerbated by other pathogens, probably the most common manifestation under field conditions, the lesions are more severe. For instance, with some strains of *E. coli,* especially in chickens about 4- to 10-weeks-old kept intensively, pericarditis and perihepatitis accompany more extensive lesions of the respiratory system.

Histologically the respiratory lesion is essentially one of hypertrophy and hyperplasia of the epithelium with deciliation, some edema, and infiltration of the subepithelial tissue with lymphocytes, reticulocytes, and plasma cells. It becomes considerably thickened in consequence. Monocytes aggregated into lymphofollicular foci with germinal centers occur throughout the respiratory system (Johnson, 1954; Jungherr, 1949, 1960; Olesiuk and Van Roekel, 1960; Barber, 1962; Kerr and Olson, 1967a). Hyperplasia of the mucous glands is seen, and in the trachea they become long and narrow, extending the whole width of the thickened mucosa (Olesiuk and Van Roekel, 1960; Garside, 1965; Grimes and Rosenfeld, 1972). In the lungs there is massive infiltration of monocytes and heterophils (Kerr and Olson, 1967a).

Salpingitis with caseous exudate in the oviduct may result from experimental infection in the chicken (Domermuth and Gross, 1962) and is not infrequently seen in female broilers at meat inspection, but in such cases it is not clear whether its appearance is solely the result of *M. gallisepticum* infection.

Arthritis and synovitis, particularly of the hocks, have been seen in chickens (Olson *et al.*, 1956; Chalquest and Fabricant, 1960; Sato *et al.*, 1972) and turkeys (Fabricant, 1969) and have been produced experimentally (Kerr and Olson, 1967a; Lamas Da Silva and Adler, 1969; Olson and Kerr, 1970; Clyde and Thomas, 1973a; Wannop *et al.*, 1971). There is swelling and edema of the periarticular tissue, inflammation of the tendovaginal sheaths, bursae, and synovial membranes, and excess joint fluid, at first clear and then turbid and later of creamy consistency. Erosion of articular surfaces and osteomyelitis may, rarely, be seen. Histologically the lesions include hyperplasia of synovial surface cells, with some cellular degeneration and marked infiltration of monocytes into synovial and adjacent tissues with lymphofollicular formation. Heterophils may be found in large numbers in joint fluid, and bursal exudate and polyarteritis of the local arteries and arterioles has been described (Lamas Da Silva and Adler, 1969).

Macroscopic lesions in the brain have only recently been reported (Varley and Jordan, 1978b,c). They appear as pale areas of 1- to 2-mm extent seen in the cerebrum; occasionally they coalesce into larger areas. Histological lesions are of focal parenchymal necrosis (Clyde and Thomas, 1973a) and vasculitis of the cerebral cortex (Cordy and Adler, 1957), resulting from arteritis of the meningeal and parenchymatous arteries and arterioles. Acute swelling of the capillary endothelium has been described (Thomas *et al.*, 1966; Manuelidis and Thomas, 1973) following intravenous inoculation with large numbers of organisms.

d. Diagnosis. The respiratory and other signs and postmortem and histological lesions are not pathognomonic for *M. gallisepticum* infection and are no more than suggestive of its presence. Diagnosis therefore depends upon isolation and identification of the casual organism, or upon examination of sera. Recovery of the causal organism may be protracted, and agar medium should be incubated for 3–4 weeks before being discarded as negative. Resort has occasionally been made to the inoculation of susceptible chickens (Bigland and Da Massa, 1963; McMartin, 1967), turkey poults, and embryonated eggs in an attempt to isolate the organism.

The identification of an isolate (see Section III) may be made based on the appearance of colonies on agar and by serological examination, unless it appears to be a new species, in which case full characterization would be necessary.

Sera may be examined by several tests (Jordan and Kulasegaram, 1968), but of these the rapid serum agglutination (RSA), tube agglutination (TA), and hemagglutination inhibition (HAI) tests are commonly used (Fabricant, 1969; Yoder, 1976). More recently the agar gel precipitation test has been used for *M. gallisepticum* and *M. synoviae* (Sahu and Olson, 1976a,b).

In the RSA test heated, inactivated serum is used, and a homologous and a negative control serum are included. It should be appreciated that several factors associated with the serum and/or the antigen can influence the specificity and sensitivity of the test (Bradbury and Jordan, 1971; Cullen and Anderton, 1974; Bigland and Matsumoto, 1975), and that the test is considered to be of greatest value for indicating flock rather than individual bird infection. The TA test (Yoder, 1976) is preferred by some to the RSA test. Serum and antigen are mixed in a ratio of 1:12.5, and tubes are incubated at 37°C overnight before reading.

More recently the agar gel precipitation test has been used for the examination of sera from flocks infected with *M. gallisepticum* or *M. synoviae* (Sahu and Olson, 1976b; Nonomura and Yoder, 1977). Its value in this respect is yet to be proved. The HAI test (Yoder, 1976) is usually performed as a microtest using 2 or 4 HA units of antigen in complete hemagglutination. Because it is more accurate (although perhaps less sensitive) but more laborious and time-consuming, it is mainly performed as a confirmatory test on sera reacting positively to the RSA test.

e. Control. Most of the epidemiological features already discussed are of significance in the consideration of control of this infection. However, there are some of particular importance. They include the short survival of the organism away from the host; its susceptibility to various drugs and bacterial disinfectants; the immune protective response following infection of the host which may collapse in the face of intercurrent infection (McMartin, 1963); and, although *M. gallisepticum* is spread through the egg and among birds in the same flock by direct and indirect transmission, it is not highly invasive and thus it may be possible with adequate management to prevent or reduce greatly spread from one flock to another at the same site.

Of the main principles of infectious disease control, namely, minimizing contact between the host and the pathogen, increasing the resistance of the host, treatment of the host, and minimizing predisposing factors, none are satisfactory in practice on their own. The first is limited because there is no satisfactory test for recognizing all the individual infected birds in a flock that would enable their segregation from the noninfected stock, although adequate management including cleaning and disinfection of buildings and equipment can preclude infection entering a flock from the environment. Increasing resistance of the host is also limited, as mentioned earlier, but it has been used at multiple-age sites as described later in this section. Treatment of stock and eggs with suitable drugs can greatly reduce infection but does not entirely eliminate it (Yoder and Hofstad, 1965), and drug therapy may be costly. Heat treatment of chicken hatching eggs may reduce *M. gallisepticum* infection but tends to reduce hatchability. The hatchability of turkey eggs is even more adversely affected by heat treatments that do not eliminate all the mycoplasmas (Jordan and Amin, 1978). Because it is possible and practicable, with adequate management, to prevent mycoplasma infection from entering a mycoplasma-free flock, the general aim has been to produce breeding flocks free of infection by the eradication of *M. gallisepticum*. This is done by a combination of methods including (1) drug treatment of breeding stock and/or hatching eggs, or heat treatment of hatching chicken eggs with the object of greatly reducing the level of infection in the progeny; (2) hatching eggs in relatively small groups (100 to 200 for chickens, or less than 50 to 100 for poults); (3) monitoring groups and eliminating a whole group from the eradication scheme when any member shows evidence of *M. gallisepticum* infection; (4) management of groups to avoid the entry of infection. Drug therapy is most economically and effectively practiced on hatching eggs. A wide variety of drugs has been used (Yoder, 1972), and of these, for the treatment of hatching eggs, tylosin tartrate and gentamycin sulfate appear to be the most effective.

Eggs can be treated either by manual injection into the air sac (Smit and Hoeckstra, 1968) or by placing them in a solution of the drug, dipping them (Yoder and Hofstad, 1965), and creating a pressure differential so that the solution enters the egg. This may be brought about by immersing eggs at 37°C in a drug solution at 5°–10°C for 15 min or more (Chalquest and Fabricant, 1959; Alls *et al.*, 1963) and perhaps repeating the process, which is known as "double dipping." An alternative method is to immerse the eggs in the drug solution and apply a vacuum to the air above the solution. The resultant drop in pressure causes air to be withdrawn from the air spaces of the eggs. Once equilibrium is reached, the pressure is slowly returned to atmospheric, and the consequent increase in pressure around the eggs causes the solution to enter them (Voeten, 1965). Although these methods are labor-saving compared with injection, there are disadvantages. For instance, the permeability of the shell of different eggs may vary considerably, and inadequate amounts of drug solution may enter some of the eggs (Alls *et al.*, 1964). In both methods some reduction in hatchability may be expected. Drug-resistant strains of *M. gallisepticum* occasionally appear (Truscott *et al.*, 1974), whatever method is used.

Heat treatment of chicken hatching eggs has been used far less widely and was pioneered by Yoder (1970). He advocated the gradual, uniform heating of hatching eggs from room temperature to 45°–46°C over a period of 12–14 hr and then allowing them to cool at room temperature. The eggs were then set for incubation. Hatchability was reduced 8–10%. Meroz *et al.* (1973) discussed some technical aspects and showed reduced hatchability of only 5.1% on apparently uninfected eggs. Jordan and Amin (1978) have not found this procedure satisfactory for turkey eggs.

There are two main methods of monitoring for infection; one is by attempting isolation of the mycoplasma by cultural means, and the other is by examination of sera for specific antibodies. Cultural examination may be applied to a variety of tissues in dead-in-shell embryos, dead or cull-day-old chicks or poults, or culls in the first few weeks of life. Swabs or tissues from the respiratory tract, esophagus, and cloaca are often examined from older birds whether showing signs of disease or lesions or not. Serological examination implies the testing of sera from individual birds in a flock by one of the methods mentioned above. The RSA test is the most frequently used because it is simple and rapid, but because of its fallibility is best used as a flock test. Such a test should be applied to all birds in a basic breeder flock at least once, usually at point of lay, and random tests of 10% or so of the flock may also be made during the rearing stage and when in lay. A flock is considered to be free of infection when serologically negative progeny are produced from negative parent birds without treatment of hatching eggs.

By these methods *M. gallisepticum* has been eradicated from a large number of turkey and chicken breeder flocks. The HAI test is often used in cases of doubt, such as a small number of "reactors" in a flock or the appearance of reactors in a supposedly uninfected flock. Cultural examination should also be attempted on such birds.

Vaccination in the control of *M. gallisepticum* is practiced (Papageorgiou, 1970, 1971; Papageorgiou and Bar, 1976; Fabricant, 1977) but suffers from the possible disadvantages associated with the superimposed infections mentioned above. The resulting production may therefore compare unfavorably with mycoplasma-free stock. Fabricant (1977) rigidly restricts its use to an autogenous vaccine used in special circumstances at multiple-age sites.

Drug therapy for affected stock alleviates the worst effects of infection and is sometimes used on infected flocks immediately after vaccination with live NDV and infectious bronchitis virus.

2. *Mycoplasma synoviae* Infection of Chickens and Turkeys

Infection with this organism may cause disease in a wide variety of organs and tissues (Sevoian *et al.*, 1958; Moorhead *et al.*, 1967; Kerr and Olson, 1970; Sells, 1971; Kleven *et al.*, 1975). However, its effect on joints, bursae, and tendon sheaths (giving rise to the name *infectious synovitis*) was first described, in the chicken, independently by Olson *et al.* (1954) and Wills (1954) in West Virginia and Texas, respectively. Snoeyenbos and Olesiuk (1955) described the disease in turkeys, and the etiological agent was first recognized and described by Chalquest and Fabricant (1960). Since that time its involvement with the viruses of Newcastle disease and infectious bronchitis in causing lesions in the respiratory tract has been indicated by Yoder (1969) and confirmed by Kleven *et al.* (1972); there were no synovial lesions. With the progressive eradication of *M. gallisepticum* the role of *M. synoviae* in causing air sacculitis in chickens is now apparent, and Goren *et al.* (1975) have reported respiratory distress and infectious sinusitis in turkeys associated with *M. synoviae*. The infection seems to be worldwide (Timms, 1978). It is of economic importance mainly because it reduces optimal production, increases food conversion rates, and causes downgrading of carcasses in chickens and turkeys (Sadler and Corstvet, 1964, 1965a,b; King *et al.*, 1973; Vardaman *et al.*, 1973a; Goren, 1978). It may also perhaps reduce the hatchability of chicken eggs (Bradbury and Howell, 1975).

a. Epidemiology. The main features of significance in the epidemiology of the disease associated with *M. synoviae* are (1) the existence of apparently only one antigenic type of organism (Olson *et al.*, 1965); (2) variation in virulence (Olson *et al.*, 1957; Chalquest and Fabricant, 1960; Kleven *et* *al.*, 1973, 1975) and perhaps tropism for joints, bursae, or respiratory tissues (Kleven *et al.*, 1975); (3) survival of the organism away from the host under field conditions has not been studied but it is probably very similar to that for *M. gallisepticum*; its susceptibility to pH below 6.9, temperatures above 39°C, and its survival at temperatures of −20°C and below have been described by Olson (1978); (4) susceptibility of the organism to various drugs (Kleven and Anderson, 1971; Olson, 1978; Hamdy *et al.*, 1976; Olson and Sahu, 1976); (5) persistence of infection in the chicken or turkey for several years (Olson, 1978).

Various factors, particularly concerning the host, may play a part in the appearance and severity of disease associated with *M. synoviae*. They include:

1. The genetic constitution: Of the natural hosts the chicken is more susceptible than the turkey, whereas the pheasant and goose can be infected by intravenous inoculation of the organism, resulting in synovitis; however, the duck was not affected by such inoculation into the tendon sheath (Sevoian *et al.*, 1958); furthermore, Amin (1977) in a survey of mycoplasma infection of British wild birds and exotic specimens from zoological gardens in no case isolated *M. synoviae*.

2. The significance of age on resistance (if any) to infection is not known, although Kerr and Olson (1964) found that chickens between 2 and 20 weeks were susceptible to experimental infection.

3. The immune status of the host may be of significance in protection. Although Cassidy and Grumbles (1959) were unable to demonstrate immunity to an earlier initial infection in chickens, Carnaghan (1962) showed that birds that had recovered from the infection were resistant to foot pad challenge, and the protective influence of immune serum, and Olson *et al.* (1964) showed that chickens exposed intranasally were resistant to foot pad challenge.

4. Intercurrent infection with NDV or infectious bronchitis virus acts synergistically with *M. synoviae* to cause air sacculitis (Kleven *et al.*, 1972). Springer *et al.* (1974) showed similar synergy between *M. synoviae* and *E. coli*, together with or without infectious bronchitis virus, in gnotobiotic chickens and Rhoades (1977) demonstrated synergy of *M. synoviae* with *M. melaegridis* in turkey sinusitis. Hinz and Luders (1969) reported infections of chickens from which *M. synoviae* and *Staphylococcus aureus* were recovered, but synergy was not shown. Bahl *et al.* (1974) suggested a synergistic effect in turkeys of *M. synoviae* and influenza A virus, and Bradbury and Garuti (1978) suggested a possible synergism with a reovirus in experimental synovitis. The inhibitory effect of *M. synoviae* on sequential infection with *M. gallisepticum* (Bradbury, 1975) has already been mentioned (Section IV,B,1,a). It is

not known whether debilitating factors, if any, are of significance in precipitating or exacerbating disease of synovial tissues, but Yoder *et al.* (1977) showed that low environmental temperatures increased the incidence and severity of air sacculitis in 3- to 4-week-old infected chickens.

The spread of *M. synoviae* is probably similar to the spread of *M. gallisepticum* within a flock and from flock to flock. It occurs mainly by direct means through the egg (Carnaghan, 1961; Hemsley, 1965; King *et al.*, 1973; Vardaman and Drott, 1977) and through droplet particles from the respiratory tract (Olson *et al.*, 1964; Olson and Kerr, 1967). This seems to be the tissue in which infection most commonly persists in carrier birds (Yoder *et al.*, 1977). Egg transmission is variable; it may occur at a low rate and is most prevalent early after the infection of adult stock (Kleven and Anderson, 1975), although exacerbating factors may modify its transmission.

b. Clinical disease. Under natural conditions the period of incubation may be as short as 6 days in chicks subsequent to infection *in ovo* (Thayer *et al.*, 1958). Periods as short as 2–3 days have been reported following foot pad or intravenous infection (Olson, 1978) although, apart from the route of infection, several factors are probably of significance, including the number and virulence of the organisms and the susceptibility of the host. Following contact exposure of infected and susceptible birds the period of incubation is about 10–20 days.

It is probable that clinical disease is the exception rather than the rule following natural invasion with *M. synoviae* in either chickens or turkeys. The disease may be seen in one or both of two forms: (1) lameness with or without generalized disease (Olson, 1978) and (2) the respiratory form.

In the locomotory form, morbidity in chickens is usually 5–15%, but exceptionally up to 75%, whereas in turkeys it is lower (10%) and rarely extends to 20% of the flock. Mortality is 1–10% unless the debilitated birds are unable to obtain food or water or are attacked by their penmates. The clinical signs vary. In severe generalized disease depression, poor growth, palor of the face and comb, and lameness are among the commoner initial signs in chickens and turkeys. Lameness is ususally associated with hot, painful, swollen hocks or foot joints, and in very severe cases there is swelling of all the joints of the body. In turkeys affected joints may not be swollen, but swollen sternal bursae are common. There may be a green diarrhea, and some birds become emaciated. The disease often becomes chronic. In the respiratory form there may be mild sneezing (snicking) following vaccination with NDV and infectious bronchitis virus (King *et al.*, 1973), and there is reduced growth and food conversion in young chickens. In turkeys sinusitis has been described (Olson and Yoder, 1968; Goren *et al.*, 1975).

c. Lesions Lesions in chickens have been described in detail by Sevoian *et al.* (1958), Moorhead *et al.* (1967), and Kerr and Olson (1970), in chickens and turkeys by Olson (1978), and in turkeys by Ghazikhanian *et al.* (1973). Lesions associated with the joints, tendon sheaths, and bursae are tendovaginitis, synovitis, and osteoarthritis and include thickening edema and exudate—at first clear, then turbid, and later caseous. Caseous exudate may also be found over the skull and dorsal surface of the neck in severe cases. The surface of affected joints becomes orange in color in chronic cases, and occasionally erosion of articular cartilage occurs.

Histologically there is edema of soft tissue with heterophil infiltration of tendon sheaths and synovial membranes followed by marked thickening caused by infiltration with mononuclear cells and plasma cells; hyperplasia of the synovial surface cells occurs and, together with inflammatory cells, these cells are shed into the joint cavities and tissue spaces. Erosion of articular cartilage, which is relatively rare, results from heterophilic inflammatory changes which eventually involve the underlying bone in fibrocystic degeneration.

In generalized disease (essentially similar in the chicken and turkey) there is hepatomegaly and splenomegaly caused by monocytic cell infiltration and an increase in reticulocytes. The kidneys also may be swollen, but the thymus and bursa of Fabricius may be shrunken as a result of lymphocyte degeneration (Sevoian *et al.*, 1958).

Changes in the blood picture have been described by Sevoian *et al.* (1958) and by Kerr and Olson (1970) and Olson (1978). In severe cases the erythrocytes showed anisocytosis, poikilocytosis, polychromatophilia, and achromia. Monocytosis and heterophilia were also observed.

Peri-, epi-, and endocarditis have been produced in inoculated (Kerr and Olson, 1967a,b) and in contact chickens (Kerr and Olson, 1970).

Lesions in the respiratory tract are similar to those seen with *M. gallisepticum* (Ghazikhanian *et al.*, 1973; King *et al.*, 1973; Kleven *et al.*, 1975). Thymus-derived lymphocytes seem to be important in the production of synovial lesions (Kume *et al.*, 1977).

d. Diagnosis. The signs and lesions are not pathognomonic, although they may be helpful. The presence of infection with *M. synoviae* thus depends upon the recovery and identification of the organism or upon serological examination. The factors influencing the recovery of *M. gallisepticum* also apply to *M. synoviae*, although the inclusion of NAD in the culture medium is essential (Chalquest, 1962; Olson *et al.*, 1963; Hinz, 1972). However, Olson (1978) has pointed out that recovery of the organism from synovial, bursal, or joint lesions of chronically affected birds may be difficult or impossible. He also suggests that inoculation of material into 5- to 7-day-old chick embryos gives the highest recovery rate.

It is now well appreciated that the organism may be recovered from the respiratory tract of apparently normal chickens and turkeys. Serological examinations by RSA tests or HAI tests indicate the infection status of a flock, but the specificity and sensitivity of the tests on individual birds are no more satisfactory than those for *M. gallisepticum*.

e. Control. The epidemiological basis and the general principles and practices for the control of *M. synoviae* infection are similar to those outlined for *M. gallisepticum,* and eradication of the infection in breeder birds is the primary objective.

The methods of eradication applied to breeding stock follow the same pattern as those used for *M. gallisepticum*. We are not aware of references in the literature to the dipping or inoculation of chicken eggs with appropriate drugs to reduce or eradicate specifically *M. synoviae* infection. Nevertheless these methods are known to be practiced commercially, and it is likely that elimination of this organism is being achieved by the process adopted for *M. gallisepticum* using such drugs as tylosin tartrate. Preincubation heat treatment of chicken hatching eggs, as advocated by Yoder (1970), has been practiced under commercial conditions.

Eggs should be hatched and the progeny reared in small groups. Should infection with *M. synoviae* be detected either by recovery of the organism or serologically, the group should be removed from the eradication scheme. A high standard of hygiene in management is essential.

There has been no study on the control of *M. synoviae* infection by vaccination.

Drug therapy may be practiced to minimize pathogenic effects of the infection, and Kleven and Anderson (1971) investigated the susceptibility of *M. synoviae* to several antibiotics and suggested that a combination of lincomycin and spectinomycin had a synergistic effect. Hamdy *et al.* (1976) demonstrated its value in experimentally infected broilers in which it reduced air sacculitis and *M. synoviae* infection. Drug therapy is probably a wise routine procedure, following vaccination with live NDV or infectious bronchitis virus if there is a likely concomitant infection with *M. synoviae*.

3. *Mycoplasma meleagridis* Infection of Turkeys

Infection with this organism was first reported by Adler *et al.* (1958), who recovered it from air sacculitis in cull-day-old poults. The organism was referred to as the N strain of PPLO. It is probably a worldwide infection of turkeys and, apart from the few breeding and experimental flocks from which the infection has been eliminated, it seems to be ubiquitous in turkeys. The organism has not been isolated from avian species other than the turkey, in which it is a primary pathogen. It is economically important because it causes suboptimal production and reduced food conversion of meat birds, downgrading of carcasses, and suboptimal hatchability and grading of day-old poults.

a. Epidemiology. The main features of significance in the epidemiology of disease associated with *M. meleagridis* are (1) the existence of only one antigenic type; (2) variation in virulence (Ghazikhanian and Yamamoto, 1974a,b) and perhaps tropism for the cloaca and bursa of Fabricius in young stock (Yamamoto and Ortmayer, 1967; Reis and Yamamoto, 1971) and the phallus and oviduct in adults (Yamamoto, 1978); (3) survival of the organism away from the host under field conditions has not been studied, but it is thought to be of short duration, as for *M. gallisepticum*; it is known to survive in the air in aerosol form for at least 6 hr (Beard and Anderson, 1967); (4) susceptibility to several antibiotics, although there is variation in this between strains (Yamamoto *et al.,* 1966a; Newman, 1967; Ghazikhanian and Yamamoto, 1969; Meroz *et al.*, 1976); tylosin tartrate and gentamycin sulfate are currently the most popular, and certain drugs are used in combination in the treatment of hatching eggs (McCapes *et al.*, 1975); (5) persistence of infection may extend well into maturity and may perhaps be lifelong.

The factors that influence the appearance and severity of disease include (1) the genetic constitution of the host; the turkey seems to be the only susceptible species; Amin (1977) undertook a survey of mycoplasma in domestic stock, wild birds, and exotic birds, but found *M. meleagridis* only in turkeys; but it may infect other avian species (Yamamoto, 1978); (2) age; this may be of significance, since lesions of the air sacs tend to be limited to birds under about 14 weeks of age and older birds are much more resistant; also chondrodystrophy of the hock seems to occur in birds infected in the egg or as young poults; (3) the immune status of the turkey may be of some significance in protection (Papageorgiou and Bar, 1976), but the degree, duration, and type of immunity following infection or vaccination have not been critically studied; (4) intercurrent infection with other avian pathogens seems to play a relatively minor role in disease caused by *M. meleagridis*, but it has been shown that synergism may exist between *M. meleagridis* and *E. coli* in respiratory disease in poults (Mohamed *et al.*, 1970a,b; Reis and Yamamoto, 1971), and with *M. synoviae* in sinusitis in turkeys (Rhoades, 1977); (5) debilitating factors seem to have received little attention, but Anderson *et al.* (1968) showed that excessive environmental dust and atmospheric ammonia exacerbated the disease condition; birds reacting to cold stress with high plasma corticosterone were also less resistant to air sacculitis.

The spread of *M. meleagridis* occurs mainly through the egg, venereally, and by lateral transmission from bird to bird through infected airborne droplets. Infection of the egg probably occurs high in the magnum (Yamamoto, 1978); egg transmission is often irregular in sequence (Mohamed and Bohl, 1967) but has been shown in some flocks to be relatively low early in lay, to reach a maximum about midlay, and to decline toward the end of lay (Bigland *et al.*, 1964; Kumar, 1967).

Both male and female turkeys may harbor the organism in the cloaca, so that if natural mating occurred, transmission of infection might be in either direction. However, under commercial conditions with artificial insemination venereal spread occurs from males to females. Nevertheless, it should be pointed out that in virgin hens *M. meleagridis* may infect the oviduct as a descending infection from air sacs or other sources of infection early in life or as an ascending infection from a focus in the cloacal region after rupture of the occluding plate at sexual maturity (Matzer and Yamamoto, 1970). Lateral spread is probably influenced by crowding, as in the hatcher and in intensive rearing, although Yamamoto and Ortmeyer (1967) found no evidence for spread in the hatcher. It is suggested (Yamamoto, 1967, 1978) that lateral transmission is not a major influence on egg transmission once sexual maturity has been reached.

b. Clinical disease. Clinical disease may or may not follow infection. The young poult seems to be much more susceptible than older birds, and acute clinical signs, probably mainly from egg-borne infection, are confined to young stock. They include reduced growth rate which might vary from very slight to marked stunting, perosis (TS 65) which may affect 10% or more of the flock, and a few birds may show crooked necks (Kleven, 1972) and abnormalities of some of the primary wing feathers which may stand out almost at right angles from the body (Bigland and Jordan, 1974); sternal bursitis is occasionally seen (Yamamoto and Bigland, 1965) and sinusitis rarely (Dierks *et al.*, 1967); very mild synovitis and arthritis may follow intravenous infection (Reis *et al.*, 1970; Yamamoto, 1978). In some birds certain features such as bone abnormalities and dwarfing may become chronic. Other signs of the infection include reduced hatchability and survival of poults and occasionally very mild respiratory signs (Yamamoto, 1978).

c. Lesions. The most common gross lesions are associated with disease of the respiratory tract, especially the air sacs, and to a lesser extent the lungs; tracheitis does not seem to be a feature. Air sacculitis, particularly of the thoracic air sacs, is a common occurrence in poults (Yamamoto,

1978) and growers and is an important cause of carcass downgrading. In uncomplicated infection the lesions have usually regressed by 16 weeks of age and frequently much earlier. The air sac walls are thickened, and there is adherent caseous exudate, although the condition is said to be less severe and extensive than *M. gallisepticum* infection (Kumar *et al.*, 1963; Dierks *et al.*, 1967). A description of the gross changes in the air sacs of poults up to 4 weeks after infection is given by Arya *et al.* (1971) and Rhoades (1971). Histologically the air sacs show a change similar to *M. gallisepticum* infection (Moorhead *et al.*, 1967; Arya *et al.*, 1971; Rhoades, 1971; see also Ghazikhanian and Yamamoto, 1974b, who showed that a nonpathogenic strain produced no gross or microscopic lesions).

Skeletal abnormalities (TS 65), including perosis, particularly affecting the tibiotarsal and tarsometatarsal bones and lateral deviation of the cervical vertebral column, are now considered to be closely associated with infection with *M. meleagridis,* although the mechanism is not understood (Wise *et al.*, 1973; Bigland and Jordan, 1974; Yamamoto *et al.*, 1974). The condition is sometimes seen in the absence of air sacculitis, but Fox and Bigland (1970) showed that *M. meleagridis* could be recovered from the air sacs in the absence of lesions. The bones are often shorter and thicker than normal, and the tarsometatarsus may show varus or valgus deformity. Histologically the initial changes are those of perosis with depressed proliferation of chondrocytes in the region of the growth plates. In long-standing cases a dyschondroplasia-like lesion is seen on the medial side of the proximal tarsometatarsal growth plate with varus deformity. Synovitis of the hock joint occasionally occurs (Bigland and Jordan, 1974). Ascites has been described by Wise *et al.* (1974) and Wise and Evans (1975) following experimental infection of embryonated hatching eggs. It is suggested that the ascites is an acute manifestation of the disease.

No gross lesions of the phallus have been observed, but Gerlach *et al.* (1968) have described extensive lymphofollicular formation in the submucosa of the lymph fold.

d. Diagnosis. A flock history of poor hatchability, second-grade poults, stunted growth, leg weakness, skeletal deformity, primary wing feather abnormalities, and air sacculitis all suggest *M. meleagridis* infection. However, the infection may occur without clinical signs or gross lesions and, in any case, there is a variety of other causes of these symptoms. Confirmation of the infection therefore depends upon isolation and identification of the organism, or serological methods.

The organism has been most frequently recovered from the air sacs, with and without lesions, the phallus and oviduct, and from the trachea and infraorbital sinus and occasionally from hock deformities in young poults.

Mycoplasma meleagridis can be readily grown from field material on a variety of mycoplasma media (Dierks *et al.*, 1967; Frey *et al.*, 1968a,b; Amin, 1977). Yamamoto (1978) advocates inoculating broth or overlay medium before plating onto agar, but Amin (1977) in a survey of mycoplasma infections obtained a greater number of recoveries by direct plating.

Identification of the organism follows the method outlined for *M. gallisepticum* and *M. synoviae*.

For the examination of sera an RSA test and a more sensitive TA test have been developed and used (Adler, 1958; Bigland and Yamamoto, 1964; Mohamed and Bohl, 1968; Yamamoto *et al.*, 1966b), and a microtiter agglutination test has been reported by Ortiz and Yamamoto (1974). The RSA test is frequently used, but its reliability, at least with some commercial antigens, is doubtful, as indicated by Wise and Fuller (1975) and by our personal observations.

A HAI test has been used and found effective (Rhoades, 1969; Wise and Fuller, 1975). However, there is difficulty in repeatedly preparing a satisfactory antigen.

e. Control. Control follows the same pattern as outlined for *M. gallisepticum*. For breeding birds eradication may be considered (Mohamed and Bohl, 1969; Yamamoto and Ortmayer, 1971; Wise and Fuller, 1975; Ghazikhanian *et al.*, 1976). In principle this is done by (1) the treatment of eggs to eradicate or very greatly reduce infection, (2) rearing birds in relatively small flocks so that, if infected birds are found in the course of monitoring, the flock may be removed from the eradication scheme without excessive economic loss, and (3) monitoring by culture or serologically. The treatment of eggs entails dipping (Kumar *et al.*, 1974), double dipping (Yamamoto, 1978), or injection with suitable drugs. Hofstad (1973) and Wise and Fuller (1975) injected tylosin into the air cell, while McCapes *et al.* (1975, 1977) used several drugs and combinations of drugs for inoculation into the small end of the egg. Heat treatment, although advocated by some, has not been found to completely eliminate *M. meleagridis*, while causing a considerable decrease in hatchability (Jordan and Amin, 1978). The monitoring consists of cultural examination of unhatched eggs, cull poults, day-old poults, and birds during the rearing and breeding stages of life. The tissues examined include the respiratory tract, esophagus, cloaca, yolk sac of embryos and young poults; and the phallus, vagina, and semen of breeding birds. Infected birds should not be used for breeding, but if it is essential to use infected males for genetic reasons, the semen may be treated with a drug such as gentamicin sulfate (Kumar *et al.*, 1968; Mohamed and Bohl, 1968; Saif and Brown, 1972), although we have not found it very satisfactory. Monitoring may also include serological examination for antibodies to *M. meleagridis* (Section IV,B,3d). Control must embrace a high standard of hygiene in management, so that lateral transmission of infection is prevented.

The worst effects of the disease can be suppressed by the treatment of poults or, preferably, hatching eggs with drugs (Yamamoto, 1978). Those most commonly used are tylosin tartrate and gentamicin sulfate.

4. *Acholeplasma axanthum* Infection in the Goose and Duck

Stipkovits *et al.* (1975), in the course of investigations on poor hatchability in goose eggs, isolated *A. axanthum* from goose embryos which had died on the thirteenth day of incubation. They also recovered the organism from peritoneal exudate and air sac lesions of laying geese which had died sporadically. In later experimental infections in 3-day-old goslings (Kisary *et al.,* 1976), the organism introduced intranasally caused air sacculitis in a proportion of infected birds. However, when such goslings were concurrently infected intraperitoneally with a goose parvovirus, very much more severe and extensive lesions occurred.

Fawzia (1976) isolated *A. axanthum* from conjunctivitis and ulceration of the cloaca of ducks and suggested a causal relationship.

5. *Mycoplasma gallinarum* Infection in the Chicken and Goose

Early in the study of avian mycoplasmas it was appreciated that there were isolates which produced no disease on inoculation (Chu, 1954; Adler *et al.*, 1957) into chickens and turkeys, and such a strain isolated by Chu was proposed by Edward and Freundt (1956) as the type strain for *M. gallinarum*. Since that time numerous workers (Kleckner, 1960; Yoder and Hofstad, 1964; Dierks *et al.*, 1967) have found the organism to be nonpathogenic for embryos, chicks, and poults.

Its apparent lack of pathogenicity has been generally accepted, and little attention seems to have been given to this feature. In a recent comparison of the virulence of several strains of *M. gallisepticum* and a strain of *M. gallinarum* by inoculation of chick embryos, chick embryo tracheal organ cultures, chicks, and poults, it was found that *M. gallinarum* caused mortality of embryos intermediate between that of a mild strain of *M. gallisepticum* and the broth controls (Power and Jordan, 1973, 1976a). In tracheal organ culture a similar effect was observed for the cessation of ciliary activity (Power and Jordan, 1976a), although the effect of the mycoplasma on chick and poult mortality was no more than that of the broth control. This was true also of the mild strain of *M. gallisepticum* for the chick but not for the poult. In a study of clinical signs, lesions, and recovery of the mycoplasma (Varley and Jordan, 1978b,c and unpublished observations) it was found that, for both chickens and turkeys, *M. gallinarum* produced no signs or gross lesions and was recovered during the first few weeks of life from relatively very few birds and tissues. The birds were kept in strict isolation, so that it was surprising that in survivor chickens at 30 weeks of age the organism was recovered relatively frequently.

It should be pointed out that only recently has a study been made of the possible role of *M. gallinarum* in multiple infection. Kleven *et al.* (1978) showed that air sacculitis could be produced in young chickens following air sac inoculation or aerosol administration of the mycoplasma along with supraconjunctival exposure to a field or vaccine strain of infectious bronchitis virus. Such lesions did not occur with the administration of either organism alone. Should this be confirmed, it would be a considerable stimulus not only to study of the epidemiological features of the disease and its control but also to investigation of the possible part played by other apparently nonpathogenic mycoplasmas in multiple infections.

Mycoplasma gallinarum is not infrequently isolated from the respiratory tract of chickens and turkeys of all ages; it is worldwide in incidence, and many of the epidemiological features of *M. gallisepticum* probably apply to it. It may be egg-transmitted. It is readily isolated on mycoplasma medium, but serological tests for the recognition of infected stock have not been developed. It is probable that in principle the control measures outlined for *M. gallisepticum* would be of value in combating this infection. Indeed, one may speculate as to its recovery being an indication of the ineffectiveness of control measures against *M. gallisepticum, M. synoviae,* and *M. meleagridis.*

In a study of mycoplasmas and acholeplasmas in geese, Stipkovits *et al.* (1975) isolated *M. gallinarum* from goose embryo fibroblast tissue cultures. They caused a cytopathic effect in the cell cultures and were suspected of being associated with disease in goslings. Further investigation (Kisary *et al.*, 1976) showed that following intranasal administration of the organism to ten 3-day-old goslings, mild air sacculitis and peritonitis occurred in four of them. However, when a goose parvovirus was administered concomitantly to ten additional birds, three died and more severe widespread lesions were seen. No mortality occurred with the mycoplasma or virus alone, and no lesions with the virus alone. The freedom of the experimental goslings from other possible participating pathogens is not mentioned. It is of interest that the strain of *M. gallinarum* caused no mortality in chick embryos.

6. *Mycoplasma anatis* Infection in the Duck

Roberts (1964) first recovered this organism from the infraorbital sinuses of ducks showing sinusitis, which were concurrently infected with influenza A virus. He attempted to reproduce the sinusitis in 2- to 3-week-old ducklings but failed both with the mycoplasma alone and mycoplasma together with influenza A virus given 14 days later. A few birds dually infected showed some respiratory distress, and only the sera of birds infected with both organisms showed positive HAI titers.

Since that time there has been little reference in the literature to this organism, although Karpas and Fabricant (1969) report its isolation from Pekin ducks and Amin (1977) isolated it frequently from ducks, particularly from the cloaca, and also from a teal (*Anas crecca*) and a scaup (*Aythya marila*).

Amin and Jordan (1978a) inoculated a culture of the type strain, 1340, into the thoracic air sac of 1- to 2-day-old susceptible ducklings and produced air sacculitis and some retardation in growth, which suggests that the organism might be pathogenic in the presence of debilitating or precipitating factors.

The problem warrants further investigation.

7. *Acholeplasma laidlawii* Infection in the Chicken, Duck, and Goose

This organism was recovered from a chicken by Adler *et al.* (1961) and Adler and Shifrine (1964), who considered it to be saprophytic. It does not appear to be frequently recovered from poultry. Amin (1977), in a survey of mycoplasma infections in avian species, recovered *A. laidlawii* from the respiratory tissue of 2 chickens and 1 duck and the cloaca of a duck out of a total of 463 tissues from which mycoplasmas or acholeplasmas were isolated. There seems to be no association with disease.

Fawzia (1976) infected 2-day-old ducklings with a culture of the organism by the supraconjunctival route and produced lachrymation and conjunctivitis. Stipkovits *et al.* (1975) isolated *A. laidlawii* from air sacculitis, peritonitis, and perihepatitis from 2- to 8-day-old goslings. However, Kisary *et al.* (1976) found that a broth culture of the organism had little effect on either chicken or goose embryos or 3-day-old goslings.

8. Ureaplasma Infection in Chickens and Turkeys

Ureaplasmas have been isolated only recently from avian species. Stipkovits (1976) recovered the organism from respiratory tissues of a chicken, and preliminary investigation suggested association with disease. Koshimizu and Magaribuchi (1977) recovered a ureaplasma from the oropharynx of three Leghorn chickens and one jungle fowl. There was no association with disease. Stipkovits *et al.* (1978) isolated a ureaplasma from turkey semen which was serologically distinct from their isolate from a chicken; it was pathogenic for chickens and turkeys.

Further investigation is necessary into the prevalence and pathogenicity of ureaplasma infections.

9. Other Avian Mycoplasmas

Of the remaining recognized serotypes [C, D, E (*M. iners*), F, I, and L] and other avian mycoplasmas, the possible role they play in disease production, if any, can only be determined by a comprehensive study of this feature for each organism acting alone or in combination with other possible pathogens (multiple infection) and also with other mycoplasmas, since recovery of more than one mycoplasma species from a tissue is not uncommon. Furthermore, the host animal (chicken, turkey, quail, or their embryos) must be defined and should preferably be specific-pathogen-free.

V. PATHOGENICITY AND PATHOGENESIS

A. General

It is well established that *M. gallisepticum, M. synoviae,* and *M. meleagridis* are associated with the production of disease in domestic poultry, but further pathogenicity studies are required for other avian mycoplasmas and acholeplasmas.

Assessment of the pathogenicity of a mycoplasma can only be made within the well-defined parameters of several influencing factors. They include many of those outlined in Section IV, and are, for the pathogen, virulence, tropism, number of organisms, and route of infection; for the host, they are species, genetic constitution, age (embryo, neonate, or older bird), immune status, intercurrent infection, and nonliving debilitating factors.

Similarly the virulence of a strain of a species of mycoplasma can only be adequately described when all the factors involved are known, and these include those mentioned for pathogenicity, except of course virulence itself.

Many of the factors influencing pathogenicity have been considered for *M. gallisepticum, M. synoviae,* and *M. meleagridis* (Sections IV,B,1,a, B,2,a, and B,3,a, respectively). In this section therefore it is proposed only to emphasize the significance of some of these factors and to indicate possible mechanisms of pathogenesis.

B. *Mycoplasma gallisepticum*

The nature and exact significance of the virulence of avian mycoplasmas are still little understood. For *M. gallisepticum* an assessment of the virulence of three strains has been made by (1) the production of mortality in chick embryos inoculated at different ages and incubated at various temperatures (Power and Jordan, 1973), (2) the cessation of movement of cilia in chick embryo tracheal organ cultures (Power and Jordan, 1976a), and (3) the effect on specific-pathogen-free chicks (Varley and Jordan, 1978b) and turkey poults (Varley and Jordan, 1978c). There was close agreement in all three methods. Variation in virulence was demonstrated and also certain proclivities. All three strains caused lesions of the respiratory system varying in degree; one strain, the most virulent, caused gross lesions in the cerebrum in the chicken and turkey; another strain caused synovitis in turkey poults, and the same strain was the only one causing unilateral enlargement of the eye in the chicken. It was also shown that continued prolonged passage of the S6 strain in laboratory media reduced virulence but not its proclivity for the brain and hock tissues.

Relatively little has been published on the influence of the number of mycoplasmas, with the exception of McMartin and Adler (1961) on the production of air sacculitis in chickens, and Clyde and Thomas (1973a) on the production of encephalopathy in turkeys.

The effect of the route of infection is known to be significant (Jordan, 1975a). For instance, although the natural route of infection with *M. gallisepticum,* transovarian or via the respiratory tract, rarely results in tendosynovitis or arthritis, they are readily produced by foot pad inoculation (Kerr and Olson, 1967a,b).

The influence of host species and age have already been mentioned (Section IV,B,1,a). It is known that the young turkey poult is more susceptible than the chicken, and Power and Jordan (1976a) showed that a yolk sac inoculation of *M. gallisepticum* organisms which was nonlethal to chick embryos killed 1-day-old turkey poults. With reference to age, chick and turkey embryos and neonates are generally more susceptible than older birds.

The protective influence of the immune response of the host (Section IV,B,1,a–c) is little understood, as is its collapse in the face of intercurrent infection.

The exacerbating effect of other pathogens in multiple infections involving *M. gallisepticum* has been mentioned (Section IV,B,1,a). In this respect Amin (1977) showed that the virulence of the strain of *M. gallisepticum* had no influence on the severity of disease following concurrent supraconjunctival infection of chicks with the mycoplasma, a mild strain of NDV, and *E. coli*.

Although one species of mycoplasma might have an ameliorating influence on another (Section IV,B,1,a), it is interesting to speculate on a possible synergistic effect in which *M. gallisepticum* is involved, since this mycoplasma and others are not infrequently isolated from field material from the same organ or tissue.

Although by no means elucidated, it has been suggested that the pathogenesis of disease caused by *M. gallisepticum* is closely associated with the activity of such factors as mycoplasmal neuraminidase, peroxide or other hemolysins, lysosomal enzyme, and/or an exotoxin. Their effect may result in cell damage followed by recovery, death, or antigenic modification. In association there may also be an inflammatory response, an immune response to the pathogen, and with antigenic modification, perhaps an autoimmune response.

Cell damage might be initiated following attachment of the mycoplasma to the host cell. Sobeslavsky *et al.* (1968) and Manchee and Taylor-Robinson (1969) showed that chicken tracheal epithelial cells adsorbed to *M. gallisepticum* colonies by means of sialic acid receptor sites on the cells. However, Cherry and Taylor-Robinson (1973) found that neither cytadsorption nor hydrogen peroxide production were essential for the cessation of ciliary movement caused by *M. gallisepticum* in chick embryo tracheal organ culture. Nevertheless, Abu-Zahr and Butler (1976), studying by electron microscopy the behavior of *M. gallisepticum* and *M. gallinarum* in chick embryo tracheal explants, observed the intimate association of *M. gallisepticum* first with epithelial cells and later with collagen fibers of the lamina propria. This organism caused deciliation and degeneration of cells into amorphous structures with desquamation of epithelium. *Mycoplasma gallinarum*, however, seemed never to be in intimate contact with cells, although it also eventually, but more slowly, invaded the lamina propria in large numbers. The degeneration produced was qualitatively different from that resulting from *M. gallisepticum*. Furthermore, Uppal and Chu (1977) showed that attachment to tracheal epithelial cells followed intratracheal infection of chickens with *M. gallisepticum*. They confirmed the observations of Zucker-Franklin *et al.* (1966a,b) that the organism was frequently attached to the plasma membrane by the bleb. It was suggested that the bleb may act as a sucker. The affected epithelial cells showed loss of cilia and slight enlargement of the mitochondria and endoplasmic reticulum. The organisms were extracellular. It seems, therefore, that although cytadsorption of the organism may not be essential in the pathogenesis of tracheitis, it may nevertheless be of significance in this respect. It seems to be essential also if the mycoplasmas become intracytoplasmic, as indicated by Boam and Sanger (1970).

Apart from attachment to cells, survival on epithelial surfaces may be important to pathogenesis, and *M. gallisepticum* seems to be capable of this, at least in the respiratory tract, since the organism can be recovered from some birds over many months. The mechanism of survival is not known.

In the respiratory tract the initial infiltration of the subepithelial tissues with monocytes may be a nonspecific inflammatory response, as seen with the injection of turpentine (Nair, 1973), but later the large numbers of lymphocytes and lymphofollicular aggregations containing germinal centers suggest a bursa-dependent immune response.

Following the intravenous inoculation of turkey poults with the S6 strain of *M. gallisepticum* Clyde and Thomas (1973a,b) showed tropism of the organism for the arterial walls of the brain, periarticular tissue, and glomeruli. Very large numbers of organisms cause acute encephalopathy, presumably by increased permeability of the vessels and swelling of the endothelium. Since no mycoplasma antigen could be detected in the brain, it has been suggested that a toxin was responsible. With smaller doses localization of *M. gallisepticum* occurs, particularly in the arteries of the brain and periarticular tissue, and the organism appears to replicate. The organisms may release toxic products, resulting in endothelial swelling and increased permeability, especially in the brain. Fibroid changes were present in the arteries. Parenchymal necrosis of the brain occurred. In birds which survived, the acute fibroid changes gave way to chronic progressive cerebral arteritis with infiltration of the vessel wall with small, round cells. At this stage mycoplasma could not be detected by immunofluorescence. Several weeks after initial infection joint lesions, especially of the legs, appeared in the turkeys which survived; a similar condition occurs in chickens (Lamas Da Silva and Adler, 1969). In both there was swelling, redness, limitation of movement, and pain, and the gross and histological lesions as described in Section IV,B,1,c, with massive invasion of lymphocytes. No mycoplasmas were detected, nor were significant amounts of IgG demonstrated in the arterial walls. The exact mechanism of production of the chronic reaction is not known, but it might result from the effect of small numbers of mycoplasmas still present in the tissue or represent an immune response to altered tissue at these sites. An immune mechanism may also be responsible for the mycoplasma antigen in the glomeruli, since concentrations of IgG were also found in the same area. Clyde and Thomas (1973a) liken the condition to human collagen-vascular disease.

It should be noted that this pathological pattern has followed infection with a strain of *M. gallisepticum* with a proclivity for certain arteries when administered intravenously. Under natural conditions infection is through the egg or the respiratory system, and the strains may vary in tropism. However, the chronic stage, with massive infiltration of lymphocytes and lymphofollicular aggregates, occurs in several tissues (Kerr and Olson, 1967a) and may result from the same pathogenic processes.

In the exacerbation of disease which occurs with certain multiple infections (Section IV,B,1,a) it is probable that the invading viruses or *E. coli* cause cell damage, releasing lysosomal enzymes which further enhance penetration by mycoplasmas.

There has been no study of the significance of biological mimicry (Cole *et al.*, 1969, 1970) in disease caused by pathogenic avian mycoplasmas, but the inability of chickens and turkeys to produce potent growth-inhibiting antibodies suggests the possibility (Yamamoto and Adler, 1958a; Jordan, 1975b).

C. *Mycoplasma synoviae*

For *M. synoviae*, variations in virulence and tropism have been mentioned (Section IV,B,2,a) and also several other factors associated with the organism and host. With reference to the influence of the number of mycoplasmas on infection and disease Ghazikhanian *et al.* (1973) showed that there was a minimum dose for the production of air sacculitis by air sac inoculation. The importance of the route of infection is well documented (Jordan, 1975a); foot pad inoculation was most likely to produce synovitis (Sevoian *et al.*, 1958; Kerr and Olson, 1970; Ghazikhanian *et al.*, 1973; Wyeth, 1974), while air sac inoculation (Ghazikhanian *et al.*, 1973) and sometimes aerosol infection (Kleven *et al.*, 1972) were most likely to produce air sacculitis, although Wyeth (1974) was unable to produce lesions by this route and infection *in ovo* produced both types of lesion (Bradbury and Howell, 1975).

The exacerbating influence of certain viruses and bacteria in the disease process has already been noted (Section IV,B,2,a).

The pathogenesis of the lesions associated with *M. synoviae* may be mediated by the same means as outlined for *M. gallisepticum*. Both Kerr and Olson (1970) and Sells (1971), in attempting to explain the mechanism for the production of anemia, have suggested that it is not associated with an immune mechanism but more likely with damage of the erythrocytes by the organism. Sells (1971) also suggested that localization of the mycoplasma in certain tissues, together with their metabolic products, attracts heterophils which when damaged release lysosomes. This could account for the progressive accumulation of caseous material around tendons and bursae and in joint cavities. These lesions, together with mycoplasma antigen, might explain the infiltration of small, round cells, plasma cells, and macrophages. Fletcher *et al.* (1976) suggest that the accumulation of lymphocytes beneath the air sac epithelium might be due to their attraction to the exudate in the air sac lumen, the mycoplasma organisms, or damaged epithelial cells. They indicate that an antibody or cell-mediated response may be involved. Recently, Kume *et al.* (1977) have shown that thymus-dependent lymphocytes are necessary for the production of joint lesions.

In discussing the alteration in serum proteins associated with infection with *M. synoviae,* Sells (1976) suggests that depletion of albumin and the variation in β-globulins are associated with hepatic disease and that elevation of γ-globulin is associated with the inflammatory response and tissue damage.

D. *Mycoplasma meleagridis*

Variation in virulence occurs (Section IV,B,3,a), but the tropism observed for reproductive tissues in mature birds does not seem to be associated with disease of these organs. This is also true for the trachea from which *M. meleagridis* is readily isolated.

The influence of the route of infection on disease does not seem to have been comprehensively studied, but it appears that air sacculitis or osteodystrophy is most likely to follow infection of the embryo under natural conditions.

Other factors influencing the organism or the host in disease production have been mentioned (Section IV,B,3,a).

Air sac lesions (Section IV,B,3,c) show a histological picture similar to that seen with *M. gallisepticum* and *M. synoviae* infection, but little has been published on the pathogenesis of the condition.

The condition of ascites described by Wise *et al.* (1974) seen in turkey poults experimentally infected with *M. meleagridis* is suggested to be a manifestation of acute disease and to result from liver damage (Wise and Evans, 1975). The osteodystrophic form seems to be caused by interference with the nutritional supply rather than the blood supply to the growth plate of the affected bones (Wise *et al.*, 1973).

VI. THE IMMUNE RESPONSE

There are several review publications on this subject. They include an outline of the antibody response to avian mycoplasmas (Kleven, 1975), a brief account of the literature on immunity to mycoplasma infections of the avian respiratory system (Jordan, 1975b), the immune response to *M. gallisepticum* infection (Adler, 1976), and agglutination tests for *M. gallisepticum* infection (Adler and Wiggins, 1973). In addition, Fabricant (1975, 1977) discusses methods for the protection of chickens against infection of the respiratory and reproductive tracts and a decrease in egg production.

Although it is undoubtedly an oversimplification of the subject, the immune response to avian mycoplasma is considered here in terms of humoral antibody, local antibody, and the cell-mediated response.

A. Humoral Antibody

The presence of humoral antibody to *M. gallisepticum* was probably first demonstrated by Van Herick and Eaton (1945) by the HAI test on chicken sera, and the value of the test for the detection of chickens infected with this organism was reported by Jungherr *et al.* (1953). Fahey (1954) first applied the test to turkey sera. Adler (1954) used the slide agglutination test for the same purpose. Since that time a wide variety of tests has been used for the detection of humoral antibodies against *M. gallisepticum* (Jordan and Kulasegaram, 1968; Yoder, 1972; Sahu and Olson, 1976a). Fewer tests have been used for *M. synoviae* (Olson, 1978) and *M. meleagridis* (Yamamoto, 1978). Antibodies against *M. gallisepticum* in chickens (Roberts, 1969) and turkeys (Kleven, 1975) have been shown to consist of an early IgM response followed by IgG (7S). This has also been shown for *M. meleagridis* infection of turkeys (Kleven and Pomeroy, 1971a,b). Cold agglutinins (isohemagglutinins) were also associated in chickens with the IgM fraction (Kuniyasu and Ando, 1966; Kuniyasu, 1969; Kuniyasu and Yoshida, 1972). Adler and Da Massa (1969) also demonstrated a warm hemagglutinin. Cold agglutinins were observed in chicken sera following *M. synoviae* infection (Sahu and Olson, 1976b). The presence of a rheumatoid factor has been demonstrated in chickens infected with *M. synoviae* (Porter and Gooderham, 1966; Sells, 1976; Cullen, 1977).

The significance of the bursa of Fabricius in the production of humoral antibody and in the protection of chickens infected with *M. gallisepticum* has been shown by Adler *et al.* (1973). Although there was no direct relationship between antibody agglutinin titer and protection against air sac challenge, bursectomized birds were more susceptible to the infection. Vardaman *et al.* (1973b) showed that for *M. synoviae* infection bursectomy at hatch resulted in more severe air sacculitis and delayed and reduced antibody titer and suggested a protective role for antibody. Giambrone *et al.* (1977) infected chickens with infectious bursal disease virus (IBDV) at 1 day old, and later with *M. synoviae* and the viruses of Newcastle disease and infectious bronchitis. IBDV damages the bursa of Fabricius, and such infected birds produced either no antibody at all or antibody of low titer against *M. synoviae,* and the disease in them was more severe than in a control group of birds that were not infected with IBDV. The role of extra bursal tissue in antibody production was shown by Bryant *et al.* (1973), who chemically bursectomized birds as 7-day-old embryos and infected the chick with *M. gallisepticum*. The appearance of agglutinins was delayed compared with controls. It was considered that lymphoid follicles in the spleen and cecal tonsils and "lymphoepithelial" tissue of the cloaca were some of the tissues responsible for this extra bursal antibody production. The observations of Kume *et al.* (1977) with bursectomized and thymectomized chickens suggest that bursa-dependent lymphocytes are correlated with resistance to *M. synoviae* and that thymus-dependent cells are necessary for the development of lesions.

B. Local Antibody

There is little reference in the literature to the appearance of local antibody in response to avian mycoplasma infection, although Parry and Aitken (1973) have pointed out that such a response may be important in protection against upper respiratory tract infection with these organisms. In an experiment involving a virulent and a mild strain of *M. gallisepticum* (Mg) and a mild vaccine strain of NDV the following supraconjunctival inoculations were made in four groups of birds: (1) Mg, mild (2) Mg, virulent (3) Mg, mild, together with NDV (4) Mg, virulent, together with NDV. When extracts of Harderian glands were examined at 6 and 12 days after infection, antibody to Mg was found in all groups infected with mycoplasma organisms whether mild or virulent and infected with or without NDV (Powell, 1977). It is of interest also that such antibody was also found on the twentieth day after infection, except in the group given mild Mg alone. Humoral antibody to Mg of either virulence, and either alone or together with NDV, did not appear until day 20. The nature of the Mg antibody extracted from the Harderian glands was not determined, but the time of its appearance relative to humoral antibody suggests that it was locally produced and may well have a component of IgA (Albini *et al.*, 1974).

C. Cell-Mediated Response

Neither passive immunity (McMartin and Adler, 1961) nor maternal immunity (Roberts *et al.*, 1967) appears to protect against *M. gallisepticum*. Adler and Lamas Da Silva (1970), Adler *et al.* (1973), and Hayatsu *et al.* (1975) showed that there was little correlation between serum titer and resistance to challenge with *M. gallisepticum*. It appears, therefore, that other immune mechanisms are involved.

In *M. gallisepticum* infection the massive infiltration of lymphocytes and the formation of cells into follicular arrangements (Johnson, 1954; McMartin, 1967; Grimes and Rosenfield, 1972) suggest a cell-mediated response, but this has not been confirmed. Timms and Cullen (1976) and Cullen (1977) described a cell-mediated response in chickens infected with *M. synoviae*. They demonstrated leukocyte migration inhibition, probably specific for *M. synoviae*, which correlated with positive skin tests in chickens infected with a virulent strain of *M. synoviae*.

VII. AVIAN MYCOPLASMAS IN EMBRYONATED EGGS, CELL CULTURE, AND ORGAN CULTURE

A. Embryonated Eggs

The infected egg is an important method of mycoplasma transmission in the domestic fowl and turkey (Sections IV,B,1,a–2a and 3a). Transmission is probably mainly by transovarian infection for *M. gallisepticum* and *M. synoviae* but chiefly venereal for *M. meleagridis*. Although the prevalence of infection varies and may be very low, the possibility of indigenous mycoplasmas inherent in the use of embryonated eggs is obvious. Furthermore, a variety of avian viruses is also egg-transmitted. To obviate these disadvantages eggs should be obtained from a specific-pathogen-free source. There are several chicken flocks of this type.

The chick embryo has been recommended as a sensitive and reliable means of recovering mycoplasmas from field material. Inoculation is usually made into the yolk sac, and the organism may or may not kill the embryo. A disadvantage of this site is that, with subculture onto mycoplasma agar, the lipids of the yolk tend to mask the mycoplasma colonies. Inoculation may therefore be made onto the chorioallantoic membrane or into the allantoic sac, but mycoplasmas may not multiply in these tissues unless the cells are concomitantly injured. For this purpose concurrent infection with a virus such as that of infectious bronchitis may be used.

Ghazikhanian and Yamamoto (1974b) have reported on a strain of *M. meleagridis* which failed to grow in chick and turkey embryos, although it grew on artificial media. The prevalence of such a phenomenon is not known, or whether it also occurs with other mycoplasmas, but the possible limitation of the embryo in this respect should be noted.

A comparative study of the value of chick embryo inoculation and artificial media in the recovery of avian mycoplasmas from the field seems to be worthwhile.

Chick embryos have been used in assessing the pathogenicity of avian mycoplasmas (Kleckner, 1960; Yoder and Hofstad, 1964) and in assessing virulence (Power and Jordan, 1973). It is important to appreciate the significance of various factors which can influence the results (Power and Jordan, 1973).

Duck and quail embryonated eggs and the eggs of other avian species have received little attention in mycoplasma studies.

It might be pointed out also that nonfertile chicken eggs do not support the growth of *M. gallisepticum* (Calnek and Levine, 1957) and that this is probably true for other avian mycoplasmas.

B. Cell Culture

There are relatively few reports on the growth of avian mycoplasmas in cell culture. Edward and Kanarek (1960) found an *M. gallisepticum*-like organism as a contaminant in tissue culture. Butler and Leach (1964) grew *M. gallisepticum* in an HEp-2 cell line with a cytopathogenic effect (CPE). Grumbles *et al.* (1964) grew two strains of *M. gallisepticum* and two untyped avian mycoplasmas in a chick embryo kidney cell culture and a human synovial fluid (McCoy) cell line. A CPE was produced by the four organisms. Barile (1974) referred to the recovery of *M. gallisepticum, M. gallinarum,* and *A. laidlawii* in a survey of uninoculated cell cultures and indicated their prevalence. He pointed out that occasionally the original tissue used to prepare the primary cell culture may be the source of contamination. This can be a particular hazard for avian cells for which only primary cultures are used.

Recently Stipkovits *et al.* (1975) showed that *M. gallinarum* and *A. axanthum,* but not *A. laidlawii,* caused a CPE in goose embryo fibroblast cultures. Sodhi *et al.* (1976) adapted *M. gallisepticum* and *M. gallinarum* and two of four local mycoplasma isolates to growth in chick embryo cell culture. The time of appearance of CPE decreased with serial passage.

Perhaps the greatest deterrent to the general use of avian cell cultures for studies on avian mycoplasma is the problem of contamination. If the source tissue for cells can be obtained from specific-pathogen-free stock and if the recommendations of Barile (1974) for preventing contamination can be practiced, cell culture may have a place in avian mycoplasma studies, particularly perhaps with reference to virulence of strains and pathogenesis.

C. Organ Culture

Most reports on studies of avian mycoplasmas in organ culture have involved chick embryo tracheal explants. The reasons for this include the involvement of respiratory tissues in various avian mycoplasma infections, the ease of preparation and maintenance of the explants, and the cessation of ciliary movement as an indication of mycoplasma growth, pathogenicity, and virulence.

Cherry and Taylor-Robinson (1973) demonstrated that *M. gallisepticum* and *M. meleagridis* organisms introduced into tracheal organ cultures stopped ciliary movement, whereas *M. gallinarum, M. iners*, serotype I (Iowa 695), and serotype F (WR1) did not. Nonomura (1973) showed interference by *M. gallisepticum* with the replication of NDV in tracheal organ culture. Power and Jordan (1976a) used the system to show that there was an indirect relationship between the virulence of strains of *M. gallisepticum* and the persistence of ciliary activity. The system has also been used in pathogenesis studies on *M. gallisepticum* (Cherry and Taylor-Robinson, 1973; Abu-Zahr and Butler, 1976).

There seems to be considerable scope for the further use of tracheal and other avian organ explants in the study of growth, pathogenicity, virulence, and pathogenesis of a variety of species of mycoplasma. It might also have a place in the recovery of organisms from field material. Investigations might involve one or more than one species of mycoplasma, with or without other pathogens or debilitating agents.

VIII. FUTURE OUTLOOK

Although it is likely that the more common mycoplasma pathogens of domestic poultry will be eradicated from basic breeder flocks within the foreseeable future, there are several problems associated with domestic poultry and other avian species worthy of attention. Some of these are:

1. Host range. Certain species of avian mycoplasmas show a distinct

proclivity for one species of host, for instance, *M. meleagridis* for the turkey. Others seem less restricted in their hosts (Section I). However, the pattern of distribution of so-called avian mycoplasmas in avian and mammalian hosts will emerge only when there has been very much more isolation and typing of these organisms. Associated with this is the necessity for characterizing untyped avian isolates and for investigating further the role of ureaplasmas in avian species.

2. Isolation of mycoplasmas from field material. Comparative studies on methods of recovery of these organisms from field material are still required and also on the factors influencing isolation. The results may be of particular value for poultry flocks in which the interpretation of serological reactions is difficult.

3. Serological identification of infected birds. The more common serological tests—agglutination and hemagglutination inhibition—have been useful in the eradication of *M. gallisepticum* and *M. synoviae* infections in chickens and turkeys. Similar tests are required, however, for *M. meleagridis*. Furthermore, the development of a reliable single-bird test would also be of value.

4. Pathogenicity of avian mycoplasmas. There is need for an assessment of the pathogenicity of several species of avian mycoplasmas under well-defined conditions. This applies to organisms isolated from domestic poultry, pigeons, and other birds.

5. Pathogenesis of the disease condition. Very little is known of the mechanism by which avian mycoplasmas cause disease, either alone or together with other pathogens or debilitating factors. Further investigation of the subject is therefore warranted. An additional incentive might be that the disease picture with certain organisms seems to parallel diseases of humans such as rheumatoid arthritis and collagen disease. Infection of the chicken or turkey might therefore provide a useful experimental model.

6. The immune response. In this field also relatively little investigation has been made. There is considerable scope therefore for a study of the mechanisms involved, as well as the significance of humoral and local antibody, and the cell-mediated response in the protection of the host and in the production of disease.

REFERENCES

Abu-Zahr, M. N., and Butler, M. (1976). *J. Comp. Pathol.* **86,** 453–463.
Adler, H. E. (1954). *Proc. Am. Vet. Med. Assoc.* pp. 346–349.

Adler, H. E. (1958). *Poult. Sci.* **37**, 1116–1125.

Adler, H. E. (1976). *Theriogenology* **6**, 87–91.

Adler, H. E., and Da Massa, A. J. (1969). *Proc. Soc. Exp. Biol. Med.* **130**, 480–483.

Adler, H. E., and Lamas Da Silva, J. M. (1970). *Avian Dis.* **14**, 763–769.

Adler, H. E., and Shifrine, M. (1964). *J. Bacteriol* **87**, 1245.

Adler, H. E., and Wiggins, A. D. (1973). *World's Poult. Sci. J.* **29**, 345–353.

Adler, H. E., and Yamamoto, R. (1956). *Cornell Vet.* **46**, 337–343.

Adler, H. E., and Yamamoto, R. (1957). *Am. J. Vet. Res.* **18**, 655–656.

Adler, H. E., Yamamoto, R., and Berg, J. (1957). *Avian Dis.* **1**, 19–27.

Adler, H. E., Fabricant, J., Yamamoto, R., and Berg, J. (1968). *Am. J. Vet. Res.* **19**, 440–447.

Adler, H. E., Shifrine, M., and Ortmayer, H. B. (1961). *J. Bacteriol.* **82**, 239–240.

Adler, H. E., McMartin, D. A., and Ortmayer, H. B. (1962). *Avian Dis.* **6**, 267–274.

Adler, H. E., Bryant, B. J., Cordy, D. R., Shifrine, M., and Da Massa, A. J. (1973). *J. Infect. Dis.* **127**, 61–66.

Aghakhan, S. M., Pattison, M., and Butler, M. (1976). *J. Comp. Pathol.* **86**, 1–9.

Albini, B., Wick, G., Rose, E., and Orlans, E. (1974). *Int. Arch. Allergy* **47**, 23–34.

Alls, A. A., Benton, W. S., Krauss, W. C., and Cover, M. S. (1963). *Avian Dis.* **7**, 89–97.

Alls, A. A., Cover, M. S., Benton, W. J., and Krauss, W. C. (1964). *Avian Dis.* **8**, 235–256.

Amin, M. M. (1977). Ph.D. Thesis, Univ. of Liverpool, Liverpool.

Amin, M. M., and Jordan, F. T. W. (1978a). *Res. Vet. Sci.* **25**, 86–88.

Amin, M. M., and Jordan, F. T. W. (1978b). *Avian Pathol.* **7**, 455–470.

Anderson, D. P., Wolfe, R. R., Cherms, F. L., and Roper, W. E. (1968). *Am. J. Vet. Res.* **29**, 1049–1058.

Arya, P. L., Sautter, J. H., and Pomeroy, B. S. (1971). *Avian Dis.* **15**, 163–176.

Aycardi, E. R., Anderson, D. P., and Hanson, R. P. (1971). *Avian Dis.* **15**, 434–447.

Bahl, A. K., Peterson, A. C., Sautter, J. H., and Pomeroy, B. S. (1974). *J. Am. Vet. Med. Assoc.* **165**, 743.

Bankowski, R. A. (1961). *Br. Vet. J.* **117**, 306–315.

Barber, C. W. (1962). *Avian Dis.* **6**, 349–358.

Barber, T. L. (1969). Ph.D. Thesis, Cornell Univ., Ithaca, New York.

Barber, T. L., and Fabricant, J. (1971). *Avian Dis.* **15**, 125–138.

Barile, M. F. (1974). *Colloq. INSERM, Mycoplasmes Homme, Anim., Veg. Insectes, Congr. Int., Bordeaux* **33**, 135–142.

Beard, G. W., and Anderson, D. P. (1967). *Avian Dis.* **11**, 54–59.

Benton, W. J., Cover, M. S., and Melchior, F. W. (1967). *Avian Dis.* **11**, 426–429.

Berry, D. M. (1969). *Vet. Rec.* **84**, 397–398.

Bezrukava, I. Y. (1965). *Veterinariya (Kiev)* **8**, 109–114.

Bigland, C. H., and Da Massa, A. J. (1963). *Proc. U.S. Livestock Sanit. Assoc., 67th, New Mexico* pp. 541–549.

Bigland, C. H., and Jordan, F. T. W. (1974). *Proc. West. Poult. Dis Conf., 23rd, Poult. Health Symp., 8th,* pp. 55–61.

Bigland, C. H., and Matsumoto, J. J. (1975). *Avian Dis.* **19**, 617–621.

Bigland, C. H., and Yamamoto, R. (1964). *Avian Dis.* **8**, 531–538.

Bigland, C. H., Dungan, W., Yamamoto, R., and Voris, J. C. (1964). *Avian Dis.* **8**, 85–92.

Blake, J. T. (1962). *Am. J. Vet. Res.* **23**, 847–854.

Boam, G. W., and Sanger, V. L. (1970). *Avian Dis.* **14**, 503–513.

Bradbury, J. M. (1975). *Proc. Conf. Taxon. Physiol. Anim. Mycoplasmas, 3rd, Brno* pp. 106–115.

Bradbury, J. M. (1978). *Vet. Rec.* **102**, 316.
Bradbury, J. M., and Garuti, A. (1978). *Avian Pathol.* **7**, 407–419.
Bradbury, J. M., and Howell, L. J. (1975). *Avian Pathol.* **4**, 277–286.
Bradbury, J. M., and Jordan, F. T. W. (1971). *J. Hyg.* **69**, 593–606.
Bradbury, J. M., Oriel, C. H., and Jordan, F. T. W. (1976). *J. Clin. Microbiol.* **3**, 449–452.
Bryant, B. J., Adler, H. E., Cordy, D. R., Shifrine, M., and Da Massa, A. J. (1973). *Eur. J. Immunol.* **3**, 9–15.
Butler, M., and Leach, R. H. (1964). *J. Gen. Microbiol.* **34**, 285–294.
Calnek, B. W., and Levine, P. P. (1957). *Avian Dis.* **1**, 208–222.
Carnaghan, R. B. A. (1961). *J. Comp. Pathol.* **71**, 279–285.
Carnaghan, R. B. A. (1962). *J. Comp. Pathol.* **72**, 433–438.
Cassidy, D. R., and Grumbles, L. C. (1959). *Avian Dis.* **3**, 126–135.
Chalquest, R. R. (1962). *Avian Dis.* **6**, 36–43.
Chalquest, R. R., and Fabricant, J. (1959). *Avian Dis.* **3**, 257–271.
Chalquest, R. R., and Fabricant, J. (1960). *Avian Dis.* **4**, 515–539.
Chandiramani, N. K., Van Roekel, H., and Olesiuk, O. M. (1966). *Poult. Sci.* **45**, 1029–1044.
Cherry, J. D., and Taylor-Robinson, D. (1973). *Ann. N.Y. Acad. Sci.* **225**, 290–303.
Chu, H. P. (1954). *Proc. World Poult. Congr., 10th, Edinburgh,* Part III, pp. 246–251.
Clyde, W. A., and Thomas, L. (1973a). *Ann. N.Y. Acad. Sci.* **225**, 413–424.
Clyde, W. A., and Thomas, L. (1973b). *Proc. Natl. Acad. Sci. U.S.A.* **70**, 1545–1549.
Cole, B. C., Cahill, J. F., Wiley, B. B., and Ward, J. R. (1969). *J. Bacteriol.* **98**, 930–937.
Cole, B. C., Golightly-Rowland, L., Ward, J. R., and Wiley, B. B. (1970). *Infect. Immun.* **2**, 419–425.
Cordy, D. R., and Adler, H. E. (1957). *Avian Dis.* **1**, 235–245.
Corstvet, R. E., and Sadler, W. W. (1966a). *Am. J. Vet. Res.* **27**, 1703–1720.
Corstvet, R. E., and Sadler, W. W. (1966b). *Am. J. Vet. Res.* **27**, 1721–1723.
Cover, M. S., and Waller, R. F. (1954). *Am. J. Vet. Res.* **15**, 119–121.
Cullen, G. A. (1977). *In* "Experimental Models of Chronic Inflammatory Diseases" Bayer-Symposium, Vol. 6, pp. 240–255. Springer-Verlag, Berlin and New York.
Cullen, G. A., and Anderton, M. F. (1974). *Avian Pathol.* **3**, 89–103.
de Blieck, L. (1948). *Tijdschr. Diergeneeskd.* **73**, 955–964.
Delaplane, J. P., and Stuart, H. O. (1943). *Am. J. Vet. Res.* **4**, 325–332.
Dierks, R. E., Newman, J. A., and Pomeroy, B. S. (1967). *Ann. N.Y. Acad. Sci.* **143**, 170–189.
Dodd, S. (1905). *J. Comp. Pathol. Ther.* **18**, 239–245.
Domermuth, C. H. (1958). *Avian Dis.* **2**, 442–449.
Domermuth, C. H. (1960). *Avian Dis.* **4**, 456–466.
Domermuth, C. H., and Gross, W. B. (1962). *Avian Dis.* **6**, 499–505.
Edward, D. G. ff., and Freundt, E. A. (1956). *J. Gen. Microbiol.* **14**, 197–207.
Edward, D. G. ff., and Freundt, E. A. (1973). *Int. J. Syst. Bacteriol.* **23**, 55–61.
Edward, D. G. ff., and Kanarek, A. D. (1960). *Ann. N.Y. Acad. Sci.* **79**, 696–702.
Ernø, H., Jurmanova, K., and Leach, R. H. (1973). *Acta Vet. Scand.* **14**, 511–523.
Fabricant, J. (1958). *Avian Dis.* **2**, 409–417.
Fabricant, J. (1969). *In* "The Mycoplasmatales and the L-Phase of Bacteria" (L. Hayflick, ed.), pp. 621–641. North-Holland Publ., Amsterdam.
Fabricant, J. (1975). *Am. J. Vet. Res.* **36**, 566–567.
Fabricant, J. (1977). *Proc. West. Poult. Dis. Conf., 26th, Poult. Health Symp., 11th, Univ. Calif., Davis,* pp. 71–74.
Fabricant, J., and Levine, P. P. (1963). *Proc. World Vet. Cong., 17th, Hanover* pp. 1469–1473.

Fahey, J. E. (1954). *Proc. Soc. Exp. Biol. Med.* **86**, 38–40.

Fahey, J. E. (1957). *Vet. Med.* **52**, 305–307.

Fahey, J. E., and Crawley, J. F. (1954). *Can. J. Comp. Med. Vet. Sci.* **18**, 67–75.

Fahey, J. E., and Crawley, J. F. (1955). *Can. J. Comp. Med. Vet. Sci.* **19**, 53–56.

Fawzia, M. M. (1976). M. V. Sci. Thesis, Cairo Univ., Cairo.

Fletcher, O. J., Anderson, D. P., and Kleven, S. H. (1976). *Vet. Pathol.* **13**, 303–314.

Fox, M. L., and Bigland, C. H. (1970). *Can. J. Comp. Med.* **34**, 285–288.

Freundt, E. A. (1955). *Int. Bull. Bacteriol. Nomencl. Taxon.* **5**, 67–78.

Frey, M. L., Hanson, R. P., and Anderson, D. P. (1968a). *Am. J. Vet. Res.* **29**, 2163–2171.

Frey, M. L., Anderson, D. P., and Hanson, R. P. (1968b). *Avian Dis.* **12**, 693–699.

Frey, M. L., Thomas, G. B., and Hale, P. A. (1973). *Ann. N.Y. Acad. Sci.* **225**, 334–346.

Friend, C., Patuleia, M. C., and Nelson, J. B. (1966). *Proc. Soc. Exp. Biol. Med.* **121**, 1009–1010.

Garside, J. S. (1965). *Vet. Rec.* **77**, 354–366.

Gerlach, H. (1977). *Berl. Muench. Tieraerztl, Wochenschr.* **90**, 140–143.

Gerlach, H., Yamamoto, R., and Ortmayer, H. B. (1968). *Arch. Gefluegelkd.* **32**, 396–399.

Ghazikhanian, G., and Yamamoto, R. (1969). *Proc. West. Poult. Dis. Conf., 18th, Poult. Health Symp., 3rd, Univ. Calif., Davis,* pp. 36–37.

Ghazikhanian, G., and Yamamoto, R. (1974a). *Am. J. Vet. Res.* **35**, 417–424.

Ghazikhanian, G., and Yamamoto, R. (1974b). *Am. J. Vet. Res.* **35**, 425–430.

Ghazikhanian, G., Yamamoto, R., and Cordy, D. R. (1973). *Avian Dis.* **17**, 122–136.

Ghazikhanian, G., Yamamoto, R., McCapes, R. H., Dungan, W. M., Larsen, C. T., and Ortmayer, H. B. (1976). *Proc. West. Poult. Dis. Conf., 25th, Poult. Health Symp., 10th, Univ. Calif., Davis,* pp. 63–64.

Giambrone, J. J., Eidson, C. S., and Kleven, S. H. (1977). *Am. J. Vet. Res.* **38**, 251–253.

Goren, E. (1978). *Tijdschr. Diergeneesk.* **103**, 361–366.

Goren, E., Litjens, J. B., and Reuten, F. M. W. J. (1975). *Tijdschr. Diergeneeskd.* **100**, 316–320.

Griffin, R. M. (1969). *J. Comp. Pathol.* **79**, 33–39.

Grimes, T. M., and Rosenfeld, L. E. (1972). *Aust. Vet. J.* **48**, 113–116.

Gross, W. B. (1956). *Poult. Sci.* **35**, 765–771.

Gross, W. B. (1958). *Am. J. Vet. Res.* **19**, 448–452.

Gross, W. B. (1961). *Avian Dis.* **5**, 431–439.

Gross, W. B., and Colmano, G. (1969). *Poult. Sci.* **43**, 514–520.

Gross, W. B., and Colmano, G. (1971). *Poult. Sci.* **50**, 1213–1217.

Gross, W. B., and Siegel, H. S. (1965). *Poult. Sci.* **44**, 998–1001.

Grumbles, L. C., Hall, C. F., and Cummings, G. (1964). *Avian Dis.* **8**, 274–280.

Hamdy, A. H., Kleven, S. H., McCune, E. L., Pomeroy, B. S., and Peterson, A. C. (1976). *Avian Dis.* **20**, 118–125.

Hayatsu, E., Sugiyama, H., Kume, K., Kawakubo, Y., Kimura, M., Yoshioka, M., Kanekos, S., Kobayashi, K., Yamasaki, T., and Nishiyama, Y. (1975). *Am. J. Vet. Res.* **36**, 217–221.

Hemsley, L. A. (1965). *Br. Vet. J.* **121**, 76–82.

Hinz, K. H. (1972). *Vet. Med. Rev.* **2**, 142–148.

Hinz, K. H., and Luders, H. (1969). *Dtsch. Tieraerztl. Wochenschr.* **76**, 88–93, 120–123.

Hofstad, M. S. (1952). *Progr. Rep., Vet. Med. Res. Inst.,* Iowa State Coll., Ames.

Hofstad, M. S. (1957). *Avian Dis.* **1**, 170–179.

Hofstad, M. S. (1973). *Poult. Sci.* **52**, 2040.

Jerstad, A. C., Hamilton, C. M., and Smith, V. E. (1949). *Vet. Med.* **44**, 272–273.

Johnson, E. P. (1954). *Cornell Vet.* **44**, 230–239.

Jordan, F. T. W. (1972). *Vet. Rec.* **90,** 556–562.

Jordan, F. T. W. (1975a). *Avian Pathol.* **4,** 165–174.

Jordan, F. T. W. (1975b). *Dev. Biol. Stand.* **28,** 590–596.

Jordan, F. T. W., and Amin, M. M. (1978). *Avian Pathol.* **7,** 349–355.

Jordan, F. T. W., and Kulasegaram, P. (1968). *J. Hyg.* **66,** 249–267.

Jungherr, E. L. (1949). *Am. J. Vet. Res.* **10,** 372–383.

Jungherr, E. L., (1960). *Ann. N.Y. Acad. Sci.* **79,** 750–755.

Jungherr, E. L., Luginbuhl, R. E., and Jacobs, R. E. (1953). *Proc. Annu. Meet. Am. Vet. Med. Assoc., 90th, Toronto* pp. 303–312.

Kaklamanis, E., Thomas, L., Stavropoulos, K., Borman, J., and Boshwitz, C. (1969). *Nature (London)* **221,** 860–862.

Kaklamanis, E., Stravropoulos, K., and Thomas, L. (1971). *In* "Mycoplasma and the L-Forms of Bacteria" (S. Madoff, ed.), pp. 27–35. Gordon & Breach, New York.

Karpas, D., and Fabricant, J. (1969). *Proc. Annu. Meet. Northeast. Conf. Avian Dis., 41st, Univ. Maine* p. 37.

Kato, K. (1965). *Natl. Inst. Anim. Health Q.* **5,** 183–189.

Katzen, S., Matsuda, K., and Reid, B. L. (1969). *Poult. Sci.* **48,** 1504–1506.

Kelton, W. H., and Van Roekel, H. (1963). *Avian Dis.* **7,** 272–286.

Kerr, K. M., and Olson, N. O. (1964). *Avian Dis.* **8,** 256–263.

Kerr, K. M., and Olson, N. O. (1967a). *Avian Dis.* **11,** 559–578.

Kerr, K. M., and Olson, N. O. (1967b). *Ann. N.Y. Acad. Sci.* **143,** 204–217.

Kerr, K. M., and Olson, N. O. (1970). *Avian Dis.* **14,** 291–320.

King, D. D., Kleven, S. H., Wenger, D. M., and Anderson, D. P. (1973). *Avian Dis.* **17,** 722–726.

Kirchhoff, H. (1974). *Zentralbl. Veterinaermed., Reihe B* **21,** 207–210.

Kisary, J., El-Ebeedy, A. A., and Stipkovits, L. (1976). *Avian Pathol.* **5,** 15–20.

Kiser, J. S. Popken, F., and Clemente, J. (1961). *Avian Dis.* **5,** 283–296.

Kleckner, A. L. (1960). *Am. J. Vet. Res.* **21,** 274–280.

Kleven, S. H. (1972). *Turkey Prod. Semin., Univ. Georgia, Athens.*

Kleven, S. H. (1975). *Am. J. Vet. Res.* **36,** 563–565.

Kleven, S. H., and Anderson, D. P. (1971). *Avian Dis.* **15,** 551–557.

Kleven, S. H., and Anderson, D. P. (1975). *Proc. West. Poult. Dis. Conf., 24th, Poult. Health Symp., 9th, Univ. Calif., Davis,* pp. 69–72.

Kleven, S. H., and Pomeroy, B. S. (1971a). *Avian Dis.* **15,** 291–298.

Kleven, S. H., and Pomeroy, B. S. (1971b). *Avian Dis.* **15,** 299–304.

Kleven, S. H., King, D. D., and Anderson, D. P. (1972). *Avian Dis.* **16,** 915–924.

Kleven, S. H., Fletcher, O. J., and Davis, R. B. (1973). *J. Am. Vet. Med. Assoc.* **163,** 1196.

Kleven, S. H., Fletcher, O. J., and Davis, R. B. (1975). *Avian Dis.* **19,** 126–135.

Kleven, S. H., Eidson, C. S., and Fletcher, O. J. (1978). *Avian Dis.* **22,** 707–716.

Koshimizu, K., and Magaribuchi, T. (1977). *Jpn. J. Vet. Sci.* **39,** 195–199.

Kumar, M. C. (1967). Ph.D. Thesis, Univ. of Minnesota, Minneapolis.

Kumar, S., Dierks, R. E., Newman, J. A., Pfow, C. L., and Pomeroy, B. S. (1963). *Avian Dis.* **7,** 376–385.

Kumar, M. C., Newman, J. A., Kleven, S. H., and Pomeroy, B. S. (1968). *Poult. Sci.* **47,** 1688. (Abstr.)

Kumar, M. C., Pomeroy, B. S., Dungan, W. M., and Larsen, C. T. (1974). *Proc. World Poult. Congr., 15th, New Orleans* pp. 353–355.

Kume, K., Kawakubo, Y., Morita, C., Hayatsu, E., and Yoshioka, M. (1977). *Am. J. Vet. Res.* **38,** 1595–1600.

Kuniyasu, C. (1969). *Natl. Inst. Anim. Health Q.* **9,** 119–128.

Kuniyasu, C., and Ando, K. (1966). *Natl. Inst. Anim. Health Q.* **6**, 136–143.
Kuniyasu, C., and Yoshida, Y. (1972). *Natl. Inst. Anim. Health Q.* **12**, 69–73.
Kuniyasu, C., Yoshida, Y., and Takano, M. (1974). *Natl. Inst. Anim. Health Q.* **14**, 48–53.
Laidlaw, P. P., and Elford, W. J. (1936). *Proc. R. Soc. London, Ser. B* **120**, 292–303.
Lamas Da Silva, J. M., and Adler, H. E. (1969). *Pathol. Vet.* **6**, 385–395.
McCapes, R. H., Yamamoto, R., Ortmayer, H. B., and Scott, W. F. (1975). *Avian Dis.* **19**, 506–514.
McCapes, R. H., Yamamoto, R., Ghazikhanian, G., Dungan, W. M., and Ortmayer, H. B. (1977). *Avian Dis.* **21**, 57–68.
McMartin, D. A. (1963). *Proc. World Vet. Congr., 17th, Hanover* **2**, 1453–1458.
McMartin, D. A. (1967). *Vet. Rec.* **81**, 317–320.
McMartin, D. A., and Adler, H. E. (1961). *J. Comp. Pathol.* **71**, 311–323.
McMartin, D. A., and Wilson, J. E. (1968). *Vet. Rec.* **82**, 392–393.
Madden, D. L., Henderson, W. H., and Moses, A. E. (1967). *Avian Dis.* **11**, 378–380.
Manchee, R. J., and Taylor-Robinson, D. (1969). *J. Bacteriol.* **98**, 914–919.
Manuelidis, E. E., and Thomas, L. (1973). *Proc. Natl. Acad. Sci. U.S.A.* **70**, 706–709.
Mårdh, P. A., and Taylor-Robinson, D. (1973). *Med. Microbiol. Immunol.* **158**, 259–266.
Markham, F. S., and Wong, S. C. (1952). *Poult. Sci.* **31**, 902–904.
Matuka, O., Aganovic, N., and Forsek, Z. (1968). *Veterinaria (Sarajevo)* **17**, 167–170.
Matzer, N., and Yamamoto, R. (1970). *Avian Dis.* **14**, 321–329.
Meroz, M., Hadash, D., and Samberg, Y. (1973). *Refu. Vet.* **30**, 101–109.
Meroz, M., Samberg, Y., Hadasah, D., and Trumper, S. (1976). *Refu. Vet.* **33**, 111–116.
Mohamed, Y. S., and Bohl, E. H. (1967). *Avian Dis.* **11**, 634–641.
Mohamed, Y. S., and Bohl, E. H. (1968). *Avian Dis.* **12**, 554–566.
Mohamed, Y. S., and Bohl, E. H. (1969). *Avian Dis.* **13**, 440–446.
Mohamed, Y. S., Moorhead, P. D., and Bohl, E. H. (1970a). *Am. J. Vet. Res.* **31**, 1637–1643.
Mohamed, Y. S., Moorhead, P. D., and Bohl, E. H. (1970b). *Avian Dis.* **14**, 410–412.
Moore, R. W., Grumbles, L. C., and Beasley, J. N. (1960). *Ann. N.Y. Acad. Sci.* **79**, 556–561.
Moorhead, P. D., Cross, R. F., and Henderson, W. (1967). *Avian Dis.* **11**, 354–365.
Nair, M. K. (1973). *Acta Vet. Scand., Suppl.* **43**, 1–103.
Nelson, J. B. (1935). *Science* **82**, 43–44.
Nelson, J. B. (1936a). *J. Exp. Med.* **63**, 509–513.
Nelson, J. B. (1936b). *J. Exp. Med.* **63**, 515–552.
Nelson, J. B. (1936c). *J. Exp. Med.* **64**, 749–758.
Nelson, J. B. (1936d). *J. Exp. Med.* **64**, 759–765.
Nelson, J. B. (1938). *J. Exp. Med.* **67**, 847–855.
Nelson, J. B. (1939). *J. Exp. Med.* **69**, 199–209.
Newman, J. A. (1967). *Diss. Abstr. B* **28**, 2254.
Newnham, A. G., and Chu, H. P. (1965). *J. Hyg.* **63**, 1–23.
Nonomura, I. (1973). *Natl. Inst. Anim. Health Q.* **13**, 105–111.
Nonomura, I., and Sato, S. (1975). *Avian Dis.* **19**, 603–607.
Nonomura, I., and Yoder, H. W. (1977). *Avian Dis.* **21**, 370–381.
Nutor, B. L. (1969). M. V. Sci. Thesis, Univ. of Liverpool, Liverpool.
Olesiuk, O. M., and Van Roekel, H. (1960). *Ann. N.Y. Acad. Sci.* **79**, 727–740.
Olson, N. O. (1978). *In* "Diseases of Poultry" (M. S. Hofstad, B. W. Calnek, C. F. Helmboldt, W. M. Reid, and H. W. Yoder, eds.), 7th Ed., pp. 261–270. Iowa State Univ. Press, Ames.
Olson, N. O., and Kerr, K. M. (1967). *Avian Dis.* **11**, 578–585.

Olson, N. O., and Kerr, K. M. (1970). *Avian Dis.* **14,** 654–664.

Olson, N. O., and Sahu, S. T. (1976). *Avian Dis.* **16,** 387–396.

Olson, N. O., and Yoder, H. W. (1968). *Proc. Poult. Pathol. Conf., 10th, Am. Cyanamide Co., Princetown, N.J.* p. 106.

Olson, N. O., Bletner, J. K., Shelton, D. C., Munro, D. A., and Anderson, G. C. (1954). *Poult. Sci.* **33,** 1075.

Olson, N. O., Shelton, D. C., Bletner, J. K., Munro, D. A., and Anderson, G. C. (1956). *Am. J. Vet. Res.* **17,** 747–754.

Olson, N. O., Shelton, D. C., and Munro, D. A. (1957). *Am. J. Vet. Res.* **18,** 735–739.

Olson, N. O., Kerr, K. M., and Campbell, A. (1963). *Avian Dis.* **7,** 310–317.

Olson, N. O., Adler, H. E., Da Massa, A. J., and Corstvet, R. E. (1964). *Avian Dis.* **8,** 623–631.

Olson, N. O., Yamamoto, R., and Ortmayer, H. (1965). *Am. J. Vet. Res.* **26,** 195–198.

Ortiz, A., and Yamamoto, R. (1974). *Proc. West. Poult. Dis. Conf., 23rd, Poult. Health Symp., 8th, Univ. Calif., Davis,* pp. 52–53.

Osborn, O. H., and Pomeroy, B. S. (1958). *Avian Dis.* **2,** 180–186.

Papageorgiou, C. (1970), *Bull. Acad. Vet. Fr.* **43,** 371–375.

Papageorgiou, C. (1971). *Bull. Acad. Vet. Fr.* **44,** 479–486.

Papageorgiou, C., and Bar, A. (1976). *Proc. Soc. Gen. Microbiol.* **3,** p. 172 (abstracts).

Parry, S. H., and Aitken, I. D. (1973). *Vet. Rec.* **93,** 258–260.

Pascucci, S., Maestrini, N., Govoni, S., and Prati, A. (1976). *Avian Pathol.* **5,** 291–297.

Polak-Vogelzang, A. A. (1977). *Avian Pathol.* **6,** 93–95.

Porter, P., and Gooderham, K. R. (1966). *Res. Vet. Sci.* **7,** 25–34.

Powell, J. R. (1977). Ph.D. Thesis, Univ. of Liverpool, Liverpool.

Power, J., and Jordan, F. T. W. (1973). *Res. Vet. Sci.* **14,** 259–261.

Power, J., and Jordan, F. T. W. (1976a). *Res. Vet. Sci.* **21,** 41–46.

Power, J., and Jordan, F. T. W. (1976b). *Vet. Rec.* **99,** 102–103.

Ranck, F. M., Grumbles, L. C., Hall, G. F., and Grimes, J. E. (1970). *Avian Dis.* **14,** 54–65.

Rashid, R. A., and Jordan, F. T. W. (1978). *Conf. Int. Org. Mycoplasmology, 2nd, Freiburg i.B., West Germany,* pp. 274–275 (abstracts).

Reis, R., and Yamamoto, R. (1971). *Am. J. Vet. Res.* **32,** 63–74.

Reis, R., Lamas Da Silva, J. M., and Yamamoto, R. (1970). *Avian Dis.* **14,** 117–125.

Rhoades, K. R. (1969). *Avian Dis.* **13,** 22–26.

Rhoades, K. R. (1971). *Avian Dis.* **15,** 910–922.

Rhoades, K. R. (1977). *Avian Dis.* **21,** 670–674.

Rhoades, K. R., Kelton, W. H., and Heddleston, K. L. (1965). *Can. J. Comp. Med. Vet. Sci.* **29,** 169–172.

Roberts, D. H. (1963). *Vet. Rec.* **75,** 665–667.

Roberts, D. H. (1964). *Vet. Rec.* **76,** 470–473.

Roberts, D. H. (1969). *J. Appl. Bacteriol.* **32,** 395–401.

Roberts, D. H., Olesiuk, O. M., and Van Roekel, H. (1967). *Am. J. Vet. Res.* **28,** 1135–1152.

Rosendal, S., and Black, F. T. (1972). *Acta Pathol. Microbiol. Scand., Sect. B* **80,** 615–622.

Sabry, M. (1968). Ph.D. Thesis, Cornell Univ., Ithaca, New York.

Sadler, W. W., and Corstvet, R. E. (1964). *Poult. Sci.* **43,** 1358.

Sadler, W. W., and Corstvet, R. E. (1965a). *Am. J. Vet. Res.* **26,** 1413–1420.

Sadler, W. W., and Corstvet, R. E. (1965b). *Am. J. Vet. Res.* **26,** 1421–1428.

Sahu, S. P., and Olson, N. O. (1976a). *Avian Dis.* **20,** 49–64.

Sahu, S. P., and Olson, N. O. (1976b). *Avian Dis.* **20,** 724–727.

Saif, Y. M., and Brown, K. I. (1972). *Turkey Res.* pp. 49–50.

Sato, S. (1970). *Jpn. Agic. Res. Q.* **5,** 48–53.
Sato, S., Nonomura, I., Shimizu, F., Shoya, S., and Horiuchi, T. (1970). *Natl. Inst. Anim. Health Q.* **10,** 58–65.
Sato, S., Shoya, S., Horiuchi, T., and Nonomura, I. (1972). *Natl. Inst. Anim. Health Q.* **12,** 54–62.
Sato, S., Shoya, S., and Kobayashi, H. (1973). *Natl. Inst. Anim. Health Q.* **13,** 45–53.
Sells, D. M. (1971). *Diss. Abstr.* **32,** 4699–4700.
Sells, D. M. (1976). *Avian Dis.* **20,** 108–113.
Sevoian, M., Snoeyenbos, G. H., Basch, H. I., and Reynolds, I. M. (1958). *Avian Dis.* **2,** 499–513.
Shimizu, T. (1978). *Conf. Int. Org. Mycoplasmology, 2nd, Freiburg, i.B., West Germany,* pp. 258–259 (abstracts).
Shimizu, T., Ernø, H., and Nagatomo, H. (1978). *Int. J. Syst. Bacteriol.* **28,** 538–546.
Simmonds, D. G., and Lukert, P. D. (1972). *Bull. Ga. Acad. Sci.* **30,** 1–10.
Smit, T. H., and Hoeckstra, J. (1968). *Neth. J. Vet. Sci.* **1,** 115–118.
Snoeyenbos, G. H., and Olesiuk, O. M. (1955). *Proc. Annu. Meet. Northeast Conf. Lab. Workers Pullorum Dis. Contrib., 27th, Durham, N.H.* p. 3.
Sobeslavsky, O., Prescott, B., and Chanock, R. M. (1968). *J. Bacteriol.* **98,** 914–919.
Sodhi, S. S., Dhillon, S. S., and Baxi, K. K. (1976). *Zentralbl. Veterinaermed., Reihe B* **23,** 609–612.
Springer, W. T., Luskus, C., and Pourciau, S. S. (1974). *Infect. Immun.* **10,** 578–589.
Stipkovits, L. (1976). *Proc. Soc. Gen. Microbiol.* **3,** p. 158 (abstracts).
Stipkovits, L., El-Ebeedy, A. A., Kisary, J., and Varga, L. (1975). *Avian Pathol.* **4,** 35–43.
Stipkovits, L., Rashwan, A., Takacs, J., and Lapis, K. (1978). *Conf. Int. Org. Mycoplasmology, 2nd, Frieburg, i.B., West Germany,* p. 257 (abstracts).
Subcommittee (1972). *Int. J. Syst. Bacteriol.* **22,** 184–188.
Subcommittee (1979). *Int. J. Syst. Bacteriol.* (in press).
Subramanyan, P., and Pomeroy, B. S. (1960). *Avian Dis.* **4,** 165–175.
Taylor-Robinson, D., and Cherry, J. D. (1972). *J. Med. Microbiol.* **5,** 291–298.
Taylor-Robinson, D., and Dinter, Z. (1968). *J. Gen. Microbiol.* **53,** 221–229.
Thayer, S. C., Strout, R. G., and Dunlop, W. R. (1958). *Poult. Sci.* **37,** 449–459.
Thomas, L., Davidson, M., and McCluskey, R. T. (1966). *J. Exp. Med.* **123,** 897–912.
Thornton, G. A. (1971). *Br. Vet. J.* **127,** 163–172.
Thornton, G. A., Wise, D. R., and Fuller, M. K. (1975). *Vet Rec.* **96,** 113–114.
Timms, L. (1967). *J. Med. Lab. Technol.* **24,** 79–89.
Timms, L. (1978). *Vet. Bull.* **48,** 187–198.
Timms, L., and Cullen, G. A. (1976). *Avian Dis.* **20,** 96–107.
Truscott, R. B., Ferguson, A. E., Ruhnke, H. L., Pettit, J. R., Robertson, A., and Speckmann, G. (1974). *Can. J. Comp. Med.* **38,** 341–343.
Tully, J. G., and Rask-Nielsen, R. (1967). *Ann. N.Y. Acad. Sci.* **143,** 345–352.
Tully, J. G., and Razin, S. (1970). *J. Bacteriol.* **103,** 751–754.
Uppal, P. K., and Chu, H. P. (1977). *Res. Vet. Sci.* **22,** 259–260.
Van Herick, W., and Eaton, M. D. (1945). *J. Bacteriol.* **50,** 47–55.
Van Roekel, H., Olesiuk, P. M., and Peck, H. A. (1952). *Am. J. Vet. Res.* **13,** 252–259.
Vardaman, T. H., and Drott, J. H. (1977). *Poult. Sci.* **56,** 72–78.
Vardaman, T. H., Reece, F. N., and Deaton, J. W. (1973a). *Poult. Sci.* **52,** 1909–1912.
Vardaman, T. H., Landreth, K., Whatley, S., Dreesen, L. J., and Glick, B. (1973b). *Infect. Immun.* **8,** 674–676.
Varley, J., and Jordan, F. T. W. (1978a). *Conf. Int. Org. Mycoplasmology, 2nd, Freiburg i.B., West Germany,* p. 216 (abstracts).

Varley, J., and Jordan, F. T. W. (1978b). *Avian Pathol.* **7,** 157–170.
Varley, J., and Jordan, F. T. W. (1978c). *Avian Pathol.* **7,** 383–395.
Voeten, A. C. (1965). Ph.D. Thesis, Univ. of Utrecht, Utrecht.
Wannop, C. C., Butler, M. A., and Pearson, A. W. (1971). *Vet. Rec.* **88,** 30–33.
Whittlestone, P. (1974). *Colloq. INSERM, Mycoplasmes Homme, Anim., Veg. Insectes, Congr. Int., Bordeaux* **33,** 143–151.
WHO/FAO Programme on Comparative Mycoplasmology (1974). Report of the Board.
Wichmann, R. W. (1957). *Avian Dis.* **1,** 222.
Wills, F. K. (1954). *Tex. Agric. Exp. Stn., Progr. Rep.* No. 1674, pp. 1–2.
Wills, F. K. (1955). *Southwest. Vet.* **8,** 258.
Wise, D. R., and Evans, E. T. R. (1975). *Res. Vet. Sci.* **18,** 190–192.
Wise, D. R., and Fuller, M. K. (1975). *Vet. Rec.* **96,** 133–134.
Wise, D. R., Fuller, J. R., and Boldero, M. K. (1970). *Vet. Rec.* **87,** 505–506.
Wise, D. R., Boldero, M. K., and Thornton, G. A. (1973). *Res. Vet. Sci.* **14,** 194–200.
Wise, D. R., Fuller, M. K., and Thornton, G. A. (1974). *Res. Vet. Sci.* **17,** 236–241.
Wright, D. N., Bailey, G. D., and Hatch, M. T. (1968). *J. Bacteriol.* **95,** 251–252.
Wyeth, P. J. (1974). *Vet. Rec.* **95,** 208–211.
Yamamoto, R. (1967). *Ann. N.Y. Acad. Sci.* **143,** 225–231.
Yamamoto, R. (1978). *In* "Diseases of Poultry" (M. S. Hofstad, B. W. Calnek, C. F. Helmboldt, W. M. Reid, and H. W. Yoder, eds.), 7th Ed., pp. 250–260. Iowa State Univ. Press, Ames.
Yamamoto, R., and Adler, H. E. (1958a). *J. Infect. Dis.* **102,** 143–152.
Yamamoto, R., and Adler, H. E. (1958b). *J. Infect. Dis.* **102,** 243–250.
Yamamoto, R., and Bigland, C. H. (1964). *Avian Dis.* **8,** 523–531.
Yamamoto, R., and Bigland, C. H. (1965). *Avian Dis.* **9,** 108–118.
Yamamoto, R., and Ortmayer, H. B. (1967). *Avian Dis.* **11,** 288–295.
Yamamoto, R., and Ortmayer, H. B. (1971). *Proc. World Vet. Congr., 19th, Mexico City* pp. 498–501.
Yamamoto, R., Bigland, C. H., and Ortmayer, H. B. (1965). *J. Bacteriol.* **90,** 47–49.
Yamamoto, R., Bigland, C. H., and Ortmayer, H. B. (1966a). *Poult. Sci.* **45,** 1139.
Yamamoto, R., Bigland, C. H., and Peterson, I. L. (1966b). *Poult. Sci.* **45,** 1245–1257.
Yamamoto, R., Kratzer, F. H., and Ortmayer, H. B. (1974). *Proc. West. Poult. Dis. Conf., 23rd, Poult. Health Symp., 8th, Univ. Calif., Davis,* pp. 53–54.
Yoder, H. W., Jr. (1969). Personal communication to N. O. Olson, 1972.
Yoder, H. W., Jr. (1970). *Avian Dis.* **14,** 75–86.
Yoder, H. W., Jr. (1976). *In* "Isolation and Identification of Avian Pathogens" (S. B. Hitchner, C. H. Domermuth, H. G. Purchase, and J. E. Williams, eds.), pp. 109–117. Arnold Print. Corp., Ithaca, New York.
Yoder, H. W., Jr. (1978). *In* "Diseases of Poultry" (M. S. Hofstad, B. W. Calnek, C. F. Helmboldt, W. M. Reid, and H. W. Yoder, eds.), 7th Ed., pp. 236–250. Iowa State Univ. Press, Ames.
Yoder, H. W., Jr., and Hofstad, M. S. (1962). *Avian Dis.* **6,** 147–160.
Yoder, H. W., Jr., and Hofstad, M. S. (1964). *Avian Dis.* **8,** 481–512.
Yoder, H. W., Jr., and Hofstad, M. S. (1965). *Avian Dis.* **9,** 291–301.
Yoder, H. W., Jr., Nelson, C. L., and Hofstad, M. S. (1961). *Vet. Med.* **56,** 178–180.
Yoder, H. W., Jr., Drury, L. N., and Hopkins, S. R. (1977). *Avian Dis.* **21,** 195–208.
Zander, D. V. (1961). *Avian Dis.* **5,** 154–156.
Zucker-Franklin, D., Davidson, M., and Thomas, L. (1966a). *J. Exp. Med.* **124,** 521–532.
Zucker-Franklin, D., Davidson, M., and Thomas, L. (1966b). *J. Exp. Med.* **124,** 533–544.

2 / BOVINE MYCOPLASMAS

R. N. Gourlay and C. J. Howard

THE MYCOPLASMAS, VOL. II

I. INTRODUCTION

Mycoplasmas of cattle enjoy a special place in the history of myco-plasma research, since the very first mycoplasma known was the agent of contagious bovine pleuropneumonia cultivated in artificial medium by Nocard and Roux (1898). This organism, now known as *Mycoplasma mycoides* subsp. *mycoides,* became the type species of the genus *Myco-plasma* (Edward and Freundt, 1956) and for 25 years was the only recog-nized mycoplasma, that is, until 1923, when it was shown that contagious agalactia of sheep was caused by a similar organism (*Mycoplasma agalac-tiae*). In the 55 years since then, mycoplasmas have become commonplace and have been isolated from almost every domestic and laboratory animal, from many wild animals, and from humans.

The great importance of *M. mycoides* subsp. *mycoides* and the disease it produces in cattle had the unfortunate effect of inhibiting the search for other bovine mycoplasmas, and it was not until 1947, half a century after the discovery of the first mycoplasma, that Edward *et al.* (1947) isolated mycoplasmas other than *M. mycoides* subsp. *mycoides* from cattle during their investigations into infertility in England. These isolates, from the genital tract, comprised two distinct types which were subsequently shown to be distinct species, *Mycoplasma bovigenitalium* and *Achole-plasma laidlawii* (Edward and Freundt, 1956).

As interest in mycoplasmas has grown, the possible role they might play in various diseases of cattle has led to numerous investigations, and mycoplasmas have been sought from many different anatomical sites. Mycoplasmas other than *M. mycoides* subsp. *mycoides* have now been isolated from the respiratory tract (Carter, 1954), the joints (Moulton *et al.*, 1956), the mammary glands (Davidson and Stuart, 1960), the eyes (Gourlay and Thomas, 1969a; Langford and Dorward, 1969), the rumen (Robinson and Hungate, 1973), the intestines (Gourlay and Wyld, 1975), and of course the urogenital tract.

Mycoplasma species are identified by biochemical and serological means and, at the time Cottew and Leach (1969) wrote their review on mycoplasmas of cattle, sheep, and goats, mycoplasma strains known to occur in cattle could be placed in eight distinct serological groups which included four named species. An indication of the progress made and knowledge gained about bovine mycoplasmas, even in the last 9 years, can be gauged by the fact that now over 20 different species or recognized serotypes of *Mycoplasma* and *Acholeplasma* have been isolated from cattle.

II. CLASSIFICATION

The general principles involved in the taxonomy of the mycoplasmas are outlined in Volume I, Chapter 1. Certain of the characteristics of the species isolated from cattle, considered to be bovine species, are given in Table I. These data are from Leach (1973), Ernø and Stipkovits (1973a,b), Al-Aubaidi and Fabricant (1971a), Askaa *et al.* (1973), Howard *et al.* (1974a), Gourlay *et al.* (1977), Langford *et al.* (1976), Langford and Leach (1973), Gourlay *et al.* (1974a), Robinson and Hungate (1973), and Robinson and Allison (1975).

III. MYCOPLASMAS OF CATTLE

A. *Mycoplasma alkalescens*

This species, although only recently named, was first isolated in Australia from the nasal passages of cattle (Hudson and Etheridge, 1963). Since then, strains of this mycoplasma have been isolated from cows with mastitis in New Zealand (Brookbanks *et al.*, 1969). Fifty cows out of 180 were affected, and 30 were subsequently culled. Mycoplasmas were isolated from milk samples from one clinical case and from 1 out of 7 recovered animals. Other isolations of this mycoplasma were from sporadic cases of mastitis, from joint and navel lesions in calves and from bulk milk samples in the Unites States (Dellinger *et al.*, 1977), and from 6 out of 7 synovial fluid samples from calves with severe arthritis (Bennett and Jasper, 1978c). Approximately 30 calves were affected, and this organism was also isolated from the liver, joint, lymph nodes, and umbilical artery of one calf. *Mycoplasma alkalescens* has also been reported from commercial bovine serum (Barile, 1973) and from the prepuce of 2 bulls in Canada (Langford, 1975a).

This species was named *M. alkalescens* by Leach (1973), and the specific epithet refers to the alkaline reaction it produces in arginine-containing medium. *Mycoplasma alkalescens* grows in conventional mycoplasma media, hydrolyzes arginine but not urea, and does not utilize glucose. It produces typical "fried egg" colonies on solid medium and does not produce film and spots.

TABLE I. General Properties of Bovine Mycoplasmas[a]

Organism	Type or reference strain	Leach group	Al-Aubaidi serotype	G + C (mole %)	Acid from glucose	Arginine catabolism	Urease activity	Film and spot production	Aerobic tetrazolium reduction	Cholesterol (serum) required	Digitonin-sensitive	Liquoid-sensitive	Growth at 22°C
Mycoplasma													
M. alvi	Ilsley			26.4	+	+	−	−	−	+	+	−	−
M. bovirhinis	PG43	4	D	27.3	+	−	−	±[b]	+ and −	+	+	+	−
M. bovoculi	M165/69			29.0	+	−	−	−	+	+	+	+	−
M. dispar	462/2			29.3	+	−	−	±[b]	+	+	+	+	−
M. mycoides subsp. mycoides	PG1	1	A	27.1	+	−	−	−	+	+	+	+	−
Group 7	PG50	7	E	25.4	+	−	−	−	+	+	+	±	±
Serotype L	B144P		L	25.4	+	−	−	−	+	+	+	+	−
M. alkalescens	PG51	8	G	25.9	−	+	−	−	−	+	+	+	−
M. arginini	G230			27.6	−	+	−	−	−	+	+	+	±
M. canadense	275C			29.0	−	+	−	−	−	+	+	+	−
M. bovigenitalium	PG11	2	B	30.2	−	−	−	+	+ and −	+	+	+	−
M. bovis	PG45	5	F	27.8	−	−	−	+	+	+	+	+	−
M. verecundum	107			29.2	−	−	−	+	−	+	+	+	+
Ureaplasma													
Ureaplasma sp.				29–29.8	−	−	+	NT	NT	+	+	NT	NT
Acholeplasma													
A. axanthum	S743		K	29.5	+	−	−	−	+	−	−	−	+
A. laidlawii	PG8	3	C	32.9	+	−	−	−	+	−	−	−	+
A. modicum	PG49	6	M	29.3	+	−	−	−	+	−	−	−	+
Anaeroplasma													
An. bactoclasticum	JR			33.7	c	−	U	U	U	+	+	?	−

[a] NT, Not tested on representative bovine strains; U, apparently unknown; ?, inconclusive results.
[b] Film and spot production, late reaction.
c Galactose utilized but not glucose.

52

Bennett and Jasper (1978c) reported that the inoculation of this mycoplasma into the joints of two calves produced a febrile response and severe fibrinopurulent arthritis. However, intravenous inoculation of two other calves failed to produce signs of arthritis and resulted in only an acute febrile reaction.

It appears that *M. alkalescens* has not been inoculated into the mammary glands of cows; however, the production of arthritis in calves inoculated intra-articularly with this mycoplasma demonstrates a pathogenic capability, even though this route of inoculation may be an excessively severe challenge. The failure to produce arthritis by intravenous inoculation may be, on the one hand, simply a result of inoculating too few organisms (10^9) or, on the other hand, a true reflection of its pathogenic limitations.

B. *Mycoplasma alvi*

Gourlay and Wyld (1975) described an apparently new species of *Mycoplasma* isolated from the intestinal tract and feces of cows in England. Further isolations were made from the lower alimentary tract (from the abomasum to the rectum), feces, bladder, and vagina of cows (Gourlay et al., 1977). In the latter study this organism was fully characterized and named *M. alvi*.

The cultural and biochemical characteristics of *M. alvi* are given in Table I. It is a slow-growing organism but can attain a high titer in broth culture ($\geq 10^{10}$ organisms/ml). The optimal pH for growth is between 6.0 and 7.0 and, although the strain can grow aerobically, it prefers reduced oxygen and increased carbon dioxide conditions. Like most *Mycoplasma* species, *M. alvi* is inhibited by 1.5% digitonin, but it is insensitive to sodium polyanethol sulfonate at concentrations normally inhibitory to *Mycoplasma* species. An interesting property of this mycoplasma is its ability to utilize both glucose and arginine, a property shown by only three currently recognized species of *Mycoplasma*, none of them of bovine origin (*Mycoplasma capricolum, M. fermentans,* and *M. moatsii*). The morphology of *M. alvi* as revealed in electron micrographs is distinctive and differs from that of all other bovine mycoplasmas; it does, however, resemble both *Mycoplasma pneumoniae* and *M. gallisepticum* in its flask or club shape and possession of a terminal structure. From the feces of a cow a strain of mycoplasma (F376) was isolated that possessed cultural, biological, and morphological characteristics similar to those of the type strain of *M. alvi*. However, it differed from *M. alvi* serologically and in possessing a G + C ratio of 27.3 mole % (compared with 26.4 mole % for *M. alvi*). Further investigations are necessary before this can be considered a similar but separate species.

Mycoplasma alvi has so far only been isolated from apparently healthy adult animals. The type strain, Ilsley, was examined for its ability to hemadsorb bovine, sheep, pig, human O-group, and guinea pig erythrocytes and calf and pig kidney cells, with negative results (R. N. Gourlay and S. G. Wyld, unpublished observations). Furthermore, this strain of *M. alvi* did not attach to calf small intestine epithelial cell brush borders but one other strain (2995) and the F376 strain did attach by their terminal structures (R. N. Gourlay, R. Sellwood, and S. G. Wyld, unpublished observations). Inoculation of the Ilsley, 2995, and F376 strains into the mammary glands of two cows resulted in moderate milk changes and excretion of the mycoplasmas for 4–5 days (R. N. Gourlay and S. G. Wyld, unpublished observations).

C. *Mycoplasma arginini*

Mycoplasma arginini was first isolated from cell cultures, sheep, and goats (Barile *et al.*, 1968). Subsequently this species was reported to have been isolated from the respiratory tract of calves with pneumonia in Switzerland, East Germany, Rumania, Czechoslovakia, the United States, and Italy (Leach, 1970; Nicolet and de Meuron, 1970; Jurmanova and Krejci, 1971; Jensen *et al.*, 1976; Pignattelli, 1978).

A mycoplasma isolated from the semen of a bull with vesiculitis was identified as *M. arginini* (Leach, 1970). This mycoplasma was also reported to be present in the semen of clinically healthy bulls by Jurmanova and Krejci (1971) and isolated from 1 of 267 preputial samples taken from different bulls examined by Langford (1975a). The isolation of *M. arginini* from the uterus of 1 infertile cow out of 80 examined has been recorded (Langford, 1975b). *Mycoplasma arginini* has also been reported to have been isolated from the eyes of cattle with keratoconjunctivitis (Leach, 1970) and from cattle with mastitis (Leach, 1970; Rinaldi *et al.*, 1971).

Mycoplasma arginini is one of the few mycoplasmas isolated from cattle that is frequently isolated from other animal species. These include sheep, goats, chamois, pigs, and certain captive wild cats (Barile *et al.*, 1968; Leach, 1970; Hill, 1972; Foggie and Angus, 1972; Orning *et al.*, 1978). It has also been suggested that this species is a common contaminant of commercial bovine sera and cell cultures (Barile and Kern, 1971).

The general properties of *M. arginini* are shown in Table I. It is distinguished from the other mycoplasmas which metabolize arginine by serological tests (Leach, 1973). It grows in broth and on solid media ranging from pH 6.2 to 7.8.

The few studies that have been made to examine the pathogenicity of *M. arginini* have involved rather few animals. Nevertheless, these studies are consistent in that they all demonstrate the relative lack of pathogenicity of this species for the respiratory tract.

No lesions were found at necropsy in the lungs of two of three calves inoculated endobronchially 11–18 days earlier with *M. arginini* (Jurmanova *et al.*, 1975). The lesions found in the remaining calf may well have been present before inoculation with mycoplasmas, as the animals were conventionally reared. *Mycoplasma arginini* was isolated from the lungs of all three animals at necropsy. Two strains of *M. arginini* were inoculated intratracheally into two gnotobiotic calves, a total of 10^9 or 10^{10} organisms into each animal. No lesions were observed at necropsy 3 weeks later, although low numbers of *M. arginini* were isolated from lung washings (R. N. Gourlay, C. J. Howard, and L. H. Thomas, unpublished observations). Further evidence for the lack of pathogenicity of this species is derived from the experiments of Foggie and Angus (1972) with specific pathogen-free lambs. Two animals were inoculated, one intranasally and one intratracheally. The pathological effects observed were minimal, and the histological lesions so slight that it was considered that they may have been induced by the broth in which the mycoplasmas were suspended. Ruffo *et al.* (1971) claimed that *M. arginini* induced experimental mastitis. However, his method of cloning the organisms is not clear, and this observation requires confirmation.

Possibly more virulent strains exist than those used in these experiments. However, the evidence presented to date indicates that this mycoplasma species is not very pathogenic. The isolations from diseased tissue may reflect its ability to invade already damaged tissue.

D. *Mycoplasma bovigenitalium*

Mycoplasma bovigenitalium is a well-established species originally isolated from the vaginas of cows and semen of bulls in England by Edward *et al.* (1947). The general features of this species were, to a great extent, known before 1969, and the literature up to this date has been thoroughly reviewed by Cottew and Leach (1969).

Mycoplasma bovigenitalium is one of the few mycoplasmas isolated from cattle which is unable to produce acid from glucose or to catabolize arginine, and which does not possess urease activity. Although a decrease in pH is evident in broth cultures, which led to earlier suggestions that it should be regarded as a glucose-fermenting species (Cottew and Leach, 1969), this was later shown not to be the case (Leach, 1973; Edward and Moore, 1975). Film and spots are produced on suitable media. Biochemically and culturally this species is rather like *Mycoplasma bovis*, from which it can be distinguished by a variety of the usual serological techniques.

As pointed out in several reviews (Cottew and Leach, 1969; Fabricant, 1973; Gourlay, 1973; Tourtellotte and Lein, 1976), numerous reports have been made confirming the presence of this species in cattle all over the world. Not only is this mycoplasma widespread, but it may be present in a large number of the animals in a particular group, although this frequency of occurrence within a group has been found to vary according to different studies. Thus Albertsen (1955) isolated *M. bovigenitalium* from the semen of 94% of the bulls studied at two artificial insemination centers in Denmark. In the majority of cases the source of the *M. bovigenitalium* was considered to be the prepuce. In this study no correlation was found with infertility. Further studies in Denmark were reported by Blom and Ernø (1970). Although the isolation rate reported by these investigators was not found to be as great as that recorded by Albertsen, up to 64% of the semen samples at a particular artificial insemination center were found to be infected with *M. bovigenitalium*. These workers also thought that in most cases *M. bovigenitalium* should be regarded as a commensal. Other surveys of the incidence of this species in bulls include the studies by Ernø *et al.* (1967), in which *M. bovigenitalium* was found in the prepuce of 12 of 45 animals, and by Langford (1975a), who reported the isolation of this mycoplasma from the semen of 15.5% of 168 animals and the prepuce of 34% of 267 animals.

Mycoplasma bovigenitalium also appears to be commonly present in the urogenital tract of cows; this may be as a result of mating, since this organism has been reported to be rare in virgin heifers (Edward and Fitzgerald, 1952). Langford (1975a) reported the isolation of *M. bovigenitalium* from the cervicovaginal mucus of 11% of 1265 animals. A much lower isolation rate was reported by Jasper *et al.* (1974), 4 of 470 samples taken from the vaginas of cows being positive.

Although the isolation of *M. bovigenitalium* from herds with infertility problems has been reported (Jain *et al.*, 1967; Cottew, 1970; Edward *et al.*, 1947; Edward and Fitzgerald, 1952; Langford, 1975b), the high isolation rates from apparently normal cows and bulls indicate that in most instances *M. bovigenitalium* is a commensal. It may be that in certain circumstances this species plays a role in diseases of the urogenital tract. Thus Ernø and Blom (1972) isolated *M. bovigenitalium* from the semen of a bull with chronic vesiculitis and induced the same disease in bulls following inoculation of the strain isolated from the diseased animal into the vesicular glands of two bulls. Strain PG11, the laboratory-adapted type strain, did not, however, produce disease following its inoculation into bulls. Similarly Al-Aubaidi *et al.* (1972b) reported that a strain of *M.*

bovigenitalium from a case of seminal vesiculitis and epididymitis, when injected into the seminal vesicles of a bull, induced disease. Parsonson *et al.* (1974), in a study involving 13 bulls, also demonstrated that the inoculation of *M. bovigenitalium* into the seminal vesicles induced lesions (epididymitis). However, because of the artificial route of these inoculations, it is difficult to decide whether the mycoplasma would cause the disease under natural conditions in the absence of some other predisposing factor.

Afshar *et al.* (1966) reported that it was possible to induce granular vulvovaginitis (nodular venereal disease) in cattle by applying *M. bovigenitalium* to scraped, but not intact, vulvoepithelium. However, these investigators doubted whether *M. bovigenitalium* was the cause of the natural outbreak of granular vulvovaginitis from which the *M. bovigenitalium* strain was isolated, because of the low isolation rate from the diseased herd. Subsequently Hirth *et al.* (1970a) reported that the infusion of *M. bovigenitalium* into the uterus, which had not been scraped, did not induce clinical disease or lesions visible at necropsy.

Occasional reports have also been made of the isolation of *M. bovigenitalium* from the aborted fetus (Langford, 1975a,b). However, the isolation rate is very low and, since *M. bovigenitalium* is frequently found in the urogenital tract of cows, the possibility of secondary invasion or contamination rather than primary cause is strong.

The problem of deciding whether a mycoplasma is the cause of the disease from which it has been isolated is especially difficult in the case of *M. bovigenitalium*. If a high isolation rate from a disease condition, absence from the same site in a similar number of normal animals, and ability to induce the disease experimentally are requisites for believing a mycoplasma is the cause of a disease, the involvement of *M. bovigenitalium* as a primary cause of urogenital tract infections should be regarded as no more than a possibility.

Occasional outbreaks of mastitis have been reported from which *M. bovigenitalium* has been isolated (Stuart *et al.*, 1963; Cho *et al.*, 1976; Jasper, 1977). The isolated mycoplasma has induced mastitis in cattle following its inoculation into the mammary gland. Isolates from the urogenital tract are also capable of inducing mastitis following their inoculation into the mammary gland (Ernø, 1967). Thus *M. bovigenitalium* can be taken to be a cause of certain cases of mastitis. Since pathogenicity has been proven at this site, pathogenicity at other sites must be considered possible.

Another feature of the pathogenicity of *M. bovigenitalium* is its ability to induce arthritis under experimental conditions. Ernø (1969) reported the induction of arthritis following the intravenous inoculation of *M.*

bovigenitalium into a single calf, and Parsonson *et al.* (1974) reported the isolation of *M. bovigenitalium* from the joint fluid of one animal following inoculation of the urogenital tract. Perhaps if *M. bovigenitalium* were causing serious outbreaks of disease under natural conditions, one might expect to find *M. bovigenitalium*-induced arthritis associated with such diseases.

Occasional references have been made to the isolation of *M. bovigenitalium* from the respiratory tract. It has been isolated from the lung of a calf with bronchopneumonia (Cottew, 1970) and from the nasal passages of an apparently normal animal (Jasper *et al.*, 1974), although the isolation was only from 1 of more than 400 animals in this latter study. Pignattelli (1978) reported the isolation of *M. bovigenitalium* from 7.5% of calves with pneumonia on 42 farms between 1975 and 1977 in Italy. Because of the proven pathogenicity of *M. bovigenitalium* for cattle, the possibility that it may occasionally be involved in pneumonia should be considered.

Finally, it should be mentioned that *M. bovigenitalium* has been isolated from an aborted equine fetus (Langford, 1974) and from the semen of a boar (Gois *et al.*, 1973). The significance of these isolations is as yet unknown.

E. *Mycoplasma bovirhinis*

Cottew and Leach (1969) reviewed the data available on *M. bovirhinis*. We therefore consider mainly work that has been done since that time.

Mycoplasma bovirhinis is a glucose-fermenting mycoplasma (see Table I) which has only been reported from cattle. It appears to be the species most commonly isolated from the bovine respiratory tract, probably because of its ubiquity and its undemanding growth requirements, as it grows in most conventional mycoplasma media. Jurmanova and Mensik (1971) reported that bovine and sheep erythrocytes adsorbed to agar-grown colonies of most strains of *M. bovirhinis,* and they recommended this characteristic as suitable for tentative identification of this organism.

This species was not named until 1967 by Leach (1967), but Harbourne *et al.* (1965) were the first to recognize it as a separate species when they isolated it from the lungs and nasal swabs of calves suffering from respiratory disease in England. Other earlier isolates from the lungs, spleen, and other tissues of cattle affected by pneumoenteritis in the Unites States were recognized as being the same, as was a single isolate from the udder in a case of mastitis (Leach, 1967). Further isolations were made in Great Britain from nasal swabs and a lung of calves with respiratory disease (Dawson *et al.*, 1966), from 17 of 47 calf lungs or tracheas (Davies, 1967), from the eyes of cattle with keratoconjunctivitis (Gourlay and Thomas, 1969a), from 23% of 65 pneumonic lungs (Gourlay *et al.*, 1970), and from 4 of 20 lungs (Pirie and Allan, 1975).

Isolations have been reported from 25% of 103 nasal swabs from pre-weaned calves and 48% of 190 calves after weaning in the United States (Hamdy and Trapp, 1967), and from a joint (Al-Aubaidi and Fabricant, 1971a). Isolations have also been reported from lungs in Holland (Cottew and Leach, 1969) and Italy (Rinaldi *et al.*, 1969), from 16 of 50 lungs in Denmark (Bitsch *et al.*, 1976), from the nose and lungs in Czechoslovakia (Jurmanova and Krejci, 1971) and Australia (Cottew, 1970), from the nasopharynx and brain in Switzerland (Nicolet and de Meuron, 1970), and from the nose, trachea, lungs, spleen, and kidneys in Japan (Shimizu *et al.*, 1973). *Mycoplasma bovirhinis* has also been reported in the USSR (Kurbanov and Gizatullin, 1975).

The first report of the isolation of *M. bovirhinis* from the genital tract of cattle was made by Langford (1975a), who reported this organism from 3 of 1265 cervicovaginal mucus samples, from 2 of 168 bull semen samples, from 7 preputial samples from 267 bulls, and from 2 of 251 fetal stomach contents. A further isolation of *M. bovirhinis* from mastitic milk was also reported (C. D. Wilson, quoted in Brownlie *et al.*, 1976).

The effect of *M. bovirhinis* in organ cultures was examined by Thomas and Howard (1974). This mycoplasma established itself and multiplied in bovine tracheal organ cultures but did not produce any cytopathic effects.

Mycoplasma bovirhinis has been isolated occasionally from mastitic milk, but reports of experimentally produced mastitis due to this organism are confusing. Langer and Carmichael (1963) reported that acute purulent mastitis followed intramammary inoculation of the 155 and 56R strains, subsequently classified by Leach (1967) as *M. bovirhinis*. However, Al-Aubaidi and Fabricant (1971b) examined strain 155 and identified it as *M. bovis*. In order to clarify the situation and evaluate the pathogenicity of these organisms, strains 155 and 56R were obtained from Carmichael, purified by "filter cloning," and subsequently identified serologically as *M. bovirhinis*, thus confirming Leach's observations (Brownlie *et al.*, 1976). Four strains of *M. bovirhinis*, including cloned 155 and 56R strains, were inoculated into the bovine mammary gland and produced only subclinical mastitis, indicated by an elevated inflammatory cell response in the milk together with multiplication of the mycoplasmas (Brownlie *et al.*, 1976). The degree of mastitis could in no way be described as acute purulent, but details of the exact severity in the earlier work are lacking for comparison. Perhaps the original cultures contained some *M. bovis*, which could account for the acute purulent mastitis reported by Langer and Carmichael (1963). The subclinical mastitis produced indicates that these *M. bovirhinis* strains were only mildly pathogenic to the mammary gland.

As noted above, the vast majority of isolations of this mycoplasma have been from the respiratory tract of cattle, and most have been made following investigations into respiratory disease. However, *M. bovirhinis* can be isolated from the apparently normal respiratory tract, mainly from the upper tract (nose and trachea), and mainly in the 3- to 4-month age group of calves (Davies, 1967; Gourlay and Thomas, 1970; Thomas and Smith, 1972). Isolations from the lung parenchyma were confined mainly to pneumonic lungs.

There are several reports that calves affected with respiratory disease develop a serological response to *M. bovirhinis* (Harbourne *et al.*, 1965; Dawson *et al.*, 1966; Jurmanova *et al.*, 1973; Shimizu *et al.*, 1973). However, as discussed in Section X, this by no means constitutes proof of etiological significance.

Inoculation of cultures of *M. bovirhinis* into colostrum-deprived calves by various routes failed to produce clinical signs of respiratory disease, although the organisms became established in the respiratory tract and induced a serological response (Langer and Carmichael, 1963; Dawson *et al.*, 1966). In contrast, Jurmanova *et al.* (1975) inoculated two conventionally reared calves endobronchially with 10^6–10^7 *M. bovirhinis*. They developed pyrexia, and one showed an ocular and nasal discharge and the organisms were reisolated from ocular and nasal swabs until slaughter 13 and 16 days after inoculation. At autopsy, only one calf had pneumonic lesions. *Mycoplasma bovirhinis* was recovered from the upper respiratory tract and other organs of both calves but not from the lungs. Three other calves were inoculated with *Pasteurella haemolytica,* and two with parainfluenza 3 virus in addition to *M. bovirhinis*. Slightly more severe signs of respiratory disease were observed in these calves, including a cough in the case of *P. haemolytica*-inoculated calves. At autopsy, 7–23 days after inoculation, four of five calves had pneumonic lesions, but *M. bovirhinis* was not recovered from the lungs of any of them. Two control calves, inoculated with heat-killed *M. bovirhinis*, did not develop clinical disease, but whether they had pneumonic lesions at autopsy was not reported. No mention was made of bacteriological examinations of the pneumonic lungs of any of these calves. Failure to reisolate *M. bovirhinis* from pneumonic lesions present at autopsy in calves inoculated with *M. bovirhinis* seems to be a common finding, as Gourlay and Thomas (1970) had reported this earlier in the case of two conventionally reared calves inoculated by the endobronchial route.

Inoculation of *M. bovirhinis* into the respiratory tract of gnotobiotic calves was reported by Gourlay and Howard (1978). Two cloned strains,

L866 (freshly isolated from a pneumonic lung) and 155 (mentioned above), were inoculated intratracheally and intraocularly into one and two gnotobiotic calves, respectively, at titers of 10^{10} organisms per calf. Signs of respiratory disease or eye infection were not observed during the 3 weeks of examination. At autopsy the lungs of two of the calves revealed no significant macroscopic lesions, while the lungs of the third calf, inoculated with strain 155, had 6% pneumonic consolidation. However, the lungs of this calf possessed high titers of four different bacterial species, whereas bacteria were not isolated from the lungs of the other two calves. *Mycoplasma bovirhinis* was not reisolated from the lungs of the two calves with insignificant lesions and only at low titer (10^2) from the other calf. *Mycoplasma bovirhinis* was reisolated, however, from nasopharyngeal swabs from all three calves 14 days after inoculation, confirming that the mycoplasmas had become established in the calves.

From all these results what conclusions can be drawn regarding the pathogenicity of *M. bovirhinis*? Work on conventionally reared calves indicating pathogenicity can be disregarded, as the significance of other microorganisms was ignored. Nevertheless in most of these reports *M. bovirhinis* does not appear to produce clinical disease. As calves were apparently not killed and autopsied in many of these earlier studies, the role of *M. bovirhinis* in subclinical pneumonia was usually not considered. The few studies with organ cultures and with gnotobiotic calves give no indication that *M. bovirhinis* is pathogenic on its own. In contrast, however, in the mammary gland *M. bovirhinis* does appear to be mildly pathogenic.

F. *Mycoplasma bovis*

Mycoplasma bovis was originally isolated from an outbreak of mastitis in cows in Connecticut (Hale *et al.*, 1962). Subsequent reports have been made of the isolation of this mycoplasma from outbreaks of mastitis in areas ranging from the east coast to the west coast of the United States (Carmichael *et al.*, 1963; Jasper *et al.*, 1966, 1974; Kehoe *et al.*, 1967a; Jasper, 1977). Isolations from mastitis outbreaks have been made in other parts of the world, including Israel (Bar-Moshe, 1964, quoted in Jasper, 1977), Italy (Guido, 1971), France (Gourlay *et al.*, 1974b), Canada (Ruhnke *et al.*, 1976; Cho *et al.*, 1976) and Great Britain (Anonymous, 1977). The clinical picture has been reviewed by Jasper (1977). The mastitis is frequently severe and results in a loss of milk secretion. Within an affected herd the mycoplasma may be isolated from apparently nonmastitic milk (Jasper *et al.*, 1966).

Mycoplasma bovis has also been isolated from the joints of animals with arthritis. Hjerpe and Knight (1972) reported the isolation, in the United States, of *M. bovis* from the joints of yearling feedlot cattle with primary polyarthritis. Mildly affected cattle recovered without treatment. Singh *et al.* (1971) reported the isolation of *M. bovis* from the joints of 6-to 9-month-old Hereford calves in Canada, 3 of 143 and 9 of 84 animals in each of two groups. Other reports of the isolation of *M. bovis* from cattle with swollen joints have been made in the United States (Jasper *et al.*, 1966; Dellinger and Jasper, 1972; Stalheim and Stone, 1975; Stalheim, 1976) and Canada (Langford, 1977). In several of these instances the arthritis was associated with either mastitis or respiratory disease from which *M. bovis* was also isolated.

Another site from which *M. bovis* is being isolated with increasing frequency is the respiratory tract. Kehoe *et al.* (1967b) reported the isolation of *M. bovis* from the nasal cavity of a cow with respiratory disease. Karst and Onoviran (1971) isolated *M. bovis* from the respiratory tract of a zebu bull in Africa, and certain of the strains studied by polyacrylamide gel electrophoresis by Dellinger and Jasper (1972) were reported to have been isolated from feedlot steer lungs. The presence of *M. bovis* in the nasal cavity of cows in herds with *M. bovis* mastitis has also been reported (Jasper *et al.*, 1974; Ruhnke *et al.*, 1976; Bennett and Jasper, 1977a).

Perhaps of more significance is the isolation of this mycoplasma from the respiratory tract, nasal cavities, and lungs of cattle with clinical respiratory disease. *Mycoplasma bovis* has now been isolated in Great Britain from several outbreaks of pneumonia in intensively reared calves (Thomas *et al.*, 1975; Anonymous, 1977). This mycoplasma was also found in 25 of 29 animals with pneumonia in 16 "lots" in Canada (Langford, 1977). Certain of these animals were found also to have arthritis, and other *Mycoplasma* species were isolated from them. The isolation of *M. bovis* from severe outbreaks of pneumonia in Italy, sometimes in association with arthritis, has also been reported (Pignattelli and Galassi, 1971; Pignattelli, 1977). The association of *M. bovis* with pneumonia in intensively reared calves has also been noted in the United States (Stalheim, 1976).

Mycoplasma bovis has also been isolated from the urogenital tract. In a large-scale survey reported by Langford (1975a), *M. bovis* was isolated from 3 of 1265 cervicovaginal mucus samples, from semen samples from 4 of 168 bulls, and from 4 of 267 washes taken from the prepuce. Six isolations were made from the stomach contents of 251 aborted fetuses but not from the lungs, liver, or spleen. A recent report (Jack *et al.*, 1977) of the isolation of *M. bovis* from cattle with infectious bovine keratoconjunctivitis associates this mycoplasma with yet another disease.

Mycoplasma bovis has at various times been called *Mycoplasma bovimastitidis* and *M. agalactiae* subsp. *bovis*. However, the studies of Askaa and Ernø (1976) involving deoxyribonucleic acid homology and serology led them to propose that this mycoplasma should not be regarded as a subspecies of *M. agalactiae* but as a distinct species.

Certain of the properties of *M. bovis* are given in Table I. It can be easily distinguished from many of the other bovine mycoplasmas by its inability to produce either an alkaline color change in medium containing arginine and urea or to produce acid from glucose. A slight fall in pH occurs in most broth cultures, but this does not seem to be due to fermentation of glucose (Leach, 1973; Edward and Moore, 1975). Most isolates produce film and spots on suitable media, a characteristic shared with *M. bovigenitalium* but not exhibited by the type strain of *M. bovis*, Donetta (PG45). *Mycoplasma bovis* is relatively easy to isolate, being capable of growth on media ranging at least from pH 6.0 to 7.8. It is undemanding in its gaseous requirements and grows under aerobic, microaerophilic, and anaerobic conditions. Isolates often grow on ox blood agar, in which case they can produce minute hemolytic colonies. Distinction from biochemically similar species, e.g., *M. bovigenitalium*, is made by serological techniques. However, inhibition of growth is sometimes difficult to demonstrate, perhaps because the organism grows so well, but inhibition of film production may be seen.

The pathogenicity of *M. bovis* has been shown for a variety of anatomical sites under controlled experimental conditions. It is, next to *M. mycoides* subsp. *mycoides*, probably the most pathogenic of the species of mycoplasma isolated from cattle.

The initial isolations of *M. bovis* were made from outbreaks of mastitis. Consequently the first pathogenicity studies under controlled experimental conditions were made to induce mastitis in cattle following inoculation of cultures into the mammary gland. Although many of these studies employed rather few cows, such experiments have been reported so many times and by so many investigators that there can be no doubt that, following its inoculation into the mammary gland of cows, *M. bovis* is capable of inducing mastitis. The clinical appearance and severity of the disease so induced is similar to that of the original natural outbreaks from which the organism has been isolated. As few as 70 colony-forming units (CFU) have been inoculated into cows and found to induce mastitis (Hale *et al.*, 1962; Kehoe *et al.*, 1967a; Jain *et al.*, 1969a,b; Stalheim and Page, 1975; Ruhnke *et al.*, 1976; Bennett and Jasper, 1977b; Jasper, 1977). Mastitis appears not to occur regularly as a result of intravenous inoculation of *M. bovis* (Jain *et al.*, 1969a).

Arthritis has been induced by *M. bovis* following its inoculation into cattle. This disease has been reported to occur following inoculation directly into the joints, intravenously, into the lung, or into the mammary gland. In the last-mentioned two cases infection was also induced at the primary site of inoculation (Stalheim and Page, 1975; Gourlay *et al.*, 1976; Singh *et al.*, 1971).

Mycoplasma bovis has been demonstrated to induce lesions in the urogenital tract following its inoculation into the posterior portion of the uterus (Hartman *et al.*, 1964). Infertility and genital lesions as a result of the inoculation of cows with semen containing *M. bovis* was reported by Hirth *et al.* (1966). The inoculation of *M. bovis* into the amniotic fluid of a fetus was found to induce abortion (Stalheim and Proctor, 1976). However, the isolation of *M. bovis* from a viable fetus has also been reported (Jain *et al.*, 1969a).

Although *M. bovis* has been isolated from outbreaks of clinical pneumonia in calves, it has not been shown to induce clinical, as opposed to subclinical, disease following its inoculation into the respiratory tract of conventionally reared calves (Onoviran, 1972) and gnotobiotic calves (Gourlay *et al.*, 1976). In the latter case subclinical cuffing pneumonia was induced with lesions extending over about 10% of the lung.

Finally there is a possibility that *M. bovis* is pathogenic for animals other than cattle. It has been isolated from the pneumonic lungs of goats (Ojo, 1976) and humans (Madoff *et al.*, 1976). Also, mastitis has been induced in goats (Redaelli *et al.*, 1969; Ojo and Ikede, 1976) and mice (Anderson *et al.*, 1976) following its inoculation into the mammary gland.

There is no doubt that *M. bovis* is the cause of certain outbreaks of mastitis in cattle and, when isolated in high titer from mastitic milk, may be regarded as the etiological agent. Similarly *M. bovis* should also be regarded as the cause of certain cases of arthritis in calves and cows. This arthritis may be associated with pneumonia or mastitis.

The possibility exists of a causal relationship between *M. bovis* and infertility and abortion in cattle. Although experimental evidence has been presented showing *M. bovis* to be capable of inducing both these conditions, insufficient survey data have been recorded to make it possible to associate, with any certainty, infertility and abortion with *M. bovis* under natural conditions. The surveys that have been made indicate that this mycoplasma is certainly a rather infrequent cause of abortion. Nevertheless, the possibility of *M. bovis* causing these conditions should be considered.

Mycoplasma bovis was almost certainly not the sole cause of the outbreaks of severe clinical pneumonia from which it has been isolated. Its association with such outbreaks indicates a role in this disease perhaps in association with other agents. On its own it is capable of inducing subclinical cuffing pneumonia, and it may cause such a disease in certain of the apparently normal animals from which it has been isolated.

G. *Mycoplasma bovoculi*

Mycoplasma bovoculi was only recently characterized and named (Langford and Leach, 1973) and, as its name implies, it comprises mycoplasma strains isolated from the eyes of cattle. The initial isolations were made from cattle suffering from infectious bovine keratoconjunctivitis (IBKC) in England (Gourlay and Thomas, 1969a) and Canada (Langford and Dorward, 1969). Since then *M. bovoculi* has been isolated from cases of IBKC in the Ivory Coast (Nicolet and Buttiker, 1974) and Switzerland (Nicolet *et al.*, 1976). This species has also been reported from commercial bovine serum (Barile, 1973).

Mycoplasma bovoculi is a glucose-fermenting mycoplasma that grows well on conventional mycoplasma media, either aerobically or under reduced oxygen tension. It fails to hydrolyze arginine or urea and does not form film and spots on horse serum agar. It produces typical "fried egg" colonies on solid medium. In other words, the cultural and biochemical characteristics of *M. bovoculi* do not distinguish it from most other glucose-fermenting mycoplasmas.

Although *M. bovoculi* has been isolated in connection with investigations into IBKC, there is very little concrete evidence for its etiological association with the disease. Langford and Dorward (1969) failed to isolate this organism from the eyes of 119 animals in a herd uninfected with IBKC, but *M. bovoculi* was isolated from 10 of 24 diseased cattle and from 1 out of 10 normal contact animals. Among these diseased animals, *M. bovoculi* was obtained from 8 of 10 acute cases and from 2 out of 14 chronic cases. These workers also suggested that the severity of IBKC may have been accentuated when both *M. bovoculi* and *Moraxella bovis* were present in the eyes. A later article by Langford and Leach (1973) reported that these two organisms, *M. bovoculi* and *Moraxella bovis*, were each isolated from only 15% of the cases of IBKC in Canada (137 swabs from 6 affected herds), about a third of the positive ones carrying both agents. Neither organism was isolated from three clinically healthy herds (370 swabs). These workers reported that preliminary transmission and infection studies indicated that *M. bovoculi* could induce symptoms of conjunctivitis in bovine eyes which may remain infected for up to 200 days. No further publication has emanated from these studies, but Nayar and Saunders (1975), as part of a study on IBKC, inoculated *M. bovoculi* into the eyes of six calves. The mycoplasma readily established itself in the eyes, and severe IBKC was produced in one calf following intracorneal inoculation. This contrasted with the lack of clinical signs of eye infection in five other calves inoculated by conjunctival instillation. These workers suggested that this indicated the need for initial damage to cells in order for infection to occur. However, the significance of this work is difficult to assess, as all the calves had been inoculated 2 weeks earlier with heat-killed or live *Moraxella bovis* and/or infectious bovine rhinotracheitis virus by conjunctival instillation or intramuscular injection.

H. *Mycoplasma canadense*

Ruhnke and Onoviran (1975) described a mycoplasma, strain 466, which they had isolated from bovine mastitic milk in Canada. This strain metabolized arginine but not glucose, and serological tests suggested that it represented a new species. Further isolations of similar strains were also made from the joint and umbilicus of a calf, from the vaginal mucus of a cow, and from the semen of bulls. Strain 466, together with two other strains isolated from the male bovine genital tract in Canada, were characterized and named *M. canadense* (Langford *et al.*, 1976). Strains of this mycoplasma have also been isolated from milk, the vagina, and the respiratory tract of cows during an epizootic of mastitis in California (Jasper, 1977; Dellinger *et al.*, 1977), and from mastitic milk in England (Gourlay *et al.*, 1978).

The cultural and biochemical characteristics of *M. canadense* are shown in Table I. Essentially it grows on conventional mycoplasma media, produces typical "fried egg" colonies on solid medium, and does not form film and spots. Its most significant features, however, are its ability to hydrolyze arginine but not urea and its failure to utilize glucose.

Strain 466 of *M. canadense* produced clinical mastitis when inoculated into the bovine mammary gland (Ruhnke and Onoviran, 1975; Bennett and Jasper, 1978b). Thus this mycoplasma must be considered a pathogenic species.

I. *Mycoplasma dispar*

This species was first isolated in England from pneumonic calf lungs (Gourlay, 1969) and was subsequently characterized and named (Gourlay and Leach, 1970). Further isolations of *M. dispar* were made from 33 of 65 pneumonic calf lungs in England (Gourlay *et al.*, 1970), from 11 tracheal ring organ cultures prepared from 29 pneumonic calf lungs in Australia

(St. George *et al.*, 1973), from 3 of 11 pneumonic bovine lungs in the United States (Ose and Muenster, 1975), from 6 of 12 pneumonic calf lungs in Scotland (Pirie and Allan, 1975), from 31 of 50 pneumonic lungs in Denmark (Bitsch *et al.*, 1976), and from 17 of 18 pneumonic lungs in Japan (Kuniyasu *et al.*, 1977).

Mycoplasma dispar has also been isolated from swabs taken from the lower respiratory tract of calves that at autopsy, 4 weeks later, showed no signs of macroscopic pneumonia (Gourlay and Thomas, 1970), and also from the respiratory tract of macroscopically nonpneumonic calves, primarily from the lower tract and lung tissue itself (Thomas and Smith, 1972). Calves in the 3- to 4-month age range appeared to have a much higher burden of these mycoplasmas than very young calves, yearlings, or adult cows (Thomas and Smith, 1972). Pirie and Allan (1975), however, reported that *M. dispar* was not recovered from 8 nonpneumonic lungs but was recovered from 6 out of 12 pneumonic lungs of calves all housed together.

Recent studies have indicated that *M. dispar* is probably the most common microbial species in the respiratory tract of calves in the Compton area, as it was isolated from nasopharyngeal swabs from 38 out of 41 (93%) apparently normal 1½- to 8-week-old Ayrshire calves between March and May 1977 (Gourlay and Howard, 1978).

Mycoplasma dispar, as its name implies (*dispar,* Latin adjective meaning "different" or "dissimilar"), has some unusual features (Gourlay and Leach, 1970). It is an exacting glucose-fermenting mycoplasma which grows poorly or not at all on conventional mycoplasma media but which produces colonies on special GS solid media (or media suitable for the growth of *Mycoplasma hyopneumoniae*) which are atypical in comparison with those of most recognized mycoplasmas. Early subcultures on GS agar produce mainly large colonies which are roughly circular and granular in appearance. They lack the "centers" characteristic of mycoplasma colonies and do not penetrate the agar. Colonies of this type cannot be subcultured by means of a wire loop. After several passages in GS broth small center-forming colonies which penetrate the agar are formed. Other unusual features of *M. dispar* include failure to pass readily through membrane filters of 450-nm pore diameter (Gourlay and Leach, 1970) and the possession of a capsule that can be visualized by electron microscopy following staining with ruthenium red (Howard and Gourlay, 1974).

In vivo pathogenicity of *M. dispar* has been clearly demonstrated by inoculation of this organism into the bovine mammary gland. Six out of seven strains of *M. dispar* produced clinical mastitis, but the seventh strain was apparently avirulent (Brownlie *et al.*, 1976). In one of these inoculated cows, preexisting leukocytosis actually enhanced the virulence of the *M. dispar* strain used. This is in contrast to bacterial mastitis where preexisting leukocytosis protects the gland.

A culture of *M. dispar* was inoculated into eight conventionally reared calves by the endobronchial route, and macroscopic lesions of pneumonia were found at autopsy in seven of them, from all of which *M. dispar* was reisolated (Gourlay and Thomas, 1969b). However, as discussed in Section X, results obtained by the inoculation of conventionally reared calves should be treated with caution. This also applies to the results obtained by St. George *et al.* (1973) in Australia, who inoculated three 1- to 2-day-old ceasarean-derived or colostrum-deprived calves with *M. dispar* culture-derived material by the intratracheal route. When the calves were killed 2–8 days later, atelectasis was observed in the lungs of all three calves, and *M. dispar* and coliform bacteria were isolated from two of them. Histologically the lesions were proliferative interstitial pneumonia. Two control calves had no macroscopic lesions.

The inoculation of gnotobiotic calves would be expected to give more meaningful results; certainly inoculation of *M. dispar* culture into these calves can produce macroscopic but subclinical pneumonia. A total of 13 gnotobiotic calves was inoculated by the intratracheal or endobronchial route, and macroscopic lesions were observed at autopsy in 11 of them involving up to 17% of the lung tissue. Even in these calves, certain nonpathogenic species of bacteria were isolated from most of the experimental calves and also from 3 control calves inoculated with sterile broth. Histologically the lesions were predominantly interstitial alveolitis centered around the bronchioles, perhaps resembling the lesions described by St. George *et al.* (1973). Peribronchial cuffing was observed in only one lung (Howard *et al.*, 1976a; Gourlay and Howard, 1978).

We can conclude therefore that some strains of *M. dispar* are undoubtedly pathogenic and are capable of producing clinical mastitis and subclinical pneumonia experimentally. Nonpathogenic strains also occur.

J. Mycoplasma mycoides subsp. mycoides

This species, the first mycoplasma isolated and the most widely known mycoplasma of cattle, is the causal agent of contagious bovine pleuropneumonia (CBPP), a disease of cattle and water buffalo characterized by fibrinous interstitial pneumonia and pleurisy. Although more widespread in the past, CBPP still exists in many countries in Africa and in parts of India. It may also be present in the Iberian Peninsula, China, and Mongolia. Sporadic outbreaks of CBPP have also been reported in the last few years in France and Jordan, probably associated with the importation of infected cattle. Australia now seems to be free of the disease after over a century of combating it.

A vast body of literature has accumulated over the years on CBPP and the causal organism. An excellent account of the present state of knowledge of the disease and *M. mycoides* subsp. *mycoides* is available (Hudson, 1971), and there is also a useful review on the diagnosis of CBPP (Windsor, 1977). We do not therefore propose to discuss this mycoplasma in any detail except to consider certain new developments.

Mycoplasma mycoides subsp. *mycoides* grows readily in conventional mycoplasma media and utilizes glucose but not urea or arginine. With most strains, inoculation of a small number of organisms into liquid medium and incubation at 37°C results in the formation of "comets" and "threads" which are whitish, translucent isles of growth joined by long threads of filamentous growth. These are visible to the naked eye, suspended in the clear medium. On further incubation, they disperse, and the culture becomes uniformly turbid. Examination of this thread phase of growth revealed that *M. mycoides* subsp. *mycoides* had a well-defined capsule which was probably carbohydrate in nature, probably galactan (Gourlay and Thrower, 1968). In a later study (Howard and Gourlay, 1974) this capsule was observed, in the electron microscope, when stained with ruthenium red.

A variant of *Mycoplasma*, the rho (ρ) form, was observed in cultures derived from the V5 strain of *M. mycoides* subsp. *mycoides* (Rodwell *et al.*, 1972, 1975). It is a relatively rigid, rodlike organism in which an intracytoplasmic striated fiber (ρ fiber) extends axially throughout the cell and terminates at the plasma membrane in a knoblike structure. The fiber appears to be composed of fibrils aligned in regular array and having a cross-banded pattern. The function, if any, of the fiber and terminal structure is unknown.

It has long been known that *M. mycoides* subsp. *mycoides* can produce natural disease in cattle (i.e., CBPP) and water buffalos (Hudson, 1971). The African or Cape Buffalo, however, does not appear to be susceptible to natural infection, although there is experimental evidence that it may develop bacteremia after subcutaneous inoculation with the mycoplasma (Shifrine *et al.*, 1970).

Strains of mycoplasma serologically and biochemically indistinguishable from *M. mycoides* subsp. *mycoides* have been isolated from goats and sheep (Al-Aubaidi *et al.*, 1972a). Whereas most pathogenicity studies performed with these caprine and ovine strains show that they are not pathogens for cattle, there are some instances in which the goat strains have been experimentally pathogenic for cattle. The O-goat strain produced a local reaction (resembling the "Willems" reaction), bacteremia, and severe polyarthritis following subcutaneous and intravenous inoculations. In one calf, sequestra were present in the lungs at autopsy (Hudson *et al.*, 1967a). Barber and Yedloutschnig (1970) reported that strains isolated in the United States were capable of producing local cellulitis or fibrinous pleuritis when inoculated intramuscularly or intratracheally into calves. Some of the calves died. Some isolations of strains of *M. mycoides* subsp. *mycoides* have been from goats and sheep in countries free of CBPP, which poses problems for those responsible for disease control regulations. Inoculation of *M. mycoides* subsp. *mycoides* of bovine origin into sheep and goats, by the subcutaneous or intravenous route, has given variable results. There is no evidence, however, that CBPP can be spread naturally or experimentally to cattle by sheep and goats (Hudson, 1971). A recent publication by Cottew and Yeats (1978) has partially resolved the problem of differentiating these goat and cattle strains. They showed that there are two types—the large and small colony formers, which are serologically indistinguishable but can be differentiated using digestion of casein, liquefaction of serum, and survival at 45°C. The large colony types are not pathogenic for cattle (also see this volume, Chapter 3).

Over the years, the inoculation of *M. mycoides* subsp. *mycoides* into small laboratory animals has not resulted in a really useful model for studies on CBPP. Local lesions can sometimes be produced, particularly if the organisms are inoculated together with agar plugs (Whittlestone, 1972), but no lung lesions result. Recent work by Lloyd (1970), who inoculated rabbits subcutaneously with a broth culture of the organisms (without agar), produced consistent transient local lesions under the skin. The virulence of the mycoplasma strains for the rabbit, however, did not correspond entirely with the virulence for cattle. Smith (1967) showed that, after intraperitoneal inoculation of mice, asymptomatic bacteremia resulted, and he subsequently used the incidence and duration of the bacteremia as an indicator in various studies on virulence and immunity. The inoculation of virulent *M. mycoides* subsp. *mycoides* strains into the mammary glands of mice induced active infection and a neutrophil response (Anderson *et al.*, 1976). The relatively avirulent KH3J strain produced minimal changes.

Other than cattle, perhaps the most satisfactory experimental "animal" is the chicken embryo which has been used for many years to grow *M. mycoides* subsp. *mycoides* and for vaccine production. The chicken embryo, however, may also play a part in studies on immunity, as chicken embryos from hens immunized with *M. mycoides* subsp. *mycoides* can survive a challenge with this organism which kills embryos from normal hens (Gourlay and Shifrine, 1966a). The mycoplasma used for this study was the Gladysdale strain. The LD_{50} calculated for this and other strains of *M. mycoides* subsp. *mycoides,* including two newly isolated strains, varied from $10^{5.5}$ to $10^{6.1}$, whereas the KH3J strain was avirulent (Gourlay and Shifrine, 1968). Only one of these strains had been specially adapted for growth in the egg embryo.

It has always been assumed that CBPP spreads by direct contact between infected and healthy cattle and, despite the fact that spread by clouds of infected droplets, carried by air currents, has been reported from time to time (Hudson, 1971), indirect spread is considered of minor importance. Recently it has been shown that indirect spread may be of more significance than hitherto thought, as it has been observed that some cattle may excrete up to 1×10^6 *M. mycoides* subsp. *mycoides* per milliliter in their urine as a result of severe kidney lesions and that the mycoplasmas can survive 72 hours in placentas and for longer periods in urine on hay (Masiga *et al.*, 1972; Windsor and Masiga, 1977). It was also possible to infect three out of six cattle by feeding them hay heavily infected with *M. mycoides* subsp. *mycoides*. Lung lesions were produced, and mycoplasmas could be reisolated from the lesions. These results suggest that indirect spread may account for some of the unexplained outbreaks of CBPP particularly when, as appears possible in the above work, there were concurrent infections.

The early work of Nocard *et al.* (1898, cited in Lloyd and Trethewie, 1970) suggested that *M. mycoides* subsp. *mycoides* might elaborate a toxin, as cultures of this organism in collodion sacs inserted into the peritoneal cavity of rabbits caused them to lose weight. Lloyd (1966) confirmed this finding but suggested that the loss of weight was associated with the laparotomy; however, he also noted that necrosis occurred around the chambers containing the mycoplasmas but not around the control chambers containing media alone. On this evidence he suggested that *M. mycoides* subsp. *mycoides* produced a diffusible toxin. Gourlay (1963) had also noted that cellophane sacs containing the mycoplasma inserted into the peritoneal cavity of cattle became embedded in a fibrinous cast. Later Lloyd (Lloyd and Trethewie, 1970) showed that, after intramuscular implantation in rabbits and also in cattle, resistant and susceptible to subcutaneous challenge with *M. mycoides* subsp. *mycoides*, the infected chambers but not the control chambers became enclosed by a jellylike clot of fibrin infiltrated with polymorphs which were later replaced by connective tissue.

The relationship of this toxin and the "endotoxin" extracted from *M. mycoides* subsp. *mycoides* by Villemot *et al.* (1962) is not clear. The endotoxin produced pyrexia and leukopenia in rabbits and fever and "blood changes" in cattle, and the intravenous injection of 2 mg into cattle caused sudden dramatic stress and collapse. This endotoxin was not purified, and the active component was not determined. Comparable sudden collapse following intravenous inoculation was later reported by Hudson *et al.* (1967b) in some cattle when galactan isolated from *M. mycoides* subsp. *mycoides* (Buttery and Plackett, 1960) was inoculated intravenously. Furthermore, the injection of at least 0.66 mg/kg of galactan into cattle subsequently infected with *M. mycoides* subsp. *mycoides* induced lesions in joints and kidneys and a prolonged mycoplasmemia (Hudson *et al.*, 1967b; Lloyd *et al.*, 1971). Several animals developed pleurisy. The same effects occurred with galactan prepared from both virulent and avirulent strains of *M. mycoides* subsp. *mycoides*. This was not unexpected, as it had been shown earlier that both virulent (T3) and avirulent (KH3J) strains of *M. mycoides* subsp. *mycoides* elaborated serologically similar galactan-containing lipopolysaccharides (Gourlay, 1965a). There could, however, be a quantitative difference, as it has been suggested that the quantity of galactan produced by a strain may vary with its virulence (Gourlay and Thrower, 1968; Lloyd *et al.*, 1971).

Lloyd *et al.* (1971) reported that galactan had no effect on the rate of clearance of *M. mycoides* subsp. *mycoides* injected intravenously into cattle, nor did it reduce the resistance of vaccinated cattle. On the contrary, the injection of galactan and Freund's adjuvant did not protect cattle against infection with *M. mycoides* subsp. *mycoides* (Hudson *et al.*, 1967b; Lloyd *et al.*, 1971). Villemot *et al.* (1962), during their endotoxin work, reported that the galactan of Buttery and Plackett (1960) was pyrogenic in large doses (1 mg), and a dose of 1 μg induced a sharp leukocyte response in rabbits. Both the endotoxin and the galactan were lethal to fowl embryos (LD_{50}, 15 μg for the endotoxin and 525 μg for the galactan). Gourlay (1965b) reported that the galactan-containing lipopolysaccharide (LPS) isolated from the urine of cattle infected with *M. mycoides* subsp. *mycoides* possessed an aggressive action when inoculated subcutaneously with the mycoplasma into immune animals and appeared to enhance the virulence of the mycoplasma in susceptible cattle. The LPS was weakly pyrogenic in rabbits and nontoxic to cattle, but lethal to fowl embryos (LD_{50}, 179 μg). Serologically the LPS and the galactan of Buttery and Plackett were very similar in the agar gel precipitin test. The endotoxin of Villemot *et al.* was very weakly antigenic, although most of the antigens present in the LPS were also present in the endotoxin (Gourlay, 1965b). Although galactan and LPS are haptens, antibodies can be produced by using Freund's complete adjuvant or by combining them with "shiga protein" or glutaraldehyde-fixed sheep erythrocytes (Hudson *et al.*, 1967b; Gourlay, 1965b; Kakoma and Kinyanjui, 1974). The antibodies fix complement, agglutinate, and give a single line in the gel precipitin test but do not inhibit growth of the mycoplasma (Kakoma and Kinyanjui, 1974).

The serological similarity between the galactan from *M. mycoides* subsp. *mycoides* and pneumogalactan isolated from normal bovine lung has been demonstrated (Shifrine and Gourlay, 1965; Gourlay and Shifrine, 1966c). It was suggested that this cross-reactivity could play a part in the pathogenesis of CBPP. A preliminary examination of this suggestion was inconclusive, but evidence was obtained suggesting that antiserum might "sensitize" the lungs so that subsequent intravenous inoculation of a virulent culture resulted in lung lesions (Gourlay and Shifrine, 1966b). Provost (1969) followed up these observations and showed that antiserum against *M. mycoides* subsp. *mycoides* possessed cytotoxic activity for bovine lung cells cultivated *in vitro*.

It has been recognized for a long time that in calves under about 6 weeks of age CBPP may manifest itself as arthritis or polyarthritis, with few or no lesions in the lungs. Joint lesions may also follow subcutaneous inoculation of viable cultures of *M. mycoides* subsp. *mycoides* (Hudson, 1971). In his studies Piercy (1972) suggested that an allergic reaction may contribute directly to the pathogenesis of this calfhood arthritis.

K. *Mycoplasma verecundum*

The original isolations were made in England from the eyes of two affected calves in a group during an apparently spontaneous outbreak of conjunctivitis (Gourlay *et al.*, 1974a). Subsequently, *M. verecundum* was demonstrated in Canadian cattle (Langford, 1975a), where it was isolated from three preputial wash samples taken from 267 different animals. It was not isolated from semen samples taken from 168 animals and cervicovaginal mucus samples taken from 1295 animals reported in the same study.

Although a slight drop in pH is observed in broth cultures as a result of the growth of *M. verecundum*, this is not considered to be due to the production of acid from glucose (Table I). Neither was any acid production demonstrated for a range of carbohydrates examined (Gourlay *et al.*, 1974a). This species also appears to be unable to catabolize arginine and not to possess urease activity. Thus on the basis of these biochemical characteristics *M. verecundum* can be distinguished from the majority of other bovine *Mycoplasma* species. Two other bovine mycoplasmas with similar biochemical properties are *M. bovigenitalium* and *M. bovis*.

Although a member of the genus *Mycoplasma*, as indicated by a requirement for cholesterol and sensitivity to growth inhibition by digitonin and sodium polyanethol sulfonate, *M. verecundum* grows at temperatures usually characteristic of the genus *Acholeplasma*. Growth at 30°C is virtually as rapid as at 37°C and growth also occurs, albeit more slowly, at temperatures down to 20°C. This mycoplasma grows on solid medium ranging from pH 4.7 to 7.8, the range tested (Gourlay *et al.*, 1974a), which is an unusually large range with an optimum, as indicated by colony size, of pH 6.0. A variety of serological tests indicates there is no antigenic relationship between this mycoplasma and other named species.

Because of its isolation from conjunctivitis the possible involvement of *M. verecundum* in this condition should be considered. Four gnotobiotic calves inoculated in each eye with 5 ml of broth culture containing 10^9 CFU/ml did not develop severe conjunctivitis, although a slight reaction may have occurred in one animal (R. N. Gourlay, C. J. Howard, and L. H. Thomas, unpublished observations). The possibility of *M. verecundum* being involved in conjunctivitis in association with other agents remains to be examined. No lesions resulted from the inoculation of 10^{10} CFU of *M. verecundum* into the lungs of two gnotobiotic calves (R. N. Gourlay, C. J. Howard, and L. H. Thomas, unpublished observations).

IV. ACHOLEPLASMAS OF CATTLE

A. *Acholeplasma axanthum*

Acholeplasma axanthum is the name given to two mycoplasma isolates recovered from a murine leukemia cell line by Tully and Razin (1970). These workers also reported that a strain of acholeplasma obtained from Olson, in the United States, from bovine nasal discharge and placed by Al-Aubaidi and Fabricant (1971a) in their group K should be classified as *A. axanthum*. This observation seems to indicate that *A. axanthum* is of bovine origin and also explains the occurrence of this acholeplasma in cell cultures (Tully and Razin, 1970). Confirmation of the bovine origin of *A. axanthum* was obtained later when it was isolated from commercial bovine serum (Barile, 1973), from kidney and peribronchial lymph glands of calves (Stipkovits *et al.*, 1975), and from mastitic milk samples (Wehnert *et al.*, 1977).

Acholeplasma axanthum has, however, also been isolated from the lung and peribronchial lymph glands of swine (Stipkovits *et al.*, 1973) and the oral cavity of a horse (Ogata *et al.*, 1974). This species is therefore one of those that are, like *Acholeplasma laidlawii* and *M. arginini*, found in several different animal hosts including cattle.

The growth of *A. axanthum* in serum-free medium was unlike that of other acholeplasmas in that only slight turbidity was noted in liquid medium unless the medium was supplemented with Tween-80, when the strains grew as well as other acholeplasmas (Tully, 1973). This was related to a requirement for some essential fatty acid. This acholeplasma, together with *Acholeplasma modicum*, also differs from the other *Acholeplasma* species in its inability to produce pigmented carotenoids (Tully, 1973). Plackett *et al.* (1970) later showed that this organism synthesized a sphingolipid, a substance rarely found in bacteria. Hydrolysis of esculin by *A. axanthum* distinguishes this acholeplasma from *A. modicum*.

It appears that the only examination of the pathogenicity or potential pathogenicity of *A. axanthum* is the work of Stipkovits *et al.* (1974) in pigs. In this work two 4- to 6-month-old specific-pathogen-free pigs were inoculated with a culture of *A. axanthum* intranasally. Mild clinical disease resulted, and at autopsy 41 days after inoculation, macroscopic and microscopic lesions of pneumonia were observed. Two control pigs revealed no clinical disease or gross pneumonia after 57 days. However, before the pathogenic properties of *A. axanthum* can be accepted, confirmation of this work is required, using a larger number of pigs and a more thorough microbiological and serological examination of the pigs and the lung lesions that may result (see also Volume I, Chapter 16).

B. *Acholeplasma laidlawii*

Mycoplasmas now classified as *A. laidlawii* were first isolated from sewage (Laidlaw and Elford, 1936) and later from soil and decayed vegetable matter. *Acholeplasma laidlawii* has also been isolated from many different animals, humans, and perhaps plants (Tully, 1973) and is also a common contaminant of tissue cultures, the most likely source of this contamination being commercial bovine serum (Barile, 1973).

Apart from the original isolations, most strains of *A. laidlawii* have been isolated from animals, particularly cattle, and from normal as well as diseased tissues. In 1950, Edward (1950) first reported its presence in the bovine genital tract, and since that date *A. laidlawii* has been frequently isolated from this site, from both male and female animals (Cottew and Leach, 1969). It has also been isolated from aborted bovine fetuses (Langford, 1975a), the bovine mammary gland (Jasper, 1967; Pan and Ogota, 1969a,b), the upper and lower respiratory tract of cattle (Harbourne *et al.*, 1965; Thomas and Smith, 1972; Pirie and Allan, 1975), and the eyes of cattle (Gourlay and Thomas, 1969a). *Acholeplasma laidlawii* has also been isolated from the visceral organs, blood, and sera of cattle (Schimmel and Pustovar, 1971; Barile, 1973).

The cultural and biochemical properties of *A. laidlawii* are given in Table I. It utilizes glucose but not arginine or urea, forms classic "fried egg" colonies on solid medium, and is distinguished from most other bovine mycoplasmas (except of course *A. axanthum* and *A. modicum*) by its ability to grow in serum-free media and at 22°C. It is also resistant to sodium polyanethol sulfonate, digitonin, and amphotericin B.

Apart from its serological differences, *A. laidlawii* can be differentiated from *A. axanthum* and *A. modicum* by its ability to produce pigmented carotenoids (Tully, 1973).

Because *A. laidlawii* was first isolated from sewage and because of its ability to grow in serum-free media at temperatures below body heat, it has usually been considered a saprophytic mycoplasma. However, there have been reports correlating isolations of *A. laidlawii* with disease situations. Hoare (1969) isolated mycoplasmas with the cultural characteristics of *A. laidlawii* from oviducts of cows, the highest rate (over 70%) being from cows with reduced fertility, and she regarded *A. laidlawii* as a potential pathogen capable at times of causing bovine infertility. *Acholeplasma laidlawii* can be isolated, not infrequently and usually at low titer, from mastitic milk (R. N. Gourlay and C. J. Howard, unpublished observations). Pan and Ogata (1969b) reported the isolation of a large number of strains from mastitic milk and genital mucus, and they suggested that they might be involved in infertility. There is, however, some doubt as to whether all their isolates were in fact *A. laidlawii*. Olson *et al.* (1960) also reported lesions in the uterus following the inoculation of a cow with a strain of this organism. There have been reports of the production of mild or subacute mastitis following the inoculation of *A. laidlawii* into the bovine mammary gland (Karbe and Mosher, 1968; Wehnert *et al.*, 1977; Erfle and Brunner, 1977). In these cases the acholeplasma was only reisolated from the milk for up to 24 hours after inoculation.

In contrast, there have also been reports of experimental inoculations of *A. laidlawii* at various sites in cattle that have given negative results. Edward (1950) inoculated a sample containing *A. laidlawii* into the uterus of a heifer, Trapp *et al.* (1966) inoculated this acholeplasma into the respiratory tract of calves, and Jain *et al.* (1969a) inoculated *A. laidlawii* into the mammary gland of a cow. In all these instances disease was not produced.

In an attempt to resolve the conflicting reports on *A. laidlawii* pathogenicity, recent work in England has shown that *A. laidlawii* can become established and multiply in bovine tracheal organ cultures but does not produce cytopathic effects (Thomas and Howard, 1974). Furthermore the inoculation of four strains of *A. laidlawii*, isolated from cattle, into bovine mammary glands failed to produce mastitis (Brownlie *et al.*, 1976), confirming the result obtained by Jain *et al.* (1969a). However, the results of inoculation of cows which had no antibody to *A. laidlawii* in either milk or serum (9 out of 12 cows had titers >4 in their sera) showed slightly exaggerated cell responses, which may explain the cell reactions reported by Karbe and Mosher (1968) and others. Inoculation of yet a further four strains of *A. laidlawii,* isolated this time from mastitic cows' milk, into cows lacking antibodies to the acholeplasmas gave similar negative results (R. N. Gourlay, C. J. Howard, and J. Brownlie, unpublished observations).

After consideration of all the data we must conclude that there is no evidence at present that *A. laidlawii,* on its own, is pathogenic to cattle (see also Volume I, Chapter 16).

C. *Acholeplasma modicum*

Langer and McEntee (1961) described certain virus isolates from cattle in the United States. These were subsequently shown to be mycoplasmas (Langer and Carmichael, 1963), and two of them, isolate 527 (from the blood of a calf with severe diarrhea, and isolate Squire (Sq) (from the bronchial lymph node of a cow that died during an outbreak of pneumonia) were similar and were assigned to distinct taxonomic groups: group 6 (Leach, 1967) and group M (Al-Aubaidi and Fabricant, 1971a). The ability of these isolates to grow in serum- or sterol-free media (Al-Aubaidi and Fabricant, 1971a; Edward, 1971) placed them within the genus *Acholeplasma,* and they were in due course named *A. modicum* (Leach, 1973).

As the original isolates 527 and Sq were grown on cell-free media only after several subcultures in bovine fetal kidney cells, some doubts remained as to whether these isolates were truly bovine in origin. However, these doubts have now been resolved, as a strain of *A. modicum* has been isolated directly into cell-free medium from the pleural exudate of a bull suffering from pneumoenteritis in Hungary (Bokori *et al.*, 1971), from the peribronchial lymph node and lung of a calf in Hungary (Stipkovits *et al.*, 1975), and also from the prepuce of a bull in Canada (Langford, 1975a).

The cultural and biochemical characteristics of *A. modicum* are shown in Table I. It resembles other recognized species of *Acholeplasma* in its main biochemical and cultural characteristics but produces colonies ("fried egg" type) distinctly smaller than those of *A. laidlawii* and *A. granularum* (Leach, 1973). *Acholeplasma modicum,* with *A. axanthum,* also differs from these other *Acholeplasma* species in giving a negative result in the carotenoid synthesis test (Tully, 1973).

Acholeplasma modicum has been isolated only rarely, but most of these isolations have been from diseased cattle. This, however, does not necessarily imply a causal relationship, and in fact attempts to reproduce disease with this organism have so far yielded no valid evidence that this species is pathogenic. Langer and Carmichael (1963) failed to reproduce pneumoenteritis when the Sq strain was inoculated into colostrum-deprived calves by "various routes." However, Bokori *et al.* (1971)

reported that experimental inoculation of two young bulls, intranasally and intratracheally, respectively, with this organism resulted in clinical signs of respiratory disease. The animals were ultimately slaughtered after 85 and 133 days, and at necropsy gross lesions of pneumonia, bronchitis, pleuritis, and pericarditis were observed. The acholeplasmas could be recovered from the affected areas. Control animals were not used, so concurrent infections cannot be excluded; furthermore, one of the bulls had bronchitis prior to infection, and also thorough virological and bacteriological examinations were not undertaken.

V. ANAEROPLASMAS OF CATTLE

Anaeroplasma bactoclasticum (originally *Acholeplasma bactoclasticum*) is the name given to a strictly anaerobic, bacteriolytic microorganism that is resistant to penicillin G and has the microscopic and colonial morphology of a mycoplasma. The type strain (ATCC 27112) was isolated from a bovine rumen by Robinson and Hungate (1973) and, although originally considered not to require sterol, was subsequently shown to be a sterol-requiring, digitonin-sensitive organism (Robinson and Allison, 1975). Bacteriolytic, sterol-requiring, strictly anaerobic mycoplasmas have also been isolated from the ovine rumen, but they have been found to be serologically distinct from the bovine strain mentioned above (Robinson and Rhoades, 1977) (see also Volume I, Chapter 19).

Robinson *et al.* (1975) reported the isolation of nonbacteriolytic anaerobic mycoplasmas from the ovine rumen. Certain of these strains require sterol, and the name *Anaeroplasma abactoclasticum* was proposed to accommodate them. Nonbacteriolytic strains that did not require sterol and which had a different mole % G + C content (40.2–40.3 mole % as compared to 29.3–29.5 mole %) were also found, but no name was proposed for them. Nonbacteriolytic anaerobic mycoplasmas were also reported to be present in the bovine rumen (Robinson *et al.*, 1975), but the relation between these strains and the nonbacteriolytic, anaerobic ovine strains remains to be examined.

No association was made between these organisms and disease.

VI. UREAPLASMAS OF CATTLE

Ureaplasmas, formerly T-strain mycoplasmas, have been isolated in various parts of the world from a variety of bovine tissues and secretions. The first isolations made from cattle were in England from the urogenital tracts of cows (Taylor-Robinson *et al.*, 1967). Subsequently, they were isolated from 16 of 49 cows, mainly from the urethra, although the bladder and vagina were also examined (Taylor-Robinson et al., 1968). Ureaplasmas have also been isolated from the urogenital tract of bulls. They were isolated from 23 of 28 seminal fluid samples and from all 8 samples of washings from the preputial cavity. In 2 of these 8 animals ureaplasmas were not isolated from seminal samples (Taylor-Robinson et al., 1969). It was suggested, because of these findings, together with the failure to isolate mycoplasmas from the testicles, vas deferens, and mucosal lining of the urethra of two bulls, that the organisms from the prepuce had contaminated the seminal fluid. There have been other reports of the isolation of ureaplasmas from the urogenital tract of cattle in countries other than England. Langford (1975b) reported the isolation of ureaplasmas from the cervicovaginal mucus of 88 of 633 animals from 110 Canadian herds. Isolations have also been reported from the urogenital tract of cattle in the United States (Livingston and Gauer, 1974), Czechoslovakia (Jurmanova and Sterbova, 1977), and Bulgaria (Savov and Buchvarova, 1976).

Ureaplasmas are also frequently present in pneumonic calf lungs. Gourlay (1968) reported their isolation from the lungs of 9 of 16 calves with pneumonia. A subsequent study, also in England, demonstrated their presence in 38 of 65 pneumonic lungs (Gourlay et al., 1970). Livingston (1972), in the United States, isolated ureaplasmas from 5 of 7 pneumonic lungs, and a ureaplasma was isolated from a calf with pneumonia in Canada in the same year (Ruhnke and van Dreumel, 1972). In Scotland, Pirie and Allan (1975) reported ureaplasmas from 8 of 12 calves with cuffing pneumonia. At about the same time isolations of ureaplasmas were made in Japan from calves with pneumonia. Shimizu et al. (1975) reported their isolation from 15 of 22 pneumonic lungs, and Oghiso et al. (1976) observed a particularly high isolation rate (90%) from pneumonic lungs from calves less than 6 months old. In Denmark ureaplasmas were found in 26 of 50 pneumonic calf lungs by Bitsch et al. (1976). Isolations of ureaplasmas have also been made from the nasopharynx and trachea of calves (Livingston and Gauer, 1974; Shimizu et al., 1975; C. J. Howard, R. N. Gourlay, and L. H. Thomas, unpublished observations), but in many of these cases the animals had pneumonia. It is worthwhile noting that ureaplasmas are rarely isolated from nonpneumonic lungs (Thomas and Smith, 1972; Shimizu et al., 1975), further evidence for the association of these organisms with pneumonia. However, it should be emphasized that in the studies mentioned above other mycoplasmas, besides ureaplasmas, and bacteria were also isolated from the pneumonic lungs. The role of ureaplasmas in the etiology of calf pneumonia cannot therefore be deduced from isolation studies alone.

Gourlay and Thomas (1969a) isolated ureaplasmas from the eyes of cattle with keratoconjunctivitis, and Morar (1969) reported the presence of organisms thought to be ureaplasmas in 10 of 17 milk samples from cows in Hungary with mastitis. A single isolation was also made in England from mastitic milk from a quarter of the udder of a cow with a damaged teat (R. N. Gourlay, C. J. Howard, and J. Brownlie, unpublished observations).

Ureaplasmas have been isolated from several species of animals, and the properties and taxonomy of bovine ureaplasmas cannot be considered in isolation (see also Volume I, Chapter 17).

T-strain mycoplasmas were first isolated from humans by Shepard, over 20 years ago. They were originally characterized by their small colony size and lower optimum pH for growth as compared to the typical mycoplasmas known at that time. Subsequently they were found to possess urease activity. A genus *Ureaplasma* was proposed for these organisms with the general characteristics of mycoplasmas that require sterol but also possess urease activity (Shepard *et al.*, 1974). A single species was proposed for human ureaplasmas, *Ureaplasma urealyticum*, the type strain being T960, and eight serotypes were included in the species. These eight serotypes were selected from a variety of strains examined by Ford (1967) and Black (1971). However, it should be noted that the serotypes of *U. urealyticum* are not as discrete as those of the various *Mycoplasma* species.

Mycoplasmas with the general characteristics of the genus *Ureaplasma* have been isolated from cattle, as noted above. However, there is some doubt as to whether they can be regarded as *U. urealyticum*.

The serology of bovine ureaplasmas is complex. Taylor-Robinson *et al.* (1971) compared 3 human and 2 bovine strains by the metabolism inhibition test. None of the strains appeared identical. A further study of 8 bovine isolates was made by Howard and Gourlay (1973a) by means of metabolism inhibition, growth inhibition, and immunofluorescence tests. None of the bovine strains was identical to any other, but the possible existence of clusters of similar, though not serologically identical, strains was noted. A subsequent examination was made of 25 bovine isolates by immunofluorescence. The existence of clusters of serologically similar but not identical strains was confirmed, and 8 strains were proposed to represent the serological diversity of the bovine isolates (Howard *et al.*, 1975a). In a study of 13 bovine isolates in the United States using the mycoplasmacidal antibody test similar conclusions were reached, and the existence of at least 8 bovine ureaplasma serotypes suggested (Livingston and Gauer, 1974).

In even more recent studies on the serology of bovine ureaplasmas (Howard *et al.*, 1978b), 77 fresh isolates were tested by the growth inhibition test with antisera to the 8 representative strains proposed previously (Howard *et al.*, 1975a). Only 5 of these 77 strains did not react with the 8 antisera, and 3 more strains were added to the list of representative bovine strains, making a total of 11. It was suggested that a variety of antigenic determinants may be synthesized by bovine ureaplasmas, and these are detected by various serological tests. These determinants may be expressed in a variety of combinations. Clusters of serologically nonidentical but related strains seem to exist.

The species *U. urealyticum* is not defined by serological means, and serologically distinct strains exist within the species. Thus lack of serological cross-reactions between a bovine isolate and the eight serotypes of *U. urealyticum* is not sufficient evidence, on its own, for proposing a new species to accommodate the bovine strain.

However, no major antigens appear to be shared by representative bovine and human ureaplasmas selected from a large number of strains studied. Also, a comparison of the G + C content of the DNA from five bovine ureaplasmas has shown them to fall within the range 29.0–29.8 mole % (Howard *et al.*, 1974a) which is outside the range 26.9–28.0 mole % found by Black *et al.*, (1972) for *U. urealyticum*, the human ureaplasmas. Other differences between ureaplasmas of human and bovine origin also occur, such as susceptibility to killing by normal rabbit serum (Howard and Gourlay, 1973b). Also, the range of animal species that can be infected by human and bovine ureaplasmas seems to differ. Thus, although bovine ureaplasmas infected cattle and goats, they did not infect simian monkeys. Also, ureaplasmas of human origin infected simian monkeys and goats, but not cows (Howard *et al.*, 1973; Gourlay *et al.*, 1973; Furr *et al.*, 1978).

It therefore seems reasonable, largely from the results of these serological and nucleic acid studies, to regard bovine ureaplasmas as belonging to a separate species or to a subspecies of *U. urealyticum*. Comparisons of a selection of strains of ureaplasmas from other animal species will show whether they are related to *U. urealyticum* or *Ureaplasma* sp. (bovine) or constitute yet another species or subspecies.

Since ureaplasmas have been isolated from a variety of diseases in cattle with some frequency, it is of considerable interest to know what role they may play in these diseases. Gourlay and Thomas (1970) reported the results of inoculating ureaplasmas into the respiratory tract of 3-week-old conventionally reared calves. Clinical signs of pneumonia were observed in 6 of 16 calves before slaughter, and pneumonic lesions found in 14 of them. Only one of 9 control calves inoculated with sterile medium showed clinical symptoms of pneumonia, and lesions were evident in the lungs of this animal and of 1 other at necropsy. Further evidence for the pathogenicity of ureaplasmas for the respiratory tract was recorded by Howard *et al.* (1976a). Two gnotobiotic calves inoculated endobronchially with a ureaplasma were found to have gross lesions involving about 10% of the lung at necropsy. This lesion consisted largely of an infiltration of round cells, and cuffing, some catarrhal bronchiolitis, and atelectasis were also evident. The pathogenicity of ureaplasmas for bovine tissue was confirmed by the finding that these organisms were capable of inducing clinical mastitis in cows following their inoculation into the mammary gland. Furthermore, these studies showed the existence of both virulent and avirulent ureaplasma strains (Gourlay *et al.*, 1972; Howard *et al.*, 1973). Bovine ureaplasmas are also capable of inducing mastitis in mice (Howard *et al.*, 1975b). In this animal, strains that appeared avirulent for the bovine mammary gland were capable of inducing disease. Thus the mammary gland of mice appears to be more easily infected than the mammary gland of cattle and may not reflect accurately the virulence of strains in cattle. However, it should be pointed out that *A. laidlawii* was not able to induce mastitis in mice (Anderson *et al.*, 1976), and thus some host resistance is shown by this organ.

Ureaplasmas have rarely been isolated from cases of bovine mastitis, therefore they cannot be considered a frequent cause of this disease. Possibly they are responsible for occasional cases. The role of ureaplasmas in keratoconjunctivitis remains to be examined. The frequent isolation of ureaplasmas from the semen of fertile bulls and the urogenital tract of normal cows suggests that at these sites they are usually commensals. As both virulent and avirulent strains have been isolated from the urogenital tract, further studies may indicate an occasional pathogenic role of particular serotypes or strains at this site.

We can conclude therefore that there is evidence suggesting that ureaplasmas are involved in the pathogenesis of certain cases of pneumonia in calves. However, evidence does not indicate that they are *the* cause of the severe pneumonia from which they are sometimes isolated. It seems more likely that they play a role in severe clinical disease in association with other agents. They should be regarded as being capable on their own of inducing only low-grade chronic pneumonia.

VII. UNUSUAL AND UNCLASSIFIED MYCOPLASMAS FROM CATTLE

There have been numerous reports of mycoplasmas isolated from cattle that have not been fully identified or indeed identified at all. Many of these isolates are probably existing bovine mycoplasma species, and some are probably other named species not usually isolated from cattle. A few, however, may represent new species not previously described.

Al-Aubaidi and Fabricant (1971a) divided bovine mycoplasmas into 13 distinct serotypes, designated A to M. Two of their serotypes, H and I, were subsequently shown to be *Mycoplasma gateae* and *M. gallinarum,* respectively (Ernø *et al.*, 1973). *Mycoplasma gateae,* normally associated only with cats, comprised 7 strains, all of which had been isolated from bovine male and female genital tracts. There were 3 strains of *M. gallinarum,* a species normally associated with birds, and all were isolated from the bovine respiratory tract. As there have been no other reported isolations of these 2 mycoplasma species from cattle, it seems unwise, at the present time, to regard them as truly bovine mycoplasmas.

In the United States Page *et al.* (1972) described the isolation and partial characterization of an unidentified glucose-fermenting mycoplasma, strain 3222. This mycoplasma was isolated from chicken embryos originally inoculated with bovine placental tissue associated with the "weak calf" syndrome. Strain 3222 was later identified as *M. gallisepticum* (Rhoades *et al.*, 1975). While it is probable that this isolate originated from the embryonated eggs and not the bovine placenta, Rhoades pointed out that similar isolates were recovered from two separate laboratories following independent inoculation of embryos with tissues from the same bovine placenta. Furthermore, there was evidence of the presence of complement-fixing antibodies to *M. gallisepticum* in many cattle in the original herd and in other herds in the area affected by the weak calf syndrome (Page *et al.*, 1972). Time will tell whether *M. gallisepticum* is a genuine inhabitant of cattle, as isolations will be made in conventional mycoplasma media. This episode, however, has been a salutary reminder to us all of the dangers of using egg embryos for primary isolation of mycoplasmas.

Polak-Vogelzang and Beuvery (1975) reported the isolation of *Mycoplasma equirhinis* from the nasopharynx of adult cattle in the Netherlands. *Mycoplasma equirhinis* is normally found in horses (Allam and Lemcke, 1975), and close contact with horses at their places of origin might be a possible explanation of this finding.

A. *Mycoplasma* Species Group 7

Until recently all isolations of strains of this group, assigned by Leach (1967) to a separate but unnamed species, were from Australia, the first isolations being from joint fluid of three calves with arthritis (Simmons and Johnston, 1963). Subsequent isolations have been from other cases of arthritis (Cottew, 1970) and mastitis (Connole *et al.*, 1967; Cottew, 1970), and two strains have been recovered from bovine lung and lymph node, respectively (Cottew, 1970).

Apart from Australia, isolations of strains of this group have recently been reported from the urogenital tract of cattle and aborted fetuses in both the United States and Canada (Al-Aubaidi and Fabricant, 1971a; Langford, 1975a). In Canada these strains were isolated from cervico-vaginal mucus (7 isolates from 1265 animals), bull semen (6 from 168 samples), prepuce (4 out of 267 samples), and from the stomach contents (2 of 251), lungs (2 of 40), liver (1 of 15), and spleen (1 of 15) of aborted fetuses. This organism has also been isolated from the urogenital tract of apparently normal animals (Langford, 1975b).

The biochemical and cultural characteristics of this group, shown in Table I, are not distinctive and resemble those of most other glucose-fermenting species. However, one consistent property of these strains was their rapid and profuse growth in conventional mycoplasma media and the production of large typical "fried egg" colonies on solid medium (Leach, 1973).

Serologically this group of *Mycoplasma* is distinct from other bovine mycoplasmas (Leach, 1967, 1973; Al-Aubaidi and Fabricant, 1971a). However, cross-reactions have been reported in serological tests between this group and some strains of *M. bovigenitalium, M. arginini*, serotype L of Al-Aubaidi and Fabricant (1971a), and *M. mycoides* subsp. *mycoides* and *M. mycoides* subsp. *capri* (Cottew, 1970; Ernø *et al.*, 1973). Leach (1973) and Ernø *et al.* (1973) concluded nevertheless that the apparent cross-reactions with *M. bovigenitalium* and *M. arginini* were probably nonspecific or of only minor antigenic significance, bearing in mind the other biochemical and cultural characteristics of these species. However, the relationship between group 7, serotype L, and the two serotypes of *M. mycoides* may be more significant and require further study. They may ultimately be shown to represent separate subspecies of *M. mycoides* (Leach, 1973; Ernø and Jurmanova, 1973). It is interesting to note that strains of group 7 produce glucan, in contrast to the galactan produced by *M. mycoides* subsp. *mycoides* (Hudson *et al.*, 1967b).

The evidence from the isolations indicates that the group-7 strains can be associated with disease; moreover evidence is also available indicating that these organisms are undoubtedly pathogenic, as clinical mastitis was reproduced by inoculation of a culture of this organism into the mammary gland of a cow (Connole *et al.*, 1967). An earlier report of Simmons and Johnston (1963) that they had produced arthritis in a calf by inoculation of a culture into a joint of a calf was suspect, as they had simultaneously inoculated another joint of the same calf with affected joint fluid. The ability to produce arthritis with this organism was confirmed later, however, following the intravenous inoculation of a culture of this organism (Cottew and Leach, 1969).

B. *Mycoplasma* Species Serotype L

During their study of bovine mycoplasmas, Al-Aubaidi and Fabricant (1971a) classified only one strain as serotype L. This was derived from a strain isolated by Moulton *et al.* (1956) from the joints, kidneys, and spleen of a calf in California showing severe arthritis and bronchopneumonia. This mycoplasma ferments glucose but not arginine or urea, requires serum for growth, and does not form film and spots. It is reported to grow at 25°C.

Although Al-Aubaidi and Fabricant considered this serotype serologically distinct from other bovine mycoplasmas, the question of its relationship to *M. mycoides* subsp. *mycoides* and *Mycoplasma* sp. group 7 (Leach, 1967) has been referred to above.

Experimental inoculation of four calves and steers intravenously or into a joint resulted in clinical signs of stiffness, lameness, and keratitis. Mycoplasmas were reisolated from the joints of two of the animals (Moulton *et al.*, 1956).

C. *Mycoplasma* Species Strain ST-6

Another interesting strain is the ST-6 strain described by Dellinger *et al.* (1977), which is representative of isolates made from several mastitis outbreaks in California. The ST-6 strain utilizes arginine but not glucose or urea and is serologically and biochemically distinct from other bovine mycoplasmas. Experimentally it induces moderately severe mastitis (Jasper, 1977).

VIII. IMMUNITY

A. Serological Tests

A variety of serological tests has been found to be capable of detecting antibody in bovine sera following infection with a mycoplasma. The sensitivities of the tests vary, certain of the tests detect different classes of immunoglobulin, most are quantitative, and some require special apparatus. These tests include complement fixation, agglutination, indirect hemagglutination, latex agglutination, metabolism inhibition, growth inhibition, inhibition of film production, radial growth precipitation, immunodiffusion, radial hemolysis, and immunofluorescence (Rurangirwa, 1976; Bennett and Jasper, 1977a; Ruhnke *et al.*, 1976; Jasper, 1977; Cho *et al.*, 1976; Jain *et al.*, 1969b; Ernø and Aalund, 1972; Ernø, 1972; Windsor, 1977; Hudson, 1971; Howard *et al.*, 1976b, 1977a; Carroll *et al.*, 1977; Bennett and Jasper, 1978a). However, it should be pointed out that a positive reaction in a serological test does not indicate the etiological significance of a particular mycoplasma in a disease, nor does it necessarily indicate the immune status of the individual animal.

B. Resistance following Recovery from Infection

Cattle that have recovered from respiratory infection with *M. mycoides* subsp. *mycoides* are immune to reinfection (Hudson, 1971; Gourlay, 1975; Whittlestone, 1976), and this immunity to respiratory disease lasts a considerable length of time. Immunity to reinfection of the mammary gland of cows also occurs. Thus Howard *et al.* (1974b) reported that cows that had recovered from mastitis induced by the intramammary inoculation of a bovine ureaplasma were immune to challenge with the same strain but not to a serologically distinct bovine ureaplasma strain. This immunity appeared to occur throughout the udder and was not limited to previously infected quarters.

Mycoplasma dispar induces clinical mastitis following its inoculation into the mammary gland. Immunity to reinfection has also been reported (Gourlay *et al.*, 1975), but there are certain differences between the immunity to *M. dispar* and to ureaplasmas. Thus immunity to reinfection with *M. dispar* appeared to be limited to the previously infected quarter only. On challenge an acute cell response, consisting mainly of neutrophils, was observed in the milk from the immune, previously infected quarter. This response was not seen in susceptible quarters not previously infected. Subsequent studies (C. J. Howard, J. Brownlie, and R. N. Gourlay, unpublished observations) have demonstrated that there may be some moderation of the infection in quarters not previously infected, but the immunity observed in the previously infected quarter is much stronger by comparison. Whether these results indicate basic differences in the mechanism of immunity to ureaplasmas and to *M. dispar,* or whether they merely reflect differences in challenge dose and pathogenicity of the strains used, is not known.

Bennett and Jasper (1978a,b) reported resistance to reinfection in cows that had previously been infected in the mammary gland with *M. bovis.* Immunity to reinfection appeared to persist longer in previously infected quarters than in previously uninfected quarters of the same cow, and an enhanced cell response, perhaps similar to that seen with *M. dispar*, was noted in previously infected immune quarters following challenge.

C. Protection by Vaccines

Vaccination against *M. mycoides* subsp. *mycoides* has been shown to be highly effective and is well documented. Live vaccines, given subcutaneously or in the tail, protect against subcutaneous challenge and also against a challenge via the respiratory route (see, e.g., Hudson, 1971; Lloyd and Trethewie, 1970; Whittlestone, 1976; Gourlay, 1975; Roberts and Windsor, 1974).

Although immunity to subcutaneous challenge has been reported to be induced with inactivated *M. mycoides* subsp. *mycoides*, it has also been noted that inactivated vaccines may induce a hypersensitivity reaction following challenge (Lindley and Abdulla, 1967; Shifrine and Beech, 1968). It seems to be generally agreed that inactivated organisms are less effective in inducing immunity than live vaccines (see reviews mentioned above).

It is possible that this is in part due to the site of the immune response. Thus following subcutaneous vaccination with *M. mycoides* subsp. *mycoides* bacteremia occurs, and it is possible that viable organisms reach the lung and induce a local response there. Systemic vaccination with inactivated *M. mycoides* subsp. *mycoides* would not be expected to stimulate a local immune response in the respiratory tract.

Resistance to *M. bovis* infection of the respiratory tract of calves has been induced by inoculating animals with Formalin-inactivated organisms (Howard *et al.*, 1977b, 1978a). Significantly less *M. bovis* was isolated, after challenge, from the lungs of calves inoculated intramuscularly and then intratracheally with inactivated *M. bovis*, compared to control calves. It was therefore suggested that local presentation of inactivated organisms is more effective in inducing resistance to respiratory infection than systemic inoculation alone.

Immunity to *M. bovis*-induced arthritis can also be induced with inactivated organisms (C. J. Howard and R. N. Gourlay, unpublished observations). Five calves were inoculated intramuscularly and then intratracheally with inactivated *M. bovis* in a manner similar to that described previously (Howard *et al.*, 1977b), except that the mycoplasmas were inactivated by exposure to 1 Mrad ^{60}Co total irradiation. These calves, and five controls inoculated with phosphate-buffered saline, were challenged intravenously with 3×10^9 CFU *M. bovis*. None of the vaccinated animals developed arthritis. All five control animals developed arthritis, the first two 6 days after challenge, the third on day 7, the fourth on day 9, and the fifth on day 12. *Mycoplasma bovis* was isolated from the swollen joints of the affected calves but not from the control calves.

D. Mechanisms of Immunity

As pointed out above, resistance to *M. mycoides* subsp. *mycoides* is observed following recovery from natural infection or vaccination with live organisms. However, recovered cattle often do not have antibody in their sera detected by the tests used. Also, a variety of serological tests has been utilized but found not to correlate with immunity following vaccination (see reviews quoted above; see also Masiga and Read, 1972; Roberts and Windsor, 1974).

Resistance to respiratory infection with *M. bovis* induced with inactivated organisms was not related to serum antibody detectable by complement fixation or single radial hemolysis (Howard *et al.*, 1977b). Bennett and Jasper (1978a) failed to find any relation between serum antibody and resistance to *M. bovis* mastitis. No relation has been found between serum levels of antibody to *M. dispar* in recovered cows and immunity to mastitis (C. J. Howard, J. Brownlie, and R. N. Gourlay, unpublished observations).

Serum antibody might be expected to be involved in protection against nonmucosal mycoplasma infections, such as the immunity to *M. bovis* arthritis induced by inactivated mycoplasmas. Also, passively transferred serum has been reported to protect against subcutaneous challenge with *M. mycoides* subsp. *mycoides*. Early work by Nocard *et al.* (1899, cited in Lloyd and Trethewie, 1970) indicated that serum from a hyperimmunized cow conferred on recipient cows some protection against subcutaneous challenge. This work was confirmed by Gourlay and Shifrine (1966b) who were able to prevent or reduce subcutaneous Willems reactions by prior administration of 100–250 ml of immune or hyperimmune serum. However, Lloyd (1967) reported that cattle inoculated with serum from cattle immune to subcutaneous challenge were not protected. Later, however, serum from a convalescent cow was found to protect recipient cattle against subcutaneous challenge (Lloyd and Trethewie, 1970). It has also been claimed that protection against respiratory infection with *M. mycoides* subsp. *mycoides* can be conferred by serum. Masiga and Windsor (1975) found that two steers inoculated intravenously with 1.5–2 liters of serum from animals that had recovered from contagious bovine pleuropneumonia, but which did not contain demonstrable serum antibody, were protected for at least 8 months to challenge from donor-diseased animals. Although the controls seem not to have been inoculated with the same volume of normal serum, it seems unlikely that any nonspecific effects due to its inoculation would have lasted as long as the protection demonstrated. The possibility of antigens from *M. mycoides* subsp. *mycoides* being present in the passively transferred serum seems not to have been excluded. In another study (Masiga *et al.*, 1975) it was reported that only one of five animals which had received serum, with no demonstrable antibody, from animals that were immune to contagious bovine pleuropneumonia, developed disease following exposure to donor-infected cattle. All five untreated control cattle developed disease. However, only three of five animals that had been inoculated with serum from cattle susceptible to contagious bovine pleuropneumonia developed disease following challenge. Thus in this instance normal serum seemed to induce some resistance to respiratory infection. Further investigations are therefore required before any definite conclusions can be reached as to whether serum can confer protection against respiratory challenge.

Dyson and Smith (1975) reported that the sera taken from cattle infected with contagious bovine pleuropneumonia or vaccinated with live or killed *M. mycoides* subsp. *mycoides,* when passively transferred into mice, protected against *M. mycoides* subsp. *mycoides* bacteremia induced by the intraperitoneal inoculation of mycoplasmas. This protective capacity of the sera seemed unrelated to antibody detectable by complement fixation or precipitation. It seems likely that the transferred bovine sera may promote phagocytosis by the reticuloendothelial system in mice and thus affect the septicemia. However, the relation between this activity, presumably due to serum antibody and immunity, must be open to doubt. Thus "antibody" detectable by this test was found at least as frequently in the sera of cattle vaccinated with inactivated *M. mycoides* subsp. *mycoides* as in the sera of cattle vaccinated with live vaccine strains, whereas it is generally considered that live vaccine strains induce a more effective immunity to respiratory infection with *M. mycoides* subsp. *mycoides* than inactivated vaccines. Also, this activity in the sera of animals naturally infected or inoculated with live vaccine was of relatively short duration compared with the length of immunity usually reported.

There is evidence that local immune mechanisms are involved in resistance to mycoplasma infections in animal species other than cattle. In cattle this possibility does not seem to have been investigated very extensively, although there is some evidence for believing that it might occur. Thus Masiga and Roberts (1973) reported the presence of antibody to galactan in the lungs of cattle vaccinated with *M. mycoides* subsp. *mycoides*. Ernø and Aalund (1972) observed the occurrence of a local antibody response in the milk of a cow with mastitis induced with *M. bovigenitalium*. The presence of locally produced antibody in the seminal fluid of animals infected with *M. bovigenitalium* and *M. bovis* has also been demonstrated (Ernø and Blom, 1973; Corbeil *et al.*, 1976). Immunity to reinfection of the udder with *M. dispar* appeared to be limited to previously infected quarters of the mammary gland and to be associated with an acute cell response in the milk from the immune quarters on challenge (Gourlay *et al.*, 1975). This indicates the existence of a local system of immunity to mycoplasmas in the udder. However, Bennett and Jasper (1978a,b) were unable to find a consistent relationship between antibody in whey and immunity to reinfection with *M. bovis*.

Delayed-type hypersensitivity reactions have been reported to occur in animals infected with *M. mycoides* subsp. *mycoides* (Gourlay, 1964). Also, lymphocyte transformation, inhibition of leukocyte migration, and an intradermal allergic reaction with *M. mycoides* subsp. *mycoides* antigen was observed in cattle, subsequent to infection, by Roberts *et al.* (1973). However, neither lymphocyte transformation, inhibition of leukocyte migration, or the intradermal allergic test was found to correlate with immunity to this mycoplasma (Roberts and Windsor, 1974). Lloyd and Trethewie (1970) found no evidence for the transfer of immunity with lymph node cells from vaccinated cattle into identical twins. Although a positive skin test reaction was found in some animals subsequent to *M. bovis* mastitis by Bennett and Jasper (1978a,b), this seems to have been an immediate antibody-mediated reaction, and it was not related to immunity. Thus there is at present no evidence for cell-mediated immunity being of prime importance in immunity to mycoplasma infections in cattle. This is in agreement with findings in other species of animals (Fernald and Clyde, 1974; Taylor and Taylor-Robinson, 1976), and might be expected in the case of infections that do not involve intracellular parasites.

It therefore seems more likely that in cattle induced resistance to mycoplasmas might be due to humoral rather than cell-mediated immunity, and local immunity is possibly of greatest importance. A local immunity need not involve just IgA, as cells synthesizing all classes of bovine immunoglobulin have been found in the lung (Morgan *et al.*, 1978).

There is a variety of ways in which antibody might be involved in inducing resistance to mycoplasma infections in cattle. Bovine alveolar macrophages and lacteal neutrophils have been shown to be capable of killing both *M. bovis* and *M. dispar* in the presence of bovine antibody (Howard *et al.*, 1976c). Thus antibody might promote phagocytosis, inhibit the attachment of mycoplasmas to mucosal surfaces, inhibit mycoplasma growth, or promote complement killing. All these effects have been demonstrated with antibody and mycoplasmas *in vitro*.

IX. VIRULENCE FACTORS

The mucosal surfaces are the sites in cattle most frequently colonized with mycoplasmas, as is the case with other animal species. Some mechanism of attachment to these surfaces therefore seems to be required for mycoplasmas to be able to persist and survive there, whether the strains are pathogenic or commensal. The ability of bovine mycoplasmas to persist and grow in cell cultures is possibly a reflection of this capacity. Many species of bovine mycoplasmas have been shown to be capable of hemagglutination or hemadsorption (Ernø and Stipkovits, 1973b). In the case of *M. dispar* bovine erythrocytes are agglutinated by means of a pronase- and trypsin-sensitive attachment site on the mycoplasma, and considerable strain variation occurs with respect to this species' ability to hemagglutinate (Howard *et al.*, 1974c). No definite relation between this property and virulence has been established. It is worth noting that the mechanism of attachment to the epithelium of tracheal organ cultures is also sensitive to proteolytic enzymes (C. J. Howard and L. H. Thomas, unpublished observations). Thus this hemagglutination mechanism might reflect attachment mechanisms *in vivo*.

The bovine mycoplasma species associated with respiratory disease do not seem to possess the terminal structure involved in attachment such as that described for *M. pneumoniae*. One bovine species, *M. alvi*, does seem to possess such a structure which may be involved in attachment to the mucosal surface of the intestine.

Certain bovine mycoplasmas have a cytopathic effect on cell cultures, e.g., *M. bovis* (Hirth *et al.*, 1970b) and *M. bovigenitalium* (Afshar, 1967). This may merely reflect their ability to grow under these conditions but is possibly related to the synthesis of toxic material. More interesting is the effect of certain species on the ciliary activity of organ cultures. *Mycoplasma dispar* destroyed the ciliated epithelium of tracheal organ cultures, so destroying ciliary activity. A variety of *A. laidlawii, M. bovirhinis,* and *Ureaplasma* sp. strains had no demonstrable effect, although they grew in the same system (Thomas and Howard, 1974). No toxin was demonstrable in supernatants of spent cultures of *M. dispar,* but the intimate association of mycoplasmas and cilia may be required for an active substance to be effective (Howard and Thomas, 1974). *Mycoplasma bovis* and *M. bovirhinis* were found to have no effect on fallopian tube organ cultures (Stalheim and Gallagher, 1975).

Stalheim *et al.* (1976) reported that bovine ureaplasmas grew in organ cultures of bovine oviducts, stopped ciliary activity, and caused histological lesions. However, subsequent studies indicated this effect to be due to the liberation of ammonia from urea by urease (Stalheim and Gallagher,

1977). Thus the potential importance of this observation on *in vivo* pathogenicity must be open to doubt.

Hemolysins are produced by most bovine mycoplasmas (Ernø and Stipkovits, 1973b) but, as they are synthesized by both pathogenic and nonpathogenic species, their importance seems limited. It has been reported that *M. bovis* synthesizes an intracellular toxin that induces an eosinophil response in the bovine mammary gland (Mosher *et al.*, 1968). However, the cell response in the mammary gland during infection seems to consist of neutrophils (Jasper *et al.*, 1966), although an eosinophil reaction has been reported during the acute stages of infection (Karbe *et al.*, 1967). Dead and avirulent mycoplasma strains can induce a cell response in the mammary gland consisting largely of neutrophils (Gourlay *et al.*, 1972; Howard *et al.*, 1973). This is presumed to be the response of the gland to foreign material. Evidence for toxin production by *M. mycoides* subsp. *mycoides* has been noted earlier.

The relation between capsules and strain virulence has been well established in bacterial infections where they have been shown to inhibit such host defense mechanisms as complement killing and phagocytosis (Glynn, 1972). A capsule is synthesized by *M. mycoides* subsp. *mycoides*, which is probably composed largely of galactan, and it has been suggested that the amount of galactan might be related to strain virulence (Gourlay and Thrower, 1968). A capsule was also seen around *M. dispar* strains stained with ruthenium red but not around a variety of other bovine species (Howard and Gourlay, 1974). Possibly such capsules affect the virulence of strains within these two species.

X. ASSOCIATION OF BOVINE MYCOPLASMAS WITH DISEASE

In the earlier part of this chapter we considered details of individual species and serotypes of bovine mycoplasmas, including their isolation, cultural and biochemical characteristics, and pathogenicity. Under this heading we attempt to summarize the data pertaining to sites of isolation and pathogenicity and endeavor to assess the role of the various species or serotypes in bovine disease.

As most mycoplasmologists are interested in the role, if any, that these organisms play in disease, most isolations have been made from diseased tissues. It is equally true that most species of mycoplasma have also been isolated from normal tissues, and this has always confused the issue. In considering the different anatomical sites from which mycoplasmas can be isolated we are only concered with sites from which the organisms are normally isolated and not those from which they can be isolated during bacteremia.

The association of a microorganism with a diseased tissue does not necessarily imply a causal relationship. It is therefore important to distinguish between mycoplasmas that play a significant role in the disease, whether as a primary or secondary agent, and those that are saprophytes or commensals. It is of course quite possible that an organism that plays a secondary role may be as important in the disease situation as the primary agent.

To prove a causal relationship between a microorganism and a disease it has sufficed, in the past, to fulfill Koch's postulates in conventionally reared animals. This was perfectly acceptable when the microorganism concerned was highly pathogenic and capable of causing serious disease or even death of the host, and when the resident microflora played an insignificant part in the disease process. However, fulfillment of Koch's postulates in conventionally reared animals becomes less meaningful when the organism concerned is less pathogenic, and especially when its significance may only be expressed fully in association with some other organism or organisms. Most pathogenic mycoplasmas fall into this category. In this case, to determine the exact role of a mycoplasma in the disease process, it is necessary to employ specific-pathogen-free, gnotobiotic, or germ-free animals. This is additionally important in studies on genital or respiratory disease, as many apparently normal animals suffer from subclinical infections.

Apart from the fulfillment of Koch's postulates, other evidence of pathogenicity or pathogenic potential may be of value in assessing the role of a mycoplasma in a disease situation. Such evidence can be the ability to cause damage to any tissue, either *in vivo* or *in vitro*, such as damage after inoculation at another anatomical site such as the mammary gland, or the inoculation of tissue or organ cultures. Certain biophysical or biochemical characteristics of the mycoplasma may be suggestive of pathogenic potential, such as the production of a toxin or the presence of a capsule or a terminal attachment structure. Incidentally, production of antibody by the animal inoculated with a particular organism does not necessarily imply etiological significance; the organism may simply be multiplying in the disease tissue. Table II lists the different anatomical sites from which the named species and recognized serotypes of bovine mycoplasmas have been isolated (under nonbacteremic situations) and also summarizes our views on the pathogenic status of these species at these sites. However, the virulence of strains within a species is not constant, and avirulent strains can exist within a pathogenic species.

From Table II we conclude that, of the 18 species or serotypes referred to, half are pathogenic to a greater or lesser degree, while the pathogenicity of the remainder has not been proved. The fact that a given species is pathogenic for one bovine tissue suggests that it is likely to play a role in a disease of any other bovine tissue from which it is isolated in large numbers.

The pathogenicity status of a given mycoplasma species is important information when considering what role it plays in the disease situation from which it is isolated. However, the fact that the species in question is undoubtedly pathogenic under experimental conditions does not necessarily imply that it is the sole cause of the disease. This must be assessed for each outbreak of disease, taking into account all the relevant informa-

TABLE II.   **Mycoplasma Species and Recognized Serotypes Isolated from Different Anatomical Sites in Cattle and Their Pathogenicity**

Site	Proved pathogen	Proved pathogen at other site	Pathogenicity not proved
Respiratory tract	M. bovis M. dispar M. mycoides subsp. mycoides Ureaplasma sp.	M. bovigenitalium M. bovirhinis M. canadense Mycoplasma sp. gp 7	M. alkalescens M. arginini A. axanthum A. laidlawii A. modicum
Urogenital tract	M. bovis	M. bovigenitalium M. bovirhinis M. canadense Ureaplasma sp. Mycoplasma sp. gp 7	M. alkalescens M. alvi M. arginini M. verecundum A. laidlawii A. modicum
Mammary gland	M. bovigenitalium M. bovirhinis M. bovis M. canadense Mycoplasma sp. gp 7	—	M. alkalescens M. arginini A. axanthum A. laidlawii
Joints	M. bovis M. mycoides subsp. mycoides Mycoplasma sp. gp 7 Mycoplasma sp. serotype L	M. bovirhinis M. canadense	M. alkalescens
Eyes	—	M. bovirhinis M. bovis Ureaplasma sp.	M. arginini M. bovoculi M. verecundum A. laidlawii
Rumen	—	—	An. bactoclasticum
Intestines	—	—	M. alvi

tion, for example, the tissue involved, the number of mycoplasmas isolated, and other possible agents present.

The bovine mammary gland is probably more susceptible to mycoplasma infections than any of the other sites, and it does not normally possess any resident microflora. Therefore any mastitis from which pathogenic mycoplasmas are isolated in large numbers can probably be safely assumed to be caused by that mycoplasma. This also applies to cases of arthritis from which a pathogenic mycoplasma is isolated. When it comes to respiratory disease, the role of mycoplasmas is not so clearcut. There is no doubt that *M. mycoides* subsp. *mycoides* is the etiological agent of CBPP, and in the last few years it has become plain that *M. bovis, M. dispar,* and *Ureaplasma* sp. play a role in bovine pneumonia. However, as the respiratory tract is colonized by and is being continuously assailed by a host of different microorganisms, some of them pathogenic, the exact role that mycoplasmas play is not yet clear. The role of mycoplasmas in diseases of the bovine urogenital tract is more controversial. That pathogenic mycoplasmas can be isolated from this tract is not questioned. *Mycoplasma bovis* is certainly capable of producing severe lesions in the genital tract but is as yet rarely incriminated in field disease. Present field data do not suggest that the majority of the other pathogenic mycoplasmas are important agents in urogenital diseases, and most have not been tested at this site. *Mycoplasma bovigenitalium* is the exception. But this mycoplasma only seems capable of producing lesions following mechanical trauma or inoculation by an abnormal route.

REFERENCES

Afshar, A. (1967). *J. Gen. Microbiol.* **47,** 103–110.
Afshar, A., Stuart, P., and Huck, R. A. (1966). *Vet. Rec.* **78,** 512–519.
Al-Aubaidi, J. M., and Fabricant, J. (1971a). *Cornell Vet.* **61,** 490–518.
Al-Aubaidi, J. M., and Fabricant, J. (1971b). *Cornell Vet.* **61,** 559–572.
Al-Aubaidi, J. M., Dardiri, A. H., and Fabricant, J. (1972a). *Int. J. Syst. Bacteriol.* **22,** 155–164.
Al-Aubaidi, J. M., McEntee, K., Lein, D. H., and Roberts, S. J. (1972b). *Cornell Vet.* **62,** 581–596.
Albertsen, B. E. (1955). *Nord. Vet. Med.* **7,** 169–201.
Allam, N. M., and Lemcke, R. M. (1975). *J. Hyg.* **74,** 385–407.
Anderson, J. C., Howard, C. J., and Gourlay, R. N. (1976). *Infect. Immun.* **13,** 1205–1208.
Anonymous (1977). *Vet. Rec.* **100,** 521.
Askaa, G., and Ernø, H. (1976). *Int. J. Syst. Bacteriol.* **26,** 323–325.
Askaa, G., Christiansen, C., and Ernø, H. (1973). *J. Gen. Microbiol.* **75,** 283–286.
Barber, T. L., and Yedloutschnig, R. J. (1970). *Cornell Vet.* **60,** 297–308.
Barile, M. F. (1973). *In* "Contamination in Tissue Culture" (J. Fogh, ed.), pp. 131–172. Academic Press, New York.

Barile, M. F., and Kern, J. (1971). *Proc. Soc. Exp. Biol. Med.* **138,** 432–437.
Barile, M. F., Del Giudice, R. A., Carski, T. R., Gibbs, C. J., and Morris, J. A. (1968). *Proc. Soc. Exp. Biol. Med.* **129,** 489–494.
Bennett, R. H., and Jasper, D. E. (1977a). *Cornell Vet.* **67,** 361–373.
Bennett, R. H., and Jasper, D. E. (1977b). *Vet. Microbiol.* **2,** 341–355.
Bennett, R. H., and Jasper, D. E. (1978a). *Am. J. Vet. Res.* **39,** 417–423.
Bennett, R. H., and Jasper, D. E. (1978b). *Am. J. Vet. Res.* **39,** 407–416.
Bennett, R. H., and Jasper, D. E. (1978c). *J. Am. Vet. Med. Assoc.* **172,** 484–488.
Bitsch, V., Friis, N. F., and Krogh, H. V. (1976). *Acta Vet. Scand.* **17,** 32–42.
Black, F. T. (1971). *Int. Congr. Infect. Dis., 5th, Vienna 1970* **1,** 407–411.
Black, F. T., Christiansen, C., and Askaa, G. (1972). *Int. J. Syst. Bacteriol.* **22,** 241–242.
Blom, E., and Ernø, H. (1970). *Proc. 11, Nord. Vet. Congr., Bergen* p. 254.
Bokori, J., Horvath, Z., Stipkovits, L., and Molnar, L. (1971). *Acta Vet. Acad. Sci. Hung.* **21,** 61–73.
Brookbanks, E. O., Carter, M. E., and Holland, J. T. S. (1969). *N.Z. Vet. J.* **17,** 179–180.
Brownlie, J., Howard, C. J., and Gourlay, R. N. (1976). *Res. Vet. Sci.* **20,** 261–266.
Buttery, S. H., and Plackett, P. (1960). *J. Gen. Microbiol.* **23,** 357–368.
Carmichael, L. E., Guthrie, R. S., Fincher, M. G., Field, L. E., Johnson, S. D., and Linquist, W. E. (1963). *Proc. Annu. Meet. U.S. Livestock Sanit. Assoc., 67th,* pp. 220–235.
Carroll, E. J., Bennett, R. H., Rollins, M., and Jasper, D. E. (1977). *Can. J. Comp. Med.* **41,** 279–286.
Carter, G. R. (1954). *Science* **120,** 113.
Cho, H. J., Ruhnke, H. L., and Langford, E. V. (1976). *Can. J. Comp. Med.* **40,** 20–29.
Connole, M. D., Laws, L., and Hart, R. K. (1967). *Aust. Vet. J.* **43,** 157–162.
Corbeil, L. B., Bier, P. J., Hall, C. E., and Duncan, J. R. (1976). *Theriogenology* **6,** 39–44.
Cottew, G. S. (1970). *Aust. Vet. J.* **46,** 378–381.
Cottew, G. S., and Leach, R. H. (1969). *In* "The Mycoplasmatales and the L-Phase of Bacteria" (L. Hayflick, ed.), pp. 527–570. North-Holland Publ. Amsterdam.
Cottew, G. S., and Yeats, F. R. (1978). *Aust. Vet. J.* **54,** 293–296.
Davidson, I., and Stuart, P. (1960). *Vet. Rec.* **72,** 766.
Davies, G. (1967). *J. Comp. Pathol.* **77,** 353–357.
Dawson, P. S., Stuart, P., Darbyshire, J. H., Parker, W. H., and McCrea, C. T. (1966). *Vet. Rec.* **78,** 543–546.
Dellinger, J. D., and Jasper, D. E. (1972). *Am. J. Vet. Res.* **33,** 769–775.
Dellinger, J. D., Jasper, D. E., and Ilic, M. (1977). *Cornell Vet.* **67,** 351–360.
Dyson, D. A., and Smith, G. R. (1975). *Res. Vet. Sci.* **19,** 8–16.
Edward, D. G. ff. (1950). *J. Gen. Microbiol.* **4,** 4–15.
Edward, D. G. ff. (1971). *J. Gen. Microbiol.* **69,** 205–210.
Edward, D. G. ff., and Fitzgerald, W. A. (1952). *Vet. Rec.* **64,** 395.
Edward, D. G. ff., and Freundt, E. A. (1956). *J. Gen. Microbiol.* **14,** 197–207.
Edward, D. G. ff., and Moore, W. B. (1975). *J. Med. Microbiol.* **8,** 451–454.
Edward, D. G. ff., Hancock, J. L., and Hignett, S. L. (1947). *Vet. Rec.* **59,** 329–330.
Erfle, Von V., and Brunner, A. (1977). *Berl. Muench. Tieraerztl. Wochenschr.* **90,** 28–34.
Ernø, H. (1967). *Acta Vet. Scand.* **8,** 184–185.
Ernø, H. (1969). *Acta Vet. Scand.* **10,** 106–107.
Ernø, H. (1972). *Infect. Immun.* **5,** 20–23.
Ernø, H., and Aalund, O. (1972). *Acta Vet. Scand.* **13,** 597–599.
Ernø, H., and Blom, E. (1972). *Acta Vet. Scand.* **13,** 161–174.
Ernø, H., and Blom, E. (1973). *Acta Vet. Scand.* **14,** 332–334.
Ernø, H., and Jurmanova, K. (1973). *Acta Vet. Scand.* **14,** 524–537.

Ernø, H., and Stipkovits, L. (1973a). *Acta Vet. Scand.* **14,** 436–449.
Ernø, H., and Stipkovits, L. (1973b). *Acta Vet. Scand.* **14,** 450–463.
Ernø, H., Plastridge, W. N., and Tourtellotte, M. E. (1967). *Acta Vet. Scand.* **8,** 123–135.
Ernø, H., Jurmanova, K., and Leach, R. H. (1973). *Acta Vet. Scand.* **14,** 511–523.
Fabricant, J. (1973). *Ann. N.Y. Acad. Sci.* **225,** 369–381.
Fernald, G. W., and Clyde, W. A. (1974). *Colloq. INSERM, Mycoplasmes Homme, Anim., Veg. Insectes, Congr. Int., Bordeaux* **33,** 421.
Foggie, A., and Angus, K. W. (1972). *Vet. Rec.* **90,** 312–313.
Ford, D. K. (1967). *Ann. N.Y. Acad. Sci.* **143,** 501–504.
Furr, P. M., Hetherington, C. M., and Taylor-Robinson, D. (1978). *J. Med. Microbiol.* **11,** 537–540.
Glynn, A. A. (1972). *Symp. Soc. Gen. Microbiol.* **22,** 75–112.
Gois, M., Kuksa, F., and Franz, J. (1973). *Vet. Rec.* **93,** 47–48.
Gourlay, R. N. (1963). *Vet. Rec.* **75,** 950–951.
Gourlay, R. N. (1964). *J. Comp. Pathol.* **74,** 286–299.
Gourlay, R. N. (1965a). *Res. Vet. Sci.* **6,** 1–8.
Gourlay, R. N. (1965b). *Res. Vet. Sci.* **6,** 263–273.
Gourlay, R. N. (1968). *Res. Vet. Sci.* **9,** 376–378.
Gourlay, R. N. (1969). *Vet. Rec.* **84,** 229–230.
Gourlay, R. N. (1973). *J. Am. Vet. Med. Assoc.* **163,** 905–909.
Gourlay, R. N. (1975). *Dev. Biol. Stand.* **28,** 586–589.
Gourlay, R. N., and Howard, C. J. (1978). *In* "Respiratory Diseases in Cattle," EEC Seminar, Edinburgh, 1977, Current Topics in Veterinary Medicine, 3. Nijhoff, The Hague (in press).
Gourlay, R. N., and Leach, R. H. (1970). *J. Med. Microbiol.* **3,** 111–123.
Gourlay, R. N., and Shifrine, M. (1966a). *Vet. Rec.* **78,** 256–257.
Gourlay, R. N., and Shifrine, M. (1966b). *Bull. Epizoot. Dis. Afr.* **14,** 369–372.
Gourlay, R. N., and Shifrine, M. (1966c). *J. Comp. Pathol.* **76,** 417–425.
Gourlay, R. N., and Shifrine, M. (1968). *Res. Vet. Sci.* **9,** 185–186.
Gourlay, R. N., and Thomas, L. H. (1969a). *Vet. Rec.* **84,** 416–417.
Gourlay, R. N., and Thomas, L. H. (1969b). *Vet. Rec.* **85,** 583.
Gourlay, R. N., and Thomas, L. H. (1970). *J. Comp. Pathol.* **80,** 585–594.
Gourlay, R. N., and Thrower, K. J. (1968). *J. Gen. Microbiol.* **54,** 155–159.
Gourlay, R. N., and Wyld, S. G. (1975). *Vet. Rec.* **97,** 370–371.
Gourlay, R. N., Mackenzie, A., and Cooper, J. E. (1970). *J. Comp. Pathol.* **80,** 575–584.
Gourlay, R. N., Howard, C. J., and Brownlie, J. (1972). *J. Hyg.* **70,** 511–521.
Gourlay, R. N., Brownlie, J., and Howard, C. J. (1973). *J. Gen. Microbiol.* **76,** 251–254.
Gourlay, R. N., Leach, R. H., and Howard, C. J. (1974a). *J. Gen. Microbiol.* **81,** 475–484.
Gourlay, R. N., Stott, E. J., Espinasse, J., and Barle, C. (1974b). *Vet. Rec.* **95,** 534–535.
Gourlay, R. N., Howard, C. J., and Brownlie, J. (1975). *Infect. Immun.* **12,** 947–950.
Gourlay, R. N., Thomas, L. H., and Howard, C. J. (1976). *Vet. Rec.* **98,** 506–507.
Gourlay, R. N., Wyld, S. G., and Leach, R. H. (1977). *Int. J. Syst. Bacteriol.* **27,** 86–96.
Gourlay, R. N., Wyld, S. G., Burke, N. F. S., and Edmonds, M. J. (1978). *Vet. Rec.* **103,** 74–75.
Guido, B. (1971). *Nuova Vet.* **47,** 202–209.
Hale, H. H., Helmboldt, C. F., Plastridge, W. N., and Stula, E. F. (1962). *Cornell Vet.* **52,** 582–591.
Hamdy, A. H., and Trapp, A. L. (1967). *Am. J. Vet. Res.* **28,** 1019–1025.
Harbourne, J. F., Hunter, D., and Leach, R. H. (1965). *Res. Vet. Sci.* **6,** 178–188.
Hartman, H. A., Tourtellotte, M. E., Nielsen, S. W., and Plastridge, W. N. (1964). *Res. Vet. Sci.* **5,** 303–309.
Hill, A. (1972). *Vet. Rec.* **91,** 224–225.

Hirth, R. S., Nielsen, S. W., and Plastridge, W. N. (1966). *Pathol. Vet.* **3**, 616–632.
Hirth, R. S., Nielsen, S. W., and Tourtellotte, M. E. (1970a). *Infect. Immun.* **2**, 101–104.
Hirth, R. S., Tourtellotte, M. E., and Nielsen, S. W. (1970b). *Infect. Immun.* **2**, 105–111.
Hjerpe, C. A., and Knight, H. D. (1972). *J. Am. Vet. Med. Assoc.* **160**, 1414–1418.
Hoare, M. (1969). *Vet. Rec.* **85**, 351–355.
Howard, C. J., and Gourlay, R. N. (1973a). *J. Gen. Microbiol.* **79**, 129–134.
Howard, C. J., and Gourlay, R. N. (1973b). *J. Gen. Microbiol.* **78**, 277–285.
Howard, C. J., and Gourlay, R. N. (1974). *J. Gen. Microbiol.* **83**, 393–398.
Howard, C. J., and Thomas, L. H. (1974). *Infect. Immun.* **10**, 405–408.
Howard, C. J., Gourlay, R. N., and Brownlie, J. (1973). *J. Hyg.* **71**, 163–170.
Howard, C. J., Gourlay, R. N., Garwes, D. J., Pocock, D. H., and Collins, J. (1974a). *Int. J. Syst. Bacteriol.* **24**, 373–374.
Howard, C. J., Gourlay, R. N., and Brownlie, J. (1974b). *Infect. Immun.* **9**, 400–403.
Howard, C. J., Gourlay, R. N., and Collins, J. (1974c). *J. Hyg.* **73**, 457–466.
Howard, C. J., Gourlay, R. N., and Collins, J. (1975a). *Int. J. Syst. Bacteriol.* **25**, 155–159.
Howard, C. J., Anderson, J. C., Gourlay, R. N., and Taylor-Robinson, D. (1975b). *J. Med. Microbiol.* **8**, 523–529.
Howard, C. J., Gourlay, R. N., Thomas, L. H., and Stott, E. J. (1976a). *Res. Vet. Sci.* **21**, 227–231.
Howard, C. J., Collins, J., and Gourlay, R. N. (1976b). *Vet. Microbiol.* **1**, 23–30.
Howard, C. J., Taylor, G., Collins, J., and Gourlay, R. N. (1976c). *Infect. Immun.* **14**, 11–17.
Howard, C. J., Collins, J., and Gourlay, R. N. (1977a). *Res. Vet. Sci.* **23**, 128–130.
Howard, C. J., Gourlay, R. N., and Taylor, G. (1977b). *Vet. Microbiol.* **2**, 29–37.
Howard, C. J., Gourlay, R. N., and Taylor, G. (1978a). *In* "Respiratory Diseases in Cattle," EEC Seminar, Edinburgh, 1977, Current Topics in Veterinary Medicine, 3. Nijhoff, The Hague (in press).
Howard, C. J., Gourlay, R. N., and Collins, J. (1978b). *Int. J. Syst. Bacteriol.* **28**, 473–477.
Hudson, J. R. (1971). "Contagious Bovine Pleuropneumonia," FAO Agricultural Studies, No. 86. FAO, Rome.
Hudson, J. R., and Etheridge, J. R. (1963). *Aust. Vet. J.* **39**, 1–5.
Hudson, J. R., Cottew, G. S., and Adler, H. E. (1967a). *Ann. N.Y. Acad. Sci.* **143**, 287–297.
Hudson, J. R., Buttery, S., and Cottew, G. S. (1967b). *J. Pathol. Bacteriol.* **94**, 257–273.
Jack, E. J., Moring, J., and Boughton, E. (1977). *Vet. Rec.* **101**, 287.
Jain, N. C., Jasper, D. E., and Dellinger, J. D. (1967). *J. Gen. Microbiol.* **49**, 401–410.
Jain, N. C., Jasper, D. E., and Dellinger, J. D. (1969a). *Cornell Vet.* **59**, 10–28.
Jain, N. C., Jasper, D. E., and Dellinger, J. D. (1969b). *Am. J. Vet. Res.* **30**, 733–742.
Jasper, D. E. (1967). *J. Am. Vet. Med. Assoc.* **151**, 1650–1655.
Jasper, D. E. (1977). *J. Am. Vet. Med. Assoc.* **170**, 1167–1172.
Jasper, D. E., Jain, N. C., and Brazil, L. H. (1966). *J. Am. Vet. Med. Assoc.* **148**, 1017–1029.
Jasper, D. E., Al-Aubaidi, J. M., and Fabricant, J. (1974). *Cornell Vet.* **64**, 407–415.
Jensen, R., Pierson, R. E., Braddy, P. M., Saari, D. A., Lauerman, L. H., Benitez, A., Christie, R. M., Horton, D. P., and McChesney, A. E. (1976). *J. Am. Vet. Med. Assoc.* **169**, 511–514.
Jurmanova, K., and Krejci, J. (1971). *Vet. Rec.* **89**, 585–586.
Jurmanova, K., and Mensik, J. (1971). *Zentralbl. Veterinaermed., Reihe B* **18**, 457–464.
Jurmanova, K., and Sterbova, J. (1977). *Vet. Rec.* **100**, 157–158.
Jurmanova, K., Mensik, J., Krejci, J., Hajkova, M., and Cerna, J. (1973). *In Vitro V CSSR* **2**, 175–185.
Jurmanova, K., Cerna, J., Sisak, F., and Hajkova, M. (1975). *In Vitro V CSSR* **4**, 167–173.
Kakoma, I., and Kinyanjui, M. (1974). *Res. Vet. Sci.* **17**, 397–399.

Karbe, E., and Mosher, A. H. (1968). *Zentralbl. Veterinaermed., Reihe B* **15,** 817–827.

Karbe, E., Nielsen, S. W., and Helmboldt, C. F. (1967). *Zentralbl. Veterinaermed., Reihe B* **14,** 7–31.

Karst, O., and Onoviran, O. (1971). *Br. Vet. J.* **127,** IX–X.

Kehoe, J. M., Norcross, N. L., Carmichael, L. E., and Strandberg, J. D. (1967a). *J. Infect. Dis.* **117,** 171–179.

Kehoe, J. M., Norcross, N. L., and Carmichael, L. E. (1967b). *Ann. N.Y. Acad. Sci.* **143,** 337–344.

Kuniyasu, C., Yoshida, Y., Ueda, H., Sugawara, H., and Ito, Y. (1977). *Nat. Inst. Anim. Hlth. Quart.* **17,** 75–78.

Kurbanov, I. A., and Gizatullin, C. G. (1975). *In Vitro V CSSR* **4,** 163.

Laidlaw, P. P., and Elford, W. J. (1936). *Proc. R. Soc. London, Ser. B* **120,** 292–303.

Langer, P. H., and Carmichael, L. E. (1963). *Proc. Annu. Meet. U.S. Livestock Sanit. Assoc., 67th,* pp. 129–139.

Langer, P. H., and McEntee, K. (1961). *Proc. Annu. Meet. U.S. Livestock Sanit. Assoc., 65th,* pp. 389–396.

Langford, E. V. (1974). *Vet. Rec.* **94,** 528.

Langford, E. V. (1975a). *Annu. Proc. Am. Assoc. Vet. Lab. Diagnosticians, 18th,* pp. 221–232.

Langford, E. V. (1975b). *Can. J. Comp. Med.* **39,** 133–138.

Langford, E. V. (1977). *Can. J. Comp. Med.* **41,** 89–94.

Langford, E. V., and Dorward, W. J. (1969). *Can. J. Comp. Med.* **33,** 275–279.

Langford, E. V., and Leach, R. H. (1973). *Can. J. Microbiol.* **19,** 1435–1444.

Langford, E. V., Ruhnke, H. L., and Onoviran, O. (1976). *Int. J. Syst. Bacteriol.* **26,** 212–219.

Leach, R. H. (1967). *Ann. N.Y. Acad. Sci.* **143,** 305–316.

Leach, R. H. (1970). *Vet. Rec.* **87,** 319–320.

Leach, R. H. (1973). *J. Gen. Microbiol.* **75,** 135–153.

Lindley, E. P., and Abdulla, A. E. D. (1967). *Sudan J. Vet. Sci. Anim. Husb.* **8,** 78–87.

Livingston, C. W. (1972). *Am. J. Vet. Res.* **33,** 1925–1929.

Livingston, C. W., and Gauer, B. B. (1974). *Am. J. Vet. Res.* **35,** 1469–1471.

Lloyd, L. C. (1966). *J. Pathol. Bacteriol.* **92,** 225–229.

Lloyd, L. C. (1967). *Bull. Epizoot. Dis. Afr.* **15,** 11–17.

Lloyd, L. C. (1970). *J. Comp. Pathol.* **80,** 195–209.

Lloyd, L. C., and Trethewie, E. R. (1970). *In* "The Role of Mycoplasmas and L-Forms of Bacteria in Disease" (J. T. Sharp, ed.), pp. 172–197. Thomas, Springfield, Illinois.

Lloyd, L. C., Buttery, S. H., and Hudson, J. R. (1971). *J. Med. Microbiol.* **4,** 425–439.

Madoff, S., Pixley, B. Q., Moellering, R. C., and Del Giudice, R. A. (1976). *Proc. Soc. Gen. Microbiol.* **3,** 142–143.

Masiga, W. N., and Read, W. C. S. (1972). *Vet. Rec.* **90,** 499–502.

Masiga, W. N., and Roberts, D. H. (1973). *Bull. Epizoot. Dis. Afr.* **21,** 325–329.

Masiga, W. N., and Windsor, R. S. (1975). *Vet. Rec.* **97,** 350–351.

Masiga, W. N., Windsor, R. S., and Read, W. C. S. (1972). *Vet. Rec.* **90,** 247–248.

Masiga, W. N., Roberts, D. H., Kakoma, I., and Rurangirwa, F. R. (1975). *Res. Vet. Sci.* **19,** 330–332.

Morar, R. (1969). *Rev. Zooteh. Med. Vet.* **19,** 76–77.

Morgan, K., Bradley, P., and Bourne, F. J. (1978). *In* "Respiratory Diseases in Cattle," EEC Seminar, Edinburgh, 1977, Current Topics in Veterinary Medicine, 3. Nijhoff, The Hague (in press).

Mosher, A. H., Plastridge, W. N., Tourtellotte, M. E., and Helmboldt, C. F. (1968). *Am. J. Vet. Res.* **29,** 517–522.

Moulton, J. E., Boidin, A. G., and Rhode, E. A. (1956). *J. Am. Vet. Med. Assoc.* **129**, 364–367.

Nayar, P. S. G., and Saunders, J. R. (1975). *Can. J. Comp. Med.* **39**, 22–31.

Nicolet, J., and Buttiker, W. (1974). *Vet. Rec.* **92**, 442–443.

Nicolet, J., and de Meuron, P. A. (1970). *Zentralbl. Veterinaermed., Reihe B* **17**, 1031–1042.

Nicolet, J., Dauwalder, M., Boss, P. H., and Anetzhofer, J. (1976). *Schweiz. Arch. Tierheilkd.* **118**, 141–150.

Nocard, E., and Roux, E. (1898). *Ann. Inst. Pasteur, Paris* **12**, 240–262.

Ogata, M., Watabe, J., and Koshimizu, K. (1974). *Jpn. J. Vet. Sci.* **36**, 43–51.

Oghiso, Y., Yamamoto, K., Goto, N., Takahashi, R., Fujiwara, K., and Miura, T. (1976). *Jpn. J. Vet. Sci.* **38**, 15–24.

Ojo, M. O. (1976). *Trop. Anim. Health Prod.* **8**, 137–146.

Ojo, M. O., and Ikede, B. O. (1976). *Vet. Microbiol.* **1**, 19–22.

Olson, N. O., Seymour, W. R., Boothe, A. D., and Dozsa, L. (1960). *Ann. N.Y. Acad. Sci.* **79**, 677–685.

Onoviran, O. (1972). *Bull. Epizoot. Dis. Afr.* **20**, 275–279.

Orning, A. P., Ross, R. F., and Barile, M. F. (1978). *Amer. J. Vet. Res.* **39**, 1169–1174.

Ose, E. E., and Muenster, O. A. (1975). *Vet. Rec.* **97**, 97.

Page, L. A., Frey, M. L., Ward, J. K., Newman, F. S., Gerloff, R. K., and Stalheim, O. H. (1972). *J. Am. Vet. Med. Assoc.* **161**, 919–925.

Pan, J., and Ogata, M. (1969a). *Jpn. J. Vet. Sci.* **31**, 83–93.

Pan, J., and Ogata, M. (1969b). *Jpn. J. Vet. Sci.* **31**, 313–324.

Parsonson, I. M., Al-Aubaidi, J. M., and McEntee, K. (1974). *Cornell Vet.* **64**, 240–264.

Piercy, D. W. T. (1972). *J. Comp. Pathol.* **82**, 291–294.

Pignattelli, P. (1978). *In* "Respiratory Diseases in Cattle," EEC Seminar, Edinburgh, 1977, Current Topics in Veterinary Medicine, 3. Nijhoff. The Hague (in press).

Pignattelli, P., and Galassi, D. (1971). *Atti Soc. Ital. Buiatria* **3**, 544–554.

Pirie, H. M., and Allan, E. M. (1975). *Vet. Rec.* **97**, 345–349.

Plackett, P., Smith, P. F., and Mayberry, W. R. (1970). *J. Bacteriol.* **104**, 798–807.

Polak-Vogelzang, A., and Beuvery, E. C. (1975). *In Vitro V CSSR* **4**, 212–221.

Provost, A. (1969). *Rev. Immunol.* **33**, 1–6.

Redaelli, G., Ruffo, G., Rinaldi, A., Guallini, L., and Cervio, G. (1969). *Atti Soc. Ital. Sci. Vet.* **23**, 1043–1046.

Rhoades, K. R., Page, L. A., and Leach, R. H. (1975). *Vet. Rec.* **96**, 470.

Rinaldi, A., Leach, R. H., Cervio, G., Mandelli, G., and Redaelli, G. (1969). *Atti Soc. Ital. Sci. Vet.* **23**, 1001–1003.

Rinaldi, A., Biancardi, G., Cessi, D., Ruffo, G., and Bertoldini, G. (1971). *Atti Soc. Ital. Buiatria* **3**, 555–563.

Roberts, D. H., and Windsor, R. S. (1974). *Res. Vet. Sci.* **17**, 403–405.

Roberts, D. H., Windsor, R. S., Masiga, W. N., and Kariavu, C. G. (1973). *Infect. Immun.* **8**, 349–354.

Robinson, I. M., and Allison, M. J. (1975). *Int. J. Syst. Bacteriol.* **25**, 182–186.

Robinson, I. M., and Rhoades, K. (1977). *Int. J. Syst. Bacteriol.* **27**, 200–203.

Robinson, I. M., Allison, M. J., and Hartman, P. A. (1975). *Int. J. Syst. Bacteriol.* **25**, 173–181.

Robinson, J. P., and Hungate, R. E. (1973). *Int. J. Syst. Bacteriol.* **23**, 171–181.

Rodwell, A. W., Peterson, J. E., and Rodwell, E. S. (1972). *Pathogenic Mycoplasmas, Ciba Found. Symp.* pp. 123–139.

Rodwell, A. W., Peterson, J. R., and Rodwell, E. S. (1975). *J. Bacteriol.* **122**, 1216–1229.

Ruffo, G., Socci, A., Mandelli, G., and Cervio, G. (1971). *Atti Soc. Ital. Buiatria* **3**, 564–571.

Ruhnke, H. L., and Onoviran, O. (1975). *Vet. Rec.* **96**, 203.

Ruhnke, H. L., and van Dreumel, A. A. (1972). *Can. J. Comp. Med.* **36**, 317–318.

Ruhnke, H. L., Thawley, D., and Nelson, F. C. (1976). *Can. J. Comp. Med.* **40**, 142–148.

Rurangirwa, F. R. (1976). *J. Comp. Pathol.* **86**, 45–50.

Savov, N., and Buchvarova, Y. (1976). Abstracted in *Vet. Bull. (London)* **47**, 20 (1977).

Schimmel, D., and Pustovar, A. (1971). *Arch. Exp. Veterinaermed.* **25**, 863–874.

Shepard, M. C., Lunceford, C. D., Ford, D. K., Purcell, R. H., Taylor-Robinson, D., Razin, S., and Black, F. T. (1974). *Int. J. Syst. Bacteriol.* **24**, 160–171.

Shifrine, M., and Beech, J. (1968). *Bull. Epizoot. Dis. Afr.* **16**, 47–52.

Shifrine, M., and Gourlay, R. N. (1965). *Nature (London)* **208**, 498–499.

Shifrine, M., Stone, S. S., and Staak, C. (1970). *Bull. Epizoot. Dis. Afr.* **18**, 201–205.

Shimizu, T., Nosaka, D., and Nakamura, N. (1973). *Jpn. J. Vet. Sci.* **35**, 535–537.

Shimizu, T., Nosaka, D., and Nakamura, N. (1975). *Jpn. J. Vet. Sci.* **37**, 121–131.

Simmons, G. C., and Johnston, L. A. Y. (1963). *Aust. Vet. J.* **39**, 11–14.

Singh, U. M., Doig, P. A., and Ruhnke, H. L. (1971). *Can. Vet. J.* **12**, 183–185.

Smith, G. R. (1967). *J. Comp. Pathol.* **77**, 203–209.

Stalheim, O. H. V. (1976). *J. Am. Vet. Med. Assoc.* **169**, 1096–1097.

Stalheim, O. H. V., and Gallagher, J. E. (1975). *Am. J. Vet. Res.* **36**, 1077–1080.

Stalheim, O. H. V., and Gallagher, J. E. (1977). *Infect. Immun.* **15**, 995–996.

Stalheim, O. H. V., and Page, L. A. (1975). *J. Clin. Microbiol.* **2**, 165–168.

Stalheim, O. H. V., and Proctor, S. J. (1976). *Am. J. Vet. Res.* **37**, 879–883.

Stalheim, O. H. V., and Stone, S. S. (1975). *J. Clin. Microbiol.* **2**, 169–172.

Stalheim, O. H. V., Proctor, S. J., and Gallagher, J. E. (1976). *Infect. Immun.* **13**, 915–925.

Stipkovits, L., Varga, L., and Schimmel, D. (1973). *Acta Vet. Hung.* **23**, 361–368.

Stipkovits, L., Romvary, J., Nagy, Z., Bodon, L., and Varga, L. (1974). *J. Hyg.* **72**, 289–296.

Stipkovits, L., Bodon, L., Romvary, J., and Varga, L. (1975). *Acta Microbiol. Hung.* **22**, 45–51.

Stuart, P., Davidson, I., Slavin, G., Edgson, F. A., and Howell, D. (1963). *Vet. Rec.* **75**, 59–64.

St. George, T. D., Horsfall, N., and Sullivan, N. D. (1973). *Aust. Vet. J.* **49**, 580–586.

Taylor, G., and Taylor-Robinson, D. (1976). *Immunology.* **30**, 611–618.

Taylor-Robinson, D., Haig, D. A., and Williams, M. H. (1967). *Ann. N.Y. Acad. Sci.* **143**, 517–518.

Taylor-Robinson, D., Williams, M. H., and Haig, D. A. (1968). *J. Gen. Microbiol.* **54**, 33–46.

Taylor-Robinson, D., Thomas, M., and Dawson, P. L. (1969). *J. Med. Microbiol.* **2**, 527–533.

Taylor-Robinson, D., Martin-Bourgon, C., Watanabe, T., and Addey, J. P. (1971). *J. Gen. Microbiol.* **68**, 97–107.

Thomas, L. H., and Howard, C. J. (1974). *J. Comp. Pathol.* **84**, 192–201.

Thomas, L. H., and Smith, G. S. (1972). *J. Comp. Pathol.* **82**, 1–4.

Thomas, L. H., Howard, C. J., and Gourlay, R. N. (1975). *Vet. Rec.* **97**, 55–56.

Tourtellotte, M. E., and Lein, D. H. (1976). *Health Lab. Sci.* **13**, 152–158.

Trapp, A. L., Hamdy, A. H., Gale, C., and King, N. B. (1966). *Am. J. Vet. Res.* **27**, 1235–1242.

Tully, J. G. (1973). *Ann. N.Y. Acad. Sci.* **225**, 74–93.

Tully, J. G., and Razin, S. (1970). *J. Bacteriol.* **103**, 751–754.

Villemot, J. M., Provost, A., and Queval, R. (1962). *Nature (London)* **193**, 906–907.

Wehnert, Von C., Teichmann, G., Hauke, H., Schimmel, D., and Lantzsch, C. (1977). *Monatsh. Veterinaermed.* **32**, 55–59.

Whittlestone, P. (1972). *Symp. Soc. Gen. Microbiol.* **22,** 217–250.
Whittlestone, P. (1976). *Adv. Vet. Sci. Comp. Med.* **20,** 277–307.
Windsor, R. S. (1977). *In* "The Veterinary Annual" (C. S. G. Grunsell and F. W. G. Hill,
    eds.), 17th Issue, pp. 59–65. Wright-Scientechnica, Bristol, England.
Windsor, R. S., and Masiga, W. N. (1977). *Res. Vet. Sci.* **23,** 230–236.

3 / CAPRINE-OVINE MYCOPLASMAS

G. S. Cottew

I. INTRODUCTION

The first mycoplasmas isolated from sheep and goats resulted from the search for the etiological agent of contagious agalactia (CA), a disease that has affected flocks, particularly in Europe and Asia, for a very long time. Bridré and Donatien (1923) demonstrated the causal agent, now named *Mycoplasma agalactiae,* and recognized that it shared the unusual morphology and fastidious growth requirements of the causal organisms of contagious bovine pleuropneumonia (CBPP). Later Longley (1951) showed that the organism of contagious caprine pleuropneumonia (CCPP) possessed similar morphology. The similarity of these and some other organisms led them to be known as the *pleuropneumonia group,* or as *pleuropneumonia-like organisms* (PPLO), until the present classification established by Edward and Freundt (1956) came into general use. The trivial name now used for all species of Mollicutes is mycoplasmas.

THE MYCOPLASMAS, VOL. II
Copyright © 1979 by Academic Press, Inc.
All rights of reproduction in any form reserved.
ISBN 0-12-078401-7

The rate of isolation of new mycoplasmas from sheep or goats up until the early 1960s was slow, but this period saw the growth of studies on the mycoplasmas of chickens and humans and the development of methods for comparing and identifying species. Most of the species known in sheep and goats today have been isolated in the last 10 years.

Reviews describing the principal diseases and the species of Mollicutes occurring in sheep and goats (Cottew and Leach, 1969; Cottew, 1970) have already been rendered incomplete, and the purpose of this chapter is largely to describe the findings made since those reviews were prepared.

It has been traditional to combine discussion of the mycoplasmas of goats with those of sheep, and this has been justified largely because several mycoplasmas occur in both these hosts but in no other. Other mycoplasmas have been found only in goats or only in sheep. No factor has yet been discerned that determines whether a species will be restricted to sheep or goats.

Not all the mycoplasmas of sheep and goats are pathogenic for the host in which they are found, but among the pathogens are mycoplasmas causing diseases of major economic importance. Others have apparently been responsible in various countries for sporadic outbreaks of disease with little or no spread to other sheep or goats.

Progress in determination of the species of *Mycoplasma* that occur in sheep and goats was greatly assisted by the work of Al-Aubaidi (1972) who examined 151 strains from these hosts and formed 12 serologically different groups from them. Tully *et al.* (1974) and Cottew (1974) also examined many strains and extended the findings of Al-Aubaidi (1972). Table I was compiled from the findings of these workers, and forms a tentative list of sheep and goat mycoplasmas for purposes of the following discussion.

Of the species listed, 11 have been recognized in sheep or goats on more than one occasion. These are *Mycoplasma agalactiae*, *M. arginini*, *M. capricolum*, *M. conjunctivae*, *Acholeplasma granularum*, *A. laidlawii*, *M. mycoides* subsp. *capri*, *M. mycoides* subsp. *mycoides*, *A. oculi*, *M. ovipneumoniae*, and *M. putrefaciens*. Of the untyped strains, the urea-plasmas and 2D type have also been found more than once. *Mycoplasma gallinarum*, *M. bovirhinis*, and the G145 and A1343 strains have been recorded once only to our knowledge.

II. CHARACTERISTICS OF THE SPECIES OCCURRING IN SHEEP AND GOATS

In Table I the biochemical characteristics of certain strains of the species are given; most are type strains. The results for *A. granularum* are

TABLE I. Biochemical Characteristics of Sheep and Goat Mycoplasmas[a,b]

Organism	G	A	T	P	F	S	C	D
Mycoplasma								
M. agalactiae (PG2)	-	-	+	+	+	-	-	+
M. arginini (G230)	-	+	-[c]	-	-	-	-	+
M. capricolum (California kid)	+	+[d]	+	-	-	+	+	+
M. conjunctivae (HRC581)	+	-	+	-	-	-	+	+
M. mycoides subsp. mycoides (SC) (PG1)	+	-	+	W	-	+	+	+
M. mycoides subsp. mycoides (LC) (YG)	+	-	+	W	-	W	W	+
M. ovipneumoniae (Y98)	+	-	+	+	+	+	-	+
M. putrefaciens (KS1)	+	+	+	+	-	-	-	+
M. bovirhinis (QEW)[e]	+	+	+	-	+	-	-	+
M. gallinarum (EHM)[e]	-	+	+	-	-	-	-	-
Mycoplasma sp. (G145)[e]	-	-	+	+	-	-	-	-
Mycoplasma sp. (A1343)[e]	-	-	+	+	+	-	-	-
Mycoplasma sp. (2D)	-	-	+	+	-	-	-	+
Acholeplasma								
A. granularum (BTS39)	+	NT	+	-	NT	-	-	-
A. laidlawii (PG8)	+	-	+	-	-	-	-	-
A. oculi (19L)	+	-	+	-	-	-	-	-
Ureaplasma spp.	NT	NT	NT	NT	NT	NT	NT	NT

[a] This table has been adapted from Cottew (1974).
[b] G, Acid from glucose; A, hydrolysis of arginine; T, anaerobic reduction of tetrazolium chloride on solid medium; P, phosphatase production; F, film and spot formation on egg medium; S, serum liquefaction; C, digestion of casein; D, sensitivity to digitonin; W, weak reaction; NT, not tested.
[c] Other strains may be negative.
[d] Some strains may be negative.
[e] Isolated once only.

from Freundt (1974); otherwise the tests were carried out in our laboratory, and the table has been adapted from Cottew (1974). The methods used were given in Cottew (1974) and in Cottew and Yeats (1978).

A. *Mycoplasma agalactiae*

Mycoplasma agalactiae is historically notable as the first mycoplasma to be isolated from sheep and goats and is economically important as the cause of contagious agalactia in these hosts.

Although for a time classified as *M. agalactiae* subsp. *agalactiae* (from sheep and goats), along with *M. agalactiae* subsp. *bovis* (from cattle), these organisms are now regarded as distinct species, *M. agalactiae* and *Mycoplasma bovis*.

The type strain of the species is PG2, which was isolated from sheep in Spain (Edward and Freundt, 1973). Of note among the biochemical characteristics of the organism listed in Table I is its inability to metabolize glucose or arginine. Barber and Yedloutschnig (1970) found that several other carbohydrates were not metabolized.

In fermentation tests in liquid medium supplemented with glucose, the pH of cultures of *M. agalactiae* usually falls by about 0.5 pH unit. That this is not due to fermentation of glucose was demonstrated by Edward and Moore (1975).

Mycoplasma agalactiae reduces methylene blue rapidly and is actively lipolytic, as shown by the formation of film and spots. Perreau *et al.* (1975) noted that the reduction of tetrazolium was weak with freshly isolated strains. In addition to the characteristics given in Table I, no growth occurs in serum-free medium or at 25°C, and strains are sensitive to 1% sodium glycotaurocholate (Al-Aubaidi, 1972).

A characteristic type of hemolysis was seen with freshly isolated strains on sheep blood agar plates (Cottew *et al.*, 1968), and in a study of mycoplasmas from sheep and goats this was used to distinguish *M. agalactiae*. The other mycoplasmas in the same study labeled N and C types are now known to be *M. arginini* and *M. mycoides* subsp. *mycoides* (large-colony type), respectively. Foggie *et al.* (1970) distinguished between a virulent challenge strain of *M. agalactiae* that produced the characteristic hemolysis and a vaccine strain attenuated by 40 serial passages on media, in which the nature of the hemolysis produced was recognizably different.

No special growth factors appear to be required by *M. agalactiae*, which grows with a small to medium-sized colony and light to medium turbidity in liquid media. When horse serum is used in the liquid medium, an iridescent film forms on the surface of the culture. Growth in broth is characterized by the production of branching filaments easily seen by microscopic examination using dark-field illumination. Unlike the more transient filamentous forms in cultures of *M. mycoides* subsp. *mycoides,* the filaments of *M. agalactiae* usually persist for at least 8 days (Cottew and Leach, 1969).

The organism is readily identified from its biochemical characteristics and its reactivity in growth or metabolism inhibition tests with specific antiserum to PG2. Metabolic inhibition tests may be carried out using the reduction of tetrazolium chloride as an indicator of growth. Prozones may occur in this test with some antisera.

Bridré and Donatien (1925) showed that the organism survived 90 min at 50°C but was killed after 10 min at 53°C. Data on the survival of *M. agalactiae* in infected milk or exudate on surfaces could be relevant to understanding the spread of infection but does not appear to be available.

Mycoplasma agalactiae is susceptible *in vitro* to tylosin and oxytetracycline. Although there was some variation in sensitivity among strains, tylosin at a concentration of 1.0 μg/ml was bacteriostatic (Arisoy *et al.*, 1969; Hernandez, 1972), and 1.25 μg/ml (Hernandez, 1972) and 8 μg/ml (Arisoy *et al.*, 1969) were bactericidal for all strains tested.

The diseases caused by this organism can be considered in two categories.

1. Contagious Agalactia

Contagious agalactia occurs chiefly in Mediterranean countries, but the disease has been reported recently from Albania, Algeria, France, Greece, India, Iran, Iraq, Israel, Italy, Lebanon, Malaysia, Mali, Mongolia, Morocco, Peru, Portugal, Rumania, Saudi Arabia, Spain, Sudan, Switzerland, Syria, Turkey, USSR, Yemen, and Yugoslavia (Anonymous, 1975, 1976).

As the description of the disease by Curasson (1946) and reviews by Turner (1959) and Cottew (1970) remain relevant, it is described here only briefly.

Acute signs usually appear in the female just after parturition, with the onset of lactation. Some animals may develop a fever and die without other signs within a few days. More often the animals become depressed and lose their appetite, there may be a short febrile period, mastitis develops, and the milk yield declines. The milk may become yellow and, when allowed to stand, solids may settle out. Eventually milk secretion stops, and only small amounts of serous fluid can be expressed. Keratoconjunctivitis is seen occasionally.

Mycoplasmas may be recovered from the blood for a short period and usually localize in the joints, giving rise to painful arthritis, and walking becomes difficult.

In 12 infected flocks studied in Turkey (Arisoy *et al.*, 1967) containing 1160 sheep and 205 goats, the morbidity in both hosts was 22% and the mortality was less than 1%.

The definitive method of diagnosing CA is by culture and identification of *M. agalactiae* from affected animals. As the organism persists for long periods in affected animals and has no special growth requirements, isolation is relatively easy, as is identification using the characteristics discussed earlier.

Serological diagnosis has been attempted by various methods, the most promising of which appears to be complement fixation (Etheridge *et al.*, 1969; Morozzi *et al.*, 1973; Perreau *et al.*, 1976).

Arisoy *et al.* (1967) reported that treatment with oxytetracycline reduced the severity of the disease but failed to stop the excretion of organisms in milk.

Prevention based on vaccination was first considered many years ago. Encouraged by the knowledge that recovered animals had solid immunity, Bridré and Donatien (1925) attempted immunization with aged cultures and with cultures in which attenuation had been attempted by serial passage. The challenge they used, intra-articular inoculation of virulent cultures, was very severe, and it is perhaps not surprising that their vaccines were considered to be ineffective. Numerous workers have examined the question of immunization since then. Effective vaccines have been reported from Italy (Zavagli, 1951), Rumania (Popovici, 1961), Iran (Baharsefat *et al.*, 1971), and Turkey (Arisoy, 1975). From a comparison of several methods of producing vaccines, Baharsefat *et al.* (1971) concluded that a saponin-treated culture vaccine was the most efficacious, and field trials have apparently confirmed this result. Similarly in Turkey, field trials using dead and live attenuated vaccines were apparently successful in exposed animals (Arisoy, 1975).

Differences between goats and sheep in susceptibility to the disease have been described (Zavagli, 1951). Similarly, differences between these animals in respect to the protection afforded by an adsorbed vaccine were described by Baharsefat *et al.* (1971), but a saponin-treated vaccine protected both hosts for 9 months. It appears that the investigation of preventive vaccination in CA has reached a very satisfactory phase.

2. Other Diseases Associated with *Mycoplasma agalactiae*

Mycoplasma agalactiae has also been recovered from conditions unlike the classic disease.

Cottew and Lloyd (1965) described an outbreak of pleurisy and pneumonia among goats in Australia from which an organism, subsequently identified as *M. agalactiae,* was isolated. Mild lung lesions were produced in experimental animals inoculated intratracheally with the organism.

In India, Singh *et al.* (1974, 1975) described granular vulvovaginitis in goats, and a mycoplasma subsequently identified as *M. agalactiae* was isolated from 20% of the cases. There was a mucopurulent exudate in the vagina, and multiple, yellowish-white, pinhead-sized granulations were present on the surface of the vagina near the clitoris. Occasionally the granulations were intensely red and ulcerated. Experimentally, infection of a similar nature was produced in 25 of 30 kids after swabbing the vagina with cultures of *M. agalactiae* isolated from a natural case. The organism persisted at the site for 7–70 days. No antibody was detected by agglutination tests on sera collected weekly for 10 weeks after inoculation.

B. *Mycoplasma arginini*

Since the description of *M. arginini* as a new species by Barile *et al.* (1968), who cultivated it from sheep brain, human, dog, and chimpanzee cell cultures and the infected knee joint of a goat, Leach (1970) has noted its occurrence in cattle and chamois; Hill (1972) recorded it in lion, lynx, tiger, and cheetah; and Orning *et al.* (1978) recovered it from swine.

Because of its occurrence in many hosts *M. arginini* is mentioned in several chapters of this book. Whether there is any greater claim for this organism to be regarded as primarily of sheep and goat origin is debatable. It is nevertheless found with great frequency in these hosts. With hindsight it is now known that the N strains isolated by Arisoy *et al.* (1967) from the nose of goats in Turkey were *M. arginini* strains. In sheep it is found occasionally in keratoconjunctivitis (Leach, 1970), more frequently as an inhabitant of pneumonic lungs (Cottew, 1971; Alley *et al.*, 1975), and with a very high prevalence in the normal mouth and esophagus (G. S. Cottew, unpublished observations).

The isolation and testing of *M. arginini* introduced an important biochemical property to the mycoplasma field—hydrolysis of arginine. This characteristic, together with another, the metabolism of glucose, has allowed mycoplasmas to be subdivided simply into four groups according to whether they metabolize both glucose and arginine, neither, or only one of these. Other reactions of *M. arginini* to biochemical tests are given in Table I.

Mycoplasma arginini grows moderately well on and in the usual mycoplasma media. Arginine supplementation of media by the addition of 10 gm/liter (50 mM) for the purpose of detecting arginine utilization proved inhibitory to many mycoplasmas that did not utilize arginine and to one strain of *Mycoplasma orale,* an arginine-utilizing mycoplasma (Leach, 1976), hence a concentration of 2 gm/liter is recommended for this reaction.

Mycoplasma arginini is inhibited by 1.0% bile salts, 3.0% sodium chloride, and 0.02% methylene blue and fails to grow at 25°C. Most strains tested by Al-Aubaidi *et al.* (1972b) grew at pH 5.5 and 9.5.

The reduction of triphenyltetrazolium chloride is variously reported as negative aerobically (Leach, 1970), negative aerobically and positive anaerobically (Tully and Razin, 1977), and negative using liquid medium (Al-Aubaidi, 1972). In our laboratory the reaction is carried out on solid medium anaerobically and is usually negative but occasionally weakly positive.

Mycoplasma arginini was antigenically different from other mycoplasmas by immunofluorescence and growth inhibition techniques when examined by Barile *et al.* (1968). By the rather sensitive two-dimensional immunoelectrophoresis method, Thirkill and Kenny (1974) showed that there were some differences in antigenic makeup among *M. arginini* strains, and some antigens were shared with *Mycoplasma gateae* and *M. arthritidis*, both of which are arginine utilizers. Nevertheless, the same workers were unable to demonstrate cross-reactions in growth inhibition on media containing 20% serum. When the serum content of the medium was reduced to 5.0%, a slight cross-reaction was observed between *M. arginini* and *M. gateae*. In passing it should be noted that these organisms are similar biochemically.

Factors produced by lymphoblast cell lines inhibit the mixed lymphocyte culture reaction, and a particular human lymphoblast cell line studied by Callawaert *et al.* (1975) that was especially active was found to be contaminated with *M. arginini*. Further investigation showed that the culture of *M. arginini* alone inhibited the mixed lymphocyte culture reaction. The nature of the factor was not described (see this volume, Chapter 13).

Several instances have been cited in which *M. arginini* appeared to be closely associated with disease in sheep (Alley *et al.*, 1975; Leach, 1970). However, Watson *et al.* (1968) found no consistent clinical or pathological abnormality ascribable to the injection of *M. arginini* into goats, and Foggie and Angus (1972) found that the pathological effects of *M. arginini* introduced intranasally or intratracheally into specific pathogen-free lambs were minimal.

C. *Mycoplasma capricolum*

When *M. capricolum* was proposed as a new species by Tully *et al.* (1974), six strains were examined. Some of these had a common origin dating back to an outbreak of disease in goats described by Cordy *et al.* (1955) in California. The history of these strains is supplied in the paper by Tully *et al.* (1974) and is recommended reading for those interested not only in *M. capricolum* but also in *M. mycoides* subsp. *capri*. This work, along with that of Lemcke (1974), finally demolished the belief that the organism referred to as "p.p. goat" was in any way related to *M. mycoides* subsp. *capri* (PG3). Moreover, it was shown that the "p.p. goat" strain was *M. capricolum*.

The necessity for comparing new isolates with authentic type strains of species during attempted identification could not be better illustrated than by this example. Much time was wasted, and erroneous findings have been left permanently in the literature as a result of not following this principle.

Recently *M. capricolum* was isolated in France (Perreau, 1974), in Rhodesia from sheep (Swanepoel *et al.*, 1977), and in Australia from goats (Littlejohns and Cottew, 1977). These appear to be the first reported occurrences of the organism for about 20 years, which for an organism as pathogenic as *M. capricolum* is difficult to understand.

The growth of *M. capricolum* is characterized by the formation of large colonies of a size similar to those of *M. mycoides* subsp. *capri*. Heavy turbidity is produced in liquid medium.

The biochemical characteristics of *M. capricolum* are listed in Table I. In addition to these, Tully *et al.* (1974) described a GC content of 25.5% and production of beta hemolysis in sheep erythrocytes, and Al-Aubaidi (1972) demonstrated growth at 25°C, reduction of methylene blue, and no growth on serum-free media.

The organism labeled "California goat mycoplasma 1958 strain" examined by Barber and Yedloutschnig (1970) was from the outbreak of disease described by Cordy *et al.* (1955) and probably was *M. capricolum* in spite of its failure to hydrolyze arginine. One of six strains of *M. capricolum* examined by Tully *et al.* (1974) also failed to split arginine, and two others gave variable results.

The strain referred to as the 1967 strain in the study of Barber and Yedloutschnig (1970) was the KS1 strain (Tully *et al.*, 1974). It differed from *M. capricolum* in that it produced film and spots and was later shown to be a new species designated *Mycoplasma putrefaciens* (Tully *et al.*, 1974).

It is not unexpected that more than one mycoplasma may be present in a herd or may even coexist in a single animal and, in view of the difficulty of identifying strains in the mid-1950s, it is not surprising that different strains have been perpetuated under a common reference. There are also examples of mixed cultures being distributed (Al-Aubaidi, 1972), and again it is not surprising that different recipients could clone out different components of the mixture so that quite different cultures would be regarded as representative of the original culture. It appears that many workers have unwittingly been involved in dispatching either mixed or improperly identified cultures. The important aim is to prevent problems from being created in the future by the oversights of the past, and it is very welcome to have in the literature the papers of Lemcke (1974), wherein the "p.p. goat" strain is shown not to be *M. mycoides* subsp. *capri*, but *M. capricolum* (Tully *et al.*, 1974), and of Perreau *et al.* (1976), wherein the *M. mycoides* subsp. *capri* reported from mastitis in goats is acknowledged to be *M. capricolum*.

Mycoplasma capricolum is pathogenic for goats and sheep (Swanepoel *et al.*, 1977; G. S. Cottew and L. A. Corner, unpublished observations). It is highly probable that *M. capricolum* was the causal organism of the disease in goats described by Cordy *et al.* (1955), despite the isolation of additional mycoplasmas from some of the animals. In that outbreak does became febrile, lactation diminished, and such painful swelling occurred in the joints that affected animals preferred to remain standing for long periods or, if down, were unable to rise. No respiratory symptoms were seen. Kids showed more severe signs, and some died within 24 hours of becoming affected. Experimental infection of 2-week-old kids by the intravenous or intraperitoneal route led to a febrile response with signs of pain in the joints; death followed within 3 days. In older kids the course was longer, but the clinical signs were similar. The pathology in experimentally infected goats was similar to that seen in natural cases. There was septicemia with lymphadenitis and splenitis, but fibrinopurulent polyarthritis was the outstanding lesion. Pneumonia was not a feature of the natural disease, although it occurred in experimental infections in some sheep and goats (Cordy *et al.*, 1955). As the commencement of disease in this closed herd was coincident with kidding and lactation, these may have been precipitating factors. Natural infections were not seen in sheep.

Although the herd in which a single lamb infected with *M. capricolum* was found (Swanepoel *et al.*, 1977) also contained 50 goats and 50 cattle, there was no infection in these animals. Sheep were shown to be susceptible to experimental infection, and calves were resistant.

The recent isolations of *M. capricolum* in Australia were made from two goats (Littlejohns and Cottew, 1977). In one, a nasopharyngeal swab of an apparently healthy buck contained the organism. Another strain was isolated from an infected joint of a doe with arthritis and mastitis, and the third was from the same goat 9 weeks later when the udder secretion was still positive. Inoculation (G. S. Cottew and L. A. Corner unpublished observations) of goats with cultures of these organisms provoked very severe, acute infections leading to death within a few days.

The puzzling feature of *M. capricolum* infection, referred to earlier, is how such a potent pathogen could remain undetected during a period of 20 years. Have outbreaks occurred that have been attributed to other causes with mycoplasmas not being sought, or have cultures obtained not been identified? Perhaps outbreaks of disease are the exception and low-grade chronic infection the rule, drawing little attention from pathologists. Alternatively, recovered animals, apparently healthy, may carry the organism for very long periods. This disease of sheep and goats is certainly worthy of further study.

D. *Mycoplasma conjunctivae*

Investigations into the etiology of ovine and caprine infectious keratoconjunctivitis led to the isolation of mycoplasmas by Surman (1968), Klingler *et al.* (1969), Langford (1971), and McCauley *et al.* (1971). As all of 14 mycoplasmas isolated from sheep and goats affected with keratoconjunctivitis by Barile *et al.* (1972) were apparently identical but differed from all known mycoplasmas, these investigators proposed that a new species, *M. conjunctivae,* be established with HRC581 as the type strain. They also found that *M. conjunctivae* and *M. arginini* had been isolated by both Surman and Langford.

Nicolet and Freundt (1975) found *M. conjunctivae* regularly in infectious keratoconjunctivitis in chamois and sheep. *Mycoplasma arginini* was present in three of these cases, twice in association with *M. conjunctivae.*

Mycoplasma conjunctivae has so far been reported only from sheep, goats, and chamois and only from Australia, Great Britain, the United States, and Switzerland. It may well be more widely distributed, but this awaits demonstration.

As there are no special growth requirements, *M. conjunctivae* is readily isolated on the usual mycoplasma media. It grows with a small colony on agar and with light turbidity in broth. Isolation is easier in the early acute stage of the disease than in chronic cases when heavy contamination with secondary invaders is encountered (Nicolet and Freundt, 1975).

The main biochemical characteristics are listed in Table I.

In our laboratory, growth of strains HRC581 and 14Z on medium containing pig serum was surrounded by a zone of milky precipitate within the agar that appeared to be different from the film and spots formed on medium containing horse serum. Jones *et al.* (1976b) found that some strains of *M. conjunctivae*, but not HRC581, formed a film and spots on medium containing 15% pig serum. Nicolet and Freundt (1975) also mentioned the production of a lipid film after prolonged incubation, but their medium contained horse serum. Further work to explore the nature and reproducibility of this reaction shown by *M. conjunctivae* on pig serum medium is indicated.

Mycoplasma conjunctivae may be identified by growth or metabolic inhibition reactions using antiserum to the HRC581 strain.

Mycoplasma conjunctivae is sensitive to several antibiotics (Jones *et al.*, 1976b) including oxytetracycline, gentamycin, and tylosin.

1. *Mycoplasma conjunctivae* and Infectious Keratoconjunctivitis

a. The natural disease. Although infectious keratoconjunctivitis occurs in cattle, there has been no report of the isolation of *M. conjunctivae* from this condition in that host. The organism appears to be restricted to sheep, goats, and chamois. *Mycoplasma arginini* (Leach, 1970), *M. ovipneumoniae* (Carmichael *et al.*, 1972; Jones *et al.*, 1976b), *A. oculi* (Al-Aubaidi *et al.*, 1973), and ureaplasmas (Spradbrow and Marley, 1971) (Section II,K) have also been isolated from infectious keratoconjunctivitis in sheep and goats.

McCauley *et al.* (1971) described the onset of the disease in goats as being accompanied by lachrymation, hyperemia of the palpebral conjunctiva followed by follicular conjunctivitis, neovascularization, pannus, iritis, and keratitis. Occasionally corneal opacity occurs, but there are no corneal ulcers and unilateral infection is usual. The disease often runs a mild course lasting a week, or a more severe course over a month. Neonatal infection occurs, and both eyes are usually involved. Infection of kids was not correlated with infection of their respective does. The natural infection in goats was examined more extensively in recent outbreaks in two separate goat herds (Baas *et al.*, 1977).

In lambs, Jones *et al.* (1976b) observed mild conjunctivitis at 6–10 days of age. Clinical signs were similar to those described above in goats, and in addition the bulbar conjunctiva was affected. Opacity and ulceration of the cornea were seen in severe cases. Jones *et al.* (1976b) differentiated two forms of infectious keratoconjunctivitis, follicular conjunctivitis and the nonfollicular form seen in the lambs from which *M. conjunctivae* was isolated.

In chamois the natural disease leads to total blindness, which is not a feature of the disease in sheep (Nicolet and Freundt, 1975). One chamois that was found dead lacked eye lesions but had pneumonic lesions in the apical and cardiac lobes of the lung from which *M. conjunctivae* was isolated.

Langford (1971) failed to isolate *M. conjunctivae* from animals in clinically healthy flocks, but culture of the eyes of clinically normal animals in infected flocks yielded *M. conjunctivae* (Jones *et al.*, 1976b).

b. Experimental infection. Several workers have succeeded in producing a mild form of the disease in experimental sheep or goats using cultures of mycoplasmas isolated from infected eyes. Surman (1968, 1973), although successful in producing experimental infection, did not clearly state that the mycoplasma used was *M. conjunctivae*. Klingler *et al.* (1969) reproduced the disease with a culture subsequently identified as *M. conjunctivae*. Despite this, Nicolet and Freundt (1975), in discussing the role of *M. conjunctivae*, considered that "some other factors" contributed to establishment of the field syndrome.

Jones *et al.* (1976b) inoculated *M. conjunctivae* intraconjunctivally and produced ocular lesions in four sheep, and Trotter *et al.* (1977) produced experimental keratoconjunctivitis in goats with purified cultures of *M. conjunctivae*. Thus there is mounting evidence that some outbreaks of keratoconjunctivitis are caused by *M. conjunctivae*, with more severe disease perhaps being attributable to the added activities of secondary organisms or other factors.

E. The Subspecies of *Mycoplasma mycoides*

If the segment of this chapter allotted to the subspecies of *M. mycoides* appears to be disproportionate, in justification let it be said that few areas of the literature on sheep and goat mycoplasmas are as confusing. As the reasons for this confusion become known, a clearer picture of the interrelationship of these mycoplasmas emerges.

The first step in attempting to clarify the situation is to describe the established subspecies, *M. mycoides* subsp. *capri* and *M. mycoides* subsp. *mycoides*. This is followed in each case by an outline of the problems associated with identification, and some recent findings on *M. mycoides* subsp. *mycoides* are described.

1. *Mycoplasma mycoides* subsp. *capri* (PG3)

Many workers contributed to the knowledge of the disease CCPP before eventual isolation of the causal agent in Nigeria by Longley (1951). At about the same time H. P. Chu and W. I. B. Beveridge (personal communication) also succeeded in isolating the causal organism from material obtained in Turkey from CCPP in goats. Both the strains of Longley and that of Chu and Beveridge were examined by Edward (1954), who selected the Turkish organism, PG3, as the type strain of *M. mycoides* subsp. *capri* (Edward and Freundt, 1956).

The characteristics described by Edward (1954) for this species have since been supplemented by others, and a list of some of the most used appears in Table I.

The work of Al-Aubaidi (1972) in particular, and also that of Cottew (1974), have established that strains known as Farcha, GPA, Smith, BQT, and N108 are identical with *M. mycoides* subsp. *capri* (PG3), and doubtless there are others that have been authenticated as *M. mycoides* subsp. *capri*.

2. Problems in the Identification of *Mycoplasma mycoides* subsp. *capri*

Had all strains suspected of being *M. mycoides* subsp. *capri* been compared directly with the type strain PG3, the number of incorrectly identified strains would have been minimized. A strain labeled "p.p. goat" was taken as being representative of PG3 and was used for comparative purposes. This occurred particularly when workers were trying to determine the degree of relationship between *M. mycoides* subsp. *mycoides* and *M. mycoides* subsp. *capri*. The strain labeled "*M. capri*" used by Hudson *et al.* (1967) was "p.p. goat," as was that used earlier by Cottew and Lloyd (1965), and it is probable that others used this strain in error. Lemcke (1974) and Tully *et al.* (1974) demonstrated the lack of relationship of "p.p. goat" to the PG3 strain and established its identity as *M. capricolum* (Section II,C).

Organisms suspected of being *M. mycoides* subsp. *capri* were also compared with a strain, Vom, which was regarded as being *M. mycoides* subsp. *capri*. This led to reports of this organism being present in Mexico (Solana and Rivera, 1967), but later it was shown (Perreau, 1971; Al-Aubaidi *et al.*, 1972a; Cottew, 1974) that the Vom strain was not *M. mycoides* subsp. *capri* but *M. mycoides* subsp. *mycoides*.

These instances are not the only ones in which identifications were influenced by the use of a mislabeled strain, but are illustrative of what has occurred and should warn readers that some earlier work may be misleading.

Another source of error has been emphasized by Al-Aubaidi (1972), who discovered two mixed cultures among those received from other laboratories.

3. *Mycoplasma mycoides* subsp. *mycoides* (PG1)

The disease of cattle CBPP occurs or has occurred in many countries, and the causal organism, *M. mycoides* subsp. *mycoides*, is well known. Furthermore, the exchange of strains between countries has never given rise to published observations on important differences in characteristics among strains, except in the degree of their pathogenicity for the host.

Thus PG1, selected as the type strain of the species (Edward and Freundt, 1956), adequately represents the known strains from cattle in all characteristics examined, except that it is no longer pathogenic for cattle, having presumably become attenuated by passage in culture (Edward and Freundt, 1973).

The characteristics of this organism are given in Table I.

4. Problems in the Identification of *Mycoplasma mycoides* subsp. *mycoides*

For years the existence of two types of *M. mycoides* subsp. *mycoides* has been obvious from their different growth characteristics, but only recently have other tests been used to support this separation.

a. The large-colony type of *M. mycoides* subsp. *mycoides*. The organisms discussed here have been the cause of some of the confusion in identification. Discussion may be conveniently introduced by mention of the first one to be adequately identified, the strain of Laws (1956), later called Y goat. The isolation of this organism from fibrinous peritonitis in a goat in Queensland proved to be a most important event. The Y-goat strain was shown (Hudson *et al.*, 1967) to be serologically very closely related to *M. mycoides* subsp. *mycoides*, differing by having a heat-labile antigen (a feature that has not been investigated in subsequent isolates). In many biochemical tests this organism behaved identically to PG1. Y goat fermented glucose, reduced tetrazolium chloride, did not form film and spots, and did not metabolize arginine. However, it grew faster and gave rise to larger colonies and greater turbidity than the bovine strains of *M. mycoides* subsp. *mycoides* and was considered to be an unusual strain of *M. mycoides* subsp. *mycoides*. Further strains of the same type have since been observed and are listed in Table II.

The advent of further strains has emphasized the problem of nomenclature. If, on the basis of close serological and biochemical relationship to PG1, strains such as Y goat are simply called *M. mycoides* subsp. *mycoides*, they may be thought of as the more usual slow-growing, small-colony-forming organisms that cause CBPP in cattle. As strains resembling Y goat do not have such characteristics, they must be differentiated in some way, especially for the benefit of disease control authorities. If they were referred to as "*M. mycoides* subsp. *mycoides* from goats" it would also be incorrect, as at least one strain of this type (801) has been recovered from cattle in our laboratory. Al-Aubaidi (1972) was aware that strains related to *M. mycoides* subsp. *mycoides* occurred in goats and allotted them to group 8 in his classification of sheep and goat strains, but he included in this group strains O goat and P goat, which had the characteristics of PG1 rather than of Y goat. It has long been consid-

TABLE II. *Mycoplasma mycoides* subsp. *mycoides* Strains from Goats

LC type	Reference[a]	SC type	Reference
Y goat[b]	Laws (1956)	Vom	Perreau (1971)
Cov 2	Arisoy et al. (1967)	O goat	Hudson et al. (1967)
OSB 42	El Nasri (1967)	P goat	Hudson et al. (1967)
Ojo 1	Ojo (1973)		
Ojo 2	Ojo (1973)		
F30	MacOwan (1976)		
74/2488	Littlejohns and Cottew (1977)		
KH1	Cottew and Yeats (1978)		
TMH	G. S. Cottew (unpublished observations)		
3172			
9214			
7510			

[a] Not necessarily that of the first isolation.

[b] The separation of *M. mycoides* subsp. *mycoides* strains into two groups on the basis of growth and biochemical characteristics was described by Cottew and Yeats (1978). Strains not included in that study, TMH, 3172, 9214, and 7510 have been characterized since in our laboratory (see also Rodwell and Rodwell, 1978).

ered in our laboratory that the Y-goat type should be differentiated from the PG1 type, and recent observations not only made this possible but also justified this separation on its relevance to the pathogenicity of the organisms in different hosts (Cottew and Yeats, 1978).

The clear distinction between the Y-goat type and *M. mycoides* subsp. *mycoides* (PG1) has been demonstrated using reactions that, although lacking novelty, appear to be effective, namely, digestion of casein, liquefaction of coagulated serum, and survival time at 45°C. The Y-goat strain and others listed in Table II actively digested casein, liquefied serum, and survived longer at 45°C than strains resembling PG1 (Cottew and Yeats, 1978). These tests, together with differences in growth characteristics, permitted differentiation of the two types of strains which were, for convenience, referred to as *M. mycoides* subsp. *mycoides* LC (large-colony) and SC (small-colony) strains. Another difference between these two groups that is not so readily used for differentiation is the quantity of galactan present in cell pellets (Rodwell et al., 1972).

b. *Mycoplasma mycoides* subsp. *mycoides* of the small-colony type. The justification for setting up this category was discussed in Section II,E,4, a. The small-colony-forming or SC type of *M. mycoides* subsp. *mycoides* includes all those that resemble PG1. By far the greatest number of these are strains of bovine origin, most if not all of which were isolated from CBPP. However, there are several well-known strains (Table II) that originated from goats.

In 1955 R. J. Olds (personal communication) isolated a mycoplasma in New Guinea from polyarthritis in goats. This strain (Olds' goat or O goat) was indistinguishable from *M. mycoides* subsp. *mycoides* (PG1) and was pathogenic for cattle (Hudson *et al.*, 1967; Cottew, 1974). A similar strain was isolated from goats in Sudan (P. Pillai, personal communication) and labeled G1/61 (or P goat). The O goat, P goat, and the Vom strain are all not only serologically identical to PG1 but are also identical in their biochemical and growth characteristics. These strains can, despite their being of goat origin, be grouped with the classic *M. mycoides* subsp. *mycoides* strains which are also SC types. Probably other strains of this type have been recovered from goats but have not yet been characterized as SC types.

5. The Relationship between *Mycoplasma mycoides* subsp. *mycoides* and *Mycoplasma mycoides* subsp. *capri*

Identification of an organism as one of the subspecies of *M. mycoides* is not assisted by its biochemical characteristics, as those of the LC types of *M. mycoides* subsp. *mycoides* are identical to those of *M. mycoides* subsp. *capri* (Table I). Growth and metabolic inhibiton reactions and immunofluorescence using antiserum to PG3 and PG1 are accepted as suitable for serological identification but are limited by the potency and specificity of the antisera used. In our experience, significant cross-reaction can occur between the subspecies with some antisera. Ojo (1976a) found four strains with biochemical characteristics common to the subspecies of *M. mycoides* but which were difficult to assign serologically to one of the subspecies of *M. mycoides*. Although the cultures could have been mixed, as suggested by Ojo, or the antisera insufficiently specific, there is also the possibility that a spectrum of antigens exists ranging from those possessed by Y goat (closely related to PG1) through the "intermediate" strains of Ojo to PG3 at the other end showing much less serological affinity with PG1. Here then is an area that requires diligent investigation, perhaps a new approach, before the identity of new isolates can be proclaimed with certainty. An important practical consequence of this is use of the correct specific preventive vaccine. There is a possibility that intermediate strains would provoke immunity to both subspecies.

6. The Pathogenicity of the *Mycoplasma mycoides* Subspecies

a. *Mycoplasma mycoides* subsp. *capri* in contagious caprine pleuropneumonia. (1) *Goats. Mycoplasma mycoides* subsp. *capri* is the classic causal agent of CCPP, as described in the extensive study of Longley (1951). This disease is one of the most important economically of all diseases in goats and is widely distributed geographically. It is not intended that CCPP be considered here in great detail, as adequate descriptions are still accessible (Longley, 1951; Turner, 1959; Cottew and Leach, 1969; Cottew, 1970) and still relevant. Briefly, CCPP is a respiratory disease confined in nature to goats, although both sheep and goats may be infected experimentally. The incubation period of 2–28 days is followed by a febrile response of up to 41°C (Turner, 1959), and signs of respiratory distress are shown. Inappetence and loss of condition are followed by prostration and, in severe cases, death. In the lung, extensive edema, hepatization, enlargement of interlobular septa, and fibrinous pleurisy are seen. Associated lymph nodes are enlarged and edematous.

Intratracheal or subcutaneous inoculation of cultures into experimental goats results in reproduction of the disease (Watson *et al.*, 1968). The histopathology observed in goats infected with *M. mycoides* subsp. *capri* was described by Longley (1951).

Although tylosin (El Nasri, 1964; Onoviran, 1974) and oxytetracycline (Onoviran, 1974) may be useful in treatment, early intervention is vital as the disease often develops rapidly. Immunity following infection was thought to be weak and of short duration (Curasson, 1946), but Onoviran (1972) demonstrated good immunity 4 months after infection. Thus preventive vaccination is a worthwhile aim and may be made more effective now that the diversity of antigenic types among causal agents is recognized.

Diagnosis of the disease on clinical and pathological grounds remains valid, but nonspecific, and isolation of the causal organism is to be preferred. Serological diagnosis is less useful in this than in some other mycoplasma infections, as death may occur before antibody can be detected.

(2) Sheep. Although the natural disease does not occur in sheep, they may be infected experimentally by intratracheal inoculation of cultures of *M. mycoides* subsp. *capri* (Watson *et al.*, 1968).

(3) Cattle. There are reports of this organism being used to infect cattle experimentally but, in retrospect, the true identity of the organisms used is still in doubt. Shirlaw (1949) indicated that cattle were not susceptible to subcutaneous inoculation or to inhalation of a nebulized culture. The Connecticut strain (Jonas and Barber, 1969) was not pathogenic for cattle by intramuscular injection, but the identity of this strain as *M. mycoides* subsp. *capri* is uncertain (Tully *et al.*, 1974).

b. Mycoplasma mycoides subsp. mycoides in CCPP. *(1) Goats.* Since about 1968 it has been realized that *M. mycoides* subsp. *mycoides* was also a causal agent of CCPP (Watson *et al.*, 1968; Cottew and Leach, 1969; Perreau, 1971), and this is further supported by the more recent work of Ojo (1976b), MacOwan (1976), and Kaliner and MacOwan (1976).

Solana and Rivera (1967), Yedloutschnig *et al.*, (1972), and later Nakagawa *et al.* (1976) demonstrated the production of CCPP with strains referred to as *M. mycoides* subsp. *capri* but which, from the examination of Al-Aubaidi (1972), were probably *M. mycoides* subsp. *mycoides* strains. In none of these cases is it possible to be certain whether LC or SC types were involved.

From the work of MacOwan (1976) and MacOwan and Minette (1976) CCPP in Kenya appears to be caused both by *M. mycoides* subsp. *mycoides* of the LC type, represented by the F30 strain, and by strains of another mycoplasma, represented by F38, which has not yet been identified. The F30 strain was isolated from chronic CCPP in which there was no spread of disease to goats in contact. The F38 strain was isolated from acute CCPP which readily spread to goats in contact. MacOwan (1976) considered that the disease caused by the F38 strain more closely resembled the natural cases seen by Kaliner and MacOwan (1976). The strain F30 and those of Ojo (1973) studied in our laboratory were LC types of *M. mycoides* subsp. *mycoides*.

For the SC types of *M. mycoides* subsp. *mycoides*, the evidence for pathogenicity in goats is not clear. Abdulla and Lindley (1967) found that a bovine isolate, presumably an SC strain, was not pathogenic for goats by endobronchial inoculation, while earlier Dick (1937), using a bovine strain, had succeeded in producing large edematous swellings at the site of subcutaneous inoculation, sometimes causing lameness, but infection by this route did not lead to lung involvement. *Mycoplasma mycoides* subsp. *mycoides* (Gladysdale) inoculated intratracheally and endobronchially caused only transient febrile responses in three goats, and the only lesion described was a small focus of red, collapsed lung tissue in one goat (Kaliner and MacOwan, 1976). The G1/61 (P goat) strain, shown to be an SC type (Cottew and Yeats, 1978), did not provoke disease in goats or sheep (El Nasri, 1967), but the O-goat strain produced polyarthritis in goats and sheep (R. J. Olds, personal communication).

(2) Sheep. CCPP is not recognized as a natural disease in sheep, and only rarely has *M. mycoides* subsp. *mycoides* been isolated from this host (Al-Aubaidi *et al.*, 1972a; Ernø *et al.*, 1972). Whether these are LC or SC types has not been established.

Experimental infections with LC types of *M. mycoides* subsp. *mycoides* led to acute fibrinous pleuropneumonia (MacOwan, 1976) or peritonitis (Hudson *et al.*, 1967). Subcutaneous injection of SC types of *M. mycoides* subsp. *mycoides* from cattle was followed by the production of characteristic edematous swellings, and the sheep often died (Turner *et al.*, 1935).

(3) Cattle. As Hudson *et al.* (1967) had shown that the Y-goat strain of *M. mycoides* subsp. *mycoides* (an LC type) was not pathogenic for cattle and that the O-goat strain (an SC type) was, and as these strains were shown to be separable using simple *in vitro* reactions (Cottew and Yeats, 1978), the working hypothesis set up was that these techniques also separated those that are pathogenic for cattle from those that are not. Further evidence for the lack of pathogenicity of the LC types was obtained with the 74/2488 (G. S. Cottew and L. C. Lloyd, unpublished observations) and the F30 (MacOwan, 1976) strains. The SC strains, on the other hand, include, as previously mentioned, all the *M. mycoides* subsp. *mycoides* strains from CBPP.

To accumulate further data relevant to this hypothesis, it is necessary to know whether a strain used for pathogenicity tests in cattle is an LC or an SC type.

Disease control authorities in countries free of CBPP in cattle may well become alarmed by reports of *M. mycoides* subsp. *mycoides* in goats in their country or may refuse entry to goats from other countries in which the organism is reported. Should further data substantiate the present belief that LC types of *M. mycoides* subsp. *mycoides* are not pathogenic for cattle, demonstration that the organism in question is an LC type should allay concern for the cattle population. At the same time it should not be overlooked that the presence of SC types of *M. mycoides* subsp. *mycoides* in goats is a potential threat to cattle.

c. Diseases of goats other than CCPP involving subspecies of *Mycoplasma mycoides*. Edema disease was described in Greece by Debonera (1937), who considered it to be a form of contagious agalactia. Characterized by extensive subcutaneous edema that usually affects the limbs and udder, hence milk production, this disease is restricted in its distribution. An organism isolated from this condition was examined by Edward (1953), who found that the mycoplasma had the same cultural and biochemical properties as the *M. mycoides* subsp. *capri* strains he had examined and was related to them serologically. Longley (1951) showed that subcutaneous or intradermal inoculation of goats with *M. mycoides* subsp. *capri* led to severe local edema which spread well away from the site of inoculation. This effect is consistent with this organism being a causal agent of edema disease. However, in Turkey (Arisoy *et al.*, 1967), field reports of a similar disease were accompanied by milk samples from which the Covenli (Cov) strains were isolated. At first only referred to as type-C strains, these were later shown to be *M. mycoides* subsp. *mycoides* of the LC type (Cottew and Yeats, 1978).

Little is known of the epidemiology of these sporadic conditions and why there are usually few animals involved in each occurrence. Yedloutschnig *et al.* (1972) speculated that many mycoplasma-associated infections may have gone undetected because of the relative unimportance of an individual goat or because mycoplasmas were not sought in such cases. In Australia the fibrinous peritonitis from which Y goat was isolated was a single episode, and about 16 years elapsed before the next strain of that type was isolated there. In the next 5 years, several strains were isolated. It is highly likely that more isolations of mycoplasmas will follow from an increased interest in the cultivation of mycoplasmas in diagnostic laboratories.

F. *Mycoplasma ovipneumoniae*

The mycoplasmas isolated from lungs of sheep with pulmonary adenomatosis in Scotland (type A of MacKay *et al.*, 1963), together with those from sheep lungs in Australia (type 2 of Cottew, 1971) and the strains described by Carmichael *et al.* (1972) as *M. ovipneumoniae,* are strains of the same species for which the proposed type strain is Y98 (Furlong and Cottew, 1973; Leach *et al.*, 1976). This organism also occurs in New Zealand (Clarke *et al.*, 1974), Hungary (Stipkovits *et al.*, 1975), and Iceland (Friis *et al.*, 1976).

Although most frequently found in the lung, trachea and nose, and occasionally the eyes of sheep with pneumonia, *M. ovipneumoniae* is also found in the respiratory tract of healthy sheep (Alley *et al.*, 1975; Jones *et al.*, 1976a).

Mycoplasma ovipneumoniae can be isolated on standard mycoplasma medium but some workers (e.g., Carmichael *et al.*, 1972) have chosen media adapted from that of Goodwin and Pryor (1970). The organism is more susceptible than most to overdrying of plates.

Colonies of *M. ovipneumoniae* on solid media containing the usual concentration of agar (1.5–2.0%) lack the central downgrowth that contributes to the "fried egg" appearance regarded as classic for mycoplasmas. Lower agar concentrations (Furlong and Cottew, 1973) permit the development of these classic colonies.

Colony impressions of the centerless colonies of *M. ovipneumoniae* stained with Giemsa have an appearance not unlike that of *Mycoplasma dispar* (Gourlay and Leach, 1970). This bizarre colony morphology appears to be restricted to these two mycoplasmas, and the reason for its unusual nature has not been explained.

The biochemical characteristics of this glycolytic mycoplasma are given in Table I.

Quinlan *et al*. (1975) determined (in liquid medium) the minimal inhibitory concentrations of several antibiotics for 40 strains of *M. ovipneumoniae*. In order of decreasing effectiveness these were tylosin (0.32 μg/
ml), oxytetracycline (0.145 μg/ml), novobiocin (6.6 μg/ml), and chloramphenicol (15.2 μg/ml).

The patterns of antibiotic sensitivity of nine Scottish strains of *M.
ovipneumoniae* studied by Jones *et al*. (1976a) were similar for each strain
and mostly agreed with the findings of Quinlan *et al*. (1975). All were
resistant to erythromycin, streptomycin, oleandomycin, nystatin, and
polymyxin B, but susceptible in varying degrees to tylosin, oxytetracycline, chlortetracycline, kanamycin, and gentamicin in sensitivity tests on
solid medium.

Polyacrylamide gel electrophoresis of proteins of the strains of *M.
ovipneumoniae*, examined by Jones *et al*. (1976a), showed that the patterns produced by each strain were similar. Some serological heterogeneity was shown among the strains in this species, and it has been suggested that tests with antiserum against more than one strain could be
required for identification. Alternatively, a test with broader specificity,
such as indirect hemagglutination, could be used (Jones *et al*., 1976a).

The natural disease associated with *M. ovipneumoniae* in sheep in
Australia was described by St. George *et al*. (1971), Carmichael *et al*.
(1972), and Sullivan *et al*. (1973). Respiratory disease in young lambs
began as occasional rales detected on careful auscultation. Severe clinical
pneumonia had its onset between 5 and 10 weeks after lambing, when the
lambs had repeated moist coughing, sneezing, and copious clear mucoid
nasal discharge. There was high morbidity, low mortality, intolerance to
exercise, and inadequate weight gain in the lambs. After 12 weeks, clinical
signs were found in fewer lambs, although all those killed at 16 weeks had
pneumonic lesions of proliferative interstitial pneumonia characterized by
septal and bronchiolar epithelial cell hyperplasia and proliferation.
Mycoplasma ovipneumoniae was isolated from lambs 6–26 weeks old.

Experimental infection of lambs has been produced with cultures of *M.
ovipneumoniae* given intravenously or by aerosol and by contact with
sheep so exposed. Gross lung lesions consisted of the lung being gray
rather than pink, with red areas of atelectasis with a lobular distribution
(Sullivan *et al*., 1973); usually the right apical lobe was affected, and next
most frequently the right and left cardiac lobes. Histologically there was a
marked thickening of alveolar septa because of proliferation of alveolar
septal cells.

Foggie *et al*. (1976) infected colostrum-deprived, specific-pathogen-free
lambs endobronchially with broth culture of *M. ovipneumoniae* and recovered the organism from the lungs of five of the six infected lambs.

Lesions were present in the lungs of three animals. In another experiment *M. ovipneumoniae* was recovered from the upper respiratory tract of six lambs in contact with two infected lambs, but no lung lesions were present in these animals.

G. *Mycoplasma putrefaciens*

Among the mycoplasmas examined by Tully *et al.* (1974) there was one, KS1, the origin of which was thought to have been the outbreak of disease in goats in California described by Cordy *et al.* (1955). This organism proved to be unlike all other mycoplasmas and was named *M. putrefaciens* because of the characteristic, peculiar to this *Mycoplasma* species, of producing in growth medium an odor of putrefaction. Only this representative was known until recently, when H. Ernø (personal communication) identified another from mastitis in goats in France.

There has been no published information on the finding of this organism in any other situation, nor on what role it plays in the host.

The biochemical characteristics are listed in Table I.

H. *Acholeplasma granularum*

Two strains of *A. granularum* from sheep lungs in India (E. A. Freundt, personal communication) and one from goat genital tracts in India (H. Ernø, personal communication) are the only records available of the presence of this organism in sheep and goats.

The biochemical characteristics were not examined in our laboratory but are reported by Freundt (1974) as acid from glucose, anaerobic reduction of tetrazolium chloride with weak reduction aerobically, negative for phosphatase, no proteolytic activity, and no hydrolysis of esculin but synthesis of carotenoid pigments.

I. *Acholeplasma laidlawii*

This organism is ubiquitous and has no special claim to be considered an organism of sheep and goats; indeed, it has been found in these hosts less frequently than in many others. Physiological and biochemical studies have often used *A. laidlawii* as a representative of a wall-less prokaryote, but this work is not sufficiently relevant to the occurrence of *A. laidlawii* in sheep and goats to warrant inclusion here.

Krauss and Wandera (1970) isolated *A. laidlawii* from the respiratory tract of sheep in Kenya but did not suggest a causal role for it in disease.

Several vaginal isolates from sheep in Australia, including the CWZ strain (Cottew, 1974), have been identified as *A. laidlawii*, as have five strains from the genital tract of goats in India (H. Ernø, personal communication).

An organism labeled "Cal. goat," originally from goats in the outbreak described by Cordy *et al.* (1955), was found to be *A. laidlawii* (Cottew, 1974).

The biochemical reactions of *A. laidlawii* are given in Table I.

J. Acholeplasma oculi

From six goats in a herd experiencing a severe outbreak of keratoconjunctivitis in Minnesota, mycoplasmas were isolated. The organisms were cultivated from conjunctival swabs from affected but not from normal animals nor from those that had recovered. When the five organisms were characterized and compared with 34 established mycoplasmas and acholeplasmas, they were found to be distinct, and Al-Aubaidi *et al.* 1973) proposed that they be the basis of a new species *Acholeplasma oculusi*. The name *A. oculusi* was subsequently changed to *A. oculi* to use the genitive of the Latin noun *oculus,* meaning "eye" (Al-Aubaidi, 1975). Tully (1973) described three strains found as contaminants in cell cultures and suggested that they may have been of bovine origin.

No further isolates were recorded until Kuksa and Gois (1975) isolated the organism from nasal swabs of pigs in Czechoslovakia.

Other recoveries (H. Ernø, personal communication) were four strains from the genital tract of goats in India.

Acholeplasma oculi grows at 22° and 37°C and produces obvious turbidity in liquid medium and a typical "fried egg" colony on solid media.

The biochemical characteristics are given in Table I. In addition, the organism hemolyzed sheep erythrocytes, did not hydrolyze urea, grew in medium without serum, did not grow in the presence of 1% bile salt, at pH 5.5 and 9.5, nor in the presence of 3% sodium chloride and 0.02% methylene blue (Al-Aubaidi *et al.*, 1973).

Acholeplasma oculi was not sensitive to 5% sodium polyanethol sulfonate, was only slightly inhibited by digitonin, and hydrolyzed esculin (Kuksa and Gois, 1975). Tully (1973) showed that the type strain, 19L, and four other strains produced carotenoids, as do strains of *A. laidlawii*.

The *A. oculi* strains tested by Al-Aubaidi *et al.* (1973) were resistant to 100 μg/ml kanamycin but were sensitive to 10 μg/ml erythromycin.

In the natural outbreak of disease in goats in Minnesota (Al-Aubaidi *et al.*, 1973) the clinical sign was severe keratoconjunctivitis. In experimental animals, intravenous inoculation of *A. oculi* led to the development of pneumonic signs, and death followed in 6 days. Congestion of the lungs, chest wall, and trachea with moderate amounts of pleural, pericardial, and peritoneal fluid was seen at autopsy. Organisms serologically and bio-chemically similar to the strain used were recovered from lungs, spleen, blood, peritoneal fluid, and conjunctiva. When *A. oculi* was given by the conjunctival route, clinical signs were induced in experimentally infected goats, including mild conjunctivitis.

K. Ureaplasmas

Organisms with tiny colonies resembling those of ureaplasmas were reported from outbreaks of keratoconjunctivitis in sheep in Australia by Spradbrow and Marley (1971). Similar organisms were cultivated from the eyes of three clinically normal sheep. Unfortunately, these organisms did not passage, nor did they survive freezing and thawing. Two sheep inocu-lated intracorneally with broth cultures developed keratoconjunctivitis within 24 hours. Serial passage of ocular fluids in sheep produced keratoconjunctivitis for nine passages, and organisms resembling urea-plasmas were isolated from all cases of the disease but also from three of the experimental sheep before inoculation. The organisms found in this study differed from classic ureaplasmas in not degrading urea, and the investigators suggested that they would be better regarded as myco-plasmas that were fastidious in their growth requirements, hence were growing with reduced colony size.

Gourlay *et al.* (1973) sought ureaplasmas in the nose and urethra of goats and succeeded in cultivating strains from the urogenital tract of two of four goats. The pathogenicity of these strains was not tested.

In a study of sheep and goats in Texas, Livingston and Gauer (1975) isolated ureaplasmas from the urine of 21 sheep and 1 goat and from the vagina of 2 goats. Sheep with granular vulvitis examined by Doig and Ruhnke (1977) contained ureaplasmas in the vulva, and similar organisms were obtained in the same region in normal sheep. Attempted transmis-sion to healthy sheep using cultures of ureaplasmas resulted in hyperemia and slight granularity of the vulva, and ureaplasmas were detected up to 7 weeks after inoculation.

The ureaplasmas found so far in sheep and goats have not been thoroughly characterized, nor have their serological relationships been investigated.

L. Miscellaneous Mycoplasmas from Sheep and Goats

1. The 2D Group

In Australia, Carmichael *et al.* (1972) described seven vaginal and three preputial isolates from sheep as being of the one biotype referred to as 2D.

Similar organisms were isolated from an outbreak of vulvovaginitis elsewhere in Australia (Cottew *et al.*, 1974). These organisms had the biochemical characteristics of *M. agalactiae* (Cottew, 1974) but were not inhibited by *M. agalactiae* antiserum. Instead, some showed a close serological relationship to *M. mycoides* subsp. *mycoides,* but this was not found for 2D by Al-Aubaidi (1972).

Descriptions by Stipkovits *et al.* (1975) and Ojo (1976a) could be interpreted as referring to similar strains in Hungary and Nigeria, respectively, but this remains to be demonstrated.

Further study of these strains is required to determine their interrelationships and what affinity they have for *M. mycoides* subsp. *mycoides*.

2. Other Organisms

Several unclassified mycoplasmas isolated from sheep and goats were described previously (Cottew, 1970, 1974). Since that time some have been shown to be distinct species and have been discussed earlier [*M. capricolum* (Kid); *M. putrefaciens* (KS1); *M. ovipneumoniae* (Y98)]. Others were identified as organisms not primarily of sheep or goat origin [(*M. bovirhinis* (QEW); *M. gallinarum* (EHM)].

The *M. dispar*-like organisms from goats described by Perreau (1973) have since been shown to be *M. ovipneumoniae* (P. Perreau, personal communication).

A mycoplasma from a lamb in the United States was identified as *M. bovis* by G. S. Cottew and by J. G. Tully (personal communication).

One mycoplasma labeled G145, and another, A1343, both from goats, were shown to be serologically distinct from other sheep and goat mycoplasmas (Al-Aubaidi, 1972) and remain the only representatives of these organisms yet found.

III. FUTURE RESEARCH

Before proceeding to discuss briefly areas for future work, it may be appropriate to indicate where type strains of mycoplasmas may be obtained. Both the National Collection of Type Cultures in England and the American Type Culture Collection hold most of the sheep and goat mycoplasmas and the FAO/WHO Collaborating Centre for Animal Mycoplasmas at the University of Aarhus in Denmark has a complete collection.

Individuals holding untyped mycoplasmas from sheep and goats should be encouraged to type their strains and publish their findings. Assistance with typing may be given by other workers in the same country who have published in this field or by laboratories in other countries. As typing is usually done as a favor, assistance is more readily forthcoming when some preliminary work has been done, for instance the biochemical characteristics described and available antisera tried in serological tests. More interest may be aroused when the isolates appear to be novel or come from a site or condition not usually associated with mycoplasmas.

Although our knowledge of the mycoplasmas of sheep and goats has increased in the last 10 years, there is still much to learn about identification, diagnosis, epidemiology, immunity, treatment, and pathogenesis.

Final identification of mycoplasmas is dependent on serology, the value of which is limited by the quality of the available antiserum. Cross-reactions between species (and subspecies) hinder identification and emphasize the need for highly specific antisera. However, within some species, strains may show antigenic differences; identification of such strains requires sera with broader specificity or the use of more than one antiserum. Good-quality antisera are in short supply, and as there are now over 50 species, determination of whether a particular strain is a new species is beyond all but a few laboratories. The use of groups of polyvalent antisera to facilitate typing was introduced by Ernø (1976) and is at present being evaluated. The immunoperoxidase test introduced by Polak-Vogelzang and Hagenaars (1976) is also being examined. Such methods should assist typing but are still dependent on the quality of the antiserum.

Identification methods that are independent of antiserum are available. One such technique is polyacrylamide gel electrophoresis of proteins. This is useful if the patterns to be compared are very similar or very different, but within the range where both similarities and differences are shown, uncertainty in interpretation lessens the value of the reaction. The more recently developed two-dimensional method overcomes the low resolving power of the one-dimensional method (Rodwell and Rodwell, 1978) and could become a valuable test, perhaps more applicable to disputed than to routine identification.

Some diseases caused by mycoplasmas are sufficiently distinctive to be diagnosed on clinical and pathological grounds, but more often demonstration of the causal organism is required. Except in contagious agalactia, little emphasis has been placed on serological diagnosis, yet adequate serological tests for these diseases would be valuable not only for the detection of disease but also for purposes of control and eradication. Similarly, the epidemiology of and immunity following the major diseases have been studied, but less is known of these aspects in diseases of more sporadic occurrence.

Little is known of the pathogenesis of mycoplasma diseases, and this large and challenging field awaits investigation.

REFERENCES

Abdulla, A. E. D., and Lindley, E. P. (1967). *Bull. Epizoot. Dis. Afr.* **15**, 313–317.

Al-Aubaidi, J. M. (1972). *D. Sci. Vet. Med.* Thesis, Cornell Univ., Ithaca, New York.

Al-Aubaidi, J. M. (1975). *Int. J. Syst. Bacteriol.* **25**, 221.

Al-Aubaidi, J. M., Dardiri, A. H., and Fabricant, J. (1972a). *Int. J. Syst. Bacteriol.* **22**, 155–164.

Al-Aubaidi, J. M., Taylor, W. D., Bubash, G. R., and Dardiri, A. H. (1972b). *Am. J. Vet. Res.* **33**, 87–90.

Al-Aubaidi, J. M., Dardiri, A. H., Muscoplatt, C. C., and McCauley, E. H. (1973). *Cornell Vet.* **63**, 117–129.

Alley, M. R., Quinlan, J. R., and Clarke, J. K. (1975). *N.Z. Vet. J.* **23**, 137–141.

Anonymous (1975). *FAO/WHO/OIE Anim. Health Yearb. 1974.*

Anonymous (1976). *FAO/WHO/OIE Anim. Health Yearb. 1975.*

Arisoy, F. (1975). *Pendik Vet. Kontrol Arastirma Enstitusu Derg.* **8**, 48–51.

Arisoy, F., Erdağ, O., Cottew, G. S., and Watson, W. A. (1967). *Turk. Vet. Hekimleri Dernegi Derg.* **37**, 11–17.

Arisoy, F., Etheridge, J. R., and Foggie, A. (1969). *Pendik Vet. Kontrol Arastirma Enstitusu Derg.* **2**, 137–149.

Baas, E. J., Trotter, S. L., Franklin, R. M., and Barile, M. F. (1977). *Infect. Immun.* **18**, 806–815.

Baharsefat, M., Yamini, B., and Ahourai, P. (1971). *Arch. Inst. Razi* **23**, 113–118.

Barber, T. L., and Yedloutschnig, R. J. (1970). *Cornell Vet.* **60**, 297–308.

Barile, M. F., Del Giudice, R. A., Carski, T. R., Gibbs, C. J., and Morris, J. A. (1968). *Proc. Soc. Exp. Biol. Med.* **129**, 489–494.

Barile, M. F., Del Giudice, R. A., and Tully, J. G. (1972). *Infect. Immun.* **5**, 70–76.

Bridré, J., and Donatien, A. (1923). *C. R. Acad. Sci.* **177**, 841–843.

Bridré, J., and Donatien, A. (1925). *Ann. Inst. Pasteur, Paris* **39**, 925–951.

Callawaert, D. M., Kaplan, J., Peterson, W. D., and Lightbody, J. J. (1975). *J. Immunol.* **115**, 1662–1664.

Carmichael, L. E., St. George, T. D., Sullivan, N. D., and Horsfall, N. (1972). *Cornell Vet.* **62**, 654–679.

Clarke, J. K., Brown, V. G., and Alley, M. R. (1974). *N.Z. Vet. J.* **22**, 117–121.

Cordy, D. R., Adler, H. E., and Yamamoto, R. (1955). *Cornell Vet.* **45**, 50–68.

Cottew, G. S. (1970). *In* "The Role of Mycoplasmas and L Forms of Bacteria in Disease" (J. T. Sharp, ed.), pp. 198–211. Thomas, Springfield, Illinois.

Cottew, G. S. (1971). *Aust. Vet. J.* **47**, 591–596.

Cottew, G. S. (1974). *Colloq. INSERM, Mycoplasmes Homme, Anim., Veg. Insectes, Congr. Int., Bordeaux* **33**, 357–362.

Cottew, G. S., and Leach, R. H. (1969). *In* "The Mycoplasmatales and the L-Phase of Bacteria" (L. Hayflick, ed.), pp. 527–570. Appleton, New York.

Cottew, G. S., and Lloyd, L. C. (1965). *J. Comp. Pathol.* **75**, 363–374.

Cottew, G. S., and Yeats, F. R. (1978). *Aust. Vet. J.* **54**, 293–296.

Cottew, G. S., Watson, W. A., Arisoy, F., Erdağ, O., and Buckley, L. S. (1968). *J. Comp. Pathol.* **78**, 275–282.

Cottew, G. S., Lloyd, L. C., Parsonson, I. M., and Hore, D. E. (1974). *Aust. Vet. J.* **50**, 576–577.

Curasson, G. (1946). "Maladies Infectieuses des Animaux Domestiques." Vigot Frères, Paris.

Debonera, G. (1937). *Recl. Med. Vet.* **113**, 79–92.

Dick, A. T. (1937). *J. Counc. Sci. Ind. Res.* **10**, 164–167.

Doig, P. A., and Ruhnke, H. L. (1977). *Vet. Rec.* **100**, 179–180.

Edward, D. G. ff. (1953). *Vet. Rec.* **65**, 873–875.

Edward, D. G. ff. (1954). *J. Gen. Microbiol.* **10,** 27–64.

Edward, D. G. ff., and Freundt, E. A. (1956). *J. Gen. Microbiol.* **14,** 197–207.

Edward, D. G. ff., and Freundt, E. A. (1973). *Int. J. Syst. Bacteriol.* **23,** 55–61.

Edward, D. G. ff., and Moore, W. B. (1975). *J. Med. Microbiol.* **8,** 451–454.

El Nasri, M. (1964). *Vet. Rec.* **76,** 876–877.

El Nasri, M. (1967). *Ann. N.Y. Acad. Sci.* **143,** 298–304.

Ernø, H. (1976). *Proc. Soc. Gen. Microbiol.* 3(4), 166.

Ernø, H., Freundt, E. A., Krogsgaard-Jensen, A., and Rosendal, S. (1972). *Acta Vet. Scand.* **13,** 263–265.

Etheridge, J. R., Foggie, A., Arisoy, F., and Erdağ, O. (1969). *Pendik Vet. Kontrol Arastirma Enstitusu Derg.* **2,** 101–119.

Foggie, A., and Angus, K. W. (1972). *Vet. Rec.* **90,** 312–313.

Foggie, A., Etheridge, J. R., Erdağ, O., and Arisoy, F. (1970). *Res. Vet. Sci.* **11,** 477–479.

Foggie, A., Jones, G. E., and Buxton, D. (1976). *Res. Vet. Sci.* **21,** 28–35.

Freundt, E. A. (1974). *In* "Bergey's Manual of Determinative Bacteriology" (R. E. Buchanan and N. E. Gibbons, eds.), 8th Ed., pp. 929–955. Williams & Wilkins, Baltimore, Maryland.

Friis, N. F., Palsson, P. A., and Petursson, G. (1976). *Acta Vet. Scand.* **17,** 255–257.

Furlong, S. L., and Cottew, G. S. (1973). *Aust. Vet. J.* **49,** 216.

Goodwin, R. F. W., and Pryor, J. E. (1970). *Vet. Rec.* **87,** 726–727.

Gourlay, R. N., and Leach, R. H. (1970). *J. Med. Microbiol.* **3,** 111–123.

Gourlay, R. N., Brownlie, J., and Howard, C. J. (1973). *J. Gen. Microbiol.* **76,** 251–254.

Hernandez, F. A. M. (1972). *Zootechnia* **21,** 485–497.

Hill, A. (1972). *Vet. Rec.* **91,** 224–225.

Hudson, J. R., Cottew, G. S., and Adler, H. E. (1967). *Ann. N.Y. Acad. Sci.* **143,** 287–297.

Jonas, A. M., and Barber, T. L. (1969). *J. Infect. Dis.* **119,** 126–131.

Jones, G. E., Foggie, A., Mould, D. L., and Livitt, S. (1976a). *J. Med. Microbiol.* **9,** 39–52.

Jones, G. E., Foggie, A., Sutherland, A., and Harker, D. B. (1976b). *Vet. Rec.* **99,** 137–141.

Kaliner, G., and MacOwan, K. J. (1976). *Zentralbl. Veterinaermed., Reihe B* **23,** 652–661.

Klingler, K., Nicolet, J., and Schipper, E. (1969). *Schweiz. Arch. Tierheilkd.* **111,** 587–602.

Krauss, H., and Wandera, J. G. (1970). *J. Comp. Pathol.* **80,** 389–397.

Kuksa, F., and Gois, M. (1975). *Proc. Conf. Taxon. Physiol. Anim. Mycoplasmas, 3rd, Brno* pp. 42–51.

Langford, E. V. (1971). *Can. J. Comp. Med.* **35,** 18–21.

Laws, L. (1956). *Aust. Vet. J.* **32,** 326–329.

Leach, R. H. (1970). *Vet. Rec.* **87,** 319–320.

Leach, R. H. (1976). *J. Appl. Bacteriol.* **41,** 259–264.

Leach, R. H., Cottew, G. S., Andrews, B. E., and Powell, D. G. (1976). *Vet. Rec.* **98,** 377–379.

Lemcke, R. M. (1974). *Res. Vet. Sci.* **16,** 119–121.

Littlejohns, I. R., and Cottew, G. S. (1977). *Aust. Vet. J.* **53,** 297–298.

Livingston, C. W., and Gauer, B. B. (1975). *Am. J. Vet. Res.* **36,** 313–314.

Longley, E. O. (1951). *Colon. Res. Publ., London* No. 7.

McCauley, E. H., Surman, P. G., and Anderson, D. R. (1971). *Am. J. Vet. Res.* **32,** 861–870.

MacKay, J. M. K., Nisbet, D. K., and Foggie, A. (1963). *Vet. Rec.* **75,** 550–551.

MacOwan, K. J. (1976). *Trop. Anim. Health Prod.* **8,** 28–36.

MacOwan, K. J., and Minette, J. E. (1976). *Trop. Anim. Health Prod.* **8,** 91–95.

Morozzi, A., Dominici, S., and Cardaras, P. (1973). *Atti Soc. Ital. Sci. Vet.* **27,** 628–632.

Nakagawa, M., Taylor, W. D., and Yedloutschnig, R. J. (1976). *Natl. Inst. Anim. Health Q.* **16,** 65–77.

Nicolet, J., and Freundt, E. A. (1975). *Zentralbl. Veterinaermed., Reihe B* **22,** 302–307.

Ojo, M. O. (1973). *Bull. Epizoot. Dis. Afr.* **21,** 319–323.

Ojo, M. O. (1976a). *Trop. Anim. Health Prod.* **8,** 137–146.

Ojo, M. O. (1976b). *J. Comp. Pathol.* **86,** 519–529.

Onoviran, O. (1972). *Res. Vet. Sci.* **13,** 599–600.

Onoviran, O. (1974). *Vet. Rec.* **94,** 418–420.

Orning, A. P., Ross, R. F., and Barile, M. F. (1978). *Amer. J. Vet. Res.* **39,** 1169–1174.

Perreau, P. (1971). *Rev. Elev. Med. Vet. Pays Trop.* **24,** 343–348.

Perreau, P. (1973). *Rev. Elev. Med. Vet. Pays Trop.* **26,** 13–25.

Perreau, P. (1974). *Bull. Acad. Vet. Fr.* **47,** 179–188.

Perreau, P., Giauffret, A., Cauzaubon, P., and Lambert, M. (1975). *Bull. Acad. Vet. Fr.* **48,** 349–357.

Perreau, P., LeGoff, C., and Giauffret, A. (1976). *Bull. Acad. Vet. Fr.* **49,** 185–192.

Polak-Vogelzang, A. A., and Hagenaars, R. (1976). *Proc. Soc. Gen. Microbiol.* **3**(4), 151.

Popovici, L. (1961). *Off. Int. Epizoot. Bull.* **56,** 880–885.

Quinlan, J. R., Alley, M. R., and Clarke, J. K. (1975). *N.Z. Vet. J.* **23,** 188–189.

Rodwell, A. W., Peterson, J. E., and Rodwell, E. S. (1972). *Pathogenic Mycoplasmas, Ciba Found. Symp.* pp. 123–144.

Rodwell, A. W., and Rodwell, E. S. (1978). *J. Gen. Microbiol.* **109,** 259–263.

Shirlaw, J. F. (1949). *Indian J. Vet. Sci. Anim. Husb.* **19,** 181–213.

Singh, N., Rajya, B. S., and Mohanty, G. C. (1974). *Cornell Vet.* **64,** 435–442.

Singh, N., Rajya, B. S., and Mohanty, G. C. (1975). *Cornell Vet.* **65,** 363–373.

Solana, P., and Rivera, E. (1967). *Ann. N.Y. Acad. Sci.* **143,** 357–363.

Spradbrow, P. B., and Marley, J. (1971). *Aust. Vet. J.* **47,** 116–118.

St. George, T. D., Sullivan, N. D., Love, J. A., and Horsfall, N. (1971). *Aust. Vet. J.* **47,** 282–283.

Stipkovits, L., Bélak, S., Pálfi, V., and Túry, E. (1975). *Acta Vet. Acad. Sci. Hung.* **25,** 267–273.

Sullivan, N. D., St. George, T. D., and Horsfall, N. (1973). *Aust. Vet. J.* **49,** 57–68.

Surman, P. G. (1968). *Aust. J. Biol. Sci.* **21,** 447–467.

Surman, P. G. (1973). *Aust. J. Exp. Biol. Med. Sci.* **51,** 589–607.

Swanepoel, R., Efstratiou, S., and Blackburn, N. K. (1977). *Vet. Rec.* **101,** 446–447.

Thirkill, C. E., and Kenny, G. E. (1974). *Infect. Immun.* **10,** 624–632.

Trotter, S. L., Franklin, R. M., Baas, E. J., and Barile, M. F. (1977). *Infect. Immun.* **18,** 816–822.

Tully, J. G. (1973). *Ann. N.Y. Acad. Sci.* **225,** 74–93.

Tully, J. G., and Razin, S. (1977). *In* "Handbook of Microbiology" (A. I. Laskin and H. A. Lechevalier, eds.), 2nd Ed., Vol. 1, p. 420. CRC Press, Cleveland, Ohio.

Tully, J. G., Barile, M. F., Edward, D. G. ff., Theodore, T. S., and Ernø, H. (1974). *J. Gen. Microbiol.* **85,** 102–120.

Turner, A. W. (1959). *In* "Infectious Diseases of Animals" (A. W. Stableforth and I. A. Galloway, eds.) Vol. 2, pp. 437–480. Butterworth, London.

Turner, A. W., Campbell, A. D., and Dick, A. T. (1935). *Aust. Vet. J.* **11,** 63–71.

Watson, W. A., Cottew, G. S., Erdağ, O., and Arisoy, F. (1968). *J. Comp. Pathol.* **78,** 283–291.

Yedloutschnig, R. J., Taylor, W. D., and Dardiri, A. H. (1972). *Proc. Meet. U.S. Anim. Health Assoc., 75th, 1971,* pp. 166–175.

Zavagli, V. (1951). *Off. Int. Epizoot., Bull.* **36,** 336–362.

4 / PORCINE MYCOPLASMAS

P. Whittlestone

THE MYCOPLASMAS, VOL. II
Copyright © 1979 by Academic Press, Inc.
All rights of reproduction in any form reserved.
ISBN 0-12-078401-7

I. INTRODUCTION

Relative Importance of the Different Porcine Mycoplasmas

There is almost general agreement that mycoplasmas play a major etiological role in porcine pneumonia. Throughout the world whenever large numbers of growing pigs are housed together within a confined air space, nonfatal pneumonia becomes a major chronic problem except in herds where effective control measures have been applied. Thus it is usual to find a significant percentage of the lungs of slaughtered market pigs with pneumonic lesions; incidences of between 12 and 81% have been reported in recent years.

Cultural examination of the porcine pneumonias seen in slaughter-houses yields several mycoplasma species, the most important ones being *Mycoplasma suipneumoniae* (also known as *Mycoplasma hyopneumoniae*) and *Mycoplasma hyorhinis. Mycoplasma hyorhinis* is by far the easier organism to cultivate, so in many laboratories it is the only mycoplasma isolated.

Within the complex of catarrhal pneumonias there is one pneumonic syndrome which stands out, in that it can be reliably transmitted to pigs of any age by respiratory tract inoculation of bacteria-free suspensions of pneumonic lung taken from affected pigs at any stage of the disease. The induced pneumonia has a characteristic serial histopathology. Earlier, this syndrome was erroneously called virus pneumonia but, since the demonstration 14 years ago that it was caused by *M. suipneumoniae,* most groups refer to this one etiological component in the complex as *enzootic pneumonia of pigs* (EPP). Thus in this chapter the abbreviation EPP is used to refer only to the pneumonic disease caused by *M. suipneumoniae.* Some groups still use the name *enzootic pneumonia* in a less restricted sense, i.e., to describe chronic catarrhal pneumonia of the growing pig. Other names used for porcine pneumonias have been discussed by Whittlestone (1973).

The precise role of the second mycoplasma, *M. hyorhinis,* is proving more difficult to determine. This organism is a common inhabitant of the nasal cavity and is very often present in pneumonic lesions with *M. suipneumoniae.* It is not known whether *M. hyorhinis* enhances the severity of EPP. It has been established that certain strains of *M. hyorhinis* alone induce pneumonia, serositis, and generalized infections experimentally in young gnotobiotic piglets (i.e., piglets produced surgically and reared with a known commensal bacterial flora). However, it is difficult to relate these experimental findings to the role of *M. hyorhinis* in the production of disease in naturally born and naturally reared piglets, which appear to be much more resistant than experimental animals to disease caused by this mycoplasma.

The other known mycoplasma pathogen of pigs is *Mycoplasma hyosynoviae,* a cause of nonsuppurative arthritis without polyserositis. This mycoplasma commonly inhabits the nasal cavity and pharynx of pigs and is recognized as one of the causes of arthritis in growing pigs in certain countries, especially the United States.

The fourth mycoplasma of interest in pigs is *Mycoplasma flocculare,* which is now found rather commonly in porcine pneumonias by two laboratories in Denmark and Great Britain. As the organism is considerably more fastidious and slower growing on primary isolation than even *M. suipneumoniae,* the absence of reports from other countries may merely be a reflection of the problem of cultivating it. It does not appear to be a pathogen.

A range of other *Mycoplasma* and *Acholeplasma* species has been isolated from pigs, but there is insufficient evidence to assess their overall importance and pathogenic significance.

II. *Mycoplasma suipneumoniae (Mycoplasma hyopneumoniae)*

A. Evidence for the Primary Etiological Role of *Mycoplasma suipneumoniae* in Enzootic Pneumonia of Pigs (EPP)

It has been known for many years that common chronic pneumonia of the growing pig, observed in many parts of the world, can be serially transmitted in pigs with bacteria-free filtrates of pneumonic lung. Because the infectivity of lung material was also unaffected by penicillin or sulfonamides, it was presumed that the causal agent was a virus. The sequence of evidence which led to the conclusion that the causal agent was *M. suipneumoniae* has been reviewed by Whittlestone (1973) and by Switzer and Ross (1975).

The main stages in the development of this evidence were as follows. First, it was demonstrated that the establishment of EPP could be prevented by prior administration of tetracycline antibiotics (Betts and

Campbell, 1956). Second, Whittlestone (1957, 1958) demonstrated that the size of the causal agent of EPP was between 0.2 and 0.45 μm and that delicate organisms of this size could be seen in Giemsa-stained EPP lung touch preparations. There was a strong association between the visible organism and the disease, and it was postulated by Whittlestone (1957, 1958) that it was the causal agent of EPP and was probably a fastidious mycoplasma that could not be cultivated at that time. Eventually the organism was grown, first in tissue culture (Betts and Whittlestone, 1963; Goodwin and Whittlestone, 1963) and then in media free of living cells (Goodwin and Whittlestone, 1964), conclusively demonstrating that the agent was nonviral. In the latter study, organisms grown in broth cultures, after repeated passage beyond the theoretical limiting dilution through which a hypothetical viral agent could have been carried, were able to induce EPP. Meanwhile, in the United States, the causative agent was propagated for a limited number of passages in cell culture (L'Ecuyer and Switzer, 1963) but lost infectivity for pigs during passage. Shortly afterwards an isolate made from EPP in the United States was shown to be cultivable in broth and to induce pneumonia, thus confirming that the EPP-inducing agent was nonviral (Maré and Switzer, 1965). From their broth cultures Maré and Switzer (1965) obtained colonies which they considered distinguishable from *M. hyorhinis* and *Acholeplasma granularum*. It was not known whether the colonial organisms, which they named *M. hyopneumoniae,* were identical to the pneumonia-inducing agent in the broth cultures. The first proof that the causal agent of EPP was a mycoplasma was provided when we obtained colonies from broth cultures, passaged them serially on agar to preclude mechanical carryover of another agent, and induced EPP in pigs with organisms from the final colonies (Goodwin *et al.*, 1965). Later we provided evidence that this mycoplasma, which was named *M. suipneumoniae,* was unrelated by the growth inhibition (GI) test to a wide range (42 strains) of other mycoplasmas (Goodwin *et al.*, 1967); we also showed that a mycoplasma isolated from the broth culture of Maré and Switzer (1965) was indistinguishable from *M. suipneumoniae.*

Since that time two names for the same mycoplasma have been used. The ICSB Subcommittee on the Taxonomy of Mycoplasmatales (Subcommittee, 1967, 1972, 1975) has commented on the taxonomic difficulties involved in this situation. The subcommittee (1975) noted that, while the designation of *M. hyopneumoniae* had priority as to date of publication, it was doubtful that the designated type strain (strain 11 or VPP11) was identical to the strain on which the description of *M. hyopneumoniae* was based. In light of this, the subcommittee (1975) recommended that a neotype strain be designated and has proposed that the J strain of the previously designated *M. suipneumoniae* (ATCC 25934 or NCTC 10110) be accepted as the neotype of *M. hyopneumoniae*.

B. Properties of *Mycoplasma suipneumoniae*

1. Isolation of *Mycoplasma suipneumoniae* from Pneumonic Tissue

a. In tissue culture. The original U.K. isolates of *M. suipneumoniae* (J strain) were made in plasma clot tissue cultures prepared from pneumonic pig lung tissue (Betts and Whittlestone, 1963; Goodwin and Whittlestone, 1963), chosen because it was free of *M. hyorhinis* (Whittlestone, 1958); subsequently we adapted the organism to pig lung monolayer cultures. The strain from the United States, VPP11, was isolated by Maré and Switzer (1966) in monolayer cell cultures prepared from pneumonic pig lung. Three Canadian strains (28, 29, and 33) were recovered by L'Ecuyer (1969) in pig testicle cell cultures. These studies have been reviewed by Whittlestone (1973). Although isolation in tissue culture has been neglected since satisfactory cell-free media became available in 1965, many workers still have great difficulty in isolating *M. suipneumoniae* in broth, and no workers isolate this mycoplasma on agar (Section II,B,1,c). Perhaps, with so many well-equipped laboratories in the world now able to employ cell culture techniques competently, attempts to isolate *M. suipneumoniae* in tissue cultures should be resumed, especially if the relevant experiences gained with selective broth media (see Section II,B,1,b) are applied.

b. In broth. Three main problems have to be overcome if *M. suipneumoniae* is to be isolated from field EPP lung tissue. First, *M. suipneumoniae* is nutritionally fastidious and has been isolated only in broths deliberately devised for this organism, although isolated and adapted strains have been propagated in other media. For the primary isolation of this mycoplasma, the degree of purity of medium constituents and the chemical cleanliness of all vessels is very critical. We have found it good practice to work at cell culture standards throughout. Second, in addition to *M. suipneumoniae* in EPP lung tissue, other mycoplasmas (especially *M. hyorhinis*) are very often present. Both these mycoplasmas are acid producers and, unfortunately, the much less fastidious *M. hyorhinis* rapidly overgrows *M. suipneumoniae*. Thus methods and media selective for *M. suipneumoniae* are required for primary isolation of the organism. Third, even if optimal isolation techniques and media are employed, it may nonetheless be difficult to recover *M. suipneumoniae* from some EPP cases (Section II,F,1,a).

To achieve isolation of *M. suipneumoniae* in the presence of *M. hyorhinis,* four main methods have been devised. First, *M. hyorhinis* antiserum (Goodwin and Hurrell, 1970; Yamamoto *et al.*, 1971) can be incorporated into the culture medium for primary isolation. Second, antibiotics, e.g., kanamycin sulfate (Yamamoto *et al.*, 1971) or cycloserine (Friis, 1971d), that have a selective action against *M. hyorhinis* can be incorporated into the medium. Third, the serum concentration can be increased to favor *M. suipneumoniae* rather than *M. hyorhinis* (Goodwin, 1976). The fourth method, used by Goiš *et al.* (1975), is to make five to seven passes at weekly intervals, after which *M. suipneumoniae* but not *M. hyorhinis* continues to multiply.

The earlier papers on selective isolation media were reviewed by Whittlestone (1973). Since then, advances have been made not only as a result of improved medium formulations but also as a consequence of increased experience which is so essential to success with this mycoplasma. For example, Goodwin (1976) found that an improved selective medium, containing 1 part *M. hyorhinis* antiserum and 9 parts Cambridge A26 medium, was a significant improvement over previous formulations and permitted the isolation of *M. suipneumoniae* from nearly all field cases of EPP. Another selective broth medium in current use is that of Friis (1971d, 1975). To 100 ml of nonselective medium (Friis, 1971a) is added 5 ml of *M. hyorhinis* rabbit antiserum and 5 ml of cycloserine (10 mg/ml), and the pH adjusted to 7.4. The tonicity should be 7–8 atm at 38°C (Friis, 1975). Friis (1971a) found that equal parts of horse and pig serum were better than pig serum alone for isolation media. Goodwin (1976) found that optimum growth of *M. suipneumoniae* was obtained in 27% serum, and Wilson (1976) found that adding 5% rabbit serum gave a stronger color change.

The method used by P. Whittlestone (unpublished observation, 1978) to isolate *M. suipneumoniae* is similar to that used by Friis (1975; personal communication, 1977) and Goodwin (1977), and is as follows. If feasible, pneumonic tissue is collected aseptically; contaminated pieces of lung tissue are surface-sterilized, e.g., by boiling in water for 8–10 sec as recommended by N. F. Friis (personal communication, 1977). A 10% suspension of lung tissue is made in nonselective broth, and dilutions made to 10^{-8} in both nonselective and selective broth. Cultures are incubated at 37°C. Cultures showing an acid pH shift are passed; with those *M. suipneumoniae* strains that grow readily, this first subculture is usually achieved after 3–10 days. Acid-producing mycoplasmas that grow slowly in selective or nonselective medium usually prove to be *M. suipneumoniae* or *M. flocculare*. These mycoplasmas can be differentiated by the metabolism inhibition (MI) test. Provided *M. hyorhinis* is not present, *M. suipneumoniae* grows slightly better in nonselective medium. Agents producing acid rapidly (within a day or two) usually prove to be *M. hyorhinis*. It should be stressed that the isolation of *M. suipneumoniae* can easily fail because of minor and often unidentified differences between various batches of media. Different batches of media of the Friis type seem to be more consistent than different batches of A26 medium. Friis (1974a) reported that the growth of *M. suipneumoniae* was strongly promoted by the roller technique. Farrington and Switzer (1976) recommend that a minimum of five to ten blind passages should be made at 3- to 5-day intervals before calling a bronchial swab or pneumonic lung tissue negative for *M. suipneumoniae*.

If isolation problems are encountered, the antibiotic content of the medium should be considered. One would not expect *M. suipneumoniae* to be sensitive to penicillin, yet Friis (1971c) demonstrated sensitivity to penicillin G and benzyl penicillin. However, others have reported no problems with these penicillins, and it seems that only certain batches are inhibitory (P. Whittlestone, unpublished observation, 1978), suggesting the occasional presence of toxic impurities. Arginine, which might be present in broth cultures used to recover *M. hyosynoviae* and other mycoplasmas, should either be omitted or reduced in concentration to 3 gm/liter or less for isolation of *M. suipneumoniae,* since the usual 10 gm/liter inhibits the growth of this organism (Leach, 1976).

c. On agar. *Mycoplasma suipneumoniae* is one of the few *Mycoplasma* species that still cannot be grown on agar during primary isolation. There seem to be only two claims in the literature that *M. suipneumoniae* can be isolated directly from pneumonic lesions from the field on solid medium, but no confirmation of these observations has appeared in later publications from either group. It seems possible that unusual and nonrepeatable batches of agar medium were employed in their apparently successful trials. N. F. Friis (personal communication, 1977) and P. Whittlestone (unpublished observation, 1978), who regularly grow *M. suipneumoniae* colonies from early broth cultures, have not obtained satisfactory colony growth directly from field cases of EPP.

d. In embryonated chicken eggs. Most of the claims that the causal agent of EPP can be isolated in embryonated chicken eggs cannot be assessed because the isolated agents were not identified; some workers were apparently even unaware of the possible complication of *M. hyorhinis*. We have succeeded in isolating *M. suipneumoniae* in yolk sacs from experimentally induced EPP (Goodwin *et al.*, 1968a), but there do not appear to be reports of such isolations from field cases of EPP.

2. Propagation and Morphology of *Mycoplasma suipneumoniae*

a. In broth. The main features of the various broth media used for propagation of adapted strains of *M. suipneumoniae* have been discussed by Whittlestone (1973). For continued propagation of *M. suipneumoniae* it is probably advisable to omit bacterial and *M. hyorhinis* inhibitors, since such inhibitors may interfere with maximal growth. For example, Goodwin (1976) suggested that cycloserine or kanamycin sulfate were inappropriate constituents of maintenance media.

Generally, *M. suipneumoniae* is cultured in broth media containing glucose, with phenol red as indicator, and growth can be readily assessed by a color shift from red (pH 7.5) to yellow (pH 6.8) on incubation. Some laboratories, however, do not obtain such clear-cut results. We find that an obvious pH change occurs within a day or two in tubes receiving inocula containing about 10^7 color-changing units (CCU), whereas tubes receiving small inocula may change color only after 20 days or more (Whittlestone, 1973). The final pH of broth cultures is 6.1 (Whittlestone, 1973; Friis, 1974a).

The morphological features of *M. suipneumoniae* grown in broth, fixed in methyl alcohol, and stained with May-Grünwald-Giemsa have been described and illustrated by Goodwin and Whittlestone (1966) and Whittlestone (1973). When the organisms are grown on the surface of glass, they form small groups or colonies composed of tiny cocci, 0.4 μm in diameter, attached to fine branching filaments 0.1–0.2 μm thick. Dried drops of culture show mainly tiny bipolar and "signet ring" organisms about 0.5–0.75 μm in diameter. Cultures also contain larger structures of unknown significance; they are especially prominent in some recently isolated strains.

b. On agar. Colonies of *M. suipneumoniae* can be obtained on agar seeded with either tissue culture or broth isolates of the organism; they can be first detected after 2–3 days' incubation and reach maximum size after about 10 days; well-adapted strains on the best batches of medium reach about 500 μm diameter. Colonies do not show a central nipple, generally appearing as convex structures with a granular surface. There is considerable variation in the ease with which different strains can be colonized, and the problems already discussed that influence the cultivation of *M. suipneumoniae* in broth are at least as relevant to cultivation on agar. The basic medium constituents are the same as those constituting nonselective broths but solidified with very pure agar. We have used 1% Ionagar No. 2 successfully since 1964; Friis (1975) confirmed the superiority of this type of agar but found 0.75% to be satisfactory. We have also used Agarose [Miles Laboratories (PTV) Ltd.] at 0.9%, as recommended by Friis (1975). Plates should be incubated at 37°C in as high a humidity as possible and in a gaseous atmosphere of between 5 and 10% carbon dioxide in air. Friis (1975) found carbon dioxide to be essential, but the air could be replaced with nitrogen.

3. Sensitivity to Antibiotics and Chemotherapeutic Drugs

Information on the *in vitro* antimicrobial sensitivity of *M. suipneumoniae* was reviewed by Whittlestone (1973), and additional evidence has been provided by Friis (1974a). Substances which have little or no effect on *M. suipneumoniae*, while controlling the growth of bacteria and fungi, include normal concentrations of penicillin (except that certain batches may be inhibitory), erythromycin, meticillin, and thallium acetate; antibiotics that allow *M. suipneumoniae* to grow while suppressing *M. hyorhinis* are discussed in Section II,B,1,b. Antibiotics that affect protein synthesis have a marked effect on *M. suipneumoniae in vitro;* Drews *et al.* (1975) found that the minimal inhibitory concentrations of tetracycline hydrochloride, tylosin tartrate, and tiamulin (14-deoxy-14-[(2-diethylaminoethyl)-mercapto-acetoxy]- mutilin hydrogen fumarate) for *M. suipneumoniae* were 1.25, 0.312, and 0.031 μg/ml, respectively.

4. Survival *in Vitro*

The evidence on the *in vitro* survival of *M. suipneumoniae* was reviewed by Whittlestone (1973, 1976b). The longest survival times of infectivity for pigs of EPP lung at different temperatures were −30°C for 20 months, −25°C for 3 months, 4°C for 4 days, 20°C for 1 day, 37°C for 4 hr, and 42.5°C for 2 hr. It is likely that there was a loss of ca. 10^6 pig infective doses per gram under these conditions, since pneumonic tissues kept for longer periods were not infective and fresh EPP lung tissue contains ca. 10^7 pig infective doses per gram. In comparison, attempted cultivation of *M. suipneumoniae* from EPP lung gave similar results: at 17°–25°C there was good survival for 3 days and some survival for 7 days, and at 1°–6°C there was no detectable loss of titer for 9 days but a slight drop by 11 days. The longest recorded survival times of *M. suipneumoniae* in broth cultures are: at −60°C for almost 9 yr, at 4°–11°C for 100 days, at 19°–26.5°C for 31 days, at 45°C for 1 hr, and at 50°C for 2 min. *Mycoplasma suipneumoniae* dried on cover slips and stored in the dark at room temperature dropped in titer from 10^5 to 10^2 in 4 days, and by 8 days no organisms could be recovered.

An x-ray dose of 300,000 to 400,000 R sterilized colostrum samples containing *M. suipneumoniae* (Schimmel *et al.*, 1974).

5. Strains of *Mycoplasma suipneumoniae*

The Cambridge J strain was isolated by Whittlestone and colleagues and is available as NCTC 10110 from the National Collection of Type Cultures, Colindale Avenue, Colindale, London, England, or from the American Type Culture Collection, 12301 Parklawn Drive, Rockville, Maryland, as ATCC 25934. Before deposition it was purified by five serial single-colony passages on agar medium. The parent strain induces EPP, but the cloned culture has not done so (P. Whittlestone, unpublished observation, 1978); no serological differences are known between the parent and the cloned culture. As noted earlier, the J strain has been proposed as the neotype strain to replace strain VPP11. Also the J strain offers several advantages in being easier to grow in broth and agar.

Strain VPP11 of *M. hyopneumoniae,* isolated by Maré and Switzer, is available from the United States collection as ATCC 25617. A closely related culture is available from the United Kingdom collection as NCTC 10127, but it was not derived directly from ATCC 25617. These latter cultures were deposited as broth cultures, and their passage history did not include any solid medium passages, so they did not derive from the colonial microorganisms actually named *M. hyopneumoniae*. As mentioned earlier, the J and VPP11 strains appear to be indistinguishable serologically.

The great majority of isolates throughout the world have been compared with the Cambridge J strain and found to be identical by one or another of the following serological tests: metabolism inhibition (MI), disc growth inhibition (DGI), immunofluorescence (IMF), complement fixation (CF), or growth precipitation (GP). References to such isolates from the United States, Great Britain, Canada, Denmark, and Japan were reviewed by Whittlestone (1973). More recent isolates, identified by reagents prepared against the J strain, have been made in Australia (Furlong and Turner, 1975a), Czechoslovakia (Goiš and Kuksa, 1975), France (Kobisch *et al.*, 1976), Hungary (Stipkovits, cited in Gois and Kuksa, 1975), Sweden (Holmgren, 1974a), and Yugoslavia (Durisic *et al.*, 1974). Thus it seems that all the isolates of *M. suipneumoniae* are closely related to each other serologically; from this point of view the organism seems to be antigenically less complex than *M. hyorhinis*.

It remains to be seen whether more sophisticated studies will reveal significant differences between the various strains of *M. suipneumoniae*. Biologically, there appear to be differences between various strains; some strains of *M. suipneumoniae* are very much more difficult to isolate in primary cultures of pneumonic lung than others (P. Whittlestone, unpublished observation, 1978). Also, some strains of the organism appear to induce much milder disease in the field; it remains to be determined whether differences are due to microorganism strain variation or whether they reflect differences in the system of management, feeding, or breed of pig.

C. The Experimental Disease

1. Induction with Lung Suspensions and Cultures

The experimental induction of pneumonia by the inoculation of EPP lung suspensions has been reviewed by Whittlestone (1973). Inoculation via the intratracheal or intranasal route produces pneumonia, and EPP lung diluted up to 10^{-7} induces gross pneumonia. All ages of pigs are equally susceptible to experimental EPP, but hysterectomy-produced, colostrum-deprived piglets are more susceptible and develop experimental pneumonia more reliably than naturally born and reared EPP-free pigs. Attempts to induce pneumonia by inoculation of EPP lung suspension by routes other than the respiratory tract have consistently failed.

The induction of EPP with cultures of *M. suipneumoniae* is less certain than with EPP lung suspensions. Our early work with broth cultures (Goodwin and Whittlestone, 1964), and that of Maré and Switzer (1965) demonstrating the pathogenicity of broth cultures, have now been confirmed by several workers. However, it seems that *M. suipneumoniae* becomes less pathogenic in broth culture, so that much greater numbers of cultured organisms are necessary to induce EPP than could possibly be present in a 10^{-7} dilution of lung suspension. Originally we successfully used repeated inoculations of broth cultures. Roberts (1974) found that more inoculated pigs developed pneumonia when a dose of 10^8 mycoplasmas was divided into two doses given on days 0 and 7, or three doses given on days 0, 3, and 7. Roberts (1974) also provided evidence that some strains of *M. suipneumoniae* were not pathogenic, but this might be related to passage level. A culture passed 19 times was shown by Mebus and Underdahl (1977) to produce quite extensive pneumonia, but the author has found that after about 30 broth passages two strains of *M. suipneumoniae* lost their ability to produce gross pneumonia. A single inoculum of a broth culture containing 2×10^9 *M. suipneumoniae* colony forming units induced EPP in specific-pathogen-free (SPF) pigs (Bruggmann et al., 1977b). A smaller dose (0.5×10^7 CCU) inoculated intranasally into gnotobiotic pigs by Goiš and Kuksa (1974a) induced symptomless gross pneumonia; this strain was used at its first broth pass after isolation from a gnotobiotic pig previously infected with a cloned culture.

There does not appear to be any confirmation by other workers of our early demonstration (Goodwin *et al.*, 1965) that EPP can be induced by colonies from agar.

A synergistic effect occurs between *M. suipneumoniae* and other agents, e.g., *Pasteurella multocida* (Smith *et al.*, 1973), *Ascaris suum* (Underdahl and Kelley, 1957; Zimmerman, 1971), *Metastronglus elongatus* (Mackenzie, 1963), and swine adenovirus (Kasza *et al.*, 1969).

2. The Pneumonic Lesions

The progressive development and resolution of EPP lesions has been described and illustrated by Whittlestone (1958, 1972) and Bertschinger *et al.* (1972). Gross lesions were detected in 7–10 days, developed to maximum extent in 20–30 days, and then gradually resolved, although residual lesions were still found 69–262 days after inoculation. Histologically, the lesions were characterized by alveolar cell pneumonia, mononuclear cell accumulations, and progressive and persistent lymphoreticular hyperplasia. The cases reported by Livingston *et al.* (1972), induced with a low dose of culture, were similar but resolved within 5–6 weeks.

A scanning electron microscope study of the changes in the trachea and bronchi of experimentally infected gnotobiotic piglets was made by Mebus and Underdahl (1977). Early in the infection, mycoplasmas occurred over normal ciliated epithelium, but later there was loss of cilia and exposure of the microvilli; leukocytes were observed with the numerous mycoplasmas on the damaged epithelial cells. By transmission electron microscopy the mycoplasmas appeared to be between the cilia rather than on the cilial surface. The lesions occurring in the trachea were more severe than those occurring in the terminal bronchioles.

The studies of Baskerville (1972), Baskerville and Wright (1973), Schuller and Abnelt (1977), and Wichert and Wilke (1976) have not been assessed, because it is not possible to be certain that the syndromes studied were EPP as defined in this chapter.

3. Distribution of *Mycoplasma suipneumoniae*

Mycoplasma suipneumoniae has been detected only in the respiratory tract and associated structures. Attempts to isolate the organism from nonrespiratory sites have been unsuccessful (Goiš and Kuksa, 1974a). This mycoplasma has a predilection for the lower respiratory tract but can also be detected in the nasal cavity (Whittlestone, 1973) and tonsils (Goiš and Kuksa, 1974a). Within the lung, *M. suipneumoniae* occurs in the greatest numbers in close association with the epithelium of the respiratory tree and often between the cilia where it can be demonstrated by

Giemsa staining, immunofluorescence, and electron microscope techniques (Whittlestone, 1958; Wegmann *et al.*, 1969; L'Ecuyer and Boulanger, 1970; Meyling, 1971; Livingston *et al.*, 1972; Mebus and Underdahl, 1977).

D. The Natural Disease

1. Incidence and Epidemiology

The incidence of chronic lung lesions characteristic of mycoplasmal pneumonia in slaughtered market-weight swine continues at about 45–70% (Woods *et al.*, 1969; Farrington, 1976; Glawischnig and Steininger, 1976); so far, little impact has been made on the overall control of this major problem. In a research herd that became infected, the incidence of pneumonia rose to 70% (Wilson, 1976).

With the wider use of selective media for the isolation of *M. suipneumoniae,* there has been repeated confirmation that *M. suipneumoniae* can be isolated from pneumonia of the growing pig. Czechoslovakian workers (Gois *et al.*, 1975) have provided much evidence of the microbial complexity of naturally occurring porcine pneumonias and seem less convinced than others about the primary etiological role of *M. suipneumoniae.* Most workers, including the author, feel that in the absence of *M. suipneumoniae* infection a majority of the continuing pneumonic problems in the growing pig disappear, although respiratory disease problems in young piglets are still common.

As far as is known, EPP spreads only by droplet infection via the airborne route. Factors affecting the spread of infection have been discussed by Whittlestone (1976b), but many questions on the spread of EPP remain unanswered. There is no evidence for the transmission of EPP via lungworm larvae-infected earthworms (Preston and Switzer, 1976). With presently available *in vitro* methods, probably about 10^3 to 10^5 wild-type *M. suipneumoniae* organisms are necessary to make an isolation (Whittlestone, 1976b). This low isolation rate is therefore a limitation on epidemiological studies requiring the detection of low numbers of organisms. The possibility that EPP might be brought into a healthy herd by boar semen used for artificial insemination (AI) was suggested by the isolation of *M. suipneumoniae* by Schulman and Estola (1974) from 1 of 101 samples. Because of this potential risk, Mandrup *et al.* (1975) cultured 169 semen samples collected from five AI centers, and R. F. W. Goodwin (personal communication, 1974) cultured 93 semen samples (as issued for AI) from 20 boars, without making any isolates of *M. suipneumoniae* (or other mycoplasmas).

The reinfection of herds previously free of EPP is a major problem within many control programs. As most breakdowns occur without any known contact with infected pigs, the likely possibilities are transmission by carrier hosts, transfer by fomites, long-distance airborne infection, or clinical expression of long-term subclinical infections. Within the Swiss SPF scheme, during a 10-yr period, Keller (1976) described three break-downs in which there were strong indications that the infection had remained subclinical for 3–15 months. Even longer subclinical infection had been indicated by the work of Goodwin (1965).

2. Effect of EPP

The effect of EPP on the productive efficiency of pigs was discussed by Whittlestone (1973). In some infected herds the disease causes at least a 20% reduction in feed/gain ratio (i.e., comparable to the effect in some experimental studies), while other herds suffer much less. Goodwin (1971) estimated that in a large, intensively managed herd, the loss attributable to EPP was about £3.50 (when converted to 1977 prices) per growing pig. A controlled study by Braude and Plonka (1975) on a large research herd which became infected with EPP showed that the feed/gain ratio was depressed by 0.15, representing a loss of £1.8 per bacon pig at 1977 food prices. The cost of EPP in the United States was estimated to be $180 million annually (Slavik, 1976).

3. Effect of Drugs on EPP

The effects of drugs on EPP have been reviewed by Switzer and Ross (1975) and Whittlestone (1973). As would be expected, penicillin and sulfonamides affect only secondary bacteria. Tetracyclines given before exposure prevent establishment of infection, but such measures have little practical value. Postexposure therapy with tetracyclines improves the clinical condition of pigs but does not eliminate the mycoplasma from the lungs. Tetracycline treatment is not economical for treatment of a herd problem but may be justified for individual valuable pigs. Tylosin is less effective than tetracyclines.

There have been several recent studies with tiamulin compounds. Naturally infected pigs receiving medicated feed containing 200 ppm of this drug for 10 days showed a reduction in clinical signs and less pneu-monia was found at slaughter (Glawischnig and Steininger, 1976; Stip-kovits et al., 1978); M. suipneumoniae could not be isolated from the lungs of treated pigs (Glawischnig and Steininger, 1976). Tiamulin injected intramuscularly (Hamm et al., 1976) or given in the drinking water (Szanto et al., 1977) was said to be very effective in the treatment of EPP, but more information is needed on the criteria for EPP diagnosis. A proper assessment of the effectiveness of tiamulin must await further work.

E. Nonspecific Methods for the Diagnosis of EPP

In recent years there have been major advances in techniques for the isolation of *M. suipneumoniae,* its serological identification, and the detection of antibody response to infection. Although in theory these specific methods could be universally applied, only the relatively small number of laboratories in the world that have concentrated on the problem have the necessary expertise to employ these techniques routinely. Therefore nonspecific methods of diagnosis must still be used (Hogg *et al.,* 1976; McKean *et al.,* 1976).

In herds previously free of respiratory disease, an outbreak of EPP is characterized by the development of chronic coughing in all age groups, the adult stock often being more severely affected with obvious malaise. A rising incidence of catarrhal pneumonia in marketed pigs even in the absence of obvious clinical signs suggests EPP, but the presence of similar pneumonic lesions in slaughtered adults is extremely suspicious. Conventional histology can be helpful if the changes seen are like those known to occur in uncomplicated EPP. Some caution in interpretation must be observed, because somewhat similar changes occur in other pneumonic conditions. A very useful rapid diagnostic method is the direct examination of Giemsa-stained pneumonic lung touch preparations for organisms with the morphology of *M. suipneumoniae* (Whittlestone, 1973). We have used this as a preliminary diagnostic method within the EPP control scheme (Goodwin and Whittlestone, 1960, 1967) run by the Pig Health Control Association in the United Kingdom. In outbreaks of pneumonia affecting pigs previously free from EPP, the presence in pneumonic lung touches of large numbers of organisms with the clear morphology of *M. suipneumoniae* indicates that the disease is virtually certain to be EPP: the absence of typical organisms in pneumonic lesions is very strong negative evidence. The method has the advantage that dried touch preparations are very stable and results can be available within a few hours of receipt of preparations. The disadvantage is that false positives can occur in lungs carrying *M. flocculare* infection (P. Whittlestone, unpublished observation, 1978); the interpretation is subjective, and some experience is essential to differentiate *M. suipneumoniae* from *M. hyorhinis* and nonspecific particles. To my knowledge, the only other group currently using this method is the one working with the Swiss control scheme (Keller and Bertschinger, 1968; Keller, 1978). There is a good correlation between this method and specific methods, e.g., isolation (Whittlestone, unpublished observation, 1978) or the IMF and immunoperoxidase tests (Giger *et al.*, 1977).

F. Specific Methods for the Diagnosis of EPP

1. Detection of the Organism or Antigen

a. Isolation of *Mycoplasma suipneumoniae* followed by its specific identification. The isolation in broth of *M. suipneumoniae* (followed by its serological identification) is the most widely used specific diagnostic method. The media, methods, problems, and solutions have been discussed in Section II,B,1,b. It should be stressed that the isolation of *M. suipneumoniae* is difficult and time-consuming (e.g., Wilson, 1976; Slavik, 1976; Schuller *et al.*, 1977b; Pijoan and Roberts, 1973). The author finds that while *M. suipneumoniae* can be isolated and identified within 7–10 days in some cases, it is not unusual for the process to take 20–30 days; semiblind passes may have to be made, and cultures should not be abandoned as negative until they have been incubated for 2 months. With some persistence it is usually possible to isolate *M. suipneumoniae* from material found positive on other evidence (P. Whittlestone, unpublished observation, 1978; Goodwin, 1977). Gois *et al.* (1975) found that, out of 39 positive *M. suipneumoniae* lungs, 11 were positive only by IMF, 18 were positive only by culture, and 10 were positive by both procedures. The author similarly finds that lungs containing a few organisms may be culture positive, while lungs containing large numbers of organisms may be culture negative.

Once the organism produces an obvious acid shift in broth, the method of choice for identification is the MI test, using hyperimmune rabbit antisera prepared against the neotype J strain. Such specific antisera, when diluted 1:40 to 1:1280 will inhibit growth of the organism (Whittlestone, unpublished observation, 1978; Goodwin, 1977).

Some workers who are able to cultivate *M. suipneumoniae* as colonies on agar use the DGI test for identification, but colony growth is so unreliable that the test is rarely used; e.g., Goiš and Kuksa (1975) found that *M. suipneumoniae* generally failed to form well-defined colonies and so could not employ the DGI test, but they found the GP test to be equal in specificity to the MI test. The GP test was also found (Friis, 1977) to identify strains readily, but cross-reactions occurred between *M. suipneumoniae* and *M. flocculare* when agar plates were incubated for prolonged periods.

b. Immunofluorescence. Since the first demonstrations of the presence of *M. suipneumoniae* on the surface of the bronchial and bronchiolar epithelium by the IMF method (L'Ecuyer and Boulanger, 1970; Meyling, 1971; Livingston, 1971), the method has become an important diagnostic test. Earlier, Meyling (1971) used the direct IMF method but, after adaptation of *M. suipneumoniae* to rabbit broth medium (N. F. Friis, personal communication, 1977), the indirect IMF method applied to frozen sections has been a reliable diagnostic method used in the Danish SPF scheme (A. Meyling, personal communication, 1977). Negative IMF results from suspicious pneumonias in important herds are checked culturally (N. F. Friis, personal communication, 1977; A. Meyling, personal communication, 1977). The IMF method has also been used in Sweden by Holmgren (1974a,b), who found it a specific and effective diagnostic method.

The indirect IMF test was used in Czechoslovakia by Goiš *et al.* (1975) to assess the presence of *M. suipneumoniae* in pneumonic lungs in slaughtered pigs from a large herd with severe respiratory disease. Of 39 positive lungs, 10 were detected by culture and IMF, 11 were positive only by IMF, and 18 were positive only by culture. This work stresses the wisdom of applying more than one diagnostic method. Giger *et al.* (1977) applied IMF methods to both frozen sections and bronchial smears; in both, *M. suipneumoniae* was identified. The bronchial smear method was considered a significant improvement in the diagnosis of EPP. There was also a good correlation between the IMF method and other diagnostic methods (Giemsa-stained touch preparations, histopathology, and the immunoperoxidase test).

c. Enzyme-linked immunoperoxidase (ELIP) technique. The ELIP technique has been used by Bruggmann *et al.* (1977a) to demonstrate *M. suipneumoniae* antigen in frozen lung sections or bronchial smears; the mycoplasma cells stained specifically and could be seen as reddish-brown pleomorphic particles. The end point of the reaction is stable and is readily visible by ordinary microscopy. Giger *et al.* (1977) found good correlation between this method and the IMF or Giemsa-stained touch preparation methods.

2. Detection of Antibody Response

a. Antibodies detected by complement fixation (CF). CF serum antibodies to *M. suipneumoniae* have been detected by the direct, modified direct, and indirect methods. The main conclusions that can be drawn from work with these tests, as reviewed by Whittlestone (1973), are that CF antibodies can be detected 2–3 weeks after infection, reach maximal titers after 1–9 months, and thereafter decline to low titers by 9–14 months. In herds clinically affected with EPP, serum CF titers are readily found. The problem from a diagnostic point of view is that false negatives and positives may occur in the test. False negatives in infected pigs have been reported by Roberts and Little (1970). False positive CF titers have been detected in pigs infected only with *M. hyorhinis* or *A. granularum,* and in some pigs from herds believed to be free of EPP (Hodges and Betts, 1969a,b; Roberts and Little, 1970). Using the microtiter CF test of Slavik and Switzer (1972) on eight SPF herds in Illinois, Woods *et al.* (1976) found that 9.4% of samples gave titers of 1:8 or higher, and only one herd was free of positive CF reactions. It is difficult to evaluate the significance of the CF work of Blackburn *et al.* (1975) and Schuller *et al.* (1977a), since data from additional methods of diagnosis were not reported. Thus the CF test cannot yet be used as a reliable check for the continuing absence of EPP in herds, since the significance of positive CF reactions cannot be readily interpreted.

b. Antibodies detected by immunofluorescence (IMF). Serum antibodies to *M. suipneumoniae* were detected by the indirect IMF method (Meyling, 1972) 3 weeks after infection, and maximum fluorescence occurred at 6–8 weeks. Sixty-seven percent of 265 slaughterhouse sera diluted 1 in 10 were IMF-positive. Of 375 sera from pneumonia-free SPF herds, 369 were negative; the 6 sera that gave trace reactions were subsequently re-evaluated and considered negative.

c. Antibodies detected by indirect hemagglutination (IHA). Although the IHA technique for the detection of serum antibodies to *M. suipneumoniae* is very sensitive, it is seldom used, probably because it is technically exacting. Holmgren (1974c) made improvements to previously described methods (reviewed in Whittlestone, 1973) by using Formalin-treated tanned swine erythrocytes and sonicated antigen. Thus large batches of red cells could be sensitized and then stored in small aliquots ready for use. Earlier we found that serum samples taken a month after infection were negative, but high titers developed later and persisted to 60 weeks (Goodwin *et al.*, 1969). Similarly, Holmgren (1974c) found that 2- to 5-week-old pigs in infected herds were negative by this test, but many 10- to 12-week old pigs were positive, as were a small proportion of sows and gilts. The IHA technique is currently used as an additional diagnostic method by A. Meyling (personal communication, 1977) within the Danish SPF scheme.

d. Antibodies detected by the indirect immunoperoxidase (IIP) test. The IIP test was used by Bruggmann *et al.* (1976) to examine sera from EPP-infected herds and primary SPF pigs; the latter were all negative, whereas 96% positives were obtained from the EPP-infected herds. No cross-reactions with *M. hyorhinis* or *M. flocculare* were obtained. The test detects all classes of antibody.

e. Antibodies detected by the enzyme-linked immunosorbent assay (ELISA) method. The ELISA method for the detection of *M. suipneumoniae* antibodies was developed by Bruggman *et al.* (1977b). Positive results were obtained 2 weeks after infection, i.e., about 3 weeks before clinical EPP developed; all sera tested between 3 and 50 weeks after inoculation were positive. The ELISA technique has the advantages that it detects all classes of immunoglobulins, gives quantitatively measurable results, and is very sensitive. Bruggmann (1978) found however that sera from pigs infected with *M. hyorhinis* gave cross-reactions with *M. suipneumoniae* antigen fractions having a molecular weight of about 300,000, whereas the specific *M. suipneumoniae* antigenic activity was located in the protein fraction having a molecular weight of between 28,000 and 60,000.

G. Immunity to EPP

Immunity to EPP has recently been reviewed by Whittlestone (1973, 1976a). The more important conclusions that can be drawn are as follows. In chronically affected herds, in which young pigs are clinically affected, clinical disease is not seen in adult stock; previously unexposed adults are, however, fully susceptible to EPP. Young pigs experimentally infected with EPP and allowed to recover resist heavy challenge for more than 1 year. Thus a strong acquired immunity develops as a result of active EPP infection. No correlation has been found between any type of serum antibody and immunity; attempts to induce immunity with inoculations of antigen which induce high levels of serum antibody have not succeeded. The only evidence suggesting that circulating antibody might contribute to immunity is that of Lam and Switzer (1971), who found that in passive protection experiments serum from hyperimmunized pigs reduced the incidence and extent of pneumonic lesions in pigs given an intranasal challenge with cultured *M. suipneumoniae*. Antibodies to *M. suipneumoniae* have been detected in tracheobronchial secretions of experimentally infected pigs (Holmgren, 1974a,d) and in the colostrum of sows inoculated with antigen and adjuvant (Durisic *et al.*, 1975), but it is not known if these antibodies are related to immunity.

The nature of the histological response in EPP (mononuclear cell accumulations and peribronchiolar lymphoreticular hyperplasia) suggests that cell-mediated immunity (CMI) could be important. This view is supported by the demonstration of lymphocyte transformation (Roberts, 1973; Adegboye, 1975); lymphocyte transformation was at maximum levels 15–44 weeks after infection (Adegboye, 1975). Other indicators of

CMI which developed during EPP infection were macrophage and leukocyte migration inhibition (Roberts, 1973; Nicolet and Rivera, 1976) and
skin reactions of the delayed hypersensitivity type (Adegboye, 1975). It
remains to be determined whether any of these responses correlate with
resistance to challenge.

H. Vaccination Attempts

The experimental vaccines for EPP have been discussed by Whittlestone (1973, 1976a). No protection against challenge was afforded by
attenuated cultures or *M. suipneumoniae* antigen given parenterally without adjuvant. Some protection against pneumonia was given by antigen
with Freund's complete adjuvant or Bayol and Arlacel (Lam and Switzer,
1971; Goodwin and Whittlestone, 1973), but a field trial of a similar
vaccine, containing a lower antigen dose, gave no protection (Goodwin,
1973). Farrington (1976) found that an antigen–peanut oil vaccine may
have given some protection. Durisic *et al.* (1975) suggested that colostral
antibodies following intramammary inoculation of antigen–Tween-80–
paraffin oil vaccine afforded protection against natural challenge, although an insufficient number of pigs was employed in the trial.

I. Control Schemes in Different Countries

Because of the economic importance of EPP and the lack of a vaccine
or satisfactory treatment, the most effective way of reducing the cost of
the disease is by establishing herds free of this disease. Healthy herds
containing the desired genetic lines can be established by a variety of
procedures including utilization of stock from others already shown to be
free of EPP, cross-suckling (onto EPP-free sows) of piglets snatched at
birth from their infected mothers, artificial rearing of piglets obtained by
surgical techniques, and artificial insemination of EPP-free sows. Following establishment, herds have to be constantly checked for the absence of
EPP. Various schemes reviewed by Whittlestone (1973) are currently
operating in many countries. These schemes have been a great stimulus to
the development of specific diagnostic methods for *M. suipneumoniae*. In
herds containing only breeding stock (i.e., with no growing pigs remaining
on the farm as indicators) there is a special problem in EPP diagnosis
(Koch and Keller, 1976).

An attempt to eliminate EPP from 10 herds in the United States by
removing CF-positive breeding stock during a period of 1 year did not
succeed in 9 of the herds as judged by the subsequent presence of

pneumonia or CF reactors (Preston, 1976), although there was a reduction in clinical signs in most of the herds.

The main problem in the European schemes has been the high breakdown rate. For example, in the United Kingdom EPP control scheme (Goodwin and Whittlestone, 1967), during the 7-year period 1960–1966, 47 herds broke down, which (with an average register of 81 herds) gives a rate of 8.3% per annum. In the 10 years to 1976, there were 43 breakdowns (Goodwin, 1977), which, with an average register of 78 herds, gives a 5.5% breakdown rate. Most of these breakdowns occurred without any known contact with unchecked pigs; the possible reasons have already been mentioned (Section II,D,1).

III. *Mycoplasma hyorhinis*

A. Introduction

The principal natural habitat of *M. hyorhinis* is the respiratory tract, especially the nasal cavity, of the young pig. Large numbers of organisms are commonly found on the nasal mucosa of the very young piglet, usually in association with other agents (such as the cytomegalovirus of inclusion body rhinitis and *Haemophilus parasuis*). Experimentally, *M. hyorhinis* readily colonizes the nasal mucosa of the piglet. Under certain conditions, it is found as the only apparent pathogen in cases of piglet pneumonia, but the organism is mainly found as an invader of preexisting pneumonic lesions of various types, notably EPP caused by *M. suipneumoniae*. It is likely that *M. hyorhinis* plays a primary role in some outbreaks of piglet pneumonia and in polyserositis and arthritis.

An important proclivity of *M. hyorhinis* is its special effectiveness in contaminating cell cultures throughout the world, which impinges on many aspects of biological research as well as the diagnosis of virus diseases and the production of uncontaminated virus vaccines.

B. Properties of *Mycoplasma hyorhinis*

1. Isolation and Morphology of *Mycoplasma hyorhinis* from Pigs

Mycoplasma hyorhinis usually grows well even on primary culture in a range of mycoplasma broths. In the porcine respiratory tract *M. hyorhinis* is often present with other mycoplasmas, but it usually rapidly outgrows other mycoplasma species provided cultures are passed before they become more acid than pH 6.9; this may require daily passage. *Mycoplasma hyorhinis* also grows well on many mycoplasma agars, both on primary isolation and on subculture, usually producing typical "fried egg" colonies; on *M. suipneumoniae* medium, *M. hyorhinis* produces large (up to 1 mm diameter), convex colonies, which are usually first visible at low-power magnification by the second day of incubation. Isolations may also be readily made by inoculation of tissue cultures or the yolk sac of embryonated hens' eggs. Although *M. hyorhinis* may sometimes be very difficult to isolate from tissue cultures, possible isolation difficulties with porcine field strains have received little attention. Goiš *et al.* (1975), however, found that they could not culture *M. hyorhinis* from 7 of 20 lungs that were IMF-positive. It is mentioned in Section III,C,2 that joints which are IMF-positive for *M. hyorhinis* may also be culture-negative. These findings suggest that the organisms were too fastidious to be isolated by the methods used or that the IMF-positive organisms were nonviable or possibly that the samples examined by the two methods were not identical microbiologically.

Mycoplasma hyorhinis organisms in broth can be demonstrated by the Giemsa staining of dried drops fixed in methyl alcohol. Individual organisms are seen as minute coccobacilli (0.3–0.6 μm long) with a fuzzy edge; only a few "signet rings" can be seen in comparison to numerous clear-edged, predominantly bipolar and "signet ring" forms observed in *M. suipneumoniae*.

2. *Mycoplasma hyorhinis* in Uninoculated Tissue Cultures

Since the isolation from tissue culture of the GDL strain and its identification as *M. hyorhinis* (Butler and Leach, 1964; Leach and Butler, 1966; Purcell *et al.*, 1966), there has been progressive recognition that *M. hyorhinis* is one of the major mycoplasmal contaminants of uninoculated cell cultures (Barile, 1973). Barile (1973) found that *M. hyorhinis* constituted 19% of a total of 1063 mycoplasmas isolated from cell culture, and in an extended series (Barile *et al.*, 1973) *M. hyorhinis* isolates constituted 16% of 1374 mycoplasma isolates from 9800 cell cultures examined. *Mycoplasma hyorhinis* contamination of cell cultures may be undetected because of the difficulty in isolating the organism as colonies on solid medium (Hopps *et al.*, 1973); agar media containing sera from different species might help to overcome this problem (MacMorine *et al.*, 1974). If *M. hyorhinis* infection is suspected but cannot be proved culturally, tissue cultures should be checked for the presence of abnormal enzyme systems (Section III,B,4) and by morphological and IMF methods (Barile *et al.*, 1973). (See also Volume II, Chapter 13.)

Although the origin of the *M. hyorhinis* contaminants is uncertain, Barile (1973) suggested that commercial pig trypsin, used in the preparation of cell cultures, might be the source. However, attempts to isolate *M. hyorhinis* from commercial trypsin failed (Barile and Del Giudice, 1972). Another possible source suggested by Barile (1973) is commercial bovine serum, from which he made one isolate of *M. hyorhinis;* the frequent processing of pigs and cattle through the same slaughterhouse suggests that bovine blood might be contaminated during collection by droplets originating from the nasal cavities of swine.

3. Strains of *Mycoplasma hyorhinis*

It has become progressively apparent, since Dinter *et al.* (1965) demonstrated that the GI test was unsatisfactory for the identification of *M. hyorhinis* strains, that this species includes a spectrum of organisms showing varying degrees and types of serological relationships to each other. Antibody-resistant strains have been studied by Hayflick and Stanbridge (1967), Goodwin *et al.* (1967), Dinter and Taylor-Robinson (1969), Goiš *et al.* (1974b), Goiš and Kuksa (1975), and Friis (1976b).

The GI-insensitive strains of Dinter and Taylor-Robinson (1969) grew in medium containing only 2% serum (compared with 4–10% for the sensitive strains) and at a lower pH (6.5); they were more resistant to colistin and polymyxin B. Strains studied by Goiš *et al.* (1974b), when examined by GI, MI, and latex agglutination tests, showed differences ranging from slight to profound, but all strains were rather similar in their polyacrylamide gel electrophoresis patterns. Goiš and Kuksa (1975) obtained some negative reactions by the GP test but found that all strains were interrelated to at least some extent.

Members of the WHO/FAO Working Team for Porcine Mycoplasmas (Whittlestone *et al.*, 1976), working in widely separated countries, examined the practicability of identifying field strains of *M. hyorhinis* by the DGI and MI tests using two reference antisera; we found that many field strains could not be identified by these techniques with these antisera. Preliminary attempts to identify colonies of *M. hyorhinis* by epifluorescence methods using fluorescein isothiocyanate conjugates prepared by M. F. Barile, suggested that this technique could identify a wider range of isolates.

It was suggested by Goiš *et al.* (1974b) that *M. hyorhinis* should be divided into subtypes, and support for this was provided by the work of Friis (1976b) who studied seven strains of *M. hyorhinis* from the conjunctiva and found them closely related to each other but either not related or only partially related to the reference strains by the DGI and MI tests. By other serological tests the relationship was closer. Further work will be needed to establish whether there is a subgroup of *M. hyorhinis* with the conjunctival sac as habitat.

Pijoan and Roberts (1972) showed that toluidine blue-stained antigens prepared from an antibody-sensitive and an antibody-resistant strain of *M. hyorhinis* were both bound to two stock antisera and could be identified by filter paper chromatography. This technique should be further explored for identifying a wider range of *M. hyorhinis* strains.

There are two main reference strains of *M. hyorhinis*. Strain BTS7, isolated by Switzer from the nasal cavity of a pig, is available from reference centers in Great Britain and the United States (see Section II,B,5 for addresses) as NCTC 10130 and ATCC 17981, respectively. Second, the tissue culture isolate, strain GDL (Leach and Butler, 1966), is available as NCTC 10121 and ATCC 23839.

4. Biochemical Properties and Antibiotic Sensitivity

Mycoplasma hyorhinis produces acid in glucose broth and is presumed to metabolize glucose. Friis (1974a) found that 214 of 216 strains, including strain BTS7, had phosphatase activity and that none metabolized arginine, thus amply confirming earlier findings on six *M. hyorhinis* cultures (Aluotto *et al.*, 1970). About half of Friis's cultures reduced tetrazolium, but others grew so poorly in the serum fraction medium that the results were uncertain. *Mycoplasma hyorhinis* (BTS7 strain) failed to show arginine deiminase activity (Barile *et al.*, 1966).

Various metabolic activities of *M. hyorhinis* have been detected in mycoplasma-infected cell cultures, some of which could provide a means of detecting mycoplasmal contamination. These activities include adenosine phosphorylase (Hatanaka *et al.*, 1975; Thomas *et al.*, 1977) and uridine phosphorylase (Levine, 1974). It was found by Grüneisen *et al.* (1975) that, in *M. hyorhinis*-infected cell cultures, the inhibitory effect of hydroxyurea on [³H]thymidine incorporation was lacking, but that cellular response returned to normal after the addition of the antimycoplasmal drug, tylosin. It was found by Hellung-Larsen and Frederiksen (1976) that *M. hyorhinis* infection prevented the identification of low-molecular-weight RNA components primarily by an effect on utilization of the added radioactive precursors.

The minimal inhibitory concentrations (MIC) of tetracycline hydrochloride, tiamulin, and tylosin tartrate for *M. hyorhinis* were studied by Drews *et al.* (1975). The MIC for tiamulin was about one-tenth of the MIC for the other antibiotics. The rate at which resistance against tiamulin emerged was much slower than that against tylosin tartrate. The greater sensitivity of *M. hyorhinis* to cycloserine and kanamycin, compared with that of *M. suipneumoniae*, has been mentioned in connection with isolation of the latter mycoplasma (Section II,B,1,b).

5. Miscellaneous Properties of *Mycoplasma hyorhinis*

Mycoplasma hyorhinis isolates that secreted hydrogen peroxide were pathogenic to cell and organ cultures (Pijoan, 1974a,b); colonies gave a positive methylene blue staining test which detects hydrogen peroxide secretion. The longest survival times of *M. hyorhinis* at different temperatures recorded by Friis (1974b) were 45°C for 30 min, 50°C for 5 min, and 55°C for 1 min. When *M. hyorhinis* was dried on coverslips, the titer fell from 10^5 to 10^2 during 5 days' storage in the dark at 20°–25°C; *M. hyorhinis* was isolated at 4 days but not at 8 days (Friis, 1973b). An x-ray dose of 300,000–400,000 R sterilized colostrum samples containing *M. hyorhinis* (Schimmel *et al.*, 1974).

The chromosome of *M. hyorhinis* was found by Teplitz (1977) to consist of loops of DNA which converged at a small locus or core. The average contour length was 220 μm, indicating an average molecular weight of 4.4 $\times$ 10^8. There was no evidence that RNA or protein was involved in maintaining the structural integrity of the DNA complex.

C. Experimental Diseases Caused by *Mycoplasma hyorhinis*

1. Experimental Induction of Pneumonia

Until about 1968 there had been no effective demonstration that *M. hyorhinis* was a primary pulmonary pathogen, and most workers, ourselves included, believed that *M. hyorhinis* merely played a secondary role in the production of chronic pneumonia in the fattening pig (Switzer, 1967; Goodwin *et al.*, 1968b; L'Ecuyer, 1969). In the light of more recent evidence it seems that our failure, and that of others, to demonstrate respiratory pathogenicity for *M. hyorhinis* was because older conventional pigs were exposed and the *M. hyorhinis* strains selected for study may have had low pathogenicity.

More recently, however, several strains of the organism isolated in Czechoslovakia, Denmark, Germany, and Great Britain were shown to induce pneumonia in piglets exposed via the respiratory tract (Goiš *et al.*, 1968, 1971; Gois and Valicek, 1968; Martin *et al.*, 1968; Friis, 1971b; Poland *et al.*, 1971). In the experiments of Friis (1971b), Goiš *et al.* (1971), and Poland *et al.* (1971) strains had been repeatedly cloned or passed beyond the point where mechanical carryover of some other agent was extremely unlikely.

There had been an indication in the work of Goiš *et al.* (1971) that different strains of *M. hyorhinis* may differ in virulence. To test this possibility, Goiš and Kuksa (1974b) used two strains to infect larger numbers of gnotobiotic piglets intranasally. Strain S218 caused clinical disease, pneumonic lesions, serositis, and arthritis in most of the piglets inoculated at 1 and 6 days of age; the mycoplasma also spread to nonrespiratory sites. Eight-week-old piglets inoculated with this strain did not develop clinical disease, and no gross lung lesions were found; mycoplasmas were generally recovered from the upper respiratory tract but also sometimes fron the lungs. Strain Ne 110 was much less pathogenic; clinical disease did not develop in the 24 gnotobiotic piglets inoculated at either 1 or 6 days of age. Only one piglet had slight pneumonic lesions, and in only one of the youngest piglets was there spread of *M. hyorhinis* to nonrespiratory sites. An extension of the work with the more pathogenic strain (S218), using a cloned, but pig-adapted, culture inoculated intranasally into twenty 5- to 6-day-old piglets (Goiš and Kuksa, 1974a) showed that 14 became clinically ill and developed arthritis or polyserositis and 12 had extensive pneumonic lesions containing *M. hyorhinis* at a mean titer of $10^{6.4}$. Piglets killed 7–28 days after inoculation yielded *M. hyorhinis* from the nasal cavity, tonsils, and lungs; most pigs killed at 14 and 21 days also yielded the organism from liver, spleen, kidney, blood, and joints.

The synergistic effect of *M. hyorhinis* and *Bordetella bronchiseptica* was studied by Goiš *et al.* (1977), since these organisms commonly occur together naturally. Strain S218 of *M. hyorhinis* alone induced temporary illness with lameness in two of three gnotobiotic piglets. *Bordetella bronchiseptica* alone caused rhinitis and bronchopneumonia. Five piglets inoculated with both organisms developed severe disease, and two died; severe fibrinous polyserositis, polyarthritis, and rhinitis were present in all piglets.

2. Experimental Induction of Serositis and Arthritis

Following intraperitoneal inoculation of *M. hyorhinis,* young piglets develop polyserositis and arthritis. It is likely that there are similarities between this experimental disease and natural situations in which young piglets are infected with an invasive and pathogenic strain of *M. hyorhinis.* Experimental polyserositis progresses for 10–14 days, and by 3 weeks there are pleural, pericardial, and peritoneal adhesions; thereafter piglets recover but are usually retarded (Switzer and Ross, 1975).

Experimental *M. hyorhinis* arthritis was studied by Duncan and Ross (1969, 1973), Barden and Decker (1971), Ennis *et al.* (1971), Barden *et al.* (1973), and Decker and Barden (1975) and had the following features. Proliferative arthritis, characterized by mononuclear cell infiltration, developed and there was pannus production with bone and cartilage erosion. Histologically, the condition was active for many months, but a progressively more inactive fibrotic scarring eventually developed. In Yorkshire pigs acute arthritis was most severe in the second and third months, which correlated with the time when *M. hyorhinis* could be readily isolated from the joints. After that time, the arthritis became chronic and persisted for the entire 18 months of the study (Decker and Barden, 1975). Pigs showed synovial swelling, reluctance to move, and limping. MI serum titers peaked 3 months after inoculation but remained fairly high to 11 months and were still detectable at 17 months (but not 18 months) in the one surviving pig. Synovial fluid MI titers greatly exceeded the serum titers, suggesting that antibody was produced by the synoviae. However, the organism could be recovered from a joint that contained a high level of antibody 3 months after inoculation. Hence synovial antibody *per se* does not necessarily prevent isolation of *M. hyorhinis*.

Cells producing IgG, IgM, and IgA were detected in the synoviae of affected pigs (some cells being positive for all three classes of immunoglobulins), but most of the lymphocytes did not stain specifically for IgG, IgM, or IgA. As the MI titers fell progressively over 8 months, so also the numbers of positive Ig cells declined. Although *M. hyorhinis* could not be isolated after the third month, *M. hyorhinis* antigen could be detected with a fluorescein-tagged anti-*M. hyorhinis* antiserum. The antigen was seen as amorphous deposits both free in the extracellular spaces and closely related to mononuclear cells. Antigen had virtually disappeared by the eighteenth month.

When miniature swine (Piney Woods strain) were inoculated intraperitoneally with *M. hyorhinis*, a much less protracted disease developed than in the Yorkshire pigs (Barden *et al.*, 1973). Both breeds developed a similar disease for the first month. Every infected pig developed some degree of arthritis and in the most severe cases had obvious joint swelling and lameness. The miniature pigs then gradually recovered over a period of several months, whereas the Yorkshire swine developed chronic arthritis. The reasons for the difference in reaction of the two breeds is unknown, but it was suggested that the breed with the more vigorous immunological response suffered the more severe polyarthritis. It seems that the capacity to develop the full-blown picture has a genetic origin (Decker and Barden, 1975).

D. The Natural Diseases Associated with *Mycoplasma hyorhinis*

Natural infection of the nasal cavity of pigs with *M. hyorhinis* has not been associated with any clinical disease, and only a mild lymphoid reaction in the submucosa occurs (Switzer and Ross, 1975). It was estimated by Switzer and Ross (1975) that in the United States 2–5% of piglets experience clinical serositis; the clinical disease progresses for 10–14 days and then usually resolves. Mortality is low, but pleural, pericardial, and peritoneal adhesions and arthritis develop.

In an attempt to assess the role of *M. hyorhinis* in naturally occurring arthritis in the Hanover area of Germany, Ross *et al.* (1977) cultured arthritic joints of 51 slaughtered pigs and made two isolations of the organism. No isolations were made from arthritic joints of 18 pigs submitted to a clinic. There seems to be no precise evidence for the occurrence of *M. hyorhinis* arthritis and polyserositis in other countries.

The author agrees with the view of Switzer and Ross (1975) that *M. hyorhinis* is a common secondary invader in preexisting pneumonia. We find the organism in many cases of EPP, and there is often no obvious difference in the severity of the pneumonia whether *M. hyorhinis* is present or not. However, occasional cases are encountered where there appears to be an association between severe *M. hyorhinis* infection and serositis, in addition to EPP lesions. In some naturally occurring piglet pneumonias examined by Meyling (1971), the surface of the bronchiolar epithelium was IMF-positive only for *M. hyorhinis*, indicating that *M. hyorhinis* alone might have induced the pneumonia.

E. Diagnosis of *Mycoplasma hyorhinis* Disease

The main method for the diagnosis of *M. hyorhinis* infection is isolation of the mycoplasma in broth or directly on agar, but the possibility that some tissues may contain *M. hyorhinis*, yet be culturally negative (Section III,B,1 and 2, and C,2) indicates that IMF methods should also be applied when appropriate. Isolates suspected to be *M. hyorhinis* on the basis of their biological characteristics should be identified serologically, preferably by an IMF method since the absence of positive reactions by the MI or DGI test does not exclude *M. hyorhinis* (Section III,B,3); if negative results are obtained by the latter tests, the use of a range of antisera to various *M. hyorhinis* strains improves the chances of a correct diagnosis. Serum antibodies detectable by CF, MI, and latex agglutination develop during *M. hyorhinis* infection; CF and MI antibodies may persist up to 6 months after inoculation (Switzer and Ross, 1975; Barden and Decker, 1971; Goiš *et al.*, 1972; Ross *et al.*, 1973; Pijoan and Boughton, 1974). Rises in serum antibodies are apparently not being used for diagnosis of *M. hyorhinis* disease.

F. Immunity to *Mycoplasma hyorhinis* Infection

The demonstration by Goiš *et al.* (1974a) that intraperitoneal inoculation of hyperimmune pig serum (or the IgG or IgM fraction) protected gnotobiotic piglets from the dissemination of *M. hyorhinis* infection to parenchymatous organs and joints suggested that in the future a vaccine might give some protection against this type of infection. Under natural conditions it is likely that piglets are partially protected by colostral antibody, but direct evidence seems to be lacking.

IV. *Mycoplasma hyosynoviae*

A. Introduction

Workers in three countries reported almost simultaneously the isolation of arginine-metabolizing mycoplasmas from pigs (Friis, 1970; Roberts and Goiš, 1970; Goiš and Taylor-Robinson, 1970; Ross and Karmon, 1970). All the isolates have proved to be the same species, and the name *M. hyosynoviae* proposed by Ross and Karmon has been adopted in preference to other proposals *(Mycoplasma suidaniae* and *Mycoplasma hyoarginini). Mycoplasma hyosynoviae* commonly inhabits the nasal cavity and pharynx of pigs and is a recognized cause of arthritis in growing pigs.

B. Properties of *Mycoplasma hyosynoviae*

1. Isolation of *Mycoplasma hyosynoviae*

The primary isolation of *M. hyosynoviae* is best accomplished in broth medium (Farrington and Switzer, 1976), the medium of choice being that of Ross and Karmon (1970) which contains mucin and turkey serum. After primary isolation, the organism can be cultivated on agar medium on which it produces colonies with a typical "fried egg" morphology, usually with a very prominent central area. Friis (1974a) used a modified Hayflick medium enriched with arginine and mucin, with equal parts of horse and pig serum. For solid medium, Friis employed 0.8% agar (Oxoid).

2. Characteristics of *Mycoplasma hyosynoviae*

The main characteristics of *M. hyosynoviae,* as summarized by Switzer and Ross (1975), are development of a granular deposit in broth, growth stimulated by swine gastric mucin or yeast autolysate but no growth stimulation by agitation, growth throughout the full depth of stab cultures and utilization of arginine, but no tetrazolium or methylene blue reduction in less than 48 hr. Microscopic examination revealed typical mycoplasmal organisms 0.3–0.6 μm in diameter, but spherical bodies 5–15 μm were seen in Giemsa-stained preparations.

The longest survival times of *M. hyosynoviae* at different temperatures recorded by Friis (1974b) were 45°C, 30 min; 50°C, 5 min; 55° and 60°C, 1 min. The resistance of *M. hyosynoviae* to drying was assessed by Friis (1973b) by allowing drops of a broth culture to dry on cover slips, storing them in the dark at room temperature (20°–25°C), and then culturing the cover slips in broth. *Mycoplasma hyosynoviae* survived considerably longer than *M. suipneumoniae* or *M. hyorhinis,* viable organisms being detected up to 32 days but not at 40 days.

3. Strains of *Mycoplasma hyosynoviae*

Although different *M. hyosynoviae* isolates (from England, the United States, and Denmark) were found to have close similarities, Goĭš and Taylor-Robinson (1972) found that the MI titers obtained showed more than a 10-fold difference when different isolates were tested against antiserum to strain A40. The strains compared by Ross *et al.* (1978) showed greater differences: homologous MI titers ranged from about 2000 to $>10^6$, but with heterologous strains the range was very wide, i.e., <2 to $>10^6$. One strain (3222) was particularly sensitive to antibody and had the greatest tendency to become nonviable during culture. By the DGI test, strains of Ross *et al.* (1978) also showed some serological heterogeneity. although all were inhibited to varying extents by antisera prepared against four of the strains. Antiserum against strain 3222 reacted well against homologous cultures and one other strain but failed to produce inhibition zones against the other cultures. By the direct epi-IMF technique applied to colonies, strains examined by Ross *et al.* (1978) gave rather close cross-reactions. Colonies were usually stained specifically by antiserum diluted 1:4 to 1:64, but heterologous reactions occurred below dilutions of 1:4. A very weak IMF reaction with S16 antiserum was found by Zimmermann (1976) when testing isolates from the tonsil, lung, and joint of a pig with arthritis. Thus none of these specific tests alone could be used with reliability to identify all field isolates of *M. hyosynoviae,* but the direct IMF test applied to colonies appeared to be most reliable.

By flat-gel polyacrylamide electrophoresis, the patterns shown by strains of *M. hyosynoviae* varied to some extent according to the strain and length of culture incubation (Wreghitt *et al.*, 1974). The strains similarly examined by Ross *et al.* (1978) gave electropherograms each with the same number and spacing of peaks.

The S16 strain of *M. hyosynoviae* is available from the United Kingdom and United States reference centers (see Section II,B,5) as NCTC 10167 and ATCC 25591, respectively.

C. Arthritis and *Mycoplasma hyosynoviae*

The information available to 1973 on arthritis caused by *M. hyosynoviae* has been reviewed by Switzer and Ross (1975); these investigators and their colleagues have contributed the greater part of the knowledge on this condition. Affected pigs are usually of 75- to 250-lb body weight; they suffer a sudden onset of acute lameness which persists for 3–10 days, which is usually followed by gradual improvement. Some pigs become progressively more lame and may be unable to rise. The arthritis in such pigs is an uncomplicated nonsuppurative arthritis involving (in order of frequency) the stifle, shoulder, elbow and hock joints. There is no polyserositis. The distension of the stifle joint is difficult to detect because of the mass of muscle in the region. Affected joints contain a yellowish-brown fluid, sometimes with flakes of fibrin present. The synovial membrane becomes yellowish and develops a velvetlike texture. In outbreaks in the United States the articular surface usually remains normal, but in the United Kingdom outbreak reported by Roberts *et al.* (1972) some pigs had erosions of the articular cartilage in the stifle joints.

The natural history of *M. hyosynoviae* infection was reviewed by Ross (1973a) and Ross and Spear (1973). Arthritic disease often occurred after new breeding stock had entered the herd, suggesting that the adult can be a carrier of the organism. *Mycoplasma hyosynoviae* was in fact found to be extremely common in pharyngeal secretions from adult pigs and from pigs convalescing after an attack of arthritis. Such pigs were probably the major reserve of infection. Once the disease occurred, it continually recurred in the herd in successive crops of pigs. *Mycoplasma hyosynoviae* was isolated from the tonsils and pharyngeal secretions of more than half the adult females, but nasal secretions contained the organism less frequently and intermittently. Surprisingly, piglets 1–6 weeks old that were suckling infected sows rarely had infected pharyngeal secretions, but *M. hyosynoviae* isolations became increasingly common as piglets became older. Separating 4- to 5-week-old noninfected piglets from their infected mothers was found to be a relatively effective method of deriving small groups of *M. hyosynoviae*-free pigs. Generally pigs first showed pharyngeal infection at 6–8 weeks of age. Pigs infected before they were 10 weeks old were apparently either subclinically affected or experienced mild disease, whereas 3- to 6-month-old pigs tended to develop arthritis (Ross, 1973a; Ross and Spear, 1973).

Cultures of *M. hyosynoviae* do not readily produce arthritis. A cloned culture inoculated intravenously into 10-week-old pigs at a dose of 2×10^{10} organism did not induce arthritis, but the organism was recovered from various joints and other sites (Furlong and Turner, 1975b). A cloned, but pig-adapted, culture inoculated intranasally into gnotobiotic piglets by Gois and Kuksa (1974a) was subsequently isolated from various organs but not from the joints. Ross *et al.* (1971) and Ross (1973b) reported that cultured organisms grown in an improved medium induced arthritis when inoculated intravenously and intranasally. There is also evidence that some strains are invasive and more likely to produce arthritis (Ross, 1973b).

During experimentally induced arthritis disease, *M. hyosynoviae* could be recovered from affected joints, blood, lymphoid tissues, and mucosal secretions. During the early stages of *M. hyosynoviae* infection, the organism was shed in vaginal, lachrymal, and preputial secretions, as well as in pharyngeal and nasal secretions (Ross *et al.*, 1971). However, after recovery from arthritis, the organism was generally found only in nasopharyngeal secretions.

There have been few surveys based on an overall assessment of the importance of *M. hyosynoviae* arthritis. In contrast to the frequent reports by workers in the United States, there are only sporadic reports of this type of arthritis occurring in other parts of the world. In the Hanover area of Germany, Ross *et al.* (1977) made one isolate of *M. hyosynoviae* from 72 joints cultured from 51 slaughtered pigs, but none from the arthritic joints of 18 pigs submitted to a clinic.

D. Diagnosis of *Mycoplasma hyosynoviae* Arthritis

Switzer and Ross (1975) suggested that a presumptive diagnosis of *M. hyosynoviae* may be based on the age of the group affected (3–6 months), the presence of serofibrinous polyarthritis (without polyserositis) and of a febrile reaction, and the typical appearance of joint lesions; the diagnosis must be verified by the isolation of *M. hyosynoviae* from arthritic joints during the acute stage of the disease, i.e., within the first 7 days. Preliminary identification of *M. hyosynoviae* is made on the basis of the following characteristics: growth with an alkaline pH shift in arginine broth medium, no acid shift in glucose medium, growth stimulation by swine gastric mucin or yeast autolysate, the development of colonies with a conspicuous central portion, and the presence of a distinct film-and-spots reaction (Switzer and Ross, 1975; Farrington and Switzer, 1976). The isolate should be identified serologically by means of DGI, MI, or IMF methods.

During *M. hyosynoviae* infection, pigs develop CF serum antibodies. However, the demonstration of a rising CF serum antibody titer alone, while suggestive of infection, is not diagnostic for joint disease, since nonarthritic infections with the organism are common. CF serum antibody has been detected in pigs experimentally infected with *M. hyosynoviae* 9–10 days previously (Ross, 1973a), and was found frequently in sows with chronic infections and in their piglets (up to 4 weeks old) (Ross and Spear, 1973). Presumably the antibody in the piglets had been passively transferred in the colostrum. Serum antibody (presumably actively induced) was detected in the sera of piglets aged 7, 8, and 12 weeks. There is a suggestion (Ross and Spear, 1973) that low levels of CF antibody to *M. hyosynoviae* may occur in swine not infected with, nor even exposed to, *M. hyosynoviae*. The test may not therefore be completely specific.

Although MI antibodies to *M. hyosynoviae* can be detected in the sera of hyperimmune rabbits, the initial attempts by Zimmermann and Ross (1977) to demonstrate MI antibodies in the sera of previously infected pigs failed. Very low MI titers were sometimes detected after supplementation with 6% unheated guinea pig serum alone, but additional supplements of 1% unheated rabbit serum gave higher MI titers. For example, serial serum samples taken from one pig gave low MI titers (1:16 to 1:32) in the 6- to 34-week specimens when the tests were performed in medium without rabbit serum; supplements of rabbit serum resulted in MI titers of 1:256 or higher (for the period of 9 days to 34 weeks), with a peak titer of 1:8192 recorded on days 12, 15, and 21.

V. *Mycoplasma flocculare*

Mycoplasma flocculare was first isolated in Denmark (Friis, 1972). The evidence of Meyling and Friis (1972) that this was a new *Mycoplasma* species has been extended and confirmed by N. F. Friis and P. Whittlestone (unpublished observation, 1978). Recently, this organism has also been isolated from British pigs (P. Whittlestone and R. F. W. Goodwin, unpublished observation, 1977). Since 1972, Friis (1976a) has made 99 isolates from pigs of all ages, 47 being from lung tissue and 52 from nasal cavities. Our United Kingdom isolates were from pneumonic lungs which were generally free of EPP. *Mycoplasma flocculare* is similar to *M. suipneumoniae* in its fastidiousness, slow acid production, reluctance to colonize on agar, and colonial morphology. *Mycoplasma flocculare* can be isolated in *M. suipneumoniae* broth (Section II,B,1) but grows even more slowly than the latter organism (Friis, 1975, 1976a; P. Whittlestone, unpublished observation, 1978). Methods of recovery, passage routine, and incubation requirements are similar to those employed in the recovery of *M. suipneumoniae*. The origin of both species from the same habitat, together with their biological similarities, stresses the importance of specific methods of identification. The MI test is probably the method of choice for this purpose. The DGI test is also satisfactory if the organism can be grown on agar. The author prefers the solid medium developed by Friis (1975), which utilizes agarose. *Mycoplasma flocculare* does not colonize on inferior media and seems to be particularly sensitive to toxic factors (P. Whittlestone, unpublished observation, 1978). Friis (1977) found that strains could be identified by the GP test, but laboratory strains tended to produce slight cross-reactions with *M. suipneumoniae* antiserum when plates were incubated for longer periods than recommended. Friis also noted that the two species cross-reacted substantially in the double immunodiffusion test, which suggested some shared antigens or the presence of antimedium antibodies in the antisera.

Piglets have been experimentally exposed to aerosols of *M. flocculare* (Friis, 1973a, 1974c). At sacrifice, 3 of 15 piglets had small pneumonic lesions in which the bronchial tree and a few alveoli showed slight mononuclear and polymorphonuclear cell accumulations. There were no gross lesions in the nasal cavities, but the nasal mucosa showed mononuclear cell accumulations and damage to the surface epithelium. These changes, which persisted to 59 days in the mucosa, were associated with high titers (10^6 or 10^7) of the organism. The brain was infected in some animals, and in one animal the pleural and pericardial cavities were infected (Friis, 1976a). The role of *M. flocculare* in the pneumonic complex of the pig is uncertain, but in Denmark infections with this mycoplasma in SPF pig herds are not associated with clinical outbreaks of pneumonia (Friis, 1976a).

The Ms 42 strain of *M. flocculare* is available from the United Kingdom and United States reference centers (see Section II,B,5) as NCTC 10143 and ATCC 27399, respectively.

VI. *Mycoplasma sualvi*

A newly recognized mycoplasma has recently been isolated from rectal swabs (Gourlay and Wyld, 1976), colon, small intestine, and vagina of pigs (Gourlay *et al.*, 1978). The name *M. sualvi* has been proposed, the Mayfield strain (clone B) has been designated the type strain and a culture deposited in the United Kingdom reference center as NCTC 10170 (Gourlay *et al.*, 1978). In its cultural and biochemical characteristics *M. sualvi* closely resembles *M. alvi,* an organism recently isolated from bovine intestinal and urogenital tracts (Gourlay *et al.*, 1977). The main features of *M. sualvi,* as described by Gourlay *et al.* (1978), in addition to those used to characterize the organism as a mycoplasma, are metabolism of glucose and arginine (in arginine broth, after an initial acid shift to pH 5.5 in 3–6 days, the medium returned to its original neutral pH of 7.0 after 2–3 weeks' incubation); better growth at 37°C than at 30°C; no pH change at 25°C; colony growth both aerobically and anaerobically, the largest colonies forming anaerobically with 10% added carbon dioxide; no utilization of urea or reduction of tetrazolium; a G + C content of the DNA of 23.7 mole %; cells coccobacillary by light microscopy; by electron microscopy, shadowed preparations showed flask- or club-shaped bodies; and in thin sections terminal structures but without a central core were visible. *Mycoplasma sualvi* was distinct by the DGI, MI, and IMF tests from 11 recognized mycoplasma and acholeplasma species previously isolated from pigs, namely, *M. hyorhinis, M. hyosynoviae, M. flocculare, M. suipneumoniae, M. arginini, M. bovigenitalium, M. buccale, Acholeplasma granularum, A. laidlawii, A. axanthum,* and *A. oculi,* as well as from the mycoplasmas also known to possess terminal structures *(M. alvi, M. pneumoniae,* and *M. gallisepticum)* and was also distinct from those metabolizing both glucose and arginine *(M. capricolum, M. fermentans,* and *M. moatsii).* Antiserum to 36 other mycoplasma species also gave negative results by the MI test.

The pathological significance of *M. sualvi* is unknown.

VII. *Acholeplasma granularum*

Several years ago *A. granularum* was said to be a cause of porcine polyarthritis, but the strains responsible for arthritis were not adequately identified. The situation was clarified by Ross and Karmon (1970), who showed that their arthritis-inducing isolates (now named *M. hyosynoviae*) were electrophoretically and serologically distinct from recognized strains of *A. granularum* known at the time, including the BTS39 strain isolated from swine nasal secretions by W. P. Switzer and characterized by Tully and Razin (1968) and the Friend strain recovered from a murine leukemia cell line (Tully, 1966). Since this clarification there have been no further claims that *A. granularum* is involved in porcine arthritis.

Porcine isolates of *A. granularum* have been reported most commonly from the nasal cavity (Goĭš *et al.*, 1969), pneumonic lungs (Goĭš *et al.*,

1969; Bannerman and Nicolet, 1971; Truszczynski and Pilaszek, 1974), puerperal metritis in sows (Draghici and Seiciu, 1973), and feces (Roberts and Little, 1976). Isolates related to *A. granularum* were made from pharyngeal secretions of sows by Ross and Spear (1973). Experimental infections of piglets via the respiratory tract provided no evidence of pathogenicity (Jericho *et al.*, 1971; Goiš and Kuksa, 1974a) and, even after intranasal inoculation into very young gnotobiotic pigs, the organism could not be recovered 7–14 days later (Goiš and Kuksa, 1974a).

The special features of *A. granularum* are described in Volume I, Chapter 16.

VIII. *Acholeplasma laidlawii*

Porcine isolates of *A. laidlawii* have been reported from the nasal cavity and lung (Goiš *et al.*, 1969), vagina and uterus (Bannerman and Nicolet, 1971), puerperal metritis (Draghici and Seiciu, 1973), pneumonic lung (Truszczynski and Pilaszek, 1974), and pharyngeal secretions of sows (Ross and Spear, 1973).

There is conflicting evidence about the pathogenicity of *A. laidlawii* for pigs. On the one hand, the isolates of Martin *et al.* (1968) appeared to be pathogenic alone, and Dzu *et al.* (1971) demonstrated pathogenicity for *A. laidlawii* in combination with *Pasteurella multocida*. It was suggested by Stipkovits *et al.* (1973a) that the pathogenicity of these isolates might correlate with the differences they found (compared with the reference strains) in their esculin-hydrolyzing and cellobiose-decomposing ability. On the other hand, there has never been any clear demonstration between the presence of *A. laidlawii* and any disease syndrome. Moreover, no evidence for a serological response (MI) was found in pigs having *A. laidlawii* in the respiratory tract (Goiš *et al.*, 1969). It was suggested by Ross (1973b) that the sporadic isolation of acholeplasmas from pigs involved exposure to the organisms in natural environments, as demonstrated by the recovery of acholeplasmas from pigpen drains.

The special features of *A. laidlawii* are described in Volume I, Chapter 16.

IX. OTHER MYCOPLASMAS ISOLATED FROM THE PIG

Several other mycoplasmas have been isolated on infrequent occasions from the pig, and there is insufficient information to judge whether they are more than chance isolations or have any pathological significance.

Some reported isolates have never been clearly characterized as myco-plasmas (Moore *et al.*, 1966a,b). Occasional isolates normally found in species other than the pig include *M. arginini* from lungs (Gois *et al.*, 1975; Galli and Leach, 1976) and from the nasal mucosa and pharynx of pigs (and from swine sewage) (Orning *et al.*, 1978), *M. bovigenitalium* from boar semen (Goiš *et al.*, 1973), *M. buccale* (formerly *M. orale* 2) from the nasal cavity of pigs (Kuksa and Goiš, 1975; M. Goiš, personal communication, 1976), *M. gallinarum* (strain B2) (Dinter *et al.*, 1965; Taylor-Robinson and Dinter, 1968), *M. iners* (strain B6) (Dinter *et al.*, 1965; Taylor-Robinson and Dinter, 1968), *M. mycoides* subsp. *mycoides* (strain B3) (Dinter *et al.*, 1965; Tully and Razin, 1968). *M. salivarium* (Friis, 1971a), *A. axanthum* (Stipkovits *et al.*, 1973b), *A. oculi* (*A. oculusi*) (Kuksa and Goiš, 1975), and *Ureaplasma* spp. (L. Stipkovits, personal communication, 1976).

The pathogenicity of *A. axanthum* for pigs was tested by Stipkovits *et al.* (1974); intranasal inoculation of a lung suspension containing the mycoplasma caused clinical respiratory disease, including gross pneumo-nia as well as a serological response. A cloned broth culture of *A. axan-thum* produced slight but similar lesions. It has been suggested by Stip-kovits (personal communication, 1976) that pigs may sometimes acquire this organism from geese, in which it is very common. More evidence is needed to know whether *A. axanthum* is a natural pig pathogen.

In cases where there has been only a single isolate of an unusual mycoplasma, the possibility of laboratory pickup must be considered. In other cases, only further work will reveal how frequently particular mycoplasmas inhabit pig tissues, how long they remain there, and whether they are commensals or pathogens.

X. FUTURE OUTLOOK WITH PORCINE MYCOPLASMAS

EPP is so widespread and causes so much economic loss that the long-term aim should be eradication of the disease, first from specific regions and then from countries. The question of whether this will be feasible, even given all possible resources, remains unanswered. Al-though the pig is the only known host of *M. suipneumoniae,* attempts to isolate the organism from other hosts have been few and inadequate, and any of the negative results obtained could reflect the insensitivity of current cultural methods. Until smaller numbers of wild-type *M. sui-pneumoniae* organisms can be cultured more readily by more workers, the necessary data on other possible hosts and on the dissemination of *M. suipneumoniae* will not emerge. Such work might lead to an understanding of the current high breakdown rate of EPP-free herds, since most breakdowns occur without any known contact with possibly infected pigs. However, we have no real assurance that such breakdowns do not originate within the herd. The possibility that herds may be subclinically infected for long periods before developing clinical disease makes it urgently necessary to develop more sensitive methods of serological diagnosis along the lines being explored by the Swiss workers.

Until the eradication is achieved, the marketing of an economical drug effective *in vivo* against *M. suipneumoniae* would be of great benefit. If such a drug could eradicate the organism from even small groups of pigs, substantial economic benefit would be realized because of the high cost of present methods for producing a new nucleus of EPP-free pigs.

An effective and inexpensive vaccine for EPP is also needed. There are no apparent prospects that a killed vaccine will be marketed in the near future, in view of the inadequate level of protection afforded by experimental vaccines and the high cost of growing an adequate antigen dose. A breakthrough might come from a different approach; work on other mycoplasmal respiratory diseases suggests that administration of antigen via the respiratory tract or the use of temperature-sensitive mutants as vaccines should be explored.

The pathogenic significance of *M. hyorhinis* under natural conditions deserves further study, since it is difficult to relate the findings of the experimental studies in the very sensitive colostrum-deprived gnotobiotic piglet to the situation in the field. Studies are needed on herds previously free from *M. hyorhinis* to see which disease syndromes follow the introduction of this organism alone or whether other agents act synergistically with *M. hyorhinis* to produce the disease syndromes from which this mycoplasma is commonly isolated. Experimental studies with *M. hyorhinis* in gnotobiotic piglets have been important in revealing strains with striking differences in pathogenicity. These strains could be used to try to identify pathogenicity markers *in vitro;* such studies could be of both fundamental and practical significance.

The main importance of *M. flocculare* appears to be in the confusion it may cause in the diagnosis of *M. suipneumoniae* infection, because of the close biological similarity of these two organisms isolated from the same habitat. Only two laboratories have reported the isolation of *M. flocculare,* and very few workers have grown even adapted cultures, so there is a paucity of information on its worldwide significance.

Similarly little information is available on *M. hyosynoviae;* although this organism is relatively easy to cultivate, it is likely that few laboratories use cultural techniques suitable for its isolation, so that data on its overall significance are not emerging.

In view of the major worldwide significance of porcine mycoplasmal infections it is surprising that so few groups of workers are able to diagnose specifically the important conditions. This situation may be rectified in the long term by the development of simpler and less subjective diagnostic methods; in the short term, however, it seems that the maximum impact on porcine mycoplasmal diseases would be produced by a more effective dissemination of the available information so that more relevant work will be encouraged.

REFERENCES

Adegboye, D. S. (1975). Ph.D. Thesis, Cambridge Univ., Cambridge, England.
Aluotto, B. B., Wittler, R. G., Williams, C. O., and Faber, J. E. (1970). *Int. J. Syst. Bacteriol.* **20,** 35–58.
Bannerman, E. S. N., and Nicolet, J. (1971). *Schweiz. Arch. Tierheilkd.* **113,** 697–710.
Barden, J. A., and Decker, J. L. (1971). *Arthritis Rheum.* **14,** 193–201.
Barden, J. A., Decker, J. L., Dalgard, D. W., and Aptekar, R. G. (1973). *Infect. Immun.* **8,** 887–890.
Barile, M. F. (1973). *In* "Contamination in Tissue Culture" (J. Fogh, ed.), pp. 131–172. Academic Press, New York.
Barile, M. F., and Del Giudice, R. A. (1972). *Pathogenic Mycoplasmas, Ciba Found. Symp.* pp. 165–185.
Barile, M. F., Schimke, R. T., and Riggs, D. B. (1966). *J. Bacteriol.* **91,** 189–192.
Barile, M. F., Hopps, H. E., Grabowski, M. W., Riggs, D. B., and Del Giudice, R. A. (1973). *Ann. N.Y. Acad. Sci.* **225,** 251–264.
Baskerville, A. (1972). *Res. Vet. Sci.* **13,** 570–578.
Baskerville, A., and Wright, C. L. (1973). *Res. Vet. Sci.* **14,** 155–160.
Bertschinger, H. U., Keller, H., Löhrer, A., and Wegmann, W. (1972). *Schweiz. Arch. Tierheilkd.* **114,** 107–116.
Betts, A. O., and Campbell, R. C. (1956). *J. Comp. Pathol. Ther.* **66,** 89–101.
Betts, A. O., and Whittlestone, P. (1963). *Res. Vet. Sci.* **4,** 471–479.
Blackburn, B. O., Wright, H. S., and Ellis, E. M. (1975). *Am. J. Vet. Res.* **36,** 1381–1382.
Braude, R., and Plonka, S. (1975). *Vet. Rec.* **96,** 359–360.
Bruggmann, S. (1978). *Zentralbl. Bakteriol., Parasitenkd., Infektionskr. Hyg., Abt. 1: Orig., Reihe A:* **241,** 245.
Bruggmann, S., Keller, H., Bertschinger, H. U., and Engberg, B. (1976). *Vet. Rec.* **99,** 101.
Bruggmann, S., Engberg, B., and Ehrensperger, F. (1977a). *Vet. Rec.* **101,** 137.
Bruggmann, S., Keller, H., Bertschinger, H. U., and Engberg, B. (1977b). *Vet. Rec.* **101,** 109–111.
Butler, M., and Leach, R. H. (1964). *J. Gen. Microbiol.* **34,** 285–294.
Decker, J. L., and Barden, J. A. (1975). *Rheumatology* **6,** 338–345.
Dinter, Z., and Taylor-Robinson, D. (1969). *J. Gen. Microbiol.* **57,** 263–272.
Dinter, Z., Danielsson, D., and Bakos, K. (1965). *J. Gen. Microbiol.* **41,** 77–84.
Draghici, D., and Seiciu, F. (1973). *Arch. Vet.* **10,** 17–26.
Drews, J., Georgopoulos, A., Laber, G., Schütze, E., and Unger, J. (1975). *Antimicrob. Agents Chemother.* **7,** 507–516.
Duncan, J. R., and Ross, R. F. (1969). *Am. J. Pathol.* **57,** 171–186.

Duncan, J. R., and Ross, R. F. (1973). *Am. J. Vet. Res.* **34**, 363–366.
Durisic, S., Knezevic, N., Markovic, S. B., Tunyogi, B. S., Maksimovic, A., and Lazic, S. (1974). *Vet. Glas.* **28**, 543–549.
Durisic, S., Knezevic, N., Markovic, B., Maksimovic, A., and Visacki, J. (1975). *Acta Vet. (Belgrade)* **25**, 189–194.
Dzu, N. M., Pustovar, A., Bathke, W., Hubrig, T., Krausse, H., and Schimmel, D. (1971). *Monatsh. Veterinaermed.* **26**, 169–181.
Ennis, R. S., Dalgard, D., Willerson, J. T., Barden, J. A., and Decker, J. L. (1971). *Arthritis Rheum.* **14**, 202–211.
Farrington, D. O. (1976). *Proc. Int. Pig Vet. Soc. Congr., Ames, Iowa,* U.S.A. PP4.
Farrington, D. O., and Switzer, W. P. (1976). *In* "Laboratory Diagnosis of Mycoplasmosis in Food Animals," Special Report of the Mycoplasmosis Committee (O. H. V. Stalheim, ed.), pp. 72–88. Am. Assoc. Vet. Lab. Diagnosticians, Madison, Wisconsin.
Friis, N. F. (1970). *Acta Vet. Scand.* **11**, 487–490.
Friis, N. F. (1971a). *Acta Vet. Scand.* **12**, 69–79.
Friis, N. F. (1971b). *Acta Vet. Scand.* **12**, 116–119.
Friis, N. F. (1971c). *Acta Vet. Scand.* **12**, 120–121.
Friis, N. F. (1971d). *Acta Vet. Scand.* **12**, 454–456.
Friis, N. F. (1972). *Acta Vet. Scand.* **13**, 284–286.
Friis, N. F. (1973a). *Acta Vet. Scand.* **14**, 344–346.
Friis, N. F. (1973b). *Acta Vet. Scand.* **14**, 489–491.
Friis, N. F. (1974a). Ph.D. Thesis, Royal Vet. Agric. Univ., Copenhagen.
Friis, N. F. (1974b). *Acta Vet. Scand.* **15**, 283–285.
Friis, N. F. (1974c). *Acta Vet. Scand.* **15**, 507–518.
Friis, N. F. (1975). *Nord. Vet. Med.* **27**, 337–339.
Friis, N. F. (1976a). *Proc. Int. Pig Vet. Soc. Congr., Ames, Iowa* PP 15.
Friis, N. F. (1976b). *Acta Vet. Scand.* **17**, 343–353.
Friis, N. F. (1977). *Acta Vet. Scand.* **18**, 168–175.
Furlong, S. L., and Turner, A. J. (1975a). *Aust. Vet. J.* **51**, 28–31.
Furlong, S. L., and Turner, A. J. (1975b). *Aust. Vet. J.* **51**, 291–293.
Galli, G., and Leach, R. H. (1976). *Clin. Vet.* **99**, 597–598.
Giger, T., Bruggmann, S., and Nicolet, J. (1977). *Schweiz. Arch. Tierheilkd.* **119**, 125–134.
Glawischnig, E., and Steininger, K. (1976). *Proc. Int. Pig Vet. Soc. Congr. Ames, Iowa* PP2.
Goiš, M., and Kuksa, F. (1974a). *Colloq. INSERM, Mycoplasmes Homme, Anim., Veg. Insectes, Congr. Int., Bordeaux* **33**, 341–348.
Goiš, M., and Kuksa, F. (1974b). *Zentralbl. Veterinaermed., Reihe B* **21**, 352-361.
Goiš, M., and Kuksa, F. (1975). *Zentralbl. Veterinaermed., Reihe B* **22**, 850–855.
Goiš, M., and Taylor-Robinson, D. (1970). *Proc. Conf. Taxonomy Bacteria Mycoplasmas, 10th, Brno* Part 2, p. 18.
Goiš, M., and Taylor-Robinson, D. (1972). *J. Med. Microbiol.* **5**, 47–54.
Goiš, M., and Valicek, L. (1968). *Doc. Vet.* **7**, 81–88.
Goiš, M., Valicek, L., and Sovadina, M. (1968). *Zentralbl. Veterinaermed., Reihe B* **15**, 230–240.
Goiš, M., Cerny, M., Rozkosny, V., and Sovadina, M. (1969). *Zentralbl. Veterinaermed., Reihe B* **16**, 253–265.
Goiš, M., Pospisil, Z., Cerny, M., and Mrva, V. (1971). *J. Comp. Pathol.* **81**, 401–410.
Goiš, M., Franz, J., Kuksa, F., Pokorny, J., and Cerny, M. (1972). *Zentralbl. Veterinaermed. Reihe B* **19**, 379–390.
Goiš, M., Kuksa, F., and Franz, J. (1973). *Vet. Rec.* **93**, 47–48.

Goiš, M., Kuksa, F., and Franz, J. (1974a). *Zentralbl. Veterinaermed., Reihe B* **21**, 176–187.
Goiš, M., Kuksa, F., Franz, J., and Taylor-Robinson, D. (1974b). *J. Med. Microbiol.* **7**, 105–115.
Goiš, M., Sisak, F., Kuksa, F., and Sovadina, M. (1975). *Zentralbl. Veterinaermed., Reihe B* **22**, 205–219.
Goiš, M., Kuksa, F., and Sisak, F. (1977). *Zentralbl. Veterinaermed., Reihe B* **24**, 89–96.
Goodwin, R. F. W. (1965). *Vet. Rec.* **77**, 383–387.
Goodwin, R. F. W. (1971). *Vet. Rec.* **89**, 77–81.
Goodwin, R. F. W. (1973). *Br. Vet. J.* **129**, 465–470.
Goodwin, R. F. W. (1976). *Vet. Rec.* **98**, 260–261.
Goodwin, R. F. W. (1977). *Vet. Rec.* **101**, 419–421.
Goodwin, R. F. W., and Hurrell, J. M. W. (1970). *J. Hyg.* **68**, 313–325.
Goodwin, R. F. W., and Whittlestone, P. (1960). *Vet. Rec.* **72**, 1029–1054.
Goodwin, R. F. W., and Whittlestone, P. (1963). *Brit. J. Exp. Pathol.* **44**, 291–299.
Goodwin, R. F. W., and Whittlestone, P. (1964). *Vet Rec.* **76**, 611–613.
Goodwin, R. F. W., and Whittlestone, P. (1966). *Brit. J. Exp. Pathol.* **47**, 518–524.
Goodwin, R. F. W., and Whittlestone, P. (1967). *Vet. Rec.* **81**, 643–647.
Goodwin, R. F. W., and Whittlestone, P. (1973). *Br. Vet. J.* **129**, 456–464.
Goodwin, R. F. W., Pomeroy, A. P., and Whittlestone, P. (1965). *Vet. Rec.* **77**, 1247–1249.
Goodwin, R. F. W., Pomeroy, A. P., and Whittlestone, P. (1967). *J. Hyg.* **65**, 85–96.
Goodwin, R. F. W., Hurrell, J. M. W., and Whittlestone, P. (1968a). *Br. J. Exp. Pathol.* **49**, 431–435.
Goodwin, R. F. W., Pomeroy, A. P., and Whittlestone, P. (1968b). *J. Hyg.* **66**, 595–603.
Goodwin, R. F. W., Hodgson, R. G., Whittlestone, P., and Woodhams, R. L. (1969). *J. Hyg.* **67**, 193–208.
Gourlay, R. N., and Wyld, S. G. (1976). *Br. Vet. J.* **132**, 652–653.
Gourlay, R. N., Wyld, S. G., and Leach, R. H. (1977). *Int. J. Syst. Bacteriol.* **27**, 86–96.
Gourlay, R. N., Wyld, S. G., and Leach, R. H. (1978). *Int. J. Syst. Bacteriol.*, **28**, 289–292.
Grüneisen, A., Rajewsky, M. F., Remmer, I., and Uschkoreit, J. (1975). *Exp. Cell Res.* **90**, 365–373.
Hamm, D., Reynolds, W. A., Szanto, J., and Maplesden, D. C. (1976). *Proc. Int. Pig Vet. Soc. Congr., Ames, Iowa* PP3.
Hatanaka, M., Del Giudice, R., and Long, C. (1975). *Proc. Natl. Acad. Sci. U.S.A.* **72**, 1401–1405.
Hayflick, L., and Stanbridge, E. (1967). *Ann. N.Y. Acad. Sci.* **143**, 608–621.
Hellung-Larsen, P., and Frederiksen, S. (1976). *Exp. Cell Res.* **99**, 295–300.
Hodges, R. T., and Betts, A. O. (1969a). *Vet. Rec.* **85**, 452–455.
Hodges, R. T., and Betts, A. O. (1969b). *Vet. Rec.* **85**, 455–458.
Hogg, A., Stair, E. L., and Underdahl, N. R. (1976). *Proc. Int. Pig Vet. Soc. Congr., Ames, Iowa* PP5.
Holmgren, N. (1974a). Ph.D. Thesis, Univ. of Stockholm, Stockholm.
Holmgren, N. (1974b). *Res. Vet. Sci.* **17**, 145–153.
Holmgren, N. (1974c). *Res. Vet. Sci.* **16**, 341–346.
Holmgren, N. (1974d). *Zentralbl. Veterinaermed., Reihe B* **21**, 131–137.
Hopps, H. E., Meyer, B. C., Barile, M. F., and Del Giudice, R. A. (1973). *Ann. N. Y. Acad. Sci.* **225**, 265–276.
Jericho, K. W. F., Austwick, P. K. C., Hodges, R. T., and Dixon, J. B. (1971). *J. Comp. Pathol.* **81**, 13–21.
Kasza, L., Hodges, R. T., Betts, A. O., and Trexler, P. C. (1969). *Vet. Rec.* **84**, 262–267.

Keller, H. (1976). *Proc. Int. Pig Vet. Soc. Congr., Ames, Iowa* PP11.

Keller, H., and Bertschinger, H. U. (1968). *Berl. Muench. Tieraerztl. Wochenschr.* **81,** 101–107.

Kobisch, M., Tillon, J.-P., Cariolet, R., and Morvan, P. (1976). *Recl. Med. Vet.* **152,** 817–827.

Koch, W., and Keller, H. (1976). *Proc. Int. Pig Vet. Soc. Congr., Ames, Iowa* PP13.

Kuksa, F., and Goiš, M. (1975). *Proc. Conf. Taxon. Physiol. Anim. Mycoplasmas, 3rd, Brno* pp. 42–51.

Lam, K. M., and Switzer, W. P. (1971). *Am. J. Vet. Res.* **32,** 1737–1741.

Leach, R. H. (1976). *J. Appl. Bacteriol.* **41,** 259–264.

Leach, R. H., and Butler, M. (1966). *J. Bacteriol.* **91,** 934–941.

L'Ecuyer, C. (1969). *Can. J. Comp. Med.* **33,** 10–19.

L'Ecuyer, C., and Boulanger, P. (1970). *Can. J. Comp. Med.* **34,** 38–46.

L'Ecuyer, C., and Switzer, W. P. (1963). *Can. J. Comp. Med. Vet. Sci.* **27,** 91–99.

Levine, E. M. (1974). *Methods Cell Biol.* **8,** 229–248.

Livingston, C. W., Jr. (1971). *Diss. Abstr. B.* **31,** 4422–4423.

Livingston, C. W., Stair, E. L., Underdahl, N. R., and Mebus, C. A. (1972). *Am. J. Vet. Res.* **33,** 2249–2258.

McKean, J. D., Andrews, J. J., and Farrington, D. O. (1976). *Proc. Int. Pig Vet. Soc. Congr., Ames, Iowa* PP9.

Mackenzie, A. (1963). *Vet. Rec.* **75,** 114–116.

MacMorine, H. C., Rankin, N., and Teleki, S. (1974). *Dev. Biol. Stand.* **23,** 120–127.

Mandrup, M., Friis, N. F., Meyling, A., and Meding, J. H. (1975). *Nord. Vet. Med.* **27,** 557–561.

Maré, C. J., and Switzer, W. P. (1965). *Vet. Med. Small Anim. Clin.* **60,** 841–846.

Maré, C. J., and Switzer, W. P. (1966). *Am. J. Vet. Res.* **27,** 1687–1693.

Martin, J., Schimmel, D., Krausse, H., and Hubrig, T. (1968). *Monatsh. Veterinaermed.* **23,** 652–658.

Mebus, C. A., and Underdahl, N. R. (1977). *Am. J. Vet. Res.* **38,** 1249–1254.

Meyling, A. (1971). *Acta Vet. Scand.* **12,** 137–141.

Meyling, A. (1972). *Proc. Int. Pig Vet. Soc. Congr., Hanover* p. 110.

Meyling, A., and Friis, N. F. (1972). *Acta Vet. Scand.* **13,** 287–289.

Moore, R. W., Redmond, H. E., and Livingston, C. W., Jr. (1966a). *Vet. Med. Small Anim. Clin.* **61,** 883–887.

Moore, R. W., Redmond, H. E., and Livingston, C. W., Jr. (1966b). *Am. J. Vet. Res.* **27,** 1649–1656.

Nicolet, J., and Rivera, E. (1976). *Proc. Int. Pig Vet. Soc. Congr., Ames, Iowa* PP8.

Orning, A. P., Ross, R. F., and Barile, M. F. (1978). *Amer. J. Vet. Res.* **39,** 1169–1174.

Pijoan, C. (1974a). *Vet. Rec.* **95,** 216–217.

Pijoan, C. (1974b). *Br. Vet. J.* **130,** xxii–xxiii.

Pijoan, C., and Boughton, E. (1974). *Br. Vet. J.* **130,** 593–598.

Pijoan, C., and Roberts, D. H. (1972). *J. Comp. Pathol.* **82,** 295–298.

Pijoan, C., and Roberts, D. H. (1973). *Med. Lab. Technol.* **30,** 123–127.

Poland, J., Edington, N., Goiš, M., and Betts, A. O. (1971). *J. Hyg.* **69,** 145–154.

Preston, K. S. (1976). *Proc. Int. Pig Vet. Soc. Congr., Ames, Iowa* PP7.

Preston, K. S., and Switzer, W. P. (1976). *Vet. Microbiol.* **1,** 15–18.

Purcell, R. H., Somerson, N. L., Fox, H., Wong, D. C., Turner, H. C., and Chanock, R. M. (1966). *J. Natl. Cancer Inst.* **37,** 251–253.

Roberts, D. H. (1973). *Br. Vet. J.* **129,** 427–438.

Roberts, D. H. (1974). *Br. Vet. J.* **130,** 68–74.

Roberts, D. H., and Gois, M. (1970). *Vet. Rec.* **87,** 214–215.

Roberts, D. H., and Little, T. W. A. (1970). *J. Comp. Pathol.* **80,** 211–220.

Roberts, D. H., and Little, T. W. A. (1976). *Vet. Rec.* **99,** 13.

Roberts, D. H., Johnson, C. T., and Tew, N. C. (1972). *Vet. Rec.* **90,** 307–309.

Ross, R. F. (1973a). *J. Infect. Dis.* **127,** S84–S86.

Ross, R. F. (1973b). *Ann. N.Y. Acad. Sci.* **225,** 347–368.

Ross, R. F., and Duncan, J. R. (1970). *J. Am. Vet. Med. Assoc.* **157,** 1515–1518.

Ross, R. F., and Karmon, J. A. (1970). *J. Bacteriol.* **103,** 707–713.

Ross, R. F., and Spear, M. L. (1973). *Am. J. Vet. Res.* **34,** 373–378.

Ross, R. F., Switzer, W. P., and Duncan, J. R. (1971). *Am. J. Vet. Res.* **32,** 1743–1749.

Ross, R. F., Dale, S. E., and Duncan, J. R. (1973). *Am. J. Vet. Res.* **34,** 367–372.

Ross, R. F., Grebe, R., and Kirchhoff, H. (1978). *Zentralbl. Veterinaermed. Reihe B* **25,** 444–451.

Ross, R. F., Weiss, R., and Kirchhoff, H. (1977). *Zentralbl. Veterinaermed. Reihe B* **24,** 741–745.

Schimmel, D., Ahlendorf, W., and Burger, E. (1974). *Z. Versuchstierkd.* **16,** 36–40.

Schuller, W., and Abnelt, P. (1977). *Wien. Tieraerztl. Monatsschr.* **64,** 37–40.

Schuller, W., Neumeister, E., and Vogl, D. (1977a). *Wien. Tieraerztl. Monatsschr.* **64,** 156–160.

Schuller, W., Swoboda, R., and Baumgartner, W. (1977b). *Wien. Tieraerztl. Monatsschr.* **64,** 236–241.

Schulman, A., and Estola, T. (1974). *Vet. Rec.* **94,** 330–331.

Slavik, M. (1976). *Proc. Int. Pig Vet. Soc. Congr., Ames, Iowa* PP6.

Slavik, M. F., and Switzer, W. P. (1972). *Iowa State J. Res.* **47,** 117–128.

Smith, I. M., Hodges, R. T., Betts, A. O., and Hayward, A. H. S. (1973). *J. Comp. Pathol.* **83,** 307–321.

Stipkovits, L., Schimmel, D., and Varga, L. (1973a). *Acta Vet. Acad. Sci. Hung.* **23,** 307–313.

Stipkovits, L., Varga, L., and Schimmel, D. (1973b). *Acta Vet. Acad. Sci. Hung.* **23,** 361–368.

Stipkovits, L., Romvary, J., Nagy, Z., Bodon, L., and Varga, L. (1974). *J. Hyg.* **72,** 289–296.

Stipkovits, L., Laber, G., and Schütze, E. (1978). *Vet. Rec.* (in press).

Subcommittee on the Taxonomy of Mycoplasmatales (1967). *Science* **155,** 1694–1696.

Subcommittee on the Taxonomy of Mycoplasmatales (1972). *Int. J. Syst. Bacteriol.* **22,** 184–188.

Subcommittee on the Taxonomy of Mycoplasmatales (1975). *Int. J. Syst. Bacteriol.* **25,** 237–239.

Switzer, W. P. (1967). *J. Am. Vet. Med. Assoc.* **151,** 1656–1661.

Switzer, W. P., and Ross, R. F. (1975). *In* "Diseases of Swine" (H. W. Dunne and A. D. Leman, eds.), 4th Ed., pp. 741–764. Iowa State Univ. Press, Ames.

Szanto, J., Guerrero, R. J., Reynolds, W. A., and Maplesden, D. C. (1977). *Proc. Panam. Vet. Congr.,* Santo Domingo **1,** 52–53.

Taylor-Robinson, D., and Dinter, Z. (1968). *J. Gen. Microbiol.* **53,** 221–229.

Teplitz, M. (1977). *Nucleic Acids Res.* **4,** 1505–1512.

Thomas, M. A., Shipman, C., Jr., Sandberg, J. N., and Drach, J. C. (1977). *In Vitro* **13,** 502–509.

Truszczynski, M., and Pilaszek, J. (1974). *Bull. Off. Int. Epizoot.* **82,** 261–269.

Tully, J. G. (1966). *Proc. Soc. Exp. Biol. Med.* **122,** 565–568.

Tully, J. G., and Razin, S. (1968). *J. Bacteriol.* **95,** 1504–1512.

Underdahl, N. R., and Kelley, G. W. (1957). *J. Am. Vet. Med. Assoc.* **130,** 173–176.
Wegmann, W., Bertschinger, H. U., and Keller, H. (1969). *Zentralbl. Veterinaermed., Reihe B* **16,** 428–447.
Whittlestone, P. (1957). *Vet. Rec.* **69,** 1354–1366.
Whittlestone, P. (1958). Ph.D. Thesis, Cambridge Univ., Cambridge.
Whittlestone, P. (1972). *Pathogenic Mycoplasmas, Ciba Found. Symp.* pp. 263–283.
Whittlestone, P. (1973). *Adv. Vet. Sci. Comp. Med.* **17,** 1–55.
Whittlestone, P. (1976a). *Adv. Vet. Sci. Comp. Med.* **20,** 277–307.
Whittlestone, P. (1976b). *Int. J. Biometeorol.* **20,** 42–48.
Whittlestone, P., Friis, N. F., Gois, M., Ogata, M., Ross, R. F., Stipkovits, L., and Taylor-Robinson, D. (1976). Report of Working team for porcine mycoplasmas. *In WHO/FAO Programme Comp. Mycoplasmol., Rep. Consultations, London* WHO/FAO Publ. VPH/MIC/77.8.
Wichert, P. V., and Wilke, A. (1976). *Scand. J. Respir. Dis.* **57,** 25–30.
Wilson, A. B. (1976). *Res. Vet. Sci.* **20,** 36–39.
Woods, G. T., Pillai, C., and Rhoades, H. E. (1969). *Ill. Res.* **11,** 14–15.
Woods, G. T., Wright, H. S., and Blackburn, B. O. (1976). *Vet. Microbiol.* **1,** 459–465.
Wreghitt, T. G., Windsor, G. D., and Butler, M. (1974). *Appl. Microbiol.* **28,** 530–533.
Yamamoto, K., Koshimizu, K., and Ogata, M. (1971). *Natl. Inst. Anim. Health Q.* **11,** 168–169.
Zimmerman, D. R. (1971). *Proc. Pork Producers Day, Iowa State Cent., Ames, Iowa* AS 370 D, pp. 1–4.
Zimmermann, B. J. (1976). Unpublished observations, quoted in Ross *et al.* (1977a).
Zimmermann, B. J., and Ross, R. F. (1977). *Am. J. Vet. Res.* **38,** 2075–2076.

5 / EQUINE MYCOPLASMAS

Ruth M. Lemcke

I. INTRODUCTION

Apart from reports by Beller (1944), Ito (1960; also cited in Ogata *et al.*, 1974), and Donker-Voet and de Bok (1968), equine mycoplasmas received little attention until the present decade. Even some recent reports deal only with occasional, mainly unidentified isolates from small numbers of horses or aborted foals (Taylor-Robinson, 1972; Dellinger and Jasper, 1972; Langford, 1974; Moorthy *et al.*, 1976, 1977b), but there are some systematic surveys of the mycoplasmal flora of the respiratory and genital tracts and of aborted fetuses (Kirchhoff *et al.*, 1972, 1973; Krabisch *et al.*, 1973; Allam *et al.*, 1973; Windsor, 1973; Allam, 1974; Kirchhoff, 1974; Allam and Lemcke, 1975; Moorthy and Spradbrow, 1976; Moorthy *et al.*, 1977a; Poland and Lemcke, 1978). It is these that provide most of the information discussed in this chapter. So far, surveys of naturally occurring antibody and investigations of the response to experimental infection

THE MYCOPLASMAS, VOL. II
Copyright © 1979 by Academic Press, Inc.
All rights of reproduction in any form reserved.
ISBN 0-12-078401-7

have also been limited (Hooker and Butler, 1976, 1978; Hooker *et al.*, 1977; Poland and Lemcke, 1978).

II. MYCOPLASMAS FROM THE RESPIRATORY TRACT

A. Prevalence

Mycoplasmas have been isolated frequently from the equine respiratory tract, even in the absence of overt respiratory disease. The results of the major surveys are summarized in Table I and show that the isolation rates have varied considerably. Undoubtedly, the results have been affected by several factors, e.g., the methods used, the nature, structure, and age distribution of the populations sampled, and the presence of respiratory illness. The relevance of most of these factors cannot yet be assessed.

Technical considerations clearly affect the frequency of isolation. Thus the isolation rates from swabs transported dry to the laboratory and those transported in fluid medium differed significantly (Poland and Lemcke, 1978). Higher rates were generally obtained from nasopharyngeal and tracheal swabs when they were preincubated in a suitable fluid medium before subculturing at intervals to solid and fluid media. Thus duplicated tracheal swabs from 21 slaughtered horses examined in two separate laboratories yielded seven mycoplasmas when preincubated (Windsor, 1973), but only two when expressed into 10 ml of infusion broth and transferred directly to solid and fluid media (Allam and Lemcke, 1975). Table I shows that, with one exception, the lowest isolation rates were recorded when preincubation was omitted. The necessity for preincubation implies that the numbers of mycoplasmas on the respiratory mucosa are often small. This may not be true of the tonsils. Mycoplasmas were detected without preincubation in 42% of the tonsils of slaughtered horses, but in only 15% of the turbinates, 10% of the tracheas, and 6% of the bronchi (Poland and Lemcke, 1978).

B. Species Detected

Representatives of five species of *Acholeplasma* and of an unnamed group of acholeplasmas have been found in the respiratory tract (Table II). Of these, *Acholeplasma laidlawii* was commonest, having been isolated from several levels of the tract but not from the bronchi. These strains may be either transitory contaminants from the environment or actually adapted to colonize the horse. Other acholeplasmas have been isolated less frequently. *Acholeplasma oculi*, originally found in the eyes

TABLE I. Prevalence of Mycoplasmas in the Respiratory Tract of Horses: Results of Major Surveys

Type of horse	Clinical or postmortem condition[a]	Region sampled	Number of horses sampled	Number of horses yielding mycoplasmas	Swabs preincubated	Reference
Living						
Not specified	NA	Pharynx, guttural pouch	83	2 (2%)	Yes	Kirchhoff et al. (1972)
Not specified	Acute respiratory disease	Pharynx, guttural pouch	21	7 (33%)	Yes	Allam (1974)
Army thoroughbred	NA	Nasopharynx	198	3 (2%)	No	Allam et al. (1973)
	Acute respiratory disease	Nasopharynx	130	10 (8%)	No	Allam and Lemcke (1975)
Thoroughbred in training	Mainly normal[b]	Nasopharynx	51	47 (92%)	Yes	Poland and Lemcke (1978)
Not specified	NA	Nasal cavity	25	0 (0%)	No	Moorthy and Spradbrow (1976)
Not specified	Respiratory disease	Nasal cavity	18	2 (11%)	No	
Slaughtered						
Not specified	NA	Trachea	18	5 (28%)	Yes	Windsor (1973)
Not specified	Respiratory disease	Trachea	3	2 (66%)	Yes	
Not specified	NA	Nasal cavity	26	4 (15%)	Yes	Ogata et al. (1974)
Not specified	NA	Trachea	21	3 (14%)	Yes	
Aged	With lung lesions	Tonsils, turbinates, trachea, bronchi	133	59 (44%)	No	Poland and Lemcke (1978)
Aged	With lung lesions	Tonsils, turbinates, trachea, bronchi	30	18 (60%)	No	
Not specified	NA	Trachea	29	1 (4%)	No	Moorthy and Spradbrow (1976)

[a] NA, No abnormalities detected clinically or at postmortem.
[b] Horses sampled on five to seven occasions over a 10–12 month period during which there were a few episodes of mild respiratory disease.

TABLE II. *Acholeplasma* Species from the Respiratory Tract of Horses

Species	Source	Condition of horses[a]	Number of isolates recorded	Isolated by:
A. laidlawii	Not specified	Not specified	2	Kirchhoff et al. (1972); Kirchhoff (1974)
	Nasal cavity, trachea	NA	7	Ogata et al. (1974)
	Nasopharynx	NA	29	Allam and Lemcke (1975); Poland and Lemcke (1978)
	Nasopharynx	Acute respiratory disease	1	Allam and Lemcke (1975)
	Tonsils, turbinates, trachea	NA	11	Poland and Lemcke (1978)
A. granularum	Tonsils, turbinates, trachea	With lung lesions	6	Poland and Lemcke (1978)
A. oculi	Nasopharynx, tonsils	NA	2	Poland and Lemcke (1978)
	Nasopharynx	NA	4	Allam and Lemcke (1975); Poland and Lemcke (1978)
	Nasal cavity	Acute febrile respiratory disease	3	Moorthy et al. (1977c)
A. equifetale	Lung	Emphysema	1	Moorthy et al. (1977c)
	Nasopharynx	Nasal discharge	1	Allam and Lemcke (1975)
A. hippikon	Trachea	NA	1	Windsor (1973)
Acholeplasma sp.	Trachea	NA	2	Poland and Lemcke (1978)
strain 881	Nasopharynx	NA	9	Poland and Lemcke (1978)

[a] NA, No abnormalities detected clinically or at postmortem.

of goats (Al-Aubaidi *et al.*, 1973), occurs occasionally in the respiratory tract as well as in other organs and in the tissues of aborted foals (see Sections III–V). *Acholeplasma granularum, A. equifetale,* and *A. hippikon* are rarer. The last two, recognized only recently as distinct species (Kirchhoff, 1974, 1978; Heitmann and Kirchhoff, 1978), were originally isolated from aborted foals (Section IV) and have not yet been found in other hosts. They may therefore be indigenous to horses. The group of nine organisms represented by strain 881 are acholeplasmas distinct from *Acholeplasma laidlawii, A. granularum, A. axanthum, A. modicum, A. oculi, A. equifetale,* and *A. hippikon* and may constitute a new species (Poland and Lemcke, 1978). This species is provisionally designated *Acholeplasma* sp. strain 881. Although it was found in only one stable, all of the six horses examined were infected at some stage during the survey.

Of the *Mycoplasma* species isolated, the arginine-degrading *Mycoplasma equirhinis* has been found most frequently in the respiratory tract (Table III). These isolations were all made in Great Britain, during four separate investigations. Most isolates were from nasopharyngeal swabs, but one was obtained from the trachea and several from the tonsils and turbinates. More recently, the recovery of *M. equirhinis* from the upper respiratory tract has been reported in Egypt (Allam *et al.*, 1978). Thus *M. equirhinis* is apparently common in the upper respiratory tract. Hooker *et al.* (1977) consider that this organism is probably a parasite of the oropharynx, because they recovered it more frequently from oropharyngeal than from nasopharyngeal swabs following experimental infection of ponies. Although originally isolated from horses, *M. equirhinis* has also been obtained from nasal swabs from cattle (A. A. Polak-Vogelzang and R. H. Leach, unpublished observations).

The other arginine-degrading species are represented by comparatively few strains (Table III). *Mycoplasma salivarium,* a normal inhabitant of the human mouth was obtained only from slaughtered horses and may have been an accidental contaminant from slaughterhouse workers. *Mycoplasma arginini,* found only once (Moorthy and Spradbrow, 1976), is a commensal of several species of domestic animal. The remaining strain belongs to a group originally found in the cervix of mares and the organs of aborted foals (Krabisch *et al.*, 1973; Kirchhoff *et al.*, 1973). These strains were at first thought to be ureaplasmas because they produced an alkaline change in urea-containing media (Kirchhoff, 1974). However, their growth characteristics are not those of ureaplasmas. Current evidence suggests that these strains comprise a new species, represented by strain TB and provisionally named *Mycoplasma subdolum* (Lemcke and Kirchhoff, 1979).

The most common group of glycolytic mycoplasmas in the equine

TABLE III. *Mycoplasma* Species from the Respiratory Tract of Horses

Species	Source	Condition of horses[a]	Number of isolates recorded	Isolated by:
Arginine-degrading species				
M. equirhinis	Nasopharynx	NA	100	Allam and Lemcke (1975); Poland and Lemcke (1978)
	Nasopharynx	Acute febrile respiratory disease	1	Allam and Lemcke (1975)
	Trachea	Mild rhinitis	1[b]	Windsor (1973)
	Tonsils, turbinates	NA	17	Poland and Lemcke (1978)
	Tonsils, turbinates	With lung lesions	6	Poland and Lemcke (1978)
M. salivarium	Tonsils	NA	3	Poland and Lemcke (1978)
M. arginini (strain NS3)	Nasal cavity	Rhinitis	1[c]	Moorthy and Spradbrow (1976)
M. subdolum	Nasopharynx	NA	1	Poland and Lemcke (1978)
Glycolytic species				
M. felis	Nasopharynx	Acute febrile respiratory disease	1	Allam and Lemcke (1975)
	Trachea	NA	4[b]	Windsor (1973)
	Trachea	Strangles	1[b]	Windsor (1973)
	Tonsils, turbinates, trachea, bronchi	NA	19	Poland and Lemcke (1978)
	Tonsils, turbinates trachea, bronchi	With lung lesions	14	Poland and Lemcke (1978)
	Nasal cavity, pharynx, treachea, guttural pouches	NA	2[d]	Kirchhoff (1974)
	Nasal cavity, pharynx trachea, guttural pouches	Acute febrile respiratory disease	15[d]	Kirchhoff (1974)
SGM strains	Nasopharynx	NA	8	Poland and Lemcke (1978)
M. pulmonis	Nasopharynx	Acute febrile respiratory disease	3	Allam and Lemcke (1975)
Strain N3[e]	Nasopharynx	Nasal discharge	2	Allam and Lemcke (1975)
M. equigenitalium (strain NSDH60)	Trachea	NA	1[c]	Moorthy and Spradbrow (1976)

[a] NA. No abnormalities detected clinically or at postmortem.
[b] Identified by Allam and Lemcke (1975).
[c] Identified by Kirchhoff (personal communication).
[d] Named *M. equipharyngis*.
[e] Cross-reacts with *M. mycoides*.

respiratory tract is related to *Mycoplasma felis*. This group includes several British isolates, represented by strains N29 A and B (Lemcke and Allam, 1974; Allam and Lemcke, 1975) and 17 strains called *Mycoplasma equipharyngis* (Kirchhoff, 1974). Allam and Lemcke (1975) consider that the biochemical and serological similarity of a representative strain of *M. equipharyngis* and four British strains to *M. felis* prohibits the recognition of the equine strains as a new species. These equine strains of *M. felis* have been isolated from the tonsils and several regions of the upper and lower respiratory tract (Table III). *Mycoplasma felis* was the only species identified in the bronchi, although eight other isolates were lost before identification (Poland and Lemcke, 1978). The species was isolated from apparently healthy horses, as well as from those with respiratory disease. Horses may become infected from cats which frequent the stables, since cats often harbor *M. felis*. However, the organism occurs sufficiently frequently in horses and in regions of the respiratory tract remote enough to suggest that it actually colonizes the equine mucosa.

Another group of glycolytic strains, designated *slow glucose-metabolizing* (SGM) mycoplasmas was encountered in one survey (Poland and Lemcke, 1978). SGM strains were isolated only in the absence of faster-growing mycoplasmas such as *A. laidlawii* and *M. equirhinis*. Eight strains were obtained from seven horses. They produce only a slow change in the pH of glucose broth, unless cultures are continuously aerated. The results of growth inhibition and indirect fluorescent antibody tests suggest that SGM strains represent a new species of *Mycoplasma* (Lemcke and Poland, 1979).

Three other types of glycolytic mycoplasmas have been isolated occasionally. One group of three strains is related to the rodent mycoplasma *Mycoplasma pulmonis* (Lemcke and Allam, 1974). Like *M. felis*, *M. pulmonis* in horses may also be derived from the natural host which infests stables. Another group, represented by strains N3 and N11, was obtained from two horses in different stables. Both had a purulent nasal discharge. The organisms were originally thought to be distinct from recognized glycolytic species (Allam and Lemcke, 1975), but cross-reactions with bovine and caprine strains of *Mycoplasma mycoides* were subsequently detected (Lemcke *et al.*, 1979). However, the classification and nomenclature of N3 and N11 must await further elucidation of the relationships between other members of the *M. mycoides* group. N3 and N11 may not be natural inhabitants of the equine respiratory tract, since N3 does not become established after intranasal inoculation (see Section II,C), but the identity of their true host is conjectural. The remaining glycolytic species is *Mycoplasma equigenitalium,* found only once in the respiratory tract (Moorthy and Spradbrow, 1976), but more frequently in the genital tract (Section III).

Of the species so far identified, *M. equirhinis*, *A. laidlawii*, and *M. felis* are the most common, the first two being particularly prevalent in the upper respiratory tract. As in other animal hosts, several species of *Acholeplasma* and/or *Mycoplasma* can coexist. Two or three different species were isolated from 22 (15%) out of 151 nasopharyngeal swabs in a recent survey, the most usual combination being *M. equirhinis* together with *A. laidlawii* or, less frequently, with another species of *Acholeplasma* (Poland and Lemcke, 1978). The same survey showed that consecutive swabs from the same horse often revealed a change in the species isolated, or a change from positive to negative. This suggests that fluctuations occur both in the type and number of mycoplasmas on the mucosa, at least in the upper respiratory tract. It follows that examination of a single nasal or nasopharyngeal swab on one occasion, as in some of the surveys, may give an erroneous impression of both the types of mycoplasma present and the prevalence of infection.

When more than one species is present, the use of an enrichment technique to detect small numbers (Section II,A) may allow rapidly developing strains to outgrow and prevent the isolation of more fastidious mycoplasmas. Thus some SGM strains and possibly also *M. pulmonis* and *M. felis* may have escaped detection in an investigation in which more than 60% of the swabs yielded *M. equirhinis* or acholeplasmas (Poland and Lemcke, 1978). No satisfactory inhibitor of the faster-growing strains has yet been found. Although all *Acholeplasma* species so far tested are inhibited by erythromycin (1 μg/ml), SGM strains are among the few *Mycoplasma* species that are also inhibited (Lewis and Poland, 1978). In the absence of a suitable selective medium, it is advisable to subculture the preincubated swab or specimen to several media of different constitution. The development of SGM strains on primary isolation plates is, for example, favored by a medium containing human serum rather than one containing swine serum (Poland and Lemcke, 1978). Ultimately, the choice of medium and methods determines which mycoplasmas are isolated.

C. Pathogenicity of Isolates

Mycoplasma equirhinis, *A. laidlawii*, and *M. felis*, the species most frequently encountered, have all been isolated from clinically normal horses as well as from those with respiratory disease. Moreover, in horses monitored over several months, there was no coincidence between the time when *M. equirhinis* or *A. laidlawii* appeared and the onset of clinical illness (Poland and Lemcke, 1978).

Other evidence supports the view that *M. equirhinis* is a common parasite of the respiratory tract but that it is not pathogenic. In parallel surveys of a population of young thoroughbreds, the prevalence of complement-fixation (CF) antibodies to *M. equirhinis* correlated with a high frequency of isolation (Hooker and Butler, 1978; Poland and Lemcke, 1978). *Mycoplasma equirhinis* soon became established in the upper respiratory tract following experimental inoculation and was rapidly transmitted to other horses in the stable, although no clinical signs developed (Hooker *et al.*, 1977). The CF antibody response to intranasal inoculation was slow, taking 6–12 weeks to appear, whereas the response to parenteral immunization appeared in 10–20 days (Hooker and Butler, 1976, 1978).

Evidence about the pathogenicity of the strains related to *M. felis* is more equivocal. They were certainly isolated from the bronchi of slaughtered horses and may therefore be capable of infecting the lower respiratory tract. There was no correlation, however, between the isolation of *M. felis* and the presence of lung lesions (Poland and Lemcke, 1978). No surveys of antibody to this species nor experimental infections have yet been carried out.

Although SGM strains were isolated from only 7 out of 18 horses in three stables, MI antibody was present in 16 of the 18 at titers between 1/40 and 1/4000. The highest titers (1/1280 to 1/4000) were found, however, in horses from the two stables where the organisms were most frequently isolated (Poland and Lemcke, 1978). Intranasal inoculation of two minimal-disease foals with an SGM strain established an infection that persisted for several weeks and elicited a rapid and strong MI antibody response (Poland and Lemcke, 1978). No signs of clinical disease developed, but the strain used was at its eighteenth passage. In addition, intranasal instillation may be unsatisfactory for producing disease, just as it is with *M. mycoides* subsp. *mycoides*.

In regard to the pathogenicity of other mycoplasma strains, *M. pulmonis* was isolated only from horses with acute febrile illness, but no other evidence is available. Inoculation of N3 into ponies (Hooker *et al.*, 1977) or minimal-disease foals (Poland and Lemcke, 1978), either by intranasal instillation or by aerosol, failed to establish infection in the upper respiratory tract. The detection of CF antibody, albeit at low levels, in a high proportion of thoroughbreds is therefore perplexing. Possibly the strains inhabit regions other than the respiratory tract in the horse. Alternatively, the antibodies detected may not be specifically directed against N3 but against another organism with related antigens, possibly glycolipid or polysaccharide in nature.

III. MYCOPLASMAS FROM THE GENITAL TRACT

Mycoplasmas have been isolated from the cervix, uterus, and vagina of mares (Beller, 1944; Krabisch *et al.*, 1973; Ogata *et al.*, 1974; Moorthy *et al.*, 1977a) ánd from the semen, urethra, prepuce, and penis of stallions (Donker-Voet and de Bok, 1968; Ogata *et al.*, 1974; Moorthy *et al.*, 1977a). Isolation rates varied from 21 (5%) out of 404 cervical swabs positive (Krabisch *et al.*, 1973) to 12 (60%) out of 19 vaginal swabs positive (Moorthy *et al.*, 1977a). As with respiratory tract infections, technical considerations probably affected the number and type of mycoplasmas isolated.

Very few of the isolates have been identified. Kirchhoff (1974) classified 18 of the 21 strains isolated from the cervix by Krabisch *et al.* (1973). Of these, 12 were assigned to a new glycolytic species, *M. equigenitalium,* and 6 to a new arginine-degrading species, *M. subdolum* (see Section II,B). The latter appears to be more widespread in the genital than in the respiratory tract, having been isolated from the cervix of normal mares (Lemcke and Kirchhoff, 1979; J. Poland, unpublished observations) and of mares with endometritis (J. Poland, unpublished observations). An isolate from the penis (Moorthy *et al.*, 1977a) and two from semen also belonged to this species (Lemcke and Kirchhoff, 1979).

Most of the strains isolated by Ogata *et al.* (1974) from the vagina, urethra, and prepuce were *A. laidlawii,* but seven clones were not identified. The apparently ubiquitous *A. oculi* (Sections II,B, IV, and V) has also been found in semen (Moorthy *et al.*, 1977c).

So far, ureaplasmas (T strains), which are found in the genital tract of other hosts, have not been isolated from horses.

In regard to pathogenicity, Donker-Voet and de Bok (1978) isolated mycoplasmas from 2 out of 6 stallions with fertility problems, but failed to isolate any from 9 normal stallions. J. Poland (unpublished observations) obtained mycoplasmas from the cervix of 9 out of 19 mares with endometritis, but from only 2 out of 16 normal mares. Most of the horses examined by Moorthy *et al.* (1977a) had genital disorders or breeding problems. Ten out of the 12 mycoplasmas they obtained from mares, and both the mycoplasmas from stallions, were isolated from such animals. Nevertheless, mycoplasmas were also found in 2 apparently healthy mares, but not in 7 others with genital abnormalities. Krabisch *et al.* (1973) found that of the 21 infertile mares that yielded mycoplasmas, 9 were in foal by the following year, although no treatment had been given to eliminate the mycoplasmas. They concluded that infertility in the mares they examined could not be ascribed to the presence of mycoplasmas.

The evidence is therefore equivocal, and the pathogenicity of mycoplasmas found in the equine genital tract cannot yet be assessed. In this connection, it would be useful to know which species constitute the mycoplasmal flora in health and disease. Ultimately, however, experimental inoculation of pure cultures will be necessary to determine whether any of the species isolated can produce lesions.

IV. MYCOPLASMAS FROM ABORTED FOALS

In the most extensive investigations yet carried out, Kirchhoff *et al.* (1973) obtained mycoplasmas from 13 (7%) of 196 fetuses. The majority of these isolates came from the lungs, although one was also found in the liver. Ten strains were identified as acholeplasmas: *A. laidlawii* (four strains), *A. equifetale* (four strains), and *A. hippikon* (two strains) (Kirchhoff, 1978). The remainder comprised one strain of *M. equigenitalium* and two of *M. subdolum* (Kirchhoff, 1974; Lemcke and Kirchhoff, 1979). Another strain from a fetal stomach (Moorthy *et al.*, 1976) was also identified as *M. subdolum* (Lemcke and Kirchhoff, 1979). The two *Mycoplasma* spp. and *A. laidlawii* have also been found in the genital tract of mares (Section III). *Acholeplasma oculi* and *Mycoplasma bovigenitalium* are two other species that have been isolated from aborted fetuses (Moorthy *et al.*, 1977c; Langford, 1974). The latter species is of interest, since it is associated with genital disease in cattle. However, the limited information currently available does not suggest any causal relationship between the presence of mycoplasmas and abortion in horses.

V. MYCOPLASMAS FROM OTHER ORGANS AND TISSUES

Mycoplasmas have been isolated from several regions other than the respiratory and genital tracts. Ogata *et al.* (1974) isolated acholeplasmas, mainly *A. laidlawii,* from the oral cavity and conjunctiva of apparently healthy horses at slaughter. *Acholeplasma laidlawii* was also found in the parotid glands of two horses with parotiditis (A. R. S. Moorthy, personal communication). A strain obtained from the brain of a dead horse with nervous signs (A. R. S. Moorthy, personal communication) was identified as *M. subdolum* (Lemcke and Kirchhoff, 1979). *Acholeplasma oculi* was isolated from an arthritic joint and also from the cerebrospinal fluid of two horses with paralysis (Moorthy *et al.*, 1977c). Three other mycoplasmas from arthritic joints have not been identified (Dellinger and Jasper, 1972; Moorthy *et al.*, 1977b). The significance of the presence of mycoplasmas in these locations cannot be assessed at present, but the preponderance of acholeplasmas renders improbable an etiological association with any of the disorders cited.

VI. CONCLUSIONS

It is obvious that our knowledge of the mycoplasmal flora of horses is still very fragmentary. Even in regard to the respiratory tract, which has been the best studied, many questions remain unanswered, especially in relation to pathogenicity. Further investigations are required of locations other than the nasopharynx to determine which mycoplasmas infect the more remote regions of the tract. Of the mycoplasmas already identified, the pathogenicity of equine strains of *M. felis* and of *M. pulmonis* needs to be explored by the inoculation of foals. The pathogenicity of the SGM strains also requires further investigation using cultures at low passage and different methods of inoculation.

It is becoming increasingly apparent that some disease syndromes are not induced by a single etiological agent. Microbial interactions may be necessary for expression of the full clinical syndrome in certain diseases. At the very least, one type of agent may modify or increase the severity of a disease produced by another. In view of this possible complexity, future investigations of equine respiratory disease should include closely coordinated bacteriological, mycological, virological, and mycoplasmal surveillance. An attempt to cover all these aspects was made by Floer (1972), but this type of approach is rare and needs to be emulated.

Investigations of mycoplasmas associated with the genital tract and abortion are at an even more elementary stage. A recent outbreak of genital disease in bloodstock at a racing center in England (Crowhurst, 1977) has served to focus attention on the microbiology of genital infections in horses. A new species of bacterium was apparently responsible for this particular outbreak (Platt *et al.*, 1977), but the episode should serve to stimulate interest in genital disease and infertility problems in horses, and consequently in the microflora of the urogenital tract.

ACKNOWLEDGMENTS

Grants from the Horse Race Betting Levy Board, London, England, which supported the work carried out at the Lister Institute of Preventive Medicine, London, England, are gratefully acknowledged. I am also indebted to Dr. J. Poland, Royal Veterinary College, London, England for reading and commenting on the manuscript and for making available unpublished results.

REFERENCES

Al-Aubaidi, J. M., Dardiri, A. H., Muscoplatt, C. C., and McCauley, E. H. (1973). *Cornell Vet.* **63**, 117–129.

Allam, N. M. (1974). M. Philos. Thesis, Univ. of London, London.

Allam, N. M., and Lemcke, R. M. (1975). *J. Hyg.* **74**, 385–408.

Allam, N. M., Powell, D. G., Andrews, B. E., and Lemcke, R. M. (1973). *Vet. Rec.* **93**, 402.

Allam, N. M., Ammar, A. M., and Sabry, M. Z. (1978). *Zentbl. Bakteriol. Parasitenkd, Infektionskr. Hyg., Abt. 1: Orig., Reihe A.* **241**, 261.

Beller, K. (1944). *Arch. Tierheilkd.* **79**, 197–210.

Crowhurst, R. C. (1977). *Vet. Rec.* **100**, 476.

Dellinger, J. D., and Jasper, D. E. (1972). *Am. J. Vet. Res.* **33**, 769–775.

Donker-Voet, J., and de Bok, J. (1968). *Tijdschr. Diergeneeskd.* **93**, 912–916.

Floer, W. (1972). Inaugural Diss., Tierärztliche Hochschule, Hanover.

Heitmann, J., and Kirchhoff, H. (1978). *Int. J. Syst. Bacteriol.* **28**, 96–98.

Hooker, J. M., and Butler, M. (1976). *J. Comp. Pathol.* **86**, 87–92.

Hooker, J. M., and Butler, M. (1978). *Proc. Int. Conf. Equine Infect. Dis., 4th, Lyon; J. Equine Med. Surg., Suppl.* **1**, 431–435.

Hooker, J. M., Butler, M., and Burrows, R. (1977). *J. Comp. Pathol.* **87**, 281–287.

Ito, S. (1960). *Nippon Saikingaku Zasshi* **15**, 1193–1199.

Kirchhoff, H. (1974). *Zentralbl. Veterinaermed., Reihe B* **21**, 207–210.

Kirchhoff, H. (1978). *Int. J. Syst. Bacteriol.* **28**, 76–81.

Kirchhoff, H., Deegen, E., Zeller, R., and Floer, W. (1972). *Dtsch. Tieraerztl. Wochenschr.* **79**, 465–468.

Kirchhoff, H., Bisping, W., and Floer, W. (1973). *Berl. Muench. Tieraerztl. Wochenschr.* **86**, 401–403.

Krabisch, P., Kirchhoff, H., and von Lepel, J. F. (1973). *Dtsch. Tieraerztl. Wochenschr.* **80**, 493–495.

Langford, E. V. (1974). *Vet. Rec.* **94**, 528.

Lemcke, R. M., and Allam, N. M. (1974). *Colloq. INSERM, Mycoplasmes Homme, Anim., Veg. Insectes, Congr. Int., Bordeaux* **33**, 153–160.

Lemcke, R. M., and Kirchhoff, H. (1979). *Int. J. Syst. Bacteriol.* **29**, 42–50.

Lemcke, R. M., and Poland, J. (1979). *Int. J. Syst. Bacteriol.* (submitted for publication).

Lemcke, R. M., Gupta, U., and Ernø, H. (1979). in preparation.

Lewis, J., and Poland, J. (1978). *Res. Vet. Sci.* **24**, 121–123.

Moorthy, A. R. S., and Spradbrow, P. B. (1976). *Vet. Rec.* **98**, 235–237.

Moorthy, A. R. S., Spradbrow, P. B., and McEvoy, T. (1976). *Aust. Vet. J.* **52**, 385.

Moorthy, A. R. S., Spradbrow, P. B., and Eisler, M. E. D. (1977a). *Aust. Vet. J.* **53**, 167–169.

Moorthy, A. R. S., Spradbrow, P. B., and Eisler, M. E. D. (1977b). *Br. Vet. J.* **133**, 320–321.

Moorthy, A. R. S., Kirchhoff, H., Heitmann, J., Plumer, J. V., and Spradbrow, P. B. (1977c). *Vet. Microbiol.* **2**, 253–256.

Ogata, M., Watabe, J., and Koshimizu, K. (1974). *Jpn. J. Vet. Sci.* **36**, 43–51.

Platt, H., Atherton, J. G., Simpson, D. J., Taylor, C. E. D., Rosenthal, R. O., Brown, D. F. J., and Wreghitt, T. G. (1977). *Vet. Rec.* **101**, 20.

Poland, J., and Lemcke, R. M. (1978). *Proc. Int. Conf. Equine Infect. Dis., 4th, Lyon; J. Equine Med. Surg., Suppl.* **1**, 437–446.

Taylor-Robinson, D. (1972). *Pathogenic Mycoplasmas, Ciba Found. Symp.* p. 181.

Windsor, G. D. (1973). *Vet. Rec.* **93**, 593–594.

6 / THE MYCOPLASMA FLORA OF HUMAN AND NONHUMAN PRIMATES

Norman L. Somerson and Barry C. Cole

I. INTRODUCTION

The first reported culture of a mycoplasma from humans was from an abscess of a Bartholin's gland (Dienes and Edsall, 1937). Five years later, there were indications that mycoplasmas were commonly found in the

THE MYCOPLASMAS, VOL. II

female genital tract (Dienes and Smith, 1942). Difficulties with medium formulations, bacterial contamination problems, and uncertainties over the relationship to L forms and bacteria delayed the recognition of mycoplasmas as resident flora of both the oral and urogenital tracts. Using improved culture media and selective inhibitors to minimize bacterial contamination, Smith and Morton (1951) succeeded in isolating and subculturing mycoplasmas from the throats and saliva of healthy individuals. These observations established mycoplasmas as part of the normal flora of humans.

II. PROBLEMS IN THE ISOLATION OF HUMAN MYCOPLASMAS

Prior to the discovery of *Mycoplasma pneumoniae*, only five mycoplasma species were recognized as organisms of human origin. These were *Mycoplasma hominis* types 1 and 2, *M. salivarium, M. fermentans,* and *Ureaplasma urealyticum,* the last-mentioned then known as T strains. Most of the recently isolated mycoplasmas are culturally fastidious, and their exact nutritional requirements are unknown. Advances in culture medium formulations have invariably preceded isolations of new mycoplasmas, and the number of human *Mycoplasma* species has increased with each improvement. *Mycoplasma pneumoniae* was isolated only after a yeast extract solution and a high concentration of horse serum were included in the culture medium. *Mycoplasma orale,* a common human oral mycoplasma, also requires a yeast factor not supplied in older formulations. The isolation of another human species, *Mycoplasma faucium,* has had a similar history, again requiring yeast extract for cultivation. A richer "basal" medium formulation, which was used to grow one of the more fastidious insect spiroplasmas (Tully *et al.*, 1977), has been found to improve the recovery of *M. pneumoniae* from human throat washings (Tully *et al.*, 1979).

Numerous studies investigating the association of human mycoplasmas with disease also have yielded information about the ecology of these organisms. Mycoplasmas vary in their nutritional requirements; the use of a single medium formulation for growing all mycoplasmas would be analogous to an attempt to grow all bacteria on blood agar medium alone. Also, some media formulations contain compounds designed to suppress bacteria. Crystal violet was used successfully as a bacterial inhibitor in the first isolations of mycoplasmas from the human oropharynx (Smith and Morton, 1951; Morton *et al.*, 1951b), but in some cases the chances of isolating mycoplasmas may be diminished by its inclusion. Thallium acetate is currently employed as an inhibitor of gram-negative bacteria, but this compound is inhibitory to ureaplasmas and, depending upon the concentration, may be toxic to *Mycoplasma* species. Polyene antibiotics have also been included in some formulations in attempts to limit contamination of clinical specimens. However, while stock mycoplasma cultures may survive the presence of a polyene used as an inhibitor, fewer mycoplasmas may be isolated from clinical specimens when polyenes are included in the culture medium formulation.

Biological components employed in culture medium formulation show lot-to-lot variations in growth-promoting activity (Hughes *et al.*, 1974). Although not always obvious in the past, it is clear now that each new lot of every medium component should be pretested for its ability to support the growth of mycoplasmas. A variety of *Mycoplasma* species should be included in these tests.

Mycoplasmologists are now aware that some tissue extracts contain mycoplasma-inhibiting substances (Tully and Rask-Nielsen, 1967). Thus tissues suspected of harboring mycoplasmas should not be subjected to grinding prior to isolation attempts.

Some species, such as *M. hominis*, grow under aerobic or anaerobic conditions, but primary isolates of other species, e.g., *Mycoplasma buccale*, *M. lipophilum*, and *M. orale*, grow better anaerobically or in an atmosphere enriched with 5–10% carbon dioxide. The number of human isolations may be increased three- to fivefold when a carbon dioxide–nitrogen environment is used in primary isolation attempts. Once the anaerobic isolation has been successful, subsequent passages under aerobic incubation are often possible.

III. UNUSUAL ISOLATIONS FROM CLINICAL MATERIALS

There are numerous references in the literature to the isolation of mycoplasmas from human malignant materials (Hayflick and Stanbridge, 1967; Murphy *et al.*, 1967). Armstrong and his associates (Armstrong *et al.*, 1971) reported on an unusual finding in which a cancer patient and members of her family were infected with *Mycoplasma canis*, a canine mycoplasma presumably transmitted from a pet dog. The isolations did not involve cell culture and were obtained by direct inoculation onto artificial medium. In another study, an attempt to link mycoplasmas directly to squamous cell dysplasia of the cervix could not be made (Lyons *et al.*, 1974).

In other experiments, leukemic marrow and blood were inoculated directly into mycoplasma broth and onto agar, or specimens were added to cell cultures from which mycoplasmas were later isolated (Barile, 1967; Murphy *et al.*, 1967). In all likelihood, the isolations from these direct inoculations were not laboratory contaminants (Barile, 1967; Hayflick and Stanbridge, 1967; Hayflick and Koprowski, 1965). Mycoplasmas that are part of the normal human flora could act as passengers or opportunists in cancer patients or in others with an impaired immune system.

However, many of the mycoplasmas supposedly isolated from cancer patients are now considered contaminants. *Mycoplasma* species normally found in the oral cavity of humans are also common cell culture contaminants. No doubt, some human mycoplasmas isolated from cell cultures inoculated with malignant tissue came from unrecognized cell culture contamination.

Numerous isolates from cell cultures inoculated with human tissue have been identified as mycoplasmas of animal origin. At the time these organisms were isolated, it was difficult to explain how the rodent species *Mycoplasma pulmonis* and the porcine species *M. hyorhinis* could be present in human neoplastic tissue. We now know that commercial sera are the source of many of these animal mycoplasmas (Barile and Kern, 1971) and, in most instances, animal mycoplasmas isolated from cell cultures inoculated with human material are cell culture contaminants (see this volume, Chapter 13).

Another point of some interest is the observation that certain strains of *M. hyorhinis* present in cell cultures cannot be routinely cultured on artificial medium (Hopps *et al.*, 1973). Therefore tests for mycoplasma contamination of infected cell cultures would be negative prior to inoculation with clinical material. As already mentioned, *M. hyorhinis* was one of the species isolated from cell cultures that received human neoplastic tissues. Perhaps the enrichment provided by the addition of blood, tumor tissue, or other human materials potentiated the growth of the *M. hyorhinis* already present in cell cultures and led to its recovery on artificial media.

Thus many of the so-called mycoplasma contaminants from human malignant tissues are probably contaminants. Cell cultures and commercial sera are the most likely sources of these organisms.

IV. CLASSIFICATION OF HUMAN MYCOPLASMAS

A. Generic Differentiation

Three mycoplasma genera have been isolated from humans (Table I). *Mycoplasma* species are predominant, and only one *Acholeplasma* species, *A. laidlawii*, is represented. Taxonomically, there is only one recognized human species of *Ureaplasma*, but among the many urea-

TABLE I. **Generic Differentiation of Mollicutes Isolated from Humans**

Genus	Cholesterol essential for growth	Urease activity	Locale of NADH oxidase	Lipid synthesis from acetate	Sensitivity to digitonin, polyenes
Mycoplasma	+	0	Cytoplasm	0	+
Acholeplasma	0	0	Membrane	+	0
Ureaplasma	+	+	Cytoplasm	0	+

plasmas isolated from humans there is a great deal of heterogeneity and a large number of serotypes.

Mycoplasma genera can be generally distinguished by biochemical tests. *Mycoplasma* species require sterol for growth, while *Acholeplasma* do not. *Ureaplasma* species are easily distinguished by their ability to hydrolyze urea. Theoretically, with just the tests for sterol requirement and urease activity, any human isolate could be assigned to the proper genus.

However, primary mycoplasma isolates may differ in cultural habit from laboratory strains, and a standardized test for the sterol requirement may be difficult to interpret. The need for exogenous sterol can be assessed by indirect means, such as sensitivity to digitonin, polyenes such as amphotericin B, and sodium polyanethol sulfonate (SPS). Three additional tests, the site of NADH oxidase activity (Pollack, 1975), the ability of these organisms to synthesize lipid from acetate (Herring and Pollack, 1974), and genome size (Bak *et al.*, 1969) are also useful in separating *Mycoplasma* and *Acholeplasma* species.

B. Classification of Species

On a practical basis, the identification of *Mycoplasma* species is based upon serological reactions. Our list includes 12 species (Table II). A mycoplasma isolate can be identified as to species by use of a growth inhibition (GI) test or immunofluorescence. Complement fixation (CF) and gel diffusion tests may aid in identifying mycoplasmas, but with both tests, human mycoplasmas show cross-reacting antigens (Taylor-Robinson *et al.*, 1963).

There are a large number of biochemical tests which are helpful in the identification of mycoplasmas. Initial subdivisions can be based on whether they ferment carbohydrate or possess the arginine dihydrolase pathway (Table III). Of the human mycoplasmas, *M. pneumoniae* ferments glucose, *M. fermentans* ferments glucose and possesses the ar-

TABLE II. Mycoplasmas Isolated from Humans

Organism	Former designation(s)	Type strain	ATTC No.	Primary location	Occurrence in humans	Reference
Acholeplasma						
A. laidlawii	M. laidlawii "saprophytes"	PG8	23026	Oropharynx	Rare	Razin et al. (1964); Laidlaw and Elford (1936)
Mycoplasma						
M. salivarium	Human type 4	PG20	23064	Oropharynx	Widespread	Nicol and Edward (1953); Edward (1955); Edward and Freundt (1956)
M. orale	M. orale type 1 or M. pharyngis	CH19299	23714	Oropharynx	Widespread	Taylor-Robinson et al. (1964); Clyde (1964)
M. buccale	M. orale type 2	CH20247	23636	Oropharynx	Uncommon	Freundt et al. (1974); Taylor-Robinson et al. (1965)
M. faucium	M. orale type 3	DC333	25293	Oropharynx	Uncommon	Freundt et al. (1974); Fox et al. (1969)
M. primatum	Navel strain	HRC292	25948	Oropharynx	Rare	Del Giudice et al. (1971); Thomsen (1974)
M. lipophilum	M. lipophiliae	MaBv	27104	Oropharynx	Rare	Ruiter and Wentholt, 1955
M. pneumoniae	Eaton agent	FH	15531	Lower respiratory tract	Subacute infection, atypical pneumonia	Del Giudice et al. (1974)
M. fermentans	Human type 3	PG18 (G)	19989	Urogenital tract	Uncommon	Chanock et al. (1962); Ruiter and Wenthold (1953); Nicol and Edward (1953)
M. hominis	Human type 1 or M. hominis type 1	PG21	23114	Urogenital tract	Widespread	Nicol and Edward (1953); Edward and Freundt (1956)
M. arthritidis (rat species)	Human type 2 or M. hominis type 2	PG6	19611	Urogenital tract?	Questionable	Edward and Freundt (1965); Morton (1970)
Ureaplasma						
U. urealyticum	T strains	960 (CX8)	27618	Urogenital	Common	Shepard et al. (1974); Shepard (1954)

TABLE III. **Differentiation of Human *Mycoplasma* Species**

Mycoplasma species	Arginine or sugar utilization	Rapid Hemolysis and hemaggluti- nation of guinea pig RBC	Aerobic reduction of tetrazolium	Production of film and spots	Phosphatase activity
M. salivarium	Arginine	0	0	+	0
M. orale	Arginine	0	0	0	0
M. buccale	Arginine	0	0	0	+
M. faucium	Arginine	0	0	+	0
M. primatum	Arginine	0	0	0	0
M. lipophilum	Arginine	0	0	+	?
M. pneumoniae	Glucose	+	+	0	0
M. fermentans	Arginine and glucose	0	0	+	+
M. hominis	Arginine	0	0	0	0
M. arthritidis	Arginine	0	0	0	+

ginine pathway, and the other human mycoplasmas do not ferment glucose but utilize arginine. *Mycoplasma pneumoniae* is easily distinguished from other *Mycoplasma* species by its ability to hemadsorb and by the production of hydrogen peroxide, causing rapid beta-type hemolysis of guinea pig red blood cells (Somerson *et al.*, 1965). In addition, *M. pneumoniae* reduces tetrazolium salts in an aerobic atmosphere; none of the other human *Mycoplasma* species share this feature. Other biochemical tests may help in differentiating one species from another, but for various reasons have limited usefulness (Bradbury, 1977; Aluotto *et al.*, 1970).

Some characteristics of mycoplasmas are variable and are difficult to control. For example, the rate of growth of *M. pneumoniae* is generally slower than that of the other human *Mycoplasma* species. Also, primary isolates of *M. pneumoniae* usually do not produce the characteristic "fried egg" morphology. These properties may vary, since the rates of growth and colonial morphology of mycoplasmas are dependent upon the quality of the nutrient components of the medium. Poor-quality components can slow growth and cause irregular morphology in any mycoplasma.

The lipid staining characteristic (Del Giudice *et al.*, 1974) and the production of film and spots on agar medium containing horse serum are useful properties in identifying *M. lipophilum*. While *M. salivarium, M. fermentans* and *M. faucium* also produce the film-and-spots reaction, they are unlikely to be confused with *M. lipophilum* because the latter species has unique lipid staining characteristics.

Aluotto and co-workers (1970) reported that a test for phosphatase activity aids in differentiating the arginine-utilizing *Mycoplasma* species of human origin. *Mycoplasma buccale* is phosphatase-positive, while *M. orale*, *M. salivarium,* and *M. primatum* are phosphatase-negative.

V. MYCOPLASMAS OF THE OROPHARYNX

Two *Mycoplasma* species, *M. salivarium* and *M. orale*, found in a large percentage of healthy individuals, can be regarded as resident flora of the oropharynx. In various studies they have been isolated from 25–80% of the normal population, but it is unclear which of these species is more common (Engel and Kenny, 1970; Hendley and Jordan, 1968; Kumagai *et al.*, 1971; Gordon *et al.*, 1967). Probably, almost every human carries at least one of these mycoplasmas, though sampling or isolation methods are usually not sensitive enough for their recovery (Stewart and Chowdray, 1968). Some reports have indicated that oral mycoplasmas are not present in edentulous subjects (Gordon *et al.*, 1967; Razin *et al.*, 1964).

Mycoplasmas have a predilection for mucosal surfaces and every oral *Mycoplasma* species at one time or another has been recovered from humans who showed no oral pathology. Even so, mycoplasmas have been isolated more often from individuals with disease, although their etiological role in these circumstances is not clear.

Kundsin and Praznik (1967) studied healthy young adults to determine the carriage of *Mycoplasma* species in the oral cavity. Their isolation rate was very high; mycoplasmas were isolated from 84% of their group. *Mycoplasma orale* was the predominant species, but *M. salivarium* was also isolated.

Mycoplasma salivarium is frequently isolated from the gingival sulci. Isolates from saliva are considered to originate from the gingival crevices, the primary sites of oral mycoplasmas (Engel and Kenny, 1970). There was a significantly higher percentage of isolations (87%) from individuals with periodontal disease, and a lower rate (32%) from a control group with healthy periodontium (Engel and Kenny, 1970). *Mycoplasma orale* was not isolated from any of the 45 subjects studied. Possibly the cultural conditions for the isolation of *M. orale* were unfavorable.

In a more recent report, Kumagai and associates (1971) determined the incidence and identity of mycoplasmas found in the oral cavity. Also, they obtained sera from their study population and attempted to correlate the presence of GI antibody to oral mycoplasmas with periodontal disease. As reported in Engel and Kenny's work, *M. salivarium* was the most common *Mycoplasma* species and the only species isolated from dental calculus and gingival crevices. *Mycoplasma orale* was also isolated. *Mycoplasma salivarium* comprised 89% of the isolates, and *M. orale* the remainder.

The antibody response to *M. salivarium* was significantly higher in individuals with periodontal disease. Levels of antibody to *M. orale* were about the same in both groups.

Mycoplasma hominis can be cultured from the oral cavity of 1–5% of normal individuals. Other *Mycoplasma* species isolated from the oropharynx, at even lower frequency, include *M. buccale*, *M. fermentans*, and *M. faucium*. *Mycoplasma buccale* is more commonly found in nonhuman primates, where often it is the predominant *Mycoplasma* species of the oropharynx. *Mycoplasma lipophilum* has been recovered from the human oropharynx, but only two isolations have been reported (Del Giudice *et al.*, 1974). Ureaplasmas are also occasionally cultured from the oral cavity. Improved medium formulations should lead to a better appreciation of their incidence. *Mycoplasma fermentans* is an infrequent isolate and probably more "at home" in the urogenital tract. A strain resembling *A. laidlawii* has been isolated from the human oral cavity (Razin *et al.*, 1964). In the past, this organism was considered a saprophyte, a soil and sewage organism; now acholeplasmas have been found in a variety of animals as well as in humans (Tully, 1973), including burn victims (Markham and Markham, 1969).

Since *M. salivarium* is the predominant mycoplasma in dental plaques and in gingival sulci, there have been attempts to determine if this organism has a role in periodontal disease. One possibility is that mycoplasmas attract polymorphonuclear leukocytes to the periodontal area and are phagocytized. Lysosomal enzymes may be released and contribute to the inflammatory process. Parkinson and Carter (1975) showed that human leukocytes effectively phagocytized *M. salivarium*. These mycoplasmas are ingested and killed even in the absence of specific antibody. Mycoplasmas located within phagocytic vacuoles lost structural integrity, an indication that they were digested by lysosomal enzymes. Another report showed that, following contact between human leukocytes and *M. salivarium*, there was a release of histamine (Parkinson, 1975), a known mediator of the inflammatory response. These studies circumstantially suggest a mechanism by which *M. salivarium* contributes to periodontal disease.

The only direct evidence for a pathogenic role for any oral mycoplasma comes from a study on human volunteers (Mufson *et al.*, 1965). In this experiment, intranasal instillation of a concentrated suspension of *M.*

hominis produced mild pharyngitis with a fourfold rise in antibody detected by the indirect hemagglutination test. Also, pharyngitis occurred more frequently in individuals with low levels of preexisting antibody.

However, there has been no association of *M. hominis* with naturally occurring sore throats or other respiratory disease. In retrospect, the pharyngitis may have been due to the extremely high inoculum. Volunteers received a minimum of 10^7 to 10^8 mycoplasma colony-forming units, but these microbes can occur in aggregates, and the inoculum may have been even larger. Furthermore, the strain of *M. hominis* used in this study could have influenced the results. *Mycoplasma hominis* strains exhibit much heterogeneity (Reich *et al.*, 1966; Purcell *et al.*, 1967). Perhaps the *M. hominis* isolate given to the volunteers had membrane antigens or other characteristics not shared with other strains and, under the conditions of the experiment, possessed a unique pathogenic potential.

VI. UROGENITAL TRACT MYCOPLASMAS

The fact that mycoplasmas are part of the normal genital tract flora makes it difficult to define their role as pathogens (see this volume, Chapter 10). Within the last 5–10 years, substantial evidence has indicated that two species of mycoplasmas can cause urogenital problems, *M. hominis* and *U. urealyticum*. *Mycoplasma hominis* is implicated in a variety of infections (Table IV). *Ureaplasma urealyticum* is associated with nonspecific urethritis and infertility. *Mycoplasma fermentans* is an infrequent isolate and probably plays no role in urogenital tract disorders.

Newborns are colonized with mycoplasmas. Apparently, in their descent through the birth canal, they become infected with these and other microbes (Klein *et al.*, 1969). In about one-fifth to one-third of newborn infants, the throat, ear canal and, in the female, urogenital tract, contain mycoplasmas. Fewer isolations are obtained from the umbilicus, perineal region, and urine.

After the first year of life, the percentage of positives declines, and it does not increase until puberty and sexual activity. In adults, the presence of genital mycoplasmas has been correlated with sexual activity. Colonization has been linked to the frequency of sexual intercourse and the number of sexual partners (Klein, 1976).

As a general rule, *M. hominis* appears to be a commensal. However, following a birth or abortion, the organism may act as an opportunist, invading the bloodstream and causing puerperal fever or localizing in the upper genital tract and producing a febrile disease (Lee and McCormack,

TABLE IV. Involvement of *M. hominis* in Human Reproductive and Urinary Tract Problems

Condition	Reference
Abortion	Harwick *et al.* (1970); Jones (1967a)
Mycoplasma Infection during pregnancy	Braun *et al.* (1970); Jones (1967b)
Neonate	
Low birth weight	Klein *et al.* (1969); Braun *et al.* (1971)
Central nervous system infection	Siber *et al.* (1977)
Skin abcess	Sacker *et al.* (1970)
Conjunctivitis	Jones and Tobin (1968)
Postabortion or postpartum fever or infection	Harwick *et al.* (1971); Tully and Smith (1968); Caspi *et al.* (1976); McCormack *et al.* (1973b); Tully *et al.* (1965); Lamey *et al.* (1974); Solomon *et al.* (1973); Jones (1967); Brunell *et al.* (1969)
Pelvic inflammatory disease	Solomon *et al.* (1973); McCormack *et al.* (1973a); Mårdh and Weström (1970)
Bacteremia in males with urogenital complications	Simberkoff and Toharsky (1976)
Presence in Bartholin's gland abcess	Solomon *et al.* (1970)

1974). *Mycoplasma hominis* has been studied extensively because it has been implicated in a variety of illnesses. As stated earlier, there are significant differences among strains of this species.

This heterogeneity has been demonstrated by tests of nucleic acid homology and DNA base ratios, and in numerous serological studies. Hollingdale and Lemcke (1970) showed that intraspecies diversities in membrane antigens were reflected in the serological differences. They also noted that the antigenic determinants of *M. hominis* were structurally different from those of fermenting mycoplasmas. In contrast to fermenting species, treatment of *M. hominis* with lipid solvents did not yield a hapten of high serological activity. Protein antigens of *M. hominis* have been shown to be involved in adsorption of the organism to tissue culture cells (Hollingdale and Manchee, 1972).

Mycoplasma fermentans is not a frequent isolate from the urogenital tract. It was first isolated by Ruiter and Wentholt (1953) from two patients with genital infections. This species also has been isolated from cell cultures inoculated with leukemic bone marrow (Murphy *et al.*, 1967), but with no evidence of any role in the induction of human disease. The membranes of *M. fermentans* are toxic for mice (Plata *et al.*, 1973; Gabridge *et al.*, 1972). Williams and Bruckner (1971) and Williams *et al.* (1970) have suggested that *M. fermentans* might play a role in rheumatoid arthritis, since the migration of leukocytes from arthritic patients was affected by *M. fermentans* (see this volume, Chapter 11). Despite these interesting features, the importance of this species to humans has not been determined.

Among the confusing aspects of the taxonomy of human mycoplasmas, the most perplexing concerns the original source of a species formerly called *M. hominis* type 2. This species designation has been discarded because of serological similarity to *Mycoplasma arthritidis* (Lemcke, 1965; Edward and Freundt, 1965) (see this volume, Chapter 8).

During an early attempt to classify mycoplasmas, Nicol and Edward (1953) showed that the Campo strain (isolated by Dienes) and some urethral mycoplasmas (sent to them by Morton, 1970) from the United States were different from the genital strains isolated in England. They tentatively called the strains from the United States Human type 2. Later, Edward and Freundt (1956) proposed a classification scheme that gained acceptance; in it they recognized two varieties of a single species, *M. hominis* type 1 and *M. hominis* type 2. The latter group included Human type 2 and was represented by the Campo strain. According to Morton (1970), Dienes had isolated the Campo strain in the 1930s from the urethra of a male patient, and the strain had been widely distributed to other laboratories.

Besides Dienes, other workers (Norman *et al.*, 1950) reported the isolation of strains which were serologically similar to the Campo strain. Morton's laboratory at the University of Pennsylvania (Morton, 1970; Morton *et al.*, 1951a) isolated various mycoplasmas from prostatic secretions, urethral discharges, and animal exudates; many of these isolates appeared to be similar to *M. hominis* type-2 strains. In the late 1940s, Morton's laboratory was in possession of the Campo strain, having obtained it from Dienes, and also strain 07, a urethral isolate sent by G. Schaub of Johns Hopkins. Over a decade later, the Campo and 07 isolates were shown to react serologically with *M. arthritidis* (Lemcke, 1965), an etiological agent of rat polyarthritis (Findlay *et al.*, 1939). This finding led to the removal of *M. hominis* type 2 from a mycoplasma classification scheme (Edward and Freundt, 1965). The ability of the Campo strain to produce experimental arthritis in rats (Cole *et al.*, 1967) supports the identity of these organisms.

It is true that mycoplasma isolates were interchanged among investigators and, since most mycoplasmas are morphologically indistinguishable, contaminating species could go unnoticed. The serological identification of mycoplasmas had not been firmly established, and cultures containing more than one *Mycoplasma* species would not be recognized. The *cloning* of isolates, the practice of subculturing and selection to ensure the purity of a strain, was not a common practice in the 1940s and 1950s. Most investigators had problems maintaining stock mycoplasma cultures and avoiding bacterial contamination. Under these circumstances, it is easy to understand how cross-contamination of human and animal mycoplasmas might have occurred.

Despite these reservations, several reported isolations of *M. arthritidis* have since been made from human clinical material. Recovery of the organism was made primarily from patients with rheumatoid arthritis (Jansson and Wager, 1967; Jansson *et al.*, 1971a,b, 1972, 1975; Brown *et al.*, 1973) (see also this volume, Chapter 11). It was suggested that modifications in the mycoplasma broth medium, involving additions of fresh pasteurized egg yolk (Jansson *et al.*, 1971a), might have accounted for the enhanced isolation of *M. arthritidis*. Several other investigators have tried to confirm the association of *M. arthritidis* with humans, with rheumatoid arthritis, or with the use of the specialized culture medium noted above, but without success (Person *et al.*, 1972; Ford and Wort, 1972; Stewart *et al.*, 1974; Middleton and Highton, 1975). *Mycoplasma arthritidis* has also been reportedly isolated on a few occasions from rhesus monkeys (M. Davidson, personal communication), from other monkeys (Smirnova *et al.*, 1975), and from bush babies (Cole *et al.*, 1972). From the above observations, it seems somewhat prudent to reserve judgment at this time as to whether *M. arthritidis* actually resides in human or nonhuman primates, either as part of the normal mycoplasma flora or during disease.

VII. MYCOPLASMAS OF THE LOWER ALIMENTARY TRACT

Most of the early work on isolation of mycoplasmas from the lower alimentary tract of humans was published between 1950 and 1960. These earlier isolation attempts have been reviewed by Morton (1970). The lower tract was not sampled adequately, since most attempts involved only examination of fecal material. We now recognize that the older culture medium formulations were inadequate for growing many *Mycoplasma* species. Also, few investigators tried to identify mycoplasmas isolated from the anal canal.

More recently, Altucci and co-workers (1971) looked for mycoplasmas in the upper small intestine. They examined mucosal biopsies, intestinal fluid aspirates, and biliary secretions. All such specimens were negative for mycoplasmas, including those obtained from individuals who had gastrointestinal pathology.

In earlier work reported by some of the same investigators (Altucci *et al.*, 1967), rectal biopsies and swabs were cultured for mycoplasmas. Fifty patients, including both males and females, participated in this study; mycoplasmas were obtained from four. By CF tests, these isolates were identified as *M. hominis*. Individuals from whom mycoplasmas were isolated did not have rectal disease and did not possess serum-specific antibody. In another study from this same institute, mycoplasmas could not be associated with chronic ulcerative colitis (Jori *et al.*, 1968).

Based on these results and on earlier reports of other workers, it has been suggested that an overall isolation rate of 8% is a reasonable figure, that rectal mycoplasmas originate in the genitourinary tract, and that these mycoplasmas are not involved in any disease.

Recent studies on the incidence and the kinds of mycoplasmas in the lower intestinal region are limited. At this time, there is no evidence that mycoplasmas are of any importance in disease of the lower alimentary tract.

VIII. DISEASES OF SUSPECTED MYCOPLASMA ETIOLOGY

The demonstration that a mycoplasma can produce pneumonia in humans has led investigators to look for other illnesses that might be produced by these agents. Recent work indicates that *M. pneumoniae* may be involved in diseases of the central nervous system. Also, Arthur and Margolis (1977) obtained electron microscope evidence of mycoplasma-like structures in brain material from two patients who had granulomatous angiitis; however, no mycoplasma was isolated. Also, *M. pneumoniae* has been implicated in skin disease or, more accurately, in the production of mucocutaneous lesions following infection. It appears to be one of many agents that may trigger erythema multiforme (Gordon and Lyell, 1970).

Another report showed that patients with sarcoidosis possessed higher titers of CF antibody to *M. pneumoniae* than the normal population (Putman *et al.*, 1975). The etiology of sarcoidosis remains uncertain, and the explanation for this finding is not clear.

One study has implicated *M. hominis* in wound infections (Lee *et al.*, 1971). Following corrections on fractured mandibles, the organism was isolated from the wound drainage of two patients. Both patients received penicillin, and these cases may represent colonization of the wound areas after the elimination of penicillin-sensitive microbes.

IX. DISTRIBUTION OF HUMAN MYCOPLASMAS IN NONHUMAN PRIMATES

In recent years it has become apparent that most human *Mycoplasma* species also can be found in nonhuman primates (Table V). The only exception appears to be *M. pneumoniae* which thus far has been isolated only from humans. Low titers of CF antibodies against *M. pneumoniae* have been detected in the sera from a wide variety of primate species (Hutchison *et al.*, 1970), but the occurrence of cross-reacting antigens (particularly in the CF test) precludes a final judgment on the distribution of *M. pneumoniae* in lower primates.

The identification of simian mycoplasmas is accomplished by serological procedures using antisera prepared against strains of human origin and, in some cases, cross-reacting antiprimate mycoplasma sera with human strains. The species with the widest distribution appears to be *M. salivarium*. It has been found mainly in the oropharynx of ten nonhuman primate species, including the great apes, as well as the more primitive prosimian species *Galago crassicaudatus* (bush baby). *Mycoplasma buccale* and *M. primatum* also appear to be widely distributed and have been found in seven and four distinct primate groups, respectively. *Mycoplasma hominis* has also been found in four primate groups, as well as in humans. Mycoplasma strains related to *M. faucium* also appear to be common, although this species appears to be serologically heterogeneous and is considered in more detail in Section X. Only single isolations have been made of *M. fermentans*, *M. lipophilum*, and *A. laidlawii*. *Mycoplasma canis*, *M. arthritidis*, and *M. orale* have been encountered only twice. Ureaplasmas have also been isolated from the oropharynx of squirrel monkeys and marmosets. Additional studies suggest that they are widely distributed in marmosets, having been detected in the testes, spinal cord, brain, and respiratory tract (A. Hill, personal communication).

Although in one study (Hutchison *et al.*, 1970) none of the mycoplasma isolated from chimpanzees, baboons, or rhesus or African green monkeys could be equated with a known human species, in most other investigations at least one human species was isolated per host and additional unidentified species not found in humans were recovered.

It is becoming apparent that some human *Mycoplasma* species occur with a much greater frequency in nonhuman primates. Thus *M. buccale* is present in only 2% of the human population (Taylor-Robinson *et al.*, 1965); whereas it is the most commonly encountered oral isolate from African green monkeys (Del Giudice *et al.*, 1969; Madden *et al.*, 1970a), rhesus

TABLE V. Distribution of Mycoplasmas in Nonhuman Primates

Mycoplasma isolated	Source of isolates	Reference
M. hominis	Chimpanzee (*Pan troglodytes*)	Cole et al. (1970a,b); Martinez-Lahoz et al. (1970)
	Baboon (*Papio* sp.)	Hill (1977)
	African Green (*Cereopithecus aethiops*)	Cole et al. (1970b)
M. fermentans	Rhesus (*Macaca mulatta*)	Madden et al. (1970b); Hill (1977)
M. salivarium	African green	Del Giudice et al. (1969)
	Chimpanzee	Cole et al. (1970a,b)
	Gorilla (*Gorilla gorilla*)	Cole et al. (1970b); Brown et al. (1970)
	Orangutan (*Pongo pygmaeus*)	Cole et al. (1970b)
	Baboon	Hill (1977)
	African green	Del Giudice et al. (1969); Madden et al. (1970a)
	Rhesus	Madden et al. (1970b); Hill (1977)
	Cynomolgous (*Macaca irus*)	Hill (1977)
	Patas (*Erythrocebus patas*)	Hill (1977)
	Squirrel (*Saimiri sciureus*)	Hill (1977)
	Bush baby (*Galago crassicaudatus*	Cole et al. (1972)
M. orale	Orangutan	Cole et al. (1970b)
	Baboon	Hill (1977)
	Chimpanzee	Martinez-Lahoz et al. (1970)
	Orangutan	Cole et al. (1970b)
	Baboon	Hill (1977); Nicol and Edward (1953)
	African green	Del Giudice et al. (1969); Madden et al. (1970a)
M. buccale	Rhesus	Madden et al. (1970b); Hill (1977)
	Cynomolgous	Hill (1977); Vogelzang and Hagenaars (1973)
	Patas	Hill (1977)

Species	Host	References
M. faucium	Chimpanzee	Cole *et al.* (1970a,b)
	Baboon	Hill (1977)
	African Green	Del Giudice *et al.* (1969)
	Rhesus	Hill (1977)
	Cynomolgous	Vogelzang and Hagenaars (1973)
	Patas	Hill (1977)
M. primatum	Baboon	Hill (1977)
	African green	Madden *et al.* (1970a); Del Giudice *et al.* (1969)
	Rhesus	Hill (1977)
	Squirrel	Hill (1977)
	Rhesus	Hill (1977)
M. lipophilum	African green	Madden *et al.* (1974)
M. moatsii	Baboon	Martinez-Lahoz *et al.* (1970)
M. canis	African green	Martinez-Lahoz *et al.* (1970)
M. arthritidis	Bush baby	Cole *et al.* (1972)
A. laidlawii	Rhesus	Madden *et al.* (1970b)
Ureaplasma sp.	Squirrel	Taylor-Robinson *et al.* (1971)
	Marmoset (*Callothrix* sp.)	Furr *et al.* (1976); Kundsin *et al.* (1973)
Unidentified	Chimpanzee	Cole *et al.* (1970a,b); Davidson and Thomas (1968); Hutchison *et al.* (1970)
	Orangutan	Cole *et al.* (1970b)
	Baboon	Davidson and Thomas (1968); Hutchison *et al.* (1970)
	African green	Davidson and Thomas (1968); Del Giudice *et al.* (1969); Hutchison *et al.* (1970); Madden *et al.* (1970a)
	Cynomolgous	Vogelzang and Hagenaars (1973)
	Rhesus	Davidson and Thomas (1968); Hill (1977); Hutchison *et al.* (1970); Madden *et al.* (1970b)
	Squirrel	Davidson and Thomas (1968)
	Bush baby	Cole *et al.* (1972)

^a For details see literature cited.

monkeys (Hill, 1977; Madden *et al.,* 1970b), baboons (Hill, 1977), patas (Hill, 1977), and cynomolgous monkeys (Hill, 1977; Vogelzang and Hagenaars, 1973). Similarly, *M. primatum* (strain Navel), which is a rare isolate from humans (Ruiter and Wentholt, 1955; Thomsen, 1974), is rather common in nonhuman primates (Hill, 1977; Madden *et al.,* 1970a; Del Giudice *et al.,* 1969) and is found at both urogenital and oropharyngeal sites.

It is difficult to provide a definitive answer to the question of the origin of human species of mycoplasma found in nonhuman primates. In most cases (Cole *et al.,* 1970a,b, 1972; Hutchison *et al.,* 1970; Madden *et al.,* 1970b) the animals examined had been in capitivity for comparatively long periods of time, potentially allowing for an exchange of flora to occur. However, other studies (Hill, 1977; Vogelzang and Hagenaars, 1973; Madden *et al.,* 1970a; Del Giudice *et al.,* 1969), which employed animals quarantined soon after capture, also resulted in the detection of human species of mycoplasmas. These observations suggest that the organisms isolated comprised part of the normal flora of the animals.

As can be seen from Table V, most nonhuman primates have been reported to harbor one or more mycoplasmas which could not be identified as any known human or animal species. In most cases detailed investigations of these strains have not been undertaken, and their taxonomic status is not known at this time.

One species, *Mycoplasma moatsii,* which was isolated from the urogenital tract and saliva of African green monkeys (Madden *et al.,* 1974), appears to be specific for these animals and is serologically distinct from a wide range of human and animal mycoplasmas. This organism metabolizes both arginine and glucose and can be adapted to grow aerobically as well as anaerobically. Neither tetrazolium nor methylene blue is reduced in either atmosphere.

Mycoplasmas isolated from the saliva and nose of six bush babies also appear to represent a new species (Cole *et al.,* 1972). The organisms comprise a closely related group of glucose-fermenting strains serologically distinct from the NIH-WHO reference antisera on the basis of metabolic inhibition (MI) and GI tests (B. C. Cole, unpublished observation). Cross-reactions are apparent with *Mycoplasma felis* in agar gel diffusion tests, and physiologically they resemble the latter species. The organisms grow rapidly under aerobic incubation. All strains are hemolytic, and most adsorb sheep erythrocytes to their colonies. Triphenyltetrazolium chloride is reduced under anaerobic conditions, but arginine is not metabolized. A film-and-spots reaction is apparent on egg yolk-containing medium.

X. RELATIONSHIP BETWEEN HUMAN AND NONHUMAN PRIMATE ISOLATES OF THE SAME SPECIES

In many studies, biological and serological comparisons of human and nonhuman primate strains were incomplete. In some cases, there was a very close similarity or identity between primate and human strains, while in others there was evidence of heterogeneity. Most workers have not differentiated human and simian isolates of *M. buccale,* although Vogelzang and Hagenaars (1973) obtained evidence of minor serological differences by GI assay. Interestingly, the medium used for cultivation appeared to alter the sensitivity of the test. Biochemically all isolates appeared to be identical.

The human and nonhuman primate strains of *M. primatum* were virtually identical in their biochemical properties, growth characteristics, and electrophoretic protein profile. Serologically all strains cross-reacted in the GI test, although some minor differences were apparent in the fluorescence antibody (FA) test (Del Giudice *et al.*, 1971).

Although simian isolates of *M. primatum* could not be differentiated from the human strain Navel on the basis of growth characteristics, biochemical reactions or protein composition, minor differences were apparent on the FA and CF antibody tests. However, the highly specific GI test failed to separate the strains (Del Giudice *et al.*, 1971).

Taylor-Robinson *et al.* (1963) showed that an oral isolate of *M. hominis* from an African green monkey could not be differentiated on the basis of the CF test from either vaginal or oral strains of *M. hominis* isolated from humans. Somerson *et al.* (1967), however, using DNA hybridization procedures, indicated that the genetic relationship between this simian isolate and a human isolate was less than that seen among different human strains of *M. hominis*. Other studies by Cole *et al.* (1970a) on *M. hominis* showed that human and chimpanzee strains could not be differentiated biochemically but could be separated by GI and MI tests. Two serological subgroups of *M. hominis* were identified within the chimpanzee strains. Strains of one of the subgroups appeared identical to the human strains, whereas the other appeared to be serologically distinct. Both subgroups were found in either the vagina or oropharynx of the chimpanzee. Interestingly, when the animals were recultured 12 months later, the chimpanzee subgroup, which contained strains more closely resembling the human isolates, was absent.

Isolates of *M. salivarium* from human, gorilla, orangutan, chimpanzee, or *Galago* sources could not be differentiated serologically. However, all three great apes were found to harbor strains which markedly differed in lipolytic activity (Cole *et al.*, 1970b). Nonlipolytic human strains of *M. salivarium* have also been reported (Cole and Pease, 1967). One chimpanzee isolate exhibited unusually coarse colonies, completely unlike those of typical *M. salivarium*. In another study, DNA hybridization between a simian and human isolate of *M. salivarium* indicated that the organisms were closely related but genetically distinct (Somerson *et al.*, 1967).

The *Galago* isolates of *M. arthritidis* were identical serologically and biochemically with a rat-passaged culture of the Campo strain from humans and were strongly arthritogenic for rats (Cole *et al.*, 1972).

Several mycoplasma isolates represented by strains HSPP chimpanzee (Cole *et al.*, 1970b), K4a cynomolgous (Vogelzang and Hagenaars, 1973), 21E cynomolgous, and 26D baboon (A. Hill, personal communication) appear to be related to *M. faucium*. They closely resemble this species in growth and physiological properties and possess characteristic mottled colonies as a result of very strong lipolytic activity (the film-and-spots reaction). They also show relatedness to *M. faucium* in CF, MI, GI, and agar gel diffusion test (B. C. Cole, A. Hill, and A. A. Vogelzang, unpublished observation). Electrophoretic analysis of cell proteins confirms the similarities among these strains, but each has a characteristic protein profile (B. C. Cole, unpublished observation).

In conclusion, whereas some primate strains of human *Mycoplasma* species appear to differ from their human counterparts, these differences are probably not due to the source of the isolates.

XI. PATHOGENIC POTENTIAL OF MYCOPLASMAS FOR NONHUMAN PRIMATES

Although mycoplasmas cause disease in a wide variety of animal species, convincing evidence of their ability to cause disease in nonhuman primates remains to be determined. Although Kundsin *et al.* (1973) reported the isolation of ureaplasmas from monkeys with reproductive failure, the etiological role of these organisms in this condition was not established. Recently, Obeck *et al.* (1976) reported a significant increase and a persisting CF antibody titer against *M. pneumoniae* in a rhesus monkey suffering from a severe polyarthritis. Although the disease resembled infectious arthritis, neither bacteria nor mycoplasmas could be cultured from the joints. Brown *et al.* (1970) have also described spontaneous rheumatoid-like arthritis in a gorilla. Not surprisingly these workers isolated *M. salivarium* from the throat of the animal but also claimed to detect *M. salivarium* in the inflamed joint tissue using indirect immunological procedures. The role of mycoplasmas in human arthritis is discussed more fully in this volume, Chapter 11.

In a few cases, simian isolates have been tested for their pathogenic effect in other hosts. The ability of *M. arthritidis* isolates from the bush baby to induce arthritis in rats has already been mentioned. Howard *et al.* (1973) showed that, whereas ureaplasma isolates from bovine lungs caused mastitis in cows following intermammary injection, an oropharyngeal simian isolate did not. Using human fallopian tube organ cultures, Taylor-Robinson and Carney (1974) demonstrated that, although a simian ureaplasma isolate grew in this system, no cytopathic effects were observed.

Studies have already been initiated to elucidate the controversial role of ureaplasmas in urogenital disease. Taylor-Robinson *et al.* (1978) inoculated human strains of ureaplasma intraurethrally into chimpanzees. A 1000-fold replication of the organisms occurred in some animals, although gross clinical pathology was not seen. These investigators have suggested considerable variation in the ability of various chimpanzees to support the growth of human ureaplasmas. The specificity of ureaplasmas is noted in the observation of Furr and Taylor-Robinson (personal communication) that human ureaplasmas infected marmoset monkeys while bovine ureaplasmas did not.

As already discussed in this chapter, the pathogenic potential of *M. hominis* for humans is equally controversial. Møller *et al.* (1978) showed that a freshly isolated strain of *M. hominis* obtained from the cervix of a patient with acute salpingitis induced a marked inflammatory response of the uterine tubes of grivet monkeys. The experimental disease was at a maximum 7–12 days after inoculation but had virtually subsided by 4–5 weeks. The ability of the organisms to persist for several months in the vagina provided further evidence that a true infection had been established.

Unfortunately, attempts to induce pneumonia in nonhuman primates using *M. pneumoniae* have not met with success. Thus Friedlaender *et al.* (1976) showed that, although rhesus monkeys responded immunologically to aerosol administration of *M. pneumoniae*, significant lower respiratory tract disease did not develop.

Several years ago cynomolgous monkeys were used to determine the ability of *Mycoplasma gallisepticum* to cause cardiac damage (Sun *et al.*, 1968). Interestingly, in one animal the mycoplasmas localized in the myocardium and were demonstrable by immunofluoresence techniques. In addition, focal myolytic inflammatory lesions were also seen in most animals.

Nonhuman primates have a great potential as experimental animals for investigating the pathogenic properties of human mycoplasmas. A necessary prerequisite for experimental studies involving these animals is characterization of the existing mycoplasma flora. Unfortunately nonhuman primates are in limited supply and their cost is prohibitive for use as routine experimental animals. Perhaps the most appropriate use of these animals may be to fulfill Koch's postulates on mycoplasma isolates for which there is already strong evidence of their disease-producing capacity in humans.

REFERENCES

Altucci, P., Jori, G. P., and De Vargas, F. (1967). *Chemotherapia* **12,** 41–46.

Altucci, P., Jori, G. P., Manguso, L., and Varone, G. L. (1971). *Pathol. Microbiol.* **37,** 181–184.

Aluotto, B. B., Wittler, R. G., Williams, C. O., and Faber, J. E. (1970). *Int. J. Syst. Bacteriol.* **20,** 35–58.

Armstrong, D., Yu, B. H., Yogoda, A., and Kagnoff, M. F. (1971). *J. Infect. Dis.* **124,** 607–609.

Arthur, G., and Margolis, G. (1977). *Arch. Pathol. Lab. Med.* **101,** 382–387.

Bak, L. B., Black, F. T., Christiansen, C., and Freundt, E. A. (1969). *Nature (London)* **224,** 1209–1210.

Barile, M. F. (1967). *Ann. N.Y. Acad. Sci.* **143,** 557–572.

Barile, M. F. (1973). *J. Infect. Dis.* **127,** Suppl., S17–S20.

Barile, M. F., and Kern, J. (1971). *Proc. Soc. Exp. Biol. Med.* **138,** 432–437.

Bradbury, J. M. (1977). *J. Clin. Microbiol.* **5,** 531–534.

Braun, P., Klein, J. O., Lee, Y. H., and Kass, E. H. (1970). *J. Infect. Dis.* **121,** 391–400.

Braun, P., Lee, Y., Klein, J. O., Marcy, S. M., Klein, T. A., Charles, D., Levy, P., and Kass, E. H. (1971). *N. Engl. J. Med.* **284,** 167–171.

Brown, T. McP., Clark, H. W., Bailey, J. S., and Gray, C. W. (1970). *Trans. Am. Clin. Climatol. Assoc.* **82,** 227–247.

Brown, T. McP., Bailey, J. S., and Clark, H. W. (1973). *Int. Congr. Rheumatol., 13th, Kyoto* p. 172.

Brunell, P. A., Dische, R. M., and Walker, M. B. (1969). *J. Am. Med. Assoc.* **207,** 2097–2099.

Caspi, E., Solomon, F., Langer, R., and Sompolinsky, D. (1976). *Obstet. Gynecol.* **48,** 682–684.

Chanock, R. M., Hayflick, L., and Barile, M. F. (1962). *Proc. Natl. Acad. Sci. U.S.A.* **48,** 41–49.

Clyde, W. A., Jr. (1964). *J. Immunol.* **92,** 958–965.

Cole, B. C., and Pease, P. E. (1967). *J. Gen. Microbiol.* **47,** 171–174.

Cole, B. C., Miller, M. L., and Ward, J. R. (1967). *Proc. Soc. Exp. Biol. Med.* **124,** 103–107.

Cole, B. C., Graham, C. E., and Ward, J. R. (1970a). *In* "The Chimpanzee" (G. H. Bourne, ed.), Vol. 2, pp. 390–409. S. Karger, Basel and New York.

Cole, B. C., Ward, J. R., Golightly-Rowland, L., and Graham, C. E. (1970b). *Can. J. Microbiol.* **16,** 1331–1339.

Cole, B. C., Graham, C. E., Golightly-Rowland, L., and Ward, J. R. (1972). *Can. J. Microbiol.* **18,** 1431–1437.

Davidson, M., and Thomas, L. (1968). *Bacteriol. Proc.* p. 79.

Del Giudice, R. A., Carski, T. R., Barile, M. F., Yamashiroya, H. M., and Verna, J. E. (1969). *Nature (London)* **222,** 1088–1089.

Del Giudice, R. A., Carski, T. R., Barile, M. F., Lemcke, R. M., and Tully, J. G. (1971). *J. Bacteriol.* **108,** 439–445.

Del Giudice, R. A., Purcell, R. H., Carski, T. R., and Chanock, R. M. (1974). *Int. J. Syst. Bacteriol.* **24,** 147–153.

Dienes, L., and Edsall, J. (1937). *Proc. Soc. Exp. Biol. Med.* **36,** 740–744.

Dienes, L., and Smith, W. E. (1942). *Proc. Soc. Exp. Biol. Med.* **50,** 99–101.

Edward, D. G. ff. (1955). *Int. Bull. Bacteriol. Nomencl. Taxon.* **5,** 85–93.

Edward, D. G. ff., and Freundt, E. A. (1956). *J. Gen. Microbiol.* **14,** 197–207.

Edward, D. G. ff., and Freundt, E. A. (1965). *J. Gen. Microbiol.* **41,** 263–265.

Engel, L. D., and Kenny, G. E. (1970). *J. Periodontal Res.* **5,** 163–171.

Findlay, G. M., Mackenzie, R. D., MacCallum, F. O., and Klieneberger, E. (1939). *Lancet* **ii,** 7–10.

Ford, D. K., and Wort, B. (1972). *Arthritis Rheum.* **15,** 650.

Fox, H., Purcell, R. H., and Chanock, R. M. (1969). *J. Bacteriol.* **98,** 36–43.

Freundt, E. A., Taylor-Robinson, D., Purcell, R. H., Chanock, R. M., and Black, F. T. (1974). *Int. J. Syst. Bacteriol.* **24,** 252–255.

Friedlaender, R. P., Grizzard, M. B., Helms, C. M., Barile, M. F., Senterfit, L., and Chanock, R. M. (1976). *J. Infect. Dis.* **133,** 343–346.

Furr, P. M., Taylor-Robinson, D., and Hetherington, C. M. (1976). *Lab. Anim.* **10,** 393–398.

Gabridge, M. G., Abrams, G. D., and Murphy, W. H. (1972). *J. Infect. Dis.* **125,** 153–160.

Gordon, A. M., and Lyell, A. (1970). *Br. J. Dermatol.* **82,** 414–416.

Gordon, A. M., Dick, H. M., Mason, D. K., Manderson, W., and Crichton, W. B. (1967). *J. Clin. Pathol.* **20,** 865–869.

Harwick, H. J., Purcell, R. H., Iuppa, J. B., and Fekety, F. R., Jr. (1970). *J. Infect. Dis.* **121,** 260–268.

Harwick, H. J., Purcell, R. H., Iuppa, J. B., and Fekety, F. R., Jr. (1971). *Obstet. Gynecol.* **37,** 765–768.

Hayflick, L., and Koprowski, H. (1965). *Nature (London)* **205,** 713–714.

Hayflick, L., and Stanbridge, E. (1967). *Ann. N.Y. Acad. Sci.* **143,** 608–621.

Hendley, J. O., and Jordan, W. S., Jr. (1968). *Am. Rev. Respir. Dis.* **97,** 524–532.

Herring, P., and Pollack, J. D. (1974). *Int. J. Syst. Bacteriol.* **24,** 73–78.

Hill, A. (1977). *Vet. Rec.* **101,** 117.

Hollingdale, M. R., and Lemcke, R. M. (1970). *J. Hyg.* **68,** 469–476.

Hollingdale, M. R., and Manchee, R. J. (1972). *J. Gen. Microbiol.* **70,** 391–393.

Hopps, H. E., Meyer, B. C., Barile, M. F., and Del Giudice, R. A. (1973). *Ann. N.Y. Acad. Sci.* **225,** 265–276.

Howard, C. J., Gourlay, R. N., and Brownlie, J. (1973). *J. Hyg.* **71,** 163–170.

Hughes, J. H., Thomas, D. C., Hamparian, V. V., and Somerson, N. L. (1974). *J. Med. Microbiol.* **7,** 35–40.

Hutchison, V. E., Pinkerton, M. E., and Kalter, S. S. (1970). *Lab. Anim. Care* **20,** 914–922.

Jansson, E., and Wager, O. (1967). *Ann. N.Y. Acad. Sci.* **143,** 535–543.

Jansson, E., Makisara, P., Vainio, K., Snellman, O., and Tuuri, S. (1971a). *Acta Rheumatol. Scand.* **17,** 227–235.

Jansson, E., Vainio, U., Snellman, O., and Tuuri, S. (1971b). *Ann. Rheum. Dis.* **30,** 413–418.

Jansson, E., Vainio, U., Lassus, A., and Tuuri, S. (1972). *Br. J. Vener. Dis.* **48,** 304–305.

Jansson, E., Reinius, S., Rimaila-Parnanen, E., and Tuuri, S. (1975). *Acta Pathol. Microbiol. Scand., Sect. B* **83,** 61–62.

Jones, D. M. (1967a). *Br. Med. J.* **1**, 338–340.

Jones, D. M. (1967b). *J. Clin. Pathol.* **20**, 633–635.

Jones, D. M., and Tobin, B. (1968). *Br. Med. J.* **iii**, 467–468.

Jori, G. P., DeVargas, F., and Altucci, P. (1968). *Pathol. Microbiol.* **31**, 209–214.

Klein, J. O. (1976). *In* "Infectious Diseases of the Fetus and Newborn Infant" (J. S. Remington and J. O. Klein, eds.), pp. 587–615. Saunders, Philadelphia, Pennsylvania.

Klein, J. O., Buckland, D., and Finland, M. (1969). *N. Engl. J. Med.* **280**, 1025–1030.

Kundsin, R. B., and Praznik, J. (1967). *Am. J. Epidemiol.* **86**, 579–583.

Kundsin, R. B., Rowell, T., and Parreno, A. (1973). *Abstr. Annu. Meet. Am. Sco. Microbiol., Washington, D.C.* p. 80.

Kumagai, K., Iwabuchi, T., Hinima, Y., Yuri, K., and Ishida, N. (1971). *J. Infect. Dis.* **123**, 16–21.

Laidlaw, P. D., and Elford, W. J. (1936). *Proc. R. Soc. Biol.* **20**, 292–303.

Lamey, J. R., Foy, H. M., and Kenny, G. E. (1974). *Obstet. Gynecol.* **44**, 703–708.

Lee, Y., and McCormack, W. M. (1974). *J. Reprod. Med.* **13**, 123–127.

Lee, Y., Nersasian, R. R., and Lan, N. K. (1971). *J. Am. Med. Assoc.* **218**, 252–253.

Lemcke, R. M. (1965). *J. Gen. Microbiol.* **38**, 91–100.

Lyons, J. F., Shepard, M. C., Daane, T. A., Wurzel, J. F., and Lunceford, C. D. (1974). *Am. J. Obstet. Gynecol.* **120**, 554–556.

McCormack, W. M., Braun, P., Lee, Y., Klein, J. O., and Kass, E. H. (1973a). *N. Engl. J. Med.* **288**, 78–89.

McCormack, W. M., Lee, Y., Lin, J., and Rankin, J. S. (1973b). *J. Infect. Dis.* **127**, 193–196.

Madden, D. L., Hildebrandt, R. J., Monif, G. R. G., London, W. T., McCullough, N. B., and Sever, J. L. (1970a). *Lab. Anim. Care* **20**, 471–473.

Madden, D. L., Hildebrandt, R. J., Monif, G. R. G., London, W. T., Sever, J. L., and McCullough, N. B. (1970b). *Lab. Anim. Care* **20**, 467–470.

Madden, D. L., Moats, K. E., London, W. T., Mathew, E. B., and Sever, J. L. (1974). *Int. J. Syst. Bacteriol.* **24**, 459–464.

Mårdh, P.-A., and Weström, L. (1970). *Br. J. Vener. Dis.* **46**, 390–397.

Markham, J. G., and Markham, N. P. (1969). *J. Bacteriol.* **98**, 827–828.

Martinez-Lahoz, A., Kalter, S. S., Pinkerton, M. E., and Hayflick, L. (1970). *Ann. N.Y. Acad. Sci.* **174**, 820–827.

Middleton, P. J., and Highton, T. C. (1975). *Ann. Rheum. Dis.* **34**, 369–372.

Millian, S. J., Leopold, I. H., and Schneierson, S. S. (1967). *Am. J. Ophthalmol.* **64**, 289–291.

Møller, B. R., Freundt, E. A., Black, F. T., and Frederiksen, P. (1978). *Infect. Immun.* **20**, 248–257.

Morton, H. E. (1970). *In* "The Role of Mycoplasmas and L Forms of Bacteria in Disease" (J. T. Sharp, ed.), pp. 147–171. Thomas, Springfield, Illinois.

Morton, H. E., Smith, P. F., and Leberman, P. R. (1951a). *Am. J. Syph., Gonorrhea, Vener. Dis.* **35**, 14–17.

Morton, H. E., Smith, P. F., Williams, N. B., and Eickenberg, C. F. (1951b). *J. Dent. Res.* **30**, 415–422.

Mufson, M. A., Ludwig, W. M., Purcell, R. H., Cate, T. R., Taylor-Robinson, D., and Chanock, R. M. (1965). *J. Am. Med. Assoc.* **192**, 1146–1152.

Murphy, W. H., Bullis, C., Ertel, I. J., and Zarafonetis, C. J. D. (1967). *Ann. N.Y. Acad. Sci.* **143**, 544–556.

Nicol, C. S., and Edward, D. G. ff. (1953). *Br. J. Vener. Dis.* **29**, 141–150.

Norman, M. C., Saslaw, S., and Kuhn, L. R. (1950). *Proc. Soc. Exp. Biol. Med.* **75,** 718–720.

Obeck, D. K., Toft, J. D., II, and Dupuy, H. J. (1976). *Lab. Anim. Sci.* **26,** 613–618.

Parkinson, C. F. (1975). *Infect. Immun.* **11,** 595–597.

Parkinson, C. F., and Carter, P. B. (1975). *Infect. Immun.* **11,** 405–414.

Person, D. A., Whitworth, M. E., and Sharp, J. T. (1972). *Arthritis Rheum.* **15,** 649–650.

Plata, E. J., Abell, M. R., and Murphy, W. H. (1973). *J. Infect. Dis.* **128,** 588–597.

Pollack, J. D. (1975). *Int. J. Syst. Bacteriol.* **25,** 108–113.

Purcell, R. H., Wong, D., Chanock, R. M., Taylor-Robinson, D., Canchola, J., and Valdesuso, J. (1967). *Ann. N.Y. Acad. Sci.* **143,** 664–675.

Putman, C. E., Baumgarten, A., and Gee, J. B. L. (1975). *Am. Rev. Respir. Dis.* **3,** 364–365.

Razin, S., Michmann, J., and Shimshoni, Z. (1964). *J. Dent. Res.* **43,** 402–405.

Reich, P. R., Somerson, N. L., Rose, J. A., and Weissman, S. (1966). *J. Bacteriol.* **91,** 153–160.

Ruiter, M., and Wentholt, H. M. M. (1953). *Acta Derm.-Venereol.* **3,** 123–129.

Ruiter, M., and Wentholt, H. M. M. (1955). *J. Invest. Dermatol.* **24,** 31–34.

Sacker, I., Walker, M., and Brunell, P. A. (1970). *Pediatrics* **46,** 303–304.

Shepard, M. C. (1954). *Am. J. Syph. Neurol.* **38,** 113–124.

Shepard, M. C., Lunceford, C. D., Ford, D. K., Purcell, R. H., Taylor-Robinson, D., Razin, S., and Black, F. T. (1974). *Int. J. Syst. Bacteriol.* **24,** 160–171.

Siber, G. R., Alpert, S., Smith, A. L., Lin, J. L., and McCormack, W. M. (1977). *J. Pediat.* **90,** 625–627.

Simberkoff, M. S., and Toharsky, B. (1976). *J. Am. Med. Assoc.* **236,** 2522–2524.

Smirnova, T. D., Yaguzhinskaya, O. E., and Balaeva, E. Y. (1975). *Zh. Mikrobiol., Epidemiol. Immunobiol.* **52,** 90–94.

Smith, P. F., and Morton, H. E. (1951). *Science* **113,** 623–624.

Solomon, F., Sompolinsky, D., Caspi, E., and Alkan, W. J. (1970). *Isr. J. Med. Sci.* **6,** 605–610.

Solomon, F., Caspi, E., Bukovsky, I., and Sompolinsky, D. (1973). *Am. J. Obstet. Gynecol.* **116,** 785–792.

Somerson, N. L., Walls, B. E., and Chanock, R. M. (1965). *Science* **150,** 226–228.

Somerson, N. L., Reich, P. R., Chanock, R. M., and Weissman, S. M. (1967). *Ann. N.Y. Acad. Sci.* **143,** 9–20.

Stewart, S. M., and Chowdray, J. E. (1968). *J. Pathol. Bacteriol.* **95,** 580–586.

Stewart, S. M., Duthie, J. J. R., Mackay, J. M. K., Marmion, B. P., and Alexander, W. R. M. (1974). *Ann. Rheum. Dis.* **33,** 346–352.

Sun, S. C., Sohal, R. S., Chu, K. C., Colcolough, H. L., Leiderman, E., and Burch, G. E. (1968). *Am. J. Pathol.* **53,** 1073–1096.

Taylor-Robinson, D., and Carney, F. E., (1974). *Br. J. Vener. Dis.* **50,** 212–216.

Taylor-Robinson, D., Somerson, N. L., Turner, H. C., and Chanock, R. M. (1963). *J. Bacteriol.* **85,** 1261–1273.

Taylor-Robinson, D., Canchola, J., Fox, H., and Chanock, R. M. (1964). *Am. J. Hyg.* **80,** 135–148.

Taylor-Robinson, D., Fox, H., and Chanock, R. M. (1965). *Am. J. Epidemiol.* **81,** 180–191.

Taylor-Robinson, D., Martin-Bourgon, C., Watanabe, T., and Addey, J. P. (1971). *J. Gen. Microbiol.* **68,** 97–107.

Taylor-Robinson, D., Purcell, R. H., London, W. T., and Sly, D. L. (1978). *J. Med. Microbiol.* **11,** 197–201.

Thomsen, A. C. (1974). *Acta Pathol. Microbiol. Scand., Sect. B* **82,** 653–656.

Tully, J. G., and Rask-Nielsen, R. (1967). *Ann. N.Y. Acad. Sci.* **143,** 345–352.

Tully, J. G. (1973). *Ann. N.Y. Acad. Sci.* **225,** 74–93.
Tully, J. G., and Smith, L. G. (1968). *J. Am. Med. Assoc.* **204,** 827–828.
Tully, J. G., Brown, M. S., Sheagren, J. N., Young, V. M., and Wolff, S. M. (1965). *N. Engl. J. Med.* **273,** 648–650.
Tully, J. G., Whitcomb, R. F., Clark, H. F., and Williamson, D. L. (1977). *Science* **195,** 892–894.
Tully, J. G., Rose, D. L., Whitcomb, R. F., and Wenzel, R. P. (1979). *J. Infect. Dis.* **139** (in press).
Vogelzang, A. A., and Hagenaars, R. (1973). *In Vitro CSSR* **2/1,** 230–235.
Williams, M. H., and Bruckner, F. E. (1971). *Ann. Rheum. Dis.* **30,** 271–273.
Williams, M. H., Brostoff, J., and Roitt, I. M. (1970). *Lancet* **2,** 277–280.

7 / CANINE AND FELINE MYCOPLASMAS

Søren Rosendal

I. INTRODUCTION

It has been over 40 years since Shoetensack (1934, 1936a,b) first reported the occurrence of mycoplasmas in dogs. These early studies were greatly hampered by difficulties in cultivating mycoplasmas in the presence of bacteria, and few techniques were available at the time to separate mixtures of mycoplasmas. It was not until 1951 that Edward and Fitzgerald (1951) provided fundamental information on the occurrence of

THE MYCOPLASMAS, VOL. II
Copyright © 1979 by Academic Press, Inc.
All rights of reproduction in any form reserved.
ISBN 0-12-078401-7

three distinct *Mycoplasma* species (*M. spumans, M. canis*, and *M. maculosum*) in dogs and established a proper taxonomic characterization.

A feline mycoplasma flora was not generally suspected until Cello (1957) and Colegrave *et al.* (1964) reported the presence of mycoplasmas in the eyes of cats with conjunctivitis. Cole and associates (Cole *et al.*, 1967) subsequently provided important data on the occurrence of two new mycoplasmas (*Mycoplasma felis* and *M. gateae*) in the eyes and oral cavity of cats. These observations were confirmed shortly thereafter, and a third distinct species (*Mycoplasma feliminutum*) was added to the list of feline mycoplasma flora (Heyward *et al.*, 1969).

Thus, at the time of the last major review of canine and feline mycoplasmas (Ward and Cole, 1970), only 6 distinct *Mycoplasma* species had been characterized. Some indication of the rapid progress in this area can be gained from the fact that now over 15 different species or recognized serotypes of mycoplasmas have been recovered from these hosts.

Most of the information in the literature on canine and feline mycoplasmas is concerned primarily with their occurrence, distribution, and taxonomy, and little definite information is known about host–parasite relationships. This chapter summarizes the current status of mycoplasmas in these hosts and records some of the observed host–parasite interactions.

II. RECOGNIZED CANINE AND FELINE MYCOPLASMAS

Table I lists the species and groups of canine and feline mycoplasmas. For each, the type strain (or reference culture) is given, as well as documentation of the taxonomic description or appropriate literature references establishing the organism in these hosts.

The list of canine species includes *Mycoplasma arginini*, since two strains isolated by Rosendal (1974b) and considered to constitute serogroup 2 within *M. gateae* have significant antigenic cross-relationships to *M. arginini*.

Tan and Miles (1974) reported on 34 feline isolates which could not be identified as either *M. felis, M. gateae, M. arginini*, or *Acholeplasma laidlawii*. Further taxonomic studies on these isolates may result in extension of this list.

III. CULTIVATION AND ISOLATION

Growth requirements of currently recognized canine and feline mycoplasmas can be satisfied by media prepared according to formulas devised

TABLE I. **Species and Groups of Canine and Feline Mycoplasmas**

Organism	Type strain	Canine isolates[a]	Feline isolates[a]
		First reported by:	
Mycoplasma			
M. spumans	PG13	Edward and Fitzgerald (1951)	NI
M. canis	PG14	Edward and Fitzgerald (1951)	NI
M. maculosum	PG15	Edward and Fitzgerald (1951)	NI
M. edwardii	PG24	Tully *et al.* (1970)	NI
M. cynos	H831	Rosendal (1973a)	NI
M. molare	H542	Rosendal (1974a)	NI
M. opalescens	MH5408	Rosendal (1975b)	NI
M. bovigenitalium	PG11	Rosendal (1974b)	NI
M. gateae	CS	Rosendal (1974b)	Cole *et al.* (1967)
M. feliminutum	BEN	Rosendal (1974b)	Heyward *et al.* (1969)
M. felis	CO	NI	Cole *et al.* (1967)
M. arginini	G230	Rosendal (1974b)	Tan and Miles (1974)
Mycoplasma group	HRC689[b]	Barile *et al.* (1970)	NI
Acholeplasma laidlawii	PG8	Rosendal and Laber (1973)	Tan and Miles (1972)
Ureaplasma	None	Taylor-Robinson *et al.* (1971)	Tan and Markham (1971a)

[a] NI, No isolates.
[b] Reference strain.

by Edward (1947) and Hayflick (1965), provided individual medium components are pretested for support of standard mycoplasma cultures. Specific details about medium preparation for recovery of canine mycoplasmas (Kato *et al.*, 1972; Rosendal, 1973c, 1975a; Kirchhoff, 1973) or feline mycoplasmas (Cole *et al.*, 1967; Tan and Miles, 1972) have been given. Ureaplasmas (formerly T strains) require specialized media for primary isolation (Taylor-Robinson *et al.*, 1971; Tan and Markham, 1971a).

None of the known canine or feline mycoplasmas are strict anaerobes. During primary isolation, normal atmospheric conditions or atmospheric air with 5% carbon dioxide seems to give satisfactory growth of mycoplasmas. The temperature range generally used for cultivation of mycoplasmas is 36°–37°C, although cultures for the specific recovery of acholeplasmas can be incubated at 22°–30°C.

Swab sampling is suitable for mycoplasma isolation from mucosal membranes. Plates are streaked directly with the swab, which is then placed in liquid or semisolid medium. The latter cultures are streaked onto plates after 3 and 6 days of incubation. In cultivation attempts from tissue, the aseptically removed sample is pushed onto plates and then placed in broth or semisolid medium. This method is preferable to homogenization, as this may cause the liberation of mycoplasmacidal factors (Tully and Rask-Nielsen, 1967; Kaklamanis *et al.*, 1969).

IV. CLASSIFICATION

A. Genus

Most canine and feline mycoplasmas have been sufficiently studied to justify classification into genus (*Mycoplasma, Acholeplasma,* or *Ureaplasma*) (Table I). However, canine and feline ureaplasmas are not well characterized at this time, and further study will be required to understand their relationship to other ureaplasmas. Data on (1) lack of a cell wall, (2) inability to revert to bacterial forms, (3) filterability, (4) cholesterol requirements for growth, and (5) biochemical properties are necessary to establish that recovered organisms belong not only to the class Mollicutes but to one of the recognized families and genera.

B. Species

1. Biochemical Properties

Biochemical reactions of canine mycoplasmas are given in Table II. Details about methods and interpretation of the tests have been reported (Kato *et al.*, 1972; Kirchhoff *et al.*, 1973; Rosendal, 1974a). Data in the latter study were based upon the examination of 240 strains with 5 strains per species as a minimum. In the case of *M. arginini* only two canine strains are known so far. The negative glucose reaction recorded for *M. feliminutum* does not agree with reports from several other laboratories (Tully and Razin, 1977; M. F. Barile, personal communication).

Biochemical data based upon the examination of a large number of feline mycoplasmas are not available. Data from the examination of one or a few strains per species are given by Cole *et al.* (1967) and by Heyward and co-workers (1969).

Canine ureaplasmas are negative for glucose fermentation and arginine hydrolysis and do not show adsorption to HeLa cells or to erythrocytes (Taylor-Robinson *et al.*, 1971). Except for positive urea hydrolysis, the biochemical properties of feline ureaplasmas are not known.

TABLE II. Biochemical Reactions of Canine Mycoplasmas[a]

Organism	Glucose fermentation	Arginine hydrolysis	Phosphatase activity	Film and spots formation	Tetrazolium chloride reduction[b]	Hemolysis
Mycoplasma						
M. spumans	0	+	+	0	0	0
M. maculosum	0	+	+	+	(+)	(+)
M. opalescens	0	+	+	+	NI	+
M. arginini	0	+	0	0	0	0
M. gateae	0	+	0	0	0	0
M. canis	+	0	0	0	(0)	+
M. edwardii	+	0	0	+	(+)	+
M. molare	+	0	+	+	+	+
M. cynos					(0)	+
Mycoplasma group HRC689	+	0	0	(+)	+	+
M. feliminutum	0	0	+	+	0	0
M. bovigenitalium	0	0		NI	NI	+
Acholeplasma laidlawii	+	0	(+)		NI	NI

[a] +, Positive; 0, negative; (+), most strains positive; (0), most strains negative; NI, no information available;
[b] 0.045% concentration used under aerobic incubation.

2. Serological Properties

Studies on the serological properties of various mycoplasmas of canine origin have been published (Armstrong *et al.*, 1970; Kato *et al.*, 1972; Rosendal, 1975b). Specific cross-reactions (as determined by growth inhibition, metabolism inhibition, and indirect immunofluorescence) were not found among individual *Mycoplasma* species of canine origin or with those from other animals, with the exception of those instances mentioned below. Studies with the double immunodiffusion test revealed antigens shared by glucose-positive species and antigens shared by arginine-positive species, whereas none were shared between these two groups (Rosendal, 1975b).

Strain HRC689 cross-reacts serologically with strains of both *Mycoplasma mycoides* subsp. *mycoides* and *M. mycoides* subsp. *capri* (Rosendal, 1975b). Further studies, including genome hybridization experiments, are needed to clarify the taxonomic position of strain HRC689.

The serological properties of feline mycoplasmas and their relationship to other *Mycoplasma* species have been reported (Cole *et al.*, 1967; Freundt *et al.*, 1973a; WHO/FAO Report, 1973). Again, no significant number of heterologous cross-reactions was apparent.

Canine ureaplasmas appear to fall into at least two serogroups when examined in the metabolism inhibition test (Taylor-Robinson *et al.*, 1971). These serogroups are not antigenically related to ureaplasmas from other hosts, or to any of the established canine *Mycoplasma* species. The serological properties of feline ureaplasmas have not been explored.

C. Serological Intraspecies Variation

When strains of a given *Mycoplasma* species can be affiliated with two or more serogroups by the use of one or more serological tests, it is considered serological intraspecies variation for purposes of this discussion.

Mycoplasma spumans appears to contain two serogroups (group I and group II), based upon information derived from indirect immunofluorescence studies (Rosendal, 1974b). Several arginine-positive canine isolates were serologically related to *M. gateae* (Rosendal, 1974b). Two serogroups (1 and 2) were proposed. However, serogroup 2 belongs to *M. arginini* based on strong cross-reactions in both growth inhibition and indirect immunofluorescence testing (Rosendal and Ernø, 1978).

Based upon growth inhibition studies, it was reported that *M. canis* strains possessed some serological variants (Armstrong *et al.*, 1970). A representative strain (MH4942) was studied in our laboratory, using both growth inhibition and immunofluorescence tests. Supportive evidence to confirm strain MH4942 as a variant of *M. canis* was not found (S. Rosendal, unpublished observations). Canine strains of *M. feliminutum* exhibit a one-way cross-reaction with the feline strain (BEN) in both growth inhibition and immunofluorescence procedures (Rosendal, 1974b). Similarly, several canine isolates of *Mycoplasma bovigenitalium* show a serological one-way cross-reaction with the type strain (PG11) of *M. bovigenitalium*, which is of bovine origin (Table III) (Bruchim *et al.*, 1978). A one-way cross-reaction may reflect quantitative differences in terms of antigen expression or a basic identical antigenic pattern with minor differences.

V. IDENTIFICATION

A. Uncloned Cultures

Agar colonies of uncloned cultures can usually be identified by use of the epi-immunofluorescence procedure (Barile *et al.*, 1970; Rosendal, 1973c). This procedure is a rapid means of determining whether a certain *Mycoplasma* or *Acholeplasma* species is present, which may be of practical importance in pathogenicity studies. The test also detects a mixed mycoplasma flora.

B. Cloned Isolates

1. Biochemical Studies

A key to the identification of canine and feline mycoplasmas through biochemical procedures is given in Table IV. The digitonin sensitivity test distinguishes among members of the families Mycoplasmataceae and Acholeplasmataceae (Freundt *et al.*, 1973b). Urease-positive strains belong to the genus *Ureaplasma*. No further identification of ureaplasmas

TABLE III. Antigenic Relationships of Two Canine Mycoplasmas (H712 and C492) to *Mycoplasma bovigenitalium* (PG11) as Determined by Indirect Immunofluorescence and Growth Inhibition

	Antiserum[a]		
Antigen	PG11	H712	C492
PG11	+	0	0
H712	+	+	0
C492	0	+	+

[a] +, Positive reaction in both tests; 0, negative reaction in both tests.

can be made until these organisms from canine and feline hosts are characterized and classified. All urease-negative strains, which may be mycoplasmas or acholeplasmas, are examined for glucose fermentation, arginine hydrolysis, phosphatase activity, and cholesterol requirements.

2. Serological Studies

The choice of specific typing antisera is made according to the pattern of biochemical activity (Table IV) (Rosendal and Laber, 1973; Rosendal, 1974b). In the case of both *M. bovigenitalium* and *M. feliminutum*, serological studies should be performed with antisera to each of the respective type strains, as well as with antisera against canine myco-plasmas of each of these species [*M. bovigenitalium* (H712) and *M. feliminutum* (H756), respectively]. This reasoning is based upon the ob-servation that H712 and H756 antisera react with both the type strains and wild strains from canines, whereas the type strain antisera does not always react with wild-type strains (see Section IV,C) (Rosendal, 1974b; Bruchim *et al.*, 1978).

The serological tests of choice are immunofluorescence and growth inhibition procedures. Proper identification is achieved when both tests give positive reactions. If only one test is positive, further serological examination with the metabolism inhibition test is recom-mended.

3. Polyacrylamide Gel Electrophoresis

Electrophoretic analysis of canine mycoplasmas may yield useful in-formation on the taxonomic separation of cloned isolates (Armstrong and Yu, 1970; Rosendal, 1973b). However, it should be noted that the cellular protein patterns of the organisms may be influenced by the composition of the medium used to grow the organisms or by cultivation time. Also, some variation in protein patterns among different strains of the same *Myco-plasma* species has been observed.

VI. CANINE AND FELINE MYCOPLASMA FLORA

A. Canine Flora

1. Occurrence in Healthy Dogs

A small percentage of dogs harbor mycoplasmas in the conjunctiva (Rosendal, 1973c). In the nasal, oral, pharyngeal, and laryngeal cavities isolation attempts are almost 100% successful (Edward and Fitzgerald,

TABLE IV. Key to Identification of Canine and Feline Mycoplasmas

Biochemical examination					Serological identification
Digitonin sensitivity[a]	Urease activity	Glucose fermentation	Arginine hydrolysis	Phosphatase activity	Typing antisera of choice
−[a]	−	+	−	+ or −	A. laidlawii (PG8)
+[b]	−	+	−	−	M. canis (PG14), M. edwardii (PG24), M. molare (H542)
+	−	+	−	+	M. cynos (H831), Mycoplasma group (HRC689)
+	−	−	+	+	M. felis (CO)
+	−	−	+	+	M. spumans group I (PG13) and group II (H764), M. maculosum (PG15), M. opalescens (MH5408)
+	−	−	+	−	M. gateae (CS) group 1 (H372) and M. arginini (G230)
+	−	−	−	+	M. bovigenitalium (PG11 and H712)
+	−	−	−	−	M. feliminutum (BEN and H756)
+	+	?	?	?	?

[a] Resistant; ≤1 mm inhibition.
[b] Sensitive; >1 mm inhibition.

1951; Barile *et al.*, 1970; Brennan and Simkins, 1970; Kato *et al.*, 1972; Kirchhoff, 1973; Rosendal, 1973c; Koshimizu and Ogata, 1974).

Mycoplasmas were not found in the lungs of 15 dogs examined by Rosendal (1973c), whereas 7% of Kirchhoff's 108 dogs were positive (Kirchhoff, 1973).

Cultures taken from the vagina are often positive. Frequencies varying between 23 and 75% have been found (Edward and Fitzgerald, 1951; Thiemann *et al.*, 1972; Kato *et al.*, 1972; Kirchhoff, 1973; Rosendal, 1973c; Koshimizu and Ogata, 1974). In the cervix, the incidence is apparently at about the same level (Barile *et al.*, 1970), in contrast to the flora of the uterus where mycoplasmas are rare and apparently unrelated to disease (Kirchhoff, 1973). In approximately 50% of the cases studied by Rosendal (1973c) and Bruchim *et al.* (1978), mycoplasmas were isolated from the canine prepuce. The prostate was observed to be less frequently infected in two independent studies, yielding isolation rates of about 14% (Barile *et al.*, 1970; Kirchhoff, 1973).

An extensive systematic investigation demonstrated that mycoplasmas occasionally may be found in liver, kidney, spleen, intestine, heart, and joints (Kato *et al.*, 1972; Kirchhoff, 1973). In several dogs various organs were positive for mycoplasmas, suggesting that mycoplasmemia had occurred.

2. Occurrence in Diseased Dogs

Pneumonia is very often associated with mycoplasmal infection (Armstrong *et al.*, 1972; Rosendal, 1973c), as opposed to the situation in healthy lungs which are either not infected (Rosendal, 1973c) or infected at a very low frequency (Kirchhoff, 1973).

Chu and Beveridge (1954) found mycoplasmas in the prepuce of 95% of dogs with balanoposthitis. This is a significantly higher incidence than found in studies on healthy dogs.

Koshimizu *et al.* (1973) isolated mycoplasmas from the spleen and lymph nodes of two dogs with malignant lymphoma. In a subsequent study, Koshimizu and Ogata (1974) compared the occurrence in several organs, including the liver, spleen, kidney, and lymph nodes of healthy dogs and of dogs with various diseases. The cultures were positive in 10–15% of the diseased dogs, whereas those from the healthy dogs were negative, suggesting that lowered resistance during disease may allow the mycoplasmas to gain entrance from the vascular system.

3. Anatomical Distribution of Species

The anatomical source of canine *Mycoplasma* species and serogroups is given in Table V. The data are based upon 233 identified isolates. Informa-

TABLE V. **Anatomical Source of Canine Mycoplasmas**

Organism	Conjunctiva	Upper respiratory tract	Pneumonic lung	Vagina and cervix	Prepuce, urethra, and prostate
Mycoplasma					
M. spumans	1	18	11	1	2
M. maculosum		2		5	
M. opalescens					6
M. gateae		2	1	1	11
M. arginini		2			
M. canis	1	28	2	46	10
M. edwardii		16	2	4	3
M. molare		5		1	
M. cynos	1	3	3	7	7
Mycoplasma sp. HRC689		1			2
M. feliminutum		1	3	1	
M. bovigenitalium and related strains	1		2	2	12
Acholeplasma laidlawii				6	

tion from the literature provides the following supplementary data. *Mycoplasma maculosum* has been isolated from the male genital tract (Skalka and Krejcir, 1968; Koshimizu and Ogata, 1974). Two of the strains of *Mycoplasma opalescens* described by Armstrong *et al.* (1970) were from the throat and bladder of dogs. Strains of *M. canis* were found in almost all cultures taken from the internal organs in one study (Koshimizu and Ogata, 1974). On one occasion, *M. canis* was reported to occur in the throat of humans, probably as a transient organism transmitted from a dog (Armstrong *et al.*, 1971). *Mycoplasma edwardii,* in addition to the sites listed in Table V, has been isolated from the pericardial cavity (S. Rosendal, unpublished observations) and from a lymph node of dogs (Koshimizu and Ogata, 1974). Canine ureaplasmas are predominant inhabitants of the lower genital tract of dogs (Taylor-Robinson and Furr, 1973).

B. Feline Flora

1. Occurrence

Cats harbor mycoplasmas in the conjunctiva, with an incidence of approximately 20% in healthy cats (Tan and Miles, 1972) and at a rate of nearly 100% in cats with conjunctivitis (Campbell *et al.*, 1973; Tan and

Miles, 1974). The vast majority of healthy as well as sick cats also have a throat mycoplasma flora (Jones and Sabine, 1970; Tan and Miles, 1972, 1974). The incidence in the trachea of healthy cats is approximately 30% (Heyward *et al.*, 1969). Tan and Miles (1974) studied cats with respiratory and urogenital tract infections and found that 27% had mycoplasmas in the trachea and 17% had mycoplasmas in the lungs. None of the cats with respiratory disease examined by Spradbrow *et al.* (1970) had mycoplasmas in the lungs. This may be due to homogenization of tissues, which can depress the recovery of mycoplasmas (see Section III).

The urogenital tract of cats is often infected with mycoplasmas. About 25% of healthy cats carry mycoplasmas in this location (Heyward *et al.*, 1969; Tan and Miles, 1972), as opposed to a recovery rate of about 42% in cats with various genital tract infections (Tan and Miles, 1974).

Only on one occasion were mycoplasmas recovered from feline organs other than those mentioned above. This isolation, which was made from the brain of a lion, was originally thought to represent a new species *(Mycoplasma leonis)* but was later identified as *M. arginini* (Heyward *et al.*, 1969; Tully *et al.*, 1972).

2. Anatomical Distribution of Species

Mycoplasma felis has been isolated from the conjunctiva, upper respiratory tract, lungs, and urogenital tract. Conjunctivitis seems often to be associated with the recovery of *M. felis* from the eyes of cats (Campbell *et al.*, 1973; Tan, 1974). *Mycoplasma gateae* has also been found in the conjunctiva but is apparently a more frequent inhabitant of the upper respiratory tract and the urogenital tract. An oral isolate of *M. feliminutum* has been recognized as the only mycoplasma of this species to be found in cats (Heyward *et al.*, 1969). The three remaining groups of feline mycoplasmas (*M. arginini, A. laidlawii,* and the ureaplasmas) have only been found in the throats of cats.

3. Host Specificity

An interesting question about host specificity arises when the same mycoplasmas occur in different animal hosts. *Mycoplasma gateae* and *M. feliminutum* seem to be part of both the canine and feline mycoplasma flora, while *M. bovigenitalium* occurs primarily in cattle but can be recovered from dogs. *Mycoplasma arginini* predominantly occurs in ruminants (sheep, goats, chamois, and cattle) but can be recovered on occasion from cats and dogs. *Acholeplasma laidlawii* has been isolated from a broad spectrum of hosts and is suspected to occur frequently in animal environments. Whether a particular strain of a *Mycoplasma* species that occurs frequently in two hosts is equally well adapted to both, or must undergo selective adaptation, is a question for future study.

VII. HOST–PARASITE INTERACTION

A. Inflammation

1. Dogs

The type strain of *Mycoplasma cynos* (H831) was initially isolated from a case of pneumonia (Rosendal, 1972). The histological findings in the lungs had many features similar to the histopathology of mycoplasmal pneumonia in naturally occurring or experimental infections of rats and pigs. It is evident from the data in Table V that many different mycoplasmas have been cultured from the pneumonic lungs of dogs and that careful experimental studies will be necessary to clarify the specific role of each of these organisms in canine pulmonary disease.

The experimental pathogenicity of five strains of representative *Mycoplasma* species of dogs was studied recently (Rosendal, 1978). *Mycoplasma cynos, M. bovigenitalium, M. canis, M. spumans* (group II), and *M. gateae* (group 1) strains were isolated from the lungs of dogs with distemper. Cloned cultures of each organism were inoculated endobronchially into 1-week-old dogs. *Mycoplasma cynos* induced focal lesions with severe bronchitis and bronchiolitis in which neutrophils were the predominant cell type. Degenerative changes and severe cilia destruction of epithelial cells were observed by electron microscopy. In addition, peribronchial and perivascular lymphoplasmacytic hyperplasia were characteristic features (Fig. 1). The alveoli were filled with neutrophils and desquamated lining cells (Fig. 2). In dogs examined at 3, 4, and 5 weeks after inoculation, the neutrophils were replaced by macrophages (Fig. 3). On many occasions, macrophages had cytoplasmic PAS-positive material. Phagolysosomes containing mycoplasmas and membrane debris were seen in macrophages examined by electron microscopy (Rosendal and Vinther, 1977). The inoculated strain of *M. cynos* could be recovered for a period of 3 weeks after inoculation.

Only one dog was challenged with *M. bovigenitalium*. This organism colonized the lungs and induced mild local bronchitis and mild inflammatory changes in adjacent tissue. Additional trials will be necessary to assess the experimental pathogenicity of canine strains of this species. *Mycoplasma canis, M. gateae* (group 1), and *M. spumans* (group II) did

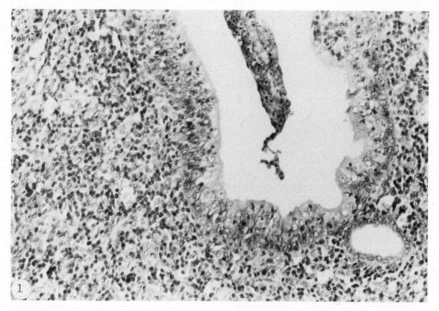

FIGURE 1. Bronchiolitis with peribronchiolar lymphoplasmacytic accumulation in dog inoculated 2 weeks previously with *M. cynos*. Hematoxylin–eosin. ×400.

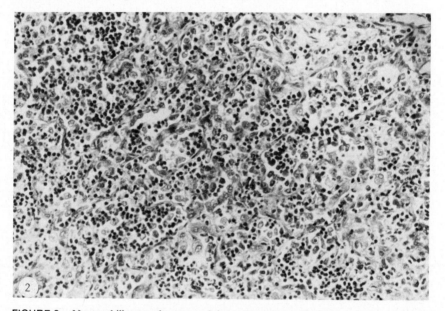

FIGURE 2. Neutrophilic granulocytes and desquamated alveolar lining cells in alveolus of dog inoculated 2 weeks previously with *M. cynos*. Hematoxylin–eosin. ×400.

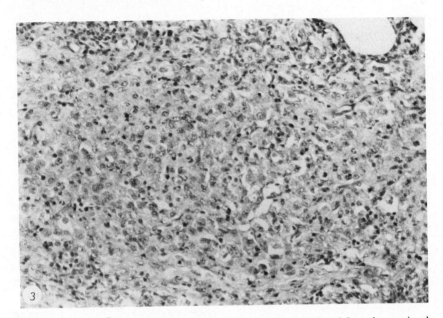

FIGURE 3. Accumulation of macrophages in lung of dog inoculated 5 weeks previously with *M. cynos*. Hematoxylin–eosin. ×400.

not induce morphological lesions, and only *M. spumans* organisms were reisolated from the experimental host (from the hilar lymph node).

2. Cats

Several investigations have established the close association of *M. felis* recovery and feline conjunctivitis (Cole *et al.*, 1967; Heyward *et al.*, 1969; Tan and Markham, 1971b; Campbell *et al.*, 1973). Some preliminary studies indicated that experimental conjunctival infections could be induced by conjunctival instillation of *M. felis* broth cultures (Cole *et al.*, 1967). Later, Tan (1974) reported the experimental production of conjunctivitis in normal 6- to 10-week-old kittens following inoculation of *M. felis* into the conjunctiva and nostrils. The ensuing conjunctivitis was characterized by edema and infiltration of lymphocytes and macrophages. In addition, two kittens developed foci of what was described as interstitial pneumonia. Although these findings suggest an etiological relationship between *M. felis* and conjunctivitis, the frequent occurrence of this organism in normal cats could complicate experimental studies in conventional animals and might also account for unsuccessful attempts to induce ocular infections with this organism (Blackmore and Hill, 1973).

A lung isolate of *M. arginini* (MT293) was examined for experimental pathogenicity by Tan *et al.* (1977). Groups of young cats (6–8 weeks old) were inoculated (1) in the conjunctiva and nostrils, (2) intraperitoneally, and (3) intrapulmonarily. The strain failed to induce inflammatory lesions but was able to colonize the upper respiratory tract.

B. Immunological Response

1. Dogs

During the course of spontaneous pneumonia in which *M. cynos* was implicated, dogs developed significant antibody titers to this organism, as measured by indirect hemagglutination (Rosendal, 1972). Spray inoculation of gnotobiotic dogs with *M. cynos* (H831) has resulted in colonization of the respiratory organs and in a specific antibody response (S. Rosendal and N. C. Juhr, unpublished observations). Dogs killed 4 and 5 weeks after endobronchial inoculation with *M. cynos* (D19) had antibody titers significantly higher than dogs killed at 1, 2, and 3 weeks. Mycoplasmas were recovered from lungs of dogs 1, 2, and 3 weeks after inoculation, but not 4 and 5 weeks after inoculation. This suggests that specific antibody might play a defensive role (Rosendal, 1978).

Serological studies with the indirect hemagglutination test (S. Rosendal, unpublished) and the work of Armstrong *et al.* (1972) have demonstrated that dogs are able to develop antibodies against most species of their mycoplasma flora. Nothing is known about the type of antibodies or what role they play in host–parasite interaction. The cellular immune response of dogs against mycoplasmas has not been studied.

2. Cats

Kittens experimentally inoculated with *M. felis* develop specific antibodies which can be measured by hemagglutination inhibition and complement fixation tests (Tan, 1974). The fact that control kittens housed close to experimental animals also responded serologically to *M. felis* suggests some transmission of mycoplasmas. Serological studies of 58 normal cats revealed that almost all possessed specific antibodies to *M. felis,* indicating a high frequency of contact with this organism (Tan and Miles, 1974). In contrast, only a few cats possessed antibodies to *M. gateae, M. arginini,* or *A. laidlawii.* For *M. gateae,* the high incidence of the organism in these hosts and the low antibody levels indicate that this organism is not very antigenic. Information on possible cellular immune responses of cats to their mycoplasma flora is not available.

C. Conclusion

The majority of canine and feline mycoplasmas are part of the normal microbial flora of the conjunctiva and of the upper respiratory and lower genital tracts. When host defenses are compromised, for whatever reason, mycoplasmas may be disseminated throughout the tissues, probably first through ductal lumina and then via the vascular system. There is strong presumptive evidence that *M. cynos* is pathogenic and probably plays a role in canine pneumonia. Of the feline mycoplasma flora, *M. felis* is strongly suspect as a potential pathogen and probably participates as one of the etiological agents in feline conjunctivitis. This organism might also play a role in feline respiratory disease. The more recent discovery of canine and feline ureaplasmas offers several other likely candidates for exploration of disease-promoting capabilities.

REFERENCES

Armstrong, D., and Yu, B. (1970). *J. Bacteriol.* **104**, 295–299.

Armstrong, D., Tully, J. G., Yu, B., Morton, V., Friedman, M. H., and Steger, L. (1970). *Infect. Immun.* **1**, 1–7.

Armstrong, D., Yu, B. H., Yagoda, A., and Kagnoff, M. F. (1971). *J. Infectious Dis.* **124**, 607–609.

Armstrong, D., Morton, V., Yu, B., Friedman, M. H., Steger, L., and Tully, J. G. (1972). *Am. J. Vet. Res.* **33**, 1471–1478.

Barile, M. F., Del Giudice, R. A., Carski, T. R., Yamashoroya, H. M., and Verna, J. A. (1970). *Proc. Soc. Exp. Biol. Med.* **134**, 146–148.

Blackmore, D. K., and Hill, A. (1973). *J. Small Anim. Pract.* **14**, 7–13.

Brennan, P. C., and Simkins, R. C. (1970). *Proc. Soc. Exp. Biol. Med.* **134**, 566–570.

Bruchim, A., Lutsky, I., and Rosendal, S. (1978). *Res. Vet. Sci.* **25**, 243–245.

Campbell, L. H., Snyder, S. B., Reed, C., and Fox, J. G. (1973). *J. Am. Vet. Med. Assoc.* **163**, 991–995.

Cello, R. M. (1957). *Am. J. Ophthalmol.* **43**, 296–297.

Chu, H. P., and Beveridge, W. I. B. (1954). *Symp. Uretrites Non Gonococciques, Monaco, Int. Union Against Vener. Dis.* pp. 61–62.

Cole, B. C., Golightly, L., and Ward, J. R. (1967). *J. Bacteriol.* **94**, 1451–1458.

Colegrave, A., Ingham, B., and Inglis, J. M. (1964). *Vet. Rec.* **76**, 68.

Edward, D. G. ff. (1947). *J. Gen. Microbiol.* **1**, 238–243.

Edward, D. G. ff., and Fitzgerald, W. A. (1951). *J. Gen. Microbiol.* **5**, 566–575.

Freundt, E. A., Ernø, H., Black, F. T., Krogsgaard-Jensen, A., and Rosendal, S. (1973a). *Ann. N.Y. Acad. Sci.* **225**, 161–171.

Freundt, E. A., Andrews, B. E., Ernø, H., Kunze, M., and Black, F. T. (1973b). *Zentralbl. Bakteriol., Parasitenkd., Infektionskr., Hyg., Abt. 1: Orig., Reihe A* **225**, 104–112.

Hayflick, L. (1965). *Tex. Rep. Biol. Med.* **23**, Suppl. 1, 285–303.

Heyward, J. T., Sabry, M. Z., and Dowdle, W. R. (1969). *Am. J. Vet. Res.* **30**, 615–622.

Jones, R. F., and Sabine, M. (1970). *Aust. Vet. J.* **46**, 343.

Kaklamanis, E., Thomas, L., Stavropoulos, K., Borman, I., and Boshwitz, C. (1969). *Nature (London)* **221**, 860–862.

Kato, H., Murakami, T., Aita, K., Takase, S., Ohmori, N., Sakaki, F., and Ono, K. (1972). *Iwate Daigaku Nogakubu Hokoku* **11**, 21–28.

Kirchhoff, H. (1973). *Zentralbl. Veterinaermed., Reihe B* **20**, 466–473.

Kirchhoff, H., Basu, A., and Loh, M. (1973). *Zentralbl. Veterinaermed., Reihe B* **20**, 474–480.

Koshimizu, K., and Ogata, M. (1974). *Jpn. J. Vet. Sci.* **36,** 391–406.

Koshimizu, K., Yamamoto, K., and Ogata, M. (1973). *Jpn. J. Vet. Sci.* **35,** 123–132.

Rosendal, S. (1972). *Acta Vet. Scand.* **13,** 137–139.

Rosendal, S. (1973a). *Int. J. Syst. Bacteriol.* **23,** 49–54.

Rosendal, S. (1973b). *Acta Pathol. Microbiol. Scand., Sect. B* **81,** 273–281.

Rosendal, S. (1973c). *Acta Pathol. Microbiol. Scand., Sect. B* **81,** 441–445.

Rosendal, S. (1974a). *Int. J. Syst. Bacteriol.* **24,** 125–130.

Rosendal, S. (1974b). *Acta Pathol. Microbiol. Scand., Sect. B* **82,** 25–32.

Rosendal, S. (1975a). *Acta Pathol. Microbiol. Scand., Sect. B* **82,** 457–462.

Rosendal, S. (1975b). *Acta Pathol. Microbiol. Scand., Sect. B.* **83,** 463–470.

Rosendal, S. (1978). *J. Infect. Dis.* **138,** 203–210.

Rosendal, S., and Laber, G. (1973). *Zentralbl. Bakteriol., Parasitenkd., Infektionskr. Hyg., Abt. 1: Orig., Reihe A* **225,** 346–349.

Rosendal, S., and Vinther, O. (1977). *Acta Pathol. Microbiol. Scand., Sect. B* **85,** 462–465.

Shoetensack, H. M. (1934). *Kitasato Arch. Exp. Med.* **11,** 277–290.

Shoetensack, H. M. (1936a). *Kitasato Arch. Exp. Med.* **13,** 175–184.

Shoetensack, H. M. (1936b). *Kitasato Arch. Exp. Med.* **13,** 269–280.

Skalka, B., and Krejcir, T. (1968). *Acta Univ. Agric. Hung.* **37,** 57–64.

Spradbrow, P. B., Marley, J., Portas, B., and Burgess, G. (1970). *Aust. Vet. J.* **46,** 109–110.

Tan, R. J. S. (1974). *Jpn. J. Exp. Med.* **44,** 235–240.

Tan, R. J. S., and Markham, J. G. (1971a). *Jpn. J. Exp. Med.* **41,** 247–248.

Tan, R. J. S., and Markham, J. G. (1971b). *N.Z. Vet. J.* **19,** 28.

Tan, R. J. S., and Miles, J. A. R. (1972). *Br. Vet. J.* **128,** 87–90.

Tan, R. J. S., and Miles, J. A. R. (1974). *Res. Vet. Sci.* **16,** 27–34.

Tan, R. J. S., Lim, E. W., and Ishak, B. (1977). *Can. J. Comp. Med.* **41,** 349–354.

Taylor-Robinson, D., and Furr, P. M. (1973). *Ann. N.Y. Acad. Sci.* **225,** 108–117.

Taylor-Robinson, D., Martin-Bourgon, C., Watanabe, T., and Addey, J. P. (1971). *J. Gen. Microbiol.* **68,** 97–107.

Thiemann, G., Laber, G., and Lorin, D. (1972). *Zentralbl. Bakteriol., Parasitenkd., Infektionskr. Hyg., Abt. 1: Orig., Reihe A* **230,** 380–381.

Tully, J. G., and Rask-Nielsen, R. (1967). *Ann. N.Y. Acad. Sci.* **143,** 345–352.

Tully, J. G., and Razin, S. (1977). *In* "Handbook of Microbiology" (A. I. Laskin and H. A. Lechevalier, eds.), 2nd Ed., Vol. 1, pp. 405–459. Chem. Rubber Publ. Co., Cleveland, Ohio.

Tully, J. G., Barile, M. F., Del Giudice, R. A., Carski, T. R., Armstrong, D., and Razin, S. (1970). *J. Bacteriol.* **101,** 346–349.

Tully, J. G., Del Giudice, R. A., and Barile, M. F. (1972). *Int. J. Syst. Bacteriol.* **22,** 47–49.

Ward, J. R., and Cole, B. C. (1970). Mycoplasmal infections of laboratory animals. *In* "The Role of Mycoplasmas and L Forms of Bacteria in Disease" (J. T. Sharp, ed.), pp. 212–239. Thomas, Springfield, Illinois.

WHO/FAO Report (1973). "Report of Working Team, International Board on Animal Mycoplasma Characterization." WHO, Geneva.

8 / MURINE AND OTHER SMALL-ANIMAL MYCOPLASMAS

Gail H. Cassell and Auriol Hill

I. INTRODUCTION

Chronic respiratory disease has been the major intercurrent disease problem encountered in laboratory rats since this species came into general use for experimental purposes. Although less common than in rats, this disease has also posed a serious problem in mice. As early as 1937, Nelson, and Klieneberger and Steabben reported the occurrence of a mycoplasma-like organism in association with the disease. This organism, later designated *Mycoplasma pulmonis* (Edward and Freundt, 1956), only recently has been conclusively shown to cause the respiratory disease (Lutsky and Organick, 1966; Kohn and Kirk, 1969; Kohn, 1971a; Lindsey *et al.*, 1971; Whittlestone *et al.*, 1972; Jersey *et al.*, 1973; Lindsey and Cassell,

THE MYCOPLASMAS, VOL. II

1973). In addition, it is now known to cause genital disease in both rats and mice (Nelson, 1954; Graham, 1963; Juhr *et al.*, 1970; Casillo and Blackmore, 1972; Ganaway *et al.*, 1973; Hill, 1974a; Cassell *et al.*, 1976, 1978a).

Shortly after Klieneberger and Steabben's (1937) report, Wolgom and Warren (1938a,b, 1939) isolated a mycoplasma from articular exudates of purulent polyarthritis in wild and laboratory rats. These isolates were subsequently classified as *Mycoplasma arthritidis* (Edward and Freundt, 1956). About the same time, Sabin (1938a,b) and Findlay *et al.* (1938) described the isolation of a neurotoxic mycoplasma, later identified as *Mycoplasma neurolyticum*, from the brains of mice.

Even today, the existence of mycoplasmas in animal facilities is practically synonymous with the presence of rats and mice (Lindsey *et al.*, 1971). With over 10 million rats and 30 million mice used yearly for research in the United States alone, the cost of mycoplasmal diseases is indeed staggering. More insidious than the direct loss is the undermining of the validity of scientific experiments that utilize these animal species (Lindsey *et al.*, 1971, 1978). Not only are murine mycoplasmal diseases a diagnostic problem, but they interact with other factors to induce extremely subtle changes in animal physiology and behavior and thereby compromise work in many different fields (Lindsey *et al.*, 1971).

Despite the economic impact of these three well-defined murine mycoplasmas, only limited efforts have been made to evaluate the true mycoplasmal flora of rats and mice. Additional species are almost certain to be recognized in the future. The mycoplasmal flora of small animals other than rats and mice is even less well defined, and even those that have been isolated have not been thoroughly evaluated for their disease-producing potential.

The present chapter reviews current knowledge of the biology of murine and other small-animal mycoplasmas and relates this knowledge to mycoplasma–host interactions, to disease pathogenesis and, subsequently, to disease detection and control.

II. MURINE MYCOPLASMAS

A. *Mycoplasma pulmonis*

1. Physiological Characteristics

Mycoplasma pulmonis is easily grown on standard mycoplasma media. On solid medium, the colonies are granular with little tendency to grow into the medium and produce typical mycoplasmal colonies. Fermenta-

tion of glucose and lack of arginine dihydrolase are biochemical characteristics useful in distinguishing this organism (Table I). It produces a
plaque-forming factor which is more likely to be a bacteriocin than a virus
(Gourlay *et al.*, 1976).

Freshly isolated strains of *M. pulmonis* demonstrate motility (Andrewes and Welch, 1946; Nelson, 1960; Bredt, 1973). Bredt and Radestock (1977) described two motile forms: (1) a round cell with a protruding
flexible stalk, often slightly thickened at the distal end, and (2) an elon-
gated cell with a tapered leading end.

Transmission and scanning electron micrographs of *M. pulmonis* show
that the predominant morphotype is spherical and ranges in size from 600
to 1500 nm (Wilborn and Cassell, 1978). An extracellular capsular matrix
can be demonstrated *in vitro* and *in vivo* by staining with ruthenium red
(Fig. 1). Surface projections morphologically similar to the "spikes" of
myxoviruses also have been observed (Hummeler *et al.*, 1965b).

2. Serological Characteristics

Early serological studies (Klieneberger, 1938; Lemcke, 1961, 1964;
Tully, 1965) failed to show any notable heterogeneity within the species
M. pulmonis. Nucleic acid homologies also failed to distinguish among
strains (Somerson *et al.*, 1967). However, recent studies using more
sensitive techniques suggest that sufficient diversity exists to justify the
establishment of subgroups (Leach and Butler, 1966; Fallon and Jackson,
1967; Deeb and Kenny, 1967a; Ogata *et al.*, 1967; Forshaw, 1972; Forshaw and Fallon, 1972; Haller *et al.*, 1973).

Mycoplasma pulmonis proteins and polysaccharides, but not lipids, are
antigenic (Deeb and Kenny, 1967b). Apparently one to three common
antigens are present (Ogata *et al.*, 1967); at least one of which may be
demonstrable by complement fixation (CF) (Haller *et al.*, 1973). Two
classes of water-soluble CF antigens have been demonstrated: (1) cross-
related, heat-labile and (2) subtype-specific, heat-stable (Deeb and
Kenny, 1967b).

3. Respiratory Disease

Few diseases of laboratory animals have been as troublesome to research workers or as enigmatic to microbiologists as chronic murine
respiratory disease (Lindsey *et al.*, 1971; Cassell *et al.*, 1973b). Its presence in most animal facilities has made study of the problem by many
investigators impractical or even impossible. Only within the last decade
have all lesions of the natural disease been successfully reproduced by
inoculation of a single agent, *M. pulmonis,* into rats (Kohn and Kirk,
1969; Lindsey *et al.*, 1971; Whittlestone *et al.*, 1972; Jersey *et al.*, 1973)

TABLE I   **Biological Characteristics of Murine and Other Small-Animal Mycoplasmas**

Mycoplasma species[a]	G + C of DNA %	Glucose catabolism	Mannose catabolism	Arginine hydrolysis	Aerobic tetrazolium reduction	Aerobic resazurin reduction	Phosphatase production
M. pulmonis	27.5–28.3	+	+	−	[b]	+	−
M. arthritidis	30.0–33.77	−	−	+	−	−	+
M. neurolyticum	23.0–26.5	+	+	−	−	−	−
M. caviae	NT	+	NT	[b]	−	+	+
A. laidlawii	31.7–35.7	+	[b]	−	[b]	+	[b]
Recently isolated strains which require further assessment							
58B (Gough)	NT	+	NT	−	+	+	−
G371	NT	+	NT	−	−	+	−
22A	NT	−	NT	−	−	+	−
117C	NT	−	NT	−	±	±	−
CH	NT	+	NT	−	+	+	+

and mice (Lutsky and Organick, 1966; Lindsey and Cassell, 1973) that were known to be free of other pathogens. Furthermore, *M. pulmonis* can consistently be demonstrated within these lesions by cultural, immunofluorescent, and ultrastructural methods (Organick *et al.*, 1966; Lindsey *et al.*, 1971). It is clear from experimental studies that the disease is an insidious, protracted process involving a variety of interrelated factors. Consequently, at various stages, lesions may exhibit a lack of uniformity. Thus it appears that the more than 20 descriptive terms advanced over the years designate a single clinicopathological entity due primarily to *M. pulmonis* (Lindsey *et al.*, 1971; Cassell *et al.*, 1973b). The more definitive term *murine respiratory mycoplasmosis* (MRM) is now preferred (Lindsey *et al.*, 1978).

  a. **The natural disease.** *(1) Epidemiology.* Evidence exists that offspring of affected mothers acquire the organisms as a result of aerosol transmission in the first few weeks of life (Lemcke, 1961; Klieneberger, 1962) and that the organism may even be acquired *in utero* (Tram and Guillon, 1970; Juhr *et al.*, 1970). Such an occurrence is probable, since

Natural host	Isolation site	Disease manifestations	Recovery from other animal species (association with disease questionable)
Mice and rats	All segments of the respiratory and urogenital tracts	Rhinitis, otitis, laryngotracheitis, bronchopneumonia, salpingitis, oophoritis, and metritis in both mice and rats; under experimental conditions the organism also produces arthritis in both rats and mice	Rabbits, guinea pigs, hamsters, horses, and humans
Rats	Joint, middle ear, oropharynx, lung, conjunctiva	Polyarthritis in rats naturally and in rats, mice, and rabbits, experimentally; association with respiratory disease and conjunctivitis in rats questionable	Humans and nonhuman primates
Mice	Brain, nasopharynx, middle ear, lung, conjunctiva	Epidemic conjunctivitis naturally and rolling disease experimentally	Rats
Guinea pigs	Nasopharynx and genital tract	Pathogenicity questionable	NT
Guinea pigs (many different animal species including rats)	Nasopharynx and genital tract of guinea pigs (many different sites in other animal species)	Not known	
Rats and mice	Nasopharynx and conjunctiva	Conjunctivitis?	NT
Guinea pigs	Genital tract	Not known	NT
Guinea pigs	Genital tract	Not known	NT
Guinea pigs	Nasopharynx	Not known	NT
Chinese hamsters	Conjunctiva, brain, nasopharynx, and lung	Not known	NT

[a] All these species except *A. laidlawii*, G371, and 22A require sterol for growth; none hydrolyze urea. They do not grow at 45°–62°C or at pH 1.0–3.0. All are sensitive to 20% sodium polyanethol sulfonate except *A. laidlawii* which is highly resistant and G371 and 22A which may be either totally resistant or show slight partial inhibition. Only *M. pulmonis* hemadsorbs. All species produce hemolysis of sheep red blood cells. *M. caviae* has not been tested for hemadsorption; and 22A and 117C have not been tested for hemolysis. All grow both aerobically and anaerobically, except 22A and 117C which grow aerobically. NT, not tested.

[b] Variable reaction.

transplacental transmission of mycoplasmas has been demonstrated in other animal species (Stone *et al.*, 1969). Once rats and mice have acquired the organism, a slowly progressing respiratory disease is initiated that may persist for life. These animals serve as reservoirs of infection and may transmit the disease to other animals via airborne transmission. Evidence is contradictory concerning the survival of *M. pulmonis* in drinking water, food, and feces and their role in disease transmission (Juhr, 1971a; Vogelzang, 1975). However, other animal species may serve as reservoirs of infection. *Mycoplasma pulmonis* has been isolated rather frequently from wild rodents (Andrewes and Niven, 1950), hamsters (Battigelli *et al.*, 1971; Hill, 1974a), guinea pigs (Juhr and Obi, 1970; Hill, unpublished observations), and infrequently from rabbits (Deeb and Kenny, 1967a).

(2) Clinical manifestations. Except for the terminal stage of the disease

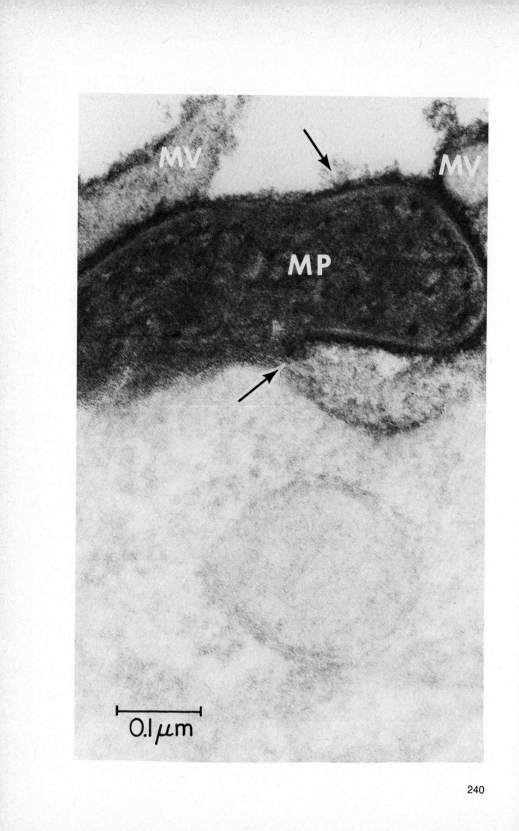

0.1 μm

when weight loss, roughened hair coat, serosanguinous nasal and ocular discharges, and dyspnea are seen, MRM is a clinically silent infection. Even in its later stages, snuffling and rales often exist without other clinical manifestations. Other signs are frequent rubbing of the eyes and, rarely, head tilt resulting from labyrinthitis. Even though clinical disease due to MRM is rare, incidence is sometimes high in epizootics. Mortality is cumulative over many months.

(3) Gross and microscopic lesions. Correlation between clinical signs and pathological alterations is almost nonexistent. Lungs, which appear normal grossly, may show extensive involvement microscopically, and the disease can involve the upper respiratory tract even when absent in the lower. One of the more noteworthy features of MRM is the lack of uniformity among lesions observed in animals of the same age, from the same cage, from the same colony and, more especially, from different colonies.

The principal lesions are acute and chronic rhinitis, otitis media, laryngotracheitis, bronchopneumonia, and bronchiectasis, and are all characterized microscopically by lymphoid hyperplasia and chronic inflammation. The anatomy of the respiratory tract in normal rats (Giddens *et al.*, 1971a,b) and the alterations seen in infected rats (Kohn and Kirk, 1969; Lindsey *et al.*, 1971; Whittlestone *et al.*, 1972) and mice (Lutsky and Organick, 1966; Lindsey and Cassell, 1973) have recently been described in detail and are not reviewed here.

b. The experimental disease. The production of MRM in mice by the intranasal inoculation of *M. pulmonis* contrasts sharply with that in rats. By varying the dose of *M. pulmonis* in mice, it is possible to produce three reasonably distinct clinicopathological syndromes (Lindsey and Cassell, 1973). When infected with less than 10^4 colony-forming units (CFU), minimal lesions develop that usually regress completely by 30 days. When greater than 10^5 CFU is given, two additional syndromes result. The first, an acute fatal disease, is characterized by the presence of edematous fluid and large numbers of neutrophils in alveolar spaces, pulmonary congestion, and hemorrhage with occasional pleuritis. Mice that survive this phase develop bronchial involvement with relatively little persistence of alveolar disease, thus giving rise to another syndrome, chronic bronchopneumonia.

The experimental disease in rats is not dose-dependent. Even when comparable numbers of organisms per gram of body weight are given,

FIGURE 1. *Mycoplasma pulmonis* (MP) between two microvilli (MV) of surface epithelial cell of rat uterus. Specimen stained with ruthenium red to show surface coat (upper arrow) of acid mucopolysaccharide associated with *M. pulmonis*. There appears to be continuity between host and mycoplasmal membranes even upon serial sectioning (lower arrow). (X227,500.)

these rats do not develop the acute alveolar phase. This difference has been explained by Cassell *et al.* (1973b) as follows: Intranasal inoculation of *M. pulmonis* in either species results in the deposition of large numbers of organisms in the lungs. Rats rapidly clear the alveoli, thus avoiding acute pneumonia, but later develop chronic lung disease. In contrast, mice are less efficient in clearing the alveoli of the initial inoculum and consequently develop both acute and chronic lung diseases, either of which may be fatal (Lindsey and Cassell, 1973). In the rat, the organisms gradually spread from the upper respiratory tract to the ciliated epithelium of the lower tract. The bronchial associated lymphoid tissue (BALT) then proliferates, mucus production increases, neutrophils accumulate in the bronchi, and eventually the full spectrum of MRM develops. This process, if unaltered by other factors (see Section II,A,6,b), can take as long as 265 days (Whittlestone *et al.*, 1972).

Quantitatively, the rat disease differs in having more hyperplasia and squamoid change of respiratory epithelium, more frequent formation of peribronchial acinar spaces, less severe accumulation of neutrophils, and predominantly lymphocytes in peribronchial infiltrates. Rat lungs normally contain BALT, which is not prominent in the lungs of normal mice. Nevertheless, the peribronchial lymphoid cuffs that develop after infection in the mouse are relatively much thicker and contain a greater preponderance of plasma cells. Similarly, local lymph nodes in the mouse tend to undergo more drastic hyperplasia and contain a higher proportion of plasma cells.

To date most pathological studies of MRM have been limited to F344 rats and CD-1 mice. Therefore, the marked differences observed may be more related to strain differences rather than species differences. Recent studies suggest that some mouse strains (particularly C57BL) respond like F344 rats, whereas Lewis rats respond more like CD-1 mice (G. Taylor, P. B. Carter, J. Davis, and G. Cassell, unpublished observations).

4. Genital Disease

a. Natural disease in rats. Females can acquire uterine infection early in life, in some cases even prior to coitus. The exact relationship of genital to respiratory mycoplasmosis is unknown; each has been detected in the absence of the other. In most cases, females harboring mycoplasmas in the upper respiratory passages probably transfer the infection to the vagina with subsequent spread to the uterus. Juhr (1971b) demonstrated a septicemic phase in *M. pulmonis* respiratory disease; thus organisms may also reach the urogenital tract via the hematogenous route.

As in the respiratory disease, genital tracts that appear normal grossly can show extensive involvement microscopically (Cassell *et al.*, 1978a). Gross lesions are limited to approximately 30% of infected females, with oophoritis and salpingitis being the most common. Microscopically, a neutrophilic exudate is seen in the oviduct lumen with hyperplasia of the epithelium and lymphoid infiltration into the submucosa.

Gross observations of uteri usually reveal no changes, except that underdeveloped or partially resorbed fetuses are occasionally seen. Histologically, lesions range from mild metritis to marked pyometra and endometritis. Epithelial changes include hyperplasia, squamous metaplasia, and polyp formation (Cassell *et al.*, 1978a).

A small percentage of male rats with epididymitis and urethritis have been shown to have positive *M. pulmonis* vas deferens cultures.

b. Experimental disease in rats. The entire spectrum of lesions seen in the natural genital disease can be reproduced by the intravenous inoculation of 10^8 CFU *M. pulmonis* into pathogen-free rats (Cassell *et al.*, 1976, 1978a). As in the natural disease, the most common lesion is salpingitis with distension of the ovarian bursae. One notable finding is that uteri from animals with salpingitis and perioophritis often appear histologically normal, although organisms can be shown to line the entire epithelial surface (Fig. 2).

Extensive surveys have not been performed on inoculated male rats, but less than 1% of vas deferens cultures are positive (Cassell *et al.*, 1978a). In such cases organisms can be demonstrated in the epididymis, associated with epididymitis and urethritis. Infrequently, infected males have testicular atrophy.

Preliminary breeding—efficiency studies indicate that 20% of experimentally infected females are sterile (Cassell *et al.*, 1978a) and at least 60% of the remainder give birth to less than half as many pups as uninfected animals. Cultural studies indicate that *M. pulmonis* is transferred to 100% of the offspring, primarily infecting the respiratory tract. The mode of transmission, however, has yet to be determined.

c. Natural and experimental disease in mice. Naturally occurring genital tract disease in mice has not been reported, but *M. pulmonis* has been isolated from vaginal and uterine washings (Hill, 1974a; Cassell, unpublished observations) and lesions similar to those in rats have been experimentally produced in mice (Nelson, 1954; Goeth and Appel, 1974). Taylor-Robinson *et al.* (1975) reported fetal wastage as a consequence of experimental infection. Others have reported that fertility is reduced by 50% and have suggested that this is due to disordered ovarian function and/or averted nidation (Goeth and Appel, 1974). *Mycoplasma pulmonis*

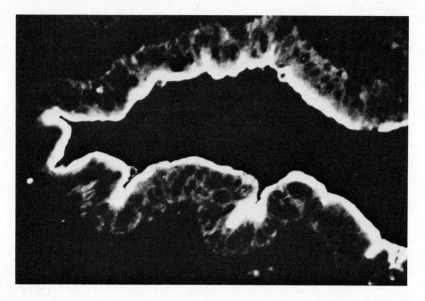

FIGURE 2. Rat endometrium 49 days after inoculation. Immunofluorescent staining shows a heavy concentration of *M. pulmonis* lining the epithelium. (X600.)

has been shown to reduce fertilization and preimplantation development *in vitro,* with relatively few embryos reaching the blastocyst stage (Fraser and Taylor-Robinson, 1977).

5. Other Disease Manifestations

Mycoplasma pulmonis inoculated intravenously produces arthritis in mice (Barden and Tully, 1969; Harwick *et al.*, 1973a; Taylor *et al.*, 1974; Cole *et al.*, 1975b) and rats (Cassell *et al.*, 1973a; Kohn *et al.*, 1977). Arthritis in rats, usually tendosynovitis, reaches maximal involvement in 10–12 days and usually dissipates within 49 days. In mice the clinical course is marked by acute onset, with maximal involvement between 2 and 4 weeks. During this stage, inflammation of the periarticular soft tissue is extensive, with an infiltration of neutrophils and mononuclear cells. Later, some mice develop a chronic disease (of possibly 12 months' duration) that is characterized by mononuclear cell infiltration and hyperplasia of synovial tissue.[1] The arthritic response varies with different mouse strains (Hannan, 1971; Taylor *et al.*, 1974). A small percentage of CD-1 mice develop flaccid hind limb paralysis associated with inflammation of the brain and spinal cord, and other visceral organs including the liver and kidneys (Cassell *et al.*, 1973a). Goeth and Appel (1974) also

[1] A detailed histological description of *M. pulmonis* arthritis is given in this volume, Chapter 11.

reported hepatitis in mice inoculated intraperitoneally. These findings are notable because similar lesions occur in humans and hamsters infected with *Mycoplasma pneumoniae* (Pachas, 1970; Mårdh *et al.*, 1974; Vitullo *et al.*, 1977). Comparable lesions have not been observed in experimentally infected rats.

Intracerebral inoculation of viable *M. pulmonis* into neonatal rats induces communicating hydrocephalus (Kohn *et al.*, 1977) which may be due to ciliary dysfunction and/or to an imbalance of cerebrospinal fluid secretion and absorption.

6. Disease Mechanisms

a. Mycoplasmal factors. The interaction of mycoplasmas with eukaryotic membranes is likely the initial event in most infections. Sobeslavsky *et al.* (1968) demonstrated that, *in vitro*, *M. pulmonis* adsorbed to red blood cells and spermatozoa but not to tracheal epithelial cells. Yet, *in vivo*, these organisms adsorb to tracheal epithelial cells and to many other cell types. In fact, this organism is almost never seen in the host unless it is attached to a cell membrane.

The specialized terminal structures of *Mycoplasma gallisepticum* and *M. pneumoniae* have been postulated to aid in both motility and cellular attachment (Collier and Clyde, 1971; Bredt, 1973). By analogy, the motility of *M. pulmonis* has led to speculation that its "stalk" or tip structure is also important for adherence (Bredt and Radestock, 1977). However, ultrastructural studies of *M. pulmonis* in infected animals show a more generalized interaction of its surface with host cell membranes (Fig. 3). It is quite possible that the nature of attachment may differ with cell type, stage of infection, and strain of *M. pulmonis*, and that a specialized tip structure may be involved in some cases.

In contrast to other mycoplasmas, neuraminic acid receptors appear not to be involved in the adsorption of *M. pulmonis* to cells (Sobeslavsky *et al.*, 1968; Manchee and Taylor-Robinson, 1969). Ultrastructural studies indicate that this organism is surrounded by a mucopolysaccharide capsule (Wilborn and Cassell, 1978). Lectin studies also suggest that *M. pulmonis* possesses a surface-bound glycoprotein (Schiefer *et al.*, 1974). The capsule and/or surface spikes (see Section II,A,1) may be correlated with this glycoprotein and may be involved in attachment.

Although adherence is a prerequisite for infection, it is unlikely that mere attachment to host cell surfaces could produce the wide variety of cellular changes reported in *M. pulmonis* infections, i.e., loss of cilia, cytoplasmic vacuolization, disruption of mitochondria (Kohn, 1971b; Organick and Lutsky, 1976), epithelial hyperplasia and metaplasia, and giant cell formation (Lindsey and Cassell, 1973). These changes are more likely due to mycoplasmal utilization of host cell components and/or release of

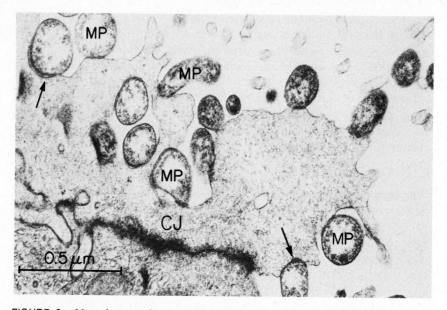

FIGURE 3. *Mycoplasma pulmonis* (MP) attached to rat oviduct epithelial cell. Note cell junction (CJ) and the morphological similarity between it and the zone of *M. pulmonis* attachment (arrows). (X84,122.)

toxic metabolic wastes. Both possibilities are compatible with known characteristics of mycoplasmal physiology. Because of its endonuclease activity, *M. pulmonis,* like certain other mycoplasmas, can use RNA and DNA as a source of nucleic acid precursors (Plackett, 1957; Razin *et al.*, 1964; Russell, 1966). Thus depletion of cellular pools may account for alterations in macromolecular synthesis and other cell injuries. Also, as in most mycoplasmas, the respiratory pathway of *M. pulmonis* is flavin-terminated, resulting in the formation of peroxides that are toxic for the host (Cole *et al.*, 1968; Brennan and Feinstein, 1969).

Like many other mycoplasmas (Hu *et al.*, 1975), *M. pulmonis* induces ciliostasis in tracheal organ cultures (Westerberg *et al.*, 1972). If paralysis of the ciliary apparatus occurs *in vivo,* it would render the host incapable of clearing inflammatory exudates from respiratory passages. Ciliostasis in the oviduct could also influence ova transport.

The nature of host cell injury suggests that communication may be established between mycoplasmas and host cells, and it is tempting to speculate that this may involve more than simple diffusion. Electron micrographs indicate that alterations of host and *M. pulmonis* membranes occur at the site of attachment (Figs. 3 and 4). The structure thus formed superficially resembles an intercellular junction, i.e., a nexus. In some instances, membrane fusion appears to occur between *M. pulmonis* and host cells (Fig. 1). Membrane fusion has been reported for other mycoplasmas (Edwards and Fogh, 1960; Hummeler *et al.*, 1965a; Zucker-Franklin *et al.*, 1966) and postulated in the interaction of *M. pneumoniae* with host cells (Gabridge *et al.*, 1977). Although positive ascertainment must await further experimental proof, continued exploration of these phenomena would appear to be particularly important for gaining insight into disease pathogenesis.

In addition to the direct molecular effects, the close association of *M. pulmonis* with host cell surfaces may lead to immunological "innocent bystander" damage (Cassell *et al.*, 1978c; Wise *et al.*, 1978). The other ways in which the host response might contribute to the lesions seen in *M. pulmonis* infection are discussed in Sections II,A,7 and 8, and also in this volume, Chapter 12.

b. Extrinsic factors. Under defined experimental conditions, *M. pulmonis* alone can produce all lesions of MRM (Lindsey *et al.*, 1971; Jersey *et al.*, 1973; Lindsey and Cassell, 1973). Nevertheless a constant finding has been that intranasal inoculation of rats most often leads only to microscopically detectable rhinitis, tracheitis, and otitis media. One key factor is that the pulmonary disease in rats progresses slowly, sometimes requiring up to 265 days for full development. Thus in many experiments infected animals were sacrificed too soon. In addition, it is now clear that many intrinsic and extrinsic factors can markedly influence the progression of respiratory tract disease. Although these factors almost certainly influence any infectious disease, their effect in MRM seems particularly pronounced.

Broderson *et al.* (1976) and Lindsey and Conner (1978) demonstrated that environmental ammonia at concentrations commonly encountered in rat cages (25–250 ppm) greatly increases the severity and incidence of the lesions of MRM throughout the respiratory tract. Although data are lacking, other environmental factors such as temperature, humidity, and degree of crowding probably also influence MRM. Environmental influences on MRM of mice have not been studied.

The influence of age upon susceptibility of mice to MRM is unknown, but older rats succumb more readily (Gay *et al.*, 1972; Jersey *et al.*, 1973; Davis and Cassell, 1978), probably because of a declining immune system. Maximal immune competence of the rat is reached at the onset of puberty and declines significantly thereafter (Bilder, 1975).

Circumstantial evidence suggests that genetic constitution influences susceptibility to MRM (Freudenberger, 1932a,b; Innes *et al.*, 1956). However, positive ascertainment is contingent upon controlled experiments with animals maintained since birth under

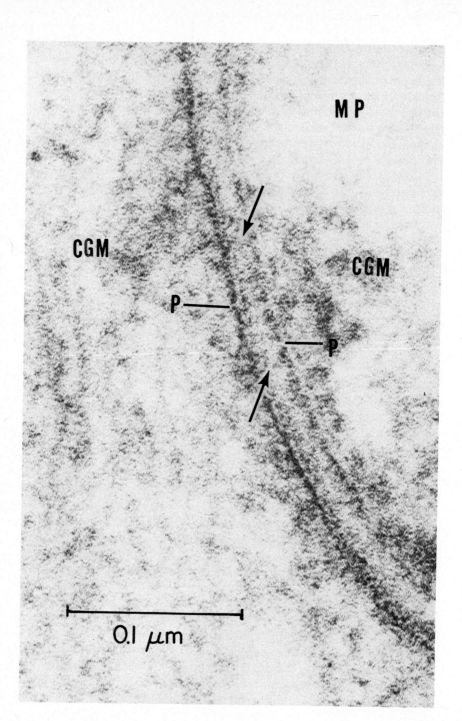

0.1 μm

identical environmental conditions, including an identical microbial flora.

Synergistic effects of concomitant infections may influence MRM in some cases. *Mycoplasma pulmonis* respiratory disease in mice has been shown to be enhanced by *Pasteurella pneumotropica* (Brennan *et al.*, 1969). The microorganism most commonly isolated in association with *M. pulmonis* in rats is *Streptococcus pneumoniae* (Giddens *et al.*, 1971 a,b) which has a synergistic effect with *M. pneumoniae* in hamsters (Liu *et al.*, 1970).

Sendai virus, which alters the phagocytic response of mouse macrophages (Goldstein and Green, 1967), has been incriminated in epizootics of MRM in rats and mice (Lane-Petter, 1970; Richter, 1970). Synergistic effects of *M. pulmonis* and viruses have also been demonstrated in tracheal organ cultures (Westerberg *et al.*, 1972).

Little is known about the possible role of ancillary factors in *M. pulmonis*-induced arthritis and genital disease. Recent reports suggest that susceptibility to arthritis may be genetically determined (Hannan, 1971; Taylor and Taylor-Robinson, 1974). Testosterone propionate given at 3 days of age increases the incidence of salpingitis and oophoritis in *M. pulmonis*-infected rats (Leader *et al.*, 1970); thus the hormonal milieu of the genital tract probably influences the progression of genital mycoplasmosis.

7. Immune Response

a. Mice. Knowledge is limited concerning the immune response of mice to naturally acquired infection. Recovery can occur, although it may take as long as a year and probably happens infrequently. It is also known that levels of CF serum antibodies increase with age and severity of lesions (Lemcke, 1961).

In experimentally infected animals, antibody titers also increase with the development of lung lesions (Cassell *et al.*, 1974; Atobe and Ogata, 1974). Antibodies of the IgM, IgG$_1$, IgG$_2$, and IgA classes are produced in the lungs and local lymph nodes and occur in both serum and tracheobronchial secretions following intranasal inoculation (Cassel *et al.*, 1974). Whereas CF antibodies are detected as early as 5–10 days after inoculation and begin to decline after 10 months, indirect hemagglutinating (IHA) antibodies no not appear until 1 month after infection and persist at high titers for up to 1 year. Metabolism-inhibition (MI) antibodies reach lower titers than CF or IHA antibodies but persist for 12 months or more (Atobe

---

FIGURE 4.   Pores (P) in membranes permit strands of granular material (arrows) to pass between *M. pulmonis* (MP) and surface epithelial cell of rat uterus. Note condensed granular material (CGM) in both host and parasite along attachment site. (X475,000.)

and Ogata, 1974). However, the level of MI antibodies may depend upon the route of injection and the strain of mouse (Cole *et al.*, 1975b).

The role of antibody in recovery from respiratory disease is uncertain. As already mentioned, antibodies are produced earlier and at higher titers in mice with more severe disease. Also, *M. pulmonis* continues to replicate even in the presence of high concentrations of specific antibody (Atobe and Ogata, 1974; Cassell *et al.*, 1974). However, development of antibody appears to correlate with a shift from acute alveolar disease to chronic bronchopneumonia. Furthermore, antibody-mediated phagocytosis probably plays a role in alveolar clearance (Jones and Hirsch, 1971; Jones *et al.*, 1973; Cole, *et al.*, 1973), but appears to be ineffective in dealing with organisms attached to respiratory epithelium (Cassell *et al.*, 1974). Whereas antimycoplasmal antibody enhances the attachment and ingestion of *M. pulmonis* by macrophages, the addition of complement to this system has no effect (Jones and Yang, 1977). This is in contrast to the effect of complement on the ingestion of *M. pneumoniae* by guinea pig macrophages (Bredt, 1975).

Although ineffective in promoting recovery from disease, antibody seems to be capable of preventing reinfection. Mice can be protected from experimental pneumonia by immunization (Cassell *et al.*, 1971; Taylor and Taylor-Robinson, 1976; Taylor *et al.*, 1977; Atobe and Ogata, 1977). Serum from these immune mice inoculated intranasally (Cassell *et al.*, 1973b) or intravenously (Taylor and Taylor-Robinson, 1974, 1976) consistently confers protection on normal mice. Passive immunization with immune serum likewise protects mice against arthritis (Taylor and Taylor-Robinson, 1977).

Classic cell-mediated immunity does not appear to play a major role against *M. pulmonis* infection in mice, since immunity cannot be passively transferred with immune cells (Taylor and Taylor-Robinson, 1976; Cassell, umpublished observations). In addition, neither congenitally athymic nude *(nu/nu)* mice (Cassell and McGhee, 1975; Cassell *et al.*, 1978b) nor neonatally thymectomized mice (Denny *et al.*, 1972; Taylor and Taylor-Robinson, 1974, 1975) are more susceptible to pneumonia than normal animals. However, T lymphocytes are essential to the generation of plasma cell infiltrates in the lung and subsequent production of anti-*M. pulmonis* antibodies (Cassell and McGhee, 1975; Cassell *et al.*, 1978b). In addition, the immune response appears necessary to limit dissemination of the mycoplasmas. Athymic mice develop arthritis following intranasal inoculation, an event which does not occur in normal animals. Reconstitution of athymic mice with congenic T cells restores the production of antimycoplasmal antibodies and the infiltration of lymphocytes into the lungs. In addition, clinical illness and microscopic lung lesions are more severe.

The anomalous lack of increased susceptibility of thymus-deficient, antibody-deficient mice may be due to the presence of a compensatory mechanism such as naturally enhanced macrophage activity or specific macrophage activation by B-cell lymphokines, or by some other mechanism. The latter hypothesis was based on observation of the infiltration of a population of undifferentiated lymphocytes into the lungs of infected athymic animals (Cassell *et al.*, 1978b). Characterization by light and immunofluorescent microscopy indicated that these were neither classic B nor T cells, but by definition were null cells. Null cells have been shown to function immunologically as killer cells in tumor cytotoxicity experiments (MacLennan, 1972), but their precise role in other immune reactions and in MRM is unknown.

b. Rats. The immunopathological character of MRM in rats and mice suggests that operative immune mechanisms differ in the two species. For example, in the rat predominantly lymphocytic hyperplasia is seen, as compared to a predominantly plasmacytic response in mice. Although more data are needed, rats appear to develop few or no MI antibodies and only low levels of CF and hemagglutinating antibodies in response to MRM (Kohn and Kirk, 1969). Neither the temporal sequence of antibody formation nor the classes involved have been defined. As in mice, CF antibody parallels the progress of infection, with the highest titers occurring in the most severely affected animals.

The local immune response of rats also appears to differ from that of mice. The strongest evidence for this is the massive proliferation of BALT. The role of BALT in respiratory immunity is undefined, but in rabbits it contains precursor cells destined to produce s-IgA (Rudzik *et al.*, 1975). BALT proliferation is associated with clearing of *Bordetella bronchiseptica* from the respiratory epithelium of the dog (Bemis *et al.*, 1977) and may be involved in the production of local immunity to *M. pulmonis* in the rat. However, it is not certain that the proliferating lymphocytes are directed against *M. pulmonis,* since this organism is known to act as a nonspecific mitogen (Ginsberg and Nicolet, 1973; Cole *et al.*, 1975b; Naot *et al.*, 1977). However, immunofluorescent studies indicated that the proliferation of BALT in MRM was accompanied by a marked increase in T and null cells. In addition, IgA-bearing B cells increased, but all other B cell populations remained unchanged, thus suggesting that the response was in fact specific (Davis and Cassell, unpublished observations).

The nonspecific local defense mechanisms of the rat seem to be more efficient than those of the mouse. Rat alveolar macrophages are capable of clearing *M. pulmonis* from the alveoli even in the absence of immune factors (Cassell *et al.*, 1973b). However, the mycoplasmas then retreat to the respiratory epithelium (as they do in mice) where they persist for the lifetime of the animal. It is evident that immune mechanisms operative in protection against *M. pulmonis* are not the same as those involved in recovery, since rats, like mice, can be effectively protected by immunization (Cassell and Davis, 1978). Surprisingly, ineffective vaccine regimens do not enhance the severity of disease upon subsequent challenge.

The hypothesis that the immune response of rats against lung disease involves cellular rather than antibody-mediated mechanisms is supported by the passive transfer of immunity using spleen cells, but not serum, from immunized rats (G. H. Cassell, P. B. Carter and J. K. Davis, unpublished observations). These results differ from those obtained in mice, once again suggesting that these species differ in response to *M. pulmonis*. Again, data thus far have been obtained using primarily CD-1 mice and F344 rats; therefore, these differences may be strain rather than species related.

No data exist concerning the immune response of rats to genital mycoplasmal infection, but the infiltration of lymphoid cells into the genital mucosa of infected females suggests that these rats mount an adaptive response. As in the respiratory tract, lymphocytes, not plasma cells, predominate in all segments of the genital tract except the oviduct, where the reverse is true.

8. Evasion of the Immune Response

Rats and mice are definitely capable of mounting responses against *M. pulmonis* that are at least theoretically capable of eliminating the organism. Yet these microorganisms survive for weeks, months, or even years in immunocompetent individuals. There are several possible mechanisms, either intrinsic to the mycoplasmas or resulting from their association with host cells, by which they could evade immunological destruction. These include organism seclusion within sites devoid of immune effector mechanisms, inefficient phagocytosis, release of soluble antigens, alteration of lymphocyte responsiveness, and antigenic variation, as well as antigenic disguise.

The most trite of these involves the seclusion of mycoplasmas at sites inaccessible to immune effector mechanisms. For example, their tendency to reside between the cilia on respiratory epithelial cells might prevent their clearance by the mucociliary escalator. Also, their partial envelopment by host cell cytoplasmic processes has been suggested to prevent phagocytosis and/or combination with antibody (Whittlestone, 1976). This association, however, is not as close as that of intracellular viruses, and immunologically competent hosts are able to rid themselves of respiratory viruses even at the cost of destroying infected cells. Therefore seclusion is not a totally satisfactory explanation.

The release of soluble antigens and formation of immune complexes may facilitate the survival of infecting organisms by blocking specific cellular or humoral effector mechanisms, by modifying immune induction through interaction with macrophages, by inducing T- or B-cell tolerance, or by activating suppressor T cells. Unfortunately, too little is known about *M. pulmonis* antigens to do more than list the areas that are worthy of further experimentation. Other mycoplasma species have already been shown to release soluble antigens (Hudson *et al.*, 1967; Eng, 1971), as well as elicit the production of "defective" mycoplasmacidal antibodies (Cole and Ward, 1973c). In addition, immune complexes have been demonstrated in human infections (Biberfeld and Norberg, 1974), and immune complex-type injury has been observed in chronic *M. pulmonis* infections of mice (Cassell *et al.*, 1971).

Alteration of lymphocyte responsiveness could be even more important. The mitogenicity of *M. pulmonis* for rat and mouse lymphocytes (Cole *et al.*, 1975b; Naot *et al.*, 1977) might misdirect the immune response by preempting helper cells or by interfering with immune regulatory mechanisms. As a consequence, inefficient effector mechanisms might be preferentially stimulated. For example, *M. pulmonis*-infected mice produce large amounts of IgG_1 (Cassell *et al.*, 1974) which is both non-complement-fixing and nonopsonizing. These probably act as "blocking antibodies," thus protecting the organism from other host defenses.

Immune escape via antigenic variation and/or antigenic disguise is perhaps the most intriguing possibility. The finding of 58 different serotypes of *M. pulmonis* within only five rat colonies (Ogata *et al.*, 1967) suggests that *M. pulmonis* may vary its antigenic makeup during the course of infection. Such antigenic drift has been shown to be involved in many persistent viral (Fenner *et al.*, 1974) and bacterial diseases (Robinet, 1962; Miller *et al.*, 1972; Bratthall and Gibbons, 1975). Mycoplasmal antigen changes could be mediated by an immune response to the initial colonizing population, thus favoring the selection of antigenically altered mutants. The persistence of viable *M. pulmonis* in immune rats and mice (Taylor and Taylor-Robinson, 1976; Cassell, unpublished observations) is consistent with this possibility.

The intimate association of *M. pulmonis* with the surface of the host cell and the ability of mycoplasmas to bind exogenous proteins readily (Razin *et al.*, 1973) suggest that the organism might avoid the lethal consequences of the immune response by disguising itself with host antigens. This would also provide for the development of autoimmune responses such as are seen in mycoplasma-infected mice (Harwick *et al.*, 1973b). Selective uptake of mouse histocompatibility and differentiation antigens by *M. hyorhinis* (Wise *et al.*, 1978) supports the thesis of mycoplasmas being capable of antigenic disguise.

The prolonged survival of *M. pulmonis* (by any of these mechanisms), leading to the release of antigenic material and continued activation of immune responses, may provide the essential basis for many of the pathological phenomena seen in MRM, genital disease, and arthritis.

B. *Mycoplasma arthritidis*

1. Serological and Physiological Characteristics

Most *M. arthritidis* isolates grow readily on conventional mycoplasma media (Hayflick, 1965) under both aerobic and anaerobic conditions. The colonial morphology is typical, with a small central area of growth into the agar and large peripheral surface growth. No pearly layer is produced. As can be seen in Table I, the characteristics most useful for distinguishing these strains from other murine mycoplasmas include their inability to ferment carbohydrates, the presence of arginine dihydrolase, and their distinct serological properties. Only limited electron microscope observations have been made, but *M. arthritidis* appears to be less filamentous than *M. pulmonis* (Morton *et al.*, 1954; Domermuth *et al.*, 1964), with no extracellular surface structures.

Differences in colonial morphology between virulent and avirulent strains have been reported (Warren, 1942; Howell and Jones, 1963), but Golightly-Rowland *et al.* (1970) could not correlate these differences with virulence. However, the less virulent strains grew faster on artificial media. CF and gel diffusion failed to reveal distinct differences, but in the growth inhibition and MI tests, the avirulent strains were more susceptible to inhibition.

Although antigenically a fairly homogeneous group, strains which differ serologically to a small degree have been described (Lemcke, 1961, 1964). The Campo (PG27) strain and a small group of related strains, originally classified as *Mycoplasma hominis* type 2, were later reclassified as *M. arthritidis* on the basis of serological observations (Lemcke, 1964; Edward and Freundt, 1965). This reclassification was subsequently justified by nucleic acid homology, enzyme analysis, examination of the electrophoretic patterns of the proteins from each of the strains involved (Razin and Rottem, 1967), and pathogenicity experiments (Cole *et al.*, 1967).

2. Naturally Occurring Polyarthritis

Spontaneous polyarthritis in laboratory and wild rats is most commonly caused by *M. arthritidis* (Collier, 1939; Klieneberger, 1940; Sokoloff, 1965, 1967; Cotchin and Roe, 1967). The infection is usually endemic in a colony, with only a few animals showing clinical disease, although this varies with individual outbreaks (Ito *et al.*, 1957). There are several detailed clinical and histological descriptions of naturally occurring arthritis in rats (Findlay *et al.*, 1939; Kleineberger, 1940; Tully, 1969). In addition, the features are described in this volume, Chapter 11.

3. Experimental Arthritis of Rats

Intravenous or foot pad inoculation of *M. arthritidis* into rats leads to mycoplasmemia that initially lasts about 5 days and occasionally reoccurs on a transient basis (Preston, 1942; Parkes and Wrigley, 1951; Ward and Jones, 1962; Cole and Ward, 1973a). Large doses (10^7 CFU) given intravenously may cause swelling and erythema of joints by 3–5 days or, if less virulent inocula are used, 7–9 days. The major lesion is acute polyarthritis which begins to subside spontaneously about 2 weeks after onset. A few animals develop flaccid paralysis of the hind limbs. Rhinitis, conjunctivitis, corneal opacities, and urethritis also have been observed in experimental infections (Ward and Cole, 1970), but it was not certain whether these lesions were actually due to *M. arthritidis*.

4. Experimental Arthritis in Mice

Although *M. arthritidis* does not naturally infect mice, it produces chronic arthritis after intravenous injection. This disease is characterized by an initial acute phase with polymorphonuclear leukocyte infiltration into the articular and periarticular tissues and mild hyperplasia of the synovial membrane, followed by chronic lesions with new areas of acute inflammation. This chronic phase persists for at least 6 months and can show massive synovial proliferation, mononuclear cell infiltration, and defects in cartilage and bone. Periods of remission are noticed during this time (Cole *et al.*, 1971b). There is a marked variation in response among mouse strains to the experimental disease. Cole *et al.* (1973) showed that DBA mice were the most severely affected of the seven strains they examined.

5. Other Disease Manifestations

Ward and Cole (1970) and Ito *et al.* (1957) have frequently isolated *M. arthritidis* from the nasopharynx of healthy rats, and Stewart and Buck (1975) have also isolated it in conjunction with *M. pulmonis* from rats suffering from MRM. It also has been recovered from subcutaneous abscesses (Klieneberger, 1938; Cole et al., 1967), otitis media (Preston, 1942), bronchiectatic lung (Cole et al., 1967), paraovarian abscesses (Preston, 1942), and conjunctivitis (Ward and Jones, 1962). In the United Kingdom, however, recovery of M. arthritidis in the absence of clinical arthritis is low (Hill, unpublished observations).

After experimental infection of rats and mice by various routes, the organism has been isolated from blood, spleen, lymph nodes, lung, liver, and brain, as well as joints (Woglom and Warren, 1938a,b; Collier, 1939; Hill and Dagnall, 1975). Although M. arthritidis produces abscesses in both rats and mice after subcutaneous injection, the lesions are quite different. A localized abscess at the site of injection forms in rats, whereas in mice the abscess enlarges and the tissue becomes necrotic (Cole et al., 1973).

Although M. arthritidis given intravenously can be toxic for mice and rats, the central nervous system does not appear to be affected. Coma and death may occur within a few hours of the injection, even though no exotoxin can be demonstrated (Cole et al., 1973). Smaller doses injected intravenously into pregnant mice cause death of the fetuses (Kaklamanis and Thomas, 1970; Cole et al., 1973). The organisms can be isolated from the fetal tissue.

Thomsen et al. (1973) produced pyelonephritis in rats with the inoculation of M. arthritidis into the kidney. Antibodies were present in the serum and urine of rats which developed inflammatory lesions in both the papilla and cortex, whereas antibodies were found only in the urine in all but one case of those with lesions in the papilla but not the cortex. Antibody was not produced in rats with no lesions (Rosendal and Thomsen, 1974).

Mycoplasma arthritidis has occasionally been isolated from the genital tract and joints (Edward and Freundt, 1965; Bartholomew, 1967; Jansson and Wager, 1967) of humans. It has even been recovered from synovial fluid of rheumatoid patients (Jansson et al., 1971), but its etiological significance in such cases has not been determined.

6. Disease Mechanisms

The natural disease occurs more frequently in young rats (from 8 to 93 days old) with no special relationship between incidence and sex (Ito et al., 1957). It appears that M. arthritidis may remain in a latent state in joints or may normally reside in the respiratory tract with occasional introduction into the joint, resulting in severe sporadic or epizootic joint disease (Cotchin and Roe, 1967). Because arthritic lesions are mostly seen on the forelimbs where rats habitually lick, mouth-to-foot inoculation has been proposed (Ito et al., 1957). However, attempts to reproduce the disease experimentally by this method have been unsuccessful (Collier, 1939; Ito *et al.*, 1957).

The disease cannot readily be transmitted by direct contact between healthy and infected animals. In view of this and of the large number of organisms required experimentally, subsidiary factors may be involved. Ward and Cole (1970) have observed that mycoplasmal arthritis seems most prevalent when rats are housed in unsuitable cages that produce injury. A synergistic effect may occur between mycoplasmas and other infectious agents or foreign material. Most early reports of the natural disease involved such a possibility. When rats have been stressed (by injections of hormones, drugs, or malignant tissues carrying latent infection) the disease is more prevalent (Preston, 1942; Hershberger *et al.*, 1960; Mielens and Rozitis, 1964; Sokoloff, 1965).

The mycoplasmal factors involved in the pathogenesis of arthritis are poorly defined. However, the organism produces gelatinases (Woolcock *et al.*, 1973). Infected animals also produce anti-DNA antibodies (Laber *et al.*, 1974; Vincze *et al.*, 1975; Klein and Wottawa, 1975; Klein, 1977) which correlate with reduced or inhibited DNA repair. In addition, *M. arthritidis* possesses antigens which cross-react with certain rat antigens (Cahill *et al.*, 1971). All these may contribute to the pathogenesis of mycoplasmal arthritis but, as Ward and Cole (1970) have concluded, pathogenic mechanisms are complex and will require much effort to unravel. Disease mechanisms are discussed in greater detail in this volume, Chapter 11, particularly those involved in eliciting chronic inflammation.

7. Immune Response

CF antibody can be detected in rats as early as 72 hr after intravenous inoculation of *M. arthritidis* (Cole *et al.*, 1969). Titers rise to 40,000 between 4 and 8 weeks (depending upon disease severity) and then drop and remain below 2000 for up to 21 weeks. MI (Cole *et al.*, 1969; Hill and Dagnall, 1975) and IHA (Cole *et al.*, 1969) antibodies cannot be detected at any time.

Although in rats CF antibody is present before the appearance of clinical arthritis, the reverse is true in mice; antibody is not present until 7 days after infection (Cole *et al.*, 1971a). In addition to the slower CF response in mice, the titers drop much faster (after 3 weeks) than in rats but persist longer (at least 6 months). Both IgM and IgG CF antibodies are detected in rats, whereas only the latter are detected in mice. Like rats, mice develop virtually no MI antibodies.

Mycoplasma arthritidis-infected rats and mice produce a defective mycoplasmacidal antibody, i.e., antibody capable of destroying only resting mycoplasmas (Cole and Ward, 1973c). These defective antibodies may play no role in immunity to *M. arthritidis* but could contribute to disease pathogenesis by giving rise to antigen–antibody complexes.

Sensitized lymphocytes develop in response to infection in both rats and mice (Cole *et al.*, 1975a), but it is not known whether these are B or T cells. *In vivo* and *in vitro*, these organisms are known to suppress immune responsiveness to other antigens (Kaklamanis and Pavlatos, 1972), and *in vitro* to inhibit transformation of lymphocytes (Copperman and Morton, 1966; Morton *et al.*, 1968; Barile and Leventhal, 1968; Simberkoff *et al.*, 1969). They also are capable of inducing cell-mediated cytotoxicity (Aldridge *et al.*, 1977a,b) and interferon production (Rinaldo *et al.*, 1974; Cole *et al.*, 1975c, 1976). The possible involvement of these phenomena in *M. arthritidis* disease pathogenesis is discussed in more detail in this volume, Chapter 11.

Rat and mouse peritoneal macrophages fail to kill *M. arthritidis*, even in the presence of homologous immune sera (Cole and Ward, 1973b). The production of defective antibodies coupled with this poor macrophage response correlates nicely with the chronicity of infection in mice. However, the same response in rats suggests that their infection should also be chronic. It is therefore surprising that the disease is self-limiting in this species.

Recovery from infection in both species is followed by resistance to reinfection (Cole *et al.*, 1969). Immunity can be passively transferred to normal animals by convalescent serum but cannot be related to the presence of CF antibodies (Cole *et al.*, 1969). Furthermore, the protective properties of the serum cannot be absorbed with washed *M. arthritidis*. Partial immunity can also be transferred in rats, but not mice, by immune spleen cells (Kahan *et al.*, 1964; Cole *et al.*, 1971b). Further evidence that the immune response is protective is shown by the enhancement of arthritis in rats treated with immunosuppressive drugs and antithymocyte serum (Jouanneau *et al.*, 1973).

C. *Mycoplasma neurolyticum*

1. Serological and Physiological Characteristics

Although minimal nutritional requirements are poorly defined, *M. neurolyticum* is apparently less exacting than most other mycoplasma species. Optimal growth is supported by as little as 1% whole or 2% agamma horse serum (Freundt, 1974). The organism ferments several carbohydrates so rapidly that viability can be quickly lost in broth cultures containing high levels of serum and carbohydrate. *Mycoplasma neurolyticum* is unique in that growth can be inhibited by moderate concentrations of penicillin G (40 units/ml and above); however, it can be adapted to growth at high levels by stepwise transfer to increasing concentrations (Wright, 1967). The effect of penicillin seems to be bacteriostatic rather than bacteriocidal. Antigenic variation among *M. neurolyticum* strains appears to be minimal, but only limited comparisons have been made. In fact, data comparing toxigenic and nontoxigenic strains are totally lacking. The glycolipid antigen of *M. neurolyticum* has been shown to cross-react with that of *M. pneumoniae* (Kenny, 1971).

2. Natural Infection

Mycoplasma neurolyticum in conventional mice seems to be as common as *M. pulmonis,* but natural infection has been associated with only one disease: conjunctivitis (Nelson, 1950a,b). Ocular lesions are seen mainly in young mice and have been transmitted to uninfected mice by direct contact or passage of ocular washings. This agent has been recovered from many tissues of latently infected mice (Nelson, 1950a,b; Tully, 1965; Tully and Rask-Nielsen, 1967). In addition to the conjunctiva and Harderian glands, the nasopharynx and central nervous system are the sites most frequently infected (A. Hill, unpublished observations). Other organisms often isolated from the conjunctiva in association with *M. neurolyticum* include *M. pulmonis, S. aureus,* and *P. pneumotropica.* The incidence of recovery of *M. neurolyticum* from sites also infected with *M. pulmonis* is lower than when *M. neurolyticum* is present alone (A. Hill, unpublished observations). This could be due to competition between the mycoplasmas *in vivo* or to difficulty in isolating *M. neurolyticum* when cultures are heavily infected with the larger, quicker-growing colonies of *M. pulmonis.* Almost the reverse is true with *M. pulmonis*-induced arthritis. Here the incidence and severity of arthritis is decreased in mice naturally infected with *M. neurolyticum* (Hannan, 1976). This effect probably does not involve immune mechanisms, since vaccination with *M. neurolyticum* provides no protection against challenge with viable *M. pulmonis* (Atobe and Ogata, 1977).

Mycoplasma neurolyticum has also been isolated from conventional rats (A. C. Thomsen, personal communication). However, these rats were in contact with infected mice, and it is possible that these were only transient infections.

3. Experimental Infection

a. Conjunctivitis. Mice are readily infected with *M. neurolyticum* when freshly isolated strains are given by the conjunctival or nasopharyngeal route (Hill, 1976). One week after inoculation, organisms can be reisolated from the inoculation site and the Harderian glands. Two to three weeks later, organisms are found in the brain, spinal cord, nasopharynx, and Harderian glands and are still present at these sites for up to 6 weeks. However, there are no detectable CF or MI antibodies, and no conjunctivitis is seen. This is in agreement with reports by investigators who have attempted to produce conjunctivitis by intranasal and intravenous inoculation of *M. neurolyticum*. Congenitally athymic mice respond similarly (A. Hill, unpublished observations). However, direct inoculation of *M. neurolyticum* into the cornea results in lesions (M. F. Barile, personal communication).

When mice are coinfected with *M. pulmonis* in the nasopharynx and *M. neurolyticum* in the conjunctiva, there is a lower incidence of recovery of the latter from the nasal passages (A. Hill, unpublished observations). These findings are similar to those in natural mixed infections, including the fact that no CF or MI anti-*M. neurolyticum* antibodies are produced. Cole *et al.* (1970) suggested that the lack of MI antibody probably plays a role in the establishment of *M. neurolyticum* infection in mice; aberrant hosts produce high titers of MI antibody.

    b. "Rolling" disease. *Mycoplasma neurolyticum* is best known for the production of rolling disease (Findlay *et al.*, 1938) in mice. Intravenous, intraperitoneal, or intracerebral inoculation of infected tissue, broth cultures containing viable organisms, or cell-free filtrates induces the rolling syndrome (Thomas and Bitensky, 1966). It is characterized by an abrupt onset of continuous rolling which persists for several hours and terminates in death (Findlay *et al.*, 1938).

Rolling disease is due to an exotoxin produced by *M. neurolyticum* (Thomas and Bitensky, 1966). The purification of the exotoxin and its biological effects have been described by Tully (1969, 1974) and Kaklamanis and Thomas (1970). It appears that mice and rats are the only animals affected. Intravenous injection produces the greatest effect. The toxin acts primarily on the vascular supply to the brain, causing cerebral edema; the severity and speed of onset are in direct proportion to the dose given (Thomas, 1969).

D. Other Murine Mycoplasmas

1. Strain 58B (Gough)

Strain 58B, a serologically distinct mycoplasma, produces typical colonies within a week on conventional mycoplasma medium (Hill, 1974b). Other known physiological characteristics are listed in Table I.

The organism was present in the conjunctiva of all the rats and in the nasopharynx of half the rats in three colonies in the United Kingdom (Young and Hill, 1974; Hill, 1974a). Natural transmission from infected parents to offspring diminished in succeeding generations (Hill, 1974b). There is some suggestion that the organism might cause conjunctivitis, since 60% of one infected colony developed the disease soon after weaning, but bacterial pathogens were also present. In addition, none of the bacterial pathogens or 58B caused conjunctivitis when inoculated into the conjunctiva of specific-pathogen-free rats (Young and Hill, 1974; Hill, 1974b). However, strain 58B organisms readily colonized the conjunctiva and brain of most animals and the nasopharynx of some and remained established at these sites for at least 6 weeks. They were not isolated from lung, liver, or spleen, and serum CF titers were negligible (A. Hill, unpublished observations). The species seems to lose infectivity and perhaps virulence rapidly upon artificial cultivation, thus possibly explaining its failure to induce conjunctivitis experimentally.

Strain 58B is serologically identical to strain Gough, which was isolated from the nasopharynx of mice in a colony known to be free of other mycoplasmas. No data on the pathogenic potential of strain 58B is available.

2. *Mycoplasma alvi* (Ilsley strain)

Gourlay and Wyld (1976) reported the isolation of mycoplasmas from the intestinal tract of wild field mice. These isolates, which resemble the Ilsley strain of *M. alvi* recovered from the intestinal tract of cattle (Gourlay *et al.*, 1977) prefer anaerobic conditions for growth, metabolize glucose, are inhibited by digitonin, and are serologically distinct from other murine mycoplasmas.

III. MYCOPLASMAS OF OTHER SMALL ANIMALS

A. Guinea Pigs

1. *Mycoplasma caviae*

a. Serological and physiological characteristics. *Mycoplasma caviae* grows readily in liquid medium, usually within a few days, but may have to be passaged through liquid medium before growing on solid medium. Colonial growth is typical and occurs under both aerobic and anaerobic conditions. A pearly layer is produced only under anaerobic conditions. Other physical characteristics are given in Table I.

Mycoplasma caviae has been isolated from guinea pigs in the United Kingdom (Hill, 1971) and in the United States (Stalheim and Matthews, 1975; M. F. Barile, personal communication). There is no evidence of strain variation; however, little serological work has been done.

b. Natural infection. *Mycoplasma caviae* is usually present in the nasopharynx or vagina, and has been isolated from the brain. In one case, the organism was isolated in pure culture from a guinea pig with metritis, but there is little other evidence of pathogenicity. The incidence of infection appears to be fairly low (Hill, 1973; Stalheim and Matthews, 1975).

   c. **Experimental infection.** *Mycoplasma caviae*, even when injected by numerous routes, has not been shown to have any pathogenic effect in normal or athymic mice, rats, guinea pigs, or rabbits, (A. Hill, unpublished observations). The organism was recovered from the nasopharynx of half the guinea pigs infected intranasally and from the vagina of a third of both pregnant and nonpregnant guinea pigs after intravaginal infection (Hill, 1973).

2. Acholeplasmas

   Acholeplasma laidlawii was recovered from the vagina of 22 out of 51 guinea pigs from a specific-pathogen-free unit, and from the vagina or nasopharynx of 25–40% of animals examined from several different conventional colonies. Rats and mice housed in the same room and on bedding taken from cages of infected guinea pigs did not become infected (Hill, 1974c). It has, however, been isolated from many other animal species (Edward, 1950; Adler and Shifrine, 1964). Stalheim and Matthews (1975) isolated glucose-fermenting acholeplasmas from the nasopharynx and vagina of guinea pigs, but they were not identified serologically. *Acholeplasma granularum* has been isolated once from the vagina of a guinea pig (A. Hill, unpublished observations).

3. *Mycoplasma pulmonis*

   Juhr and Obi (1970) reported that all 80 guinea pigs they examined were infected with *M. pulmonis* in the uterus. Recently a strain of *M. pulmonis* has been isolated from the nasopharynx and conjunctiva of one out of four guinea pigs which had no apparent contact with mice or rats (A. Hill, unpublished observation). However, there have been no other reports of *M. pulmonis* infection in guinea pigs.

4. Other Mycoplasmas in Guinea Pigs

   Strains G371 and 22A have been isolated from the vagina of guinea pigs, and strain 117C from the nasopharynx (Hill, 1974a). The latter strain colonizes the nasopharynx of mice upon intranasal inoculation, but it has not been shown to infect them naturally. All three strains are serologically distinct and have different physiological characteristics (Table I).

   A survey by Rigby and Langford (1976) suggests that genital mycoplasmosis may be common in male guinea pigs. In females, however, infection seems to be transient, but the incidence of vaginal mycoplasmas may vary widely. The organisms most frequently isolated by these investigators were a serologically distinct *Acholeplasma* sp. and *Mycoplasma* sp. (group 7 of Leach) (Leach, 1973). The latter was an unexpected finding, since this organism had previously been reported only from cattle. It would be of interest to know the relationship of this organism to the mycoplasmas isolated by Hill (1974a) and Stalheim and Matthews (1975) from guinea pigs. The spontaneous occurrence of a mycoplasma-like organism has been demonstrated in the lungs of guinea pigs by electron microscopy (Sherwin *et al.*, 1973).

B. Chinese Hamsters

1. Strain CH

This strain grows on normal mycoplasma medium under aerobic conditions and occasionally can be difficult to isolate. No pearly layer is produced; colonial growth shows a small central zone with a large clear periphery. Other characteristics are given in Table I.

a. Natural infection. Strain CH was isolated from the conjunctiva of all animals examined in one colony, from the nasopharynx and brain of most, and the lungs of a few (Hill, 1974a). One Steppe lemming housed with these hamsters was also infected. A serologically identical strain has since been isolated from another colony of Chinese hamsters in the United Kingdom and a colony in the Netherlands (A. A. Polak-Vogelzang, personal communication).

b. Experimental infection. Strain CH induced CF antibody titers of 32 to 128 in mice 3 weeks after inoculation by the intranasal, conjunctival, and intravenous routes. However, the organism could not be recovered (Hill, 1974a).

2. *Mycoplasma pulmonis*

This species was isolated from the nasopharynx of two out of six Chinese hamsters, all of which were infected in the conjunctiva, but not nasopharynx, with strain CH. It is difficult to speculate on the frequency of *M. pulmonis* in Chinese hamsters, as very few have been examined. In the case above there were, however, *M. pulmonis*-infected mice housed in the same building, although not in the same room. *Mycoplasma pulmonis* has also been isolated from Syrian hamsters (Battigelli *et al.*, 1971).

C. Rabbits

An extensive survey of conventional rabbits failed to isolate mycoplasmas, even though cultures were taken from the nasopharynx, middle ear, and vagina (Hill, 1974a). The isolation of *M. pulmonis* from rabbits (Deeb and Kenny, 1967a) has not been repeated and could have been a transient infection. However, this organism produces arthritis upon intra-articular inoculation (Cole *et al.*, 1977), and uveitis upon inoculation into the anterior chamber of the eye (Kunishi, 1974). Arthritis in rabbits can also be induced by intra-articular inoculation of *M. arthritidis* (Cole *et al.*, 1977).

D. Other Small Animals

Mycoplasmas have also been isolated from the nasopharynx and alimentary tract of voles (Gourlay and Wyld, 1976), hedgehogs (Tan *et al.*, 1971), squirrels (Katoch and Chandiramani, 1975), and tortoises (Hill, unpublished observations). In addition, strains SH1, *Mycoplasma edwardii*, and *M. alvi* (Ilsley type) have been isolated from wild shrews (Gourlay and Wyld, 1976; A. Hill, unpublished observations).

IV. DETECTION AND CONTROL: REMAINING PROBLEMS AND FUTURE OUTLOOK

As mentioned earlier in this chapter, *M. pulmonis* respiratory and genital mycoplasmoses seriously restrict the usefulness of murine species for research purposes. Although *M. arthritidis* apparently occurs less frequently, it too can have devastating effects (Tully, 1969; Ward and Cole, 1970; Lindsey *et al.*, 1971, 1978). For the naive investigator, these organisms pose a particular threat because of their subtle interactions with their mammalian host. In view of this it is imperative that effective detection and control procedures be developed. The following discussion describes the current methods and points out the remaining problems in these areas.

A. Detection

Presently, it is necessary to use several time-consuming procedures in conjunction with one another to diagnose mycoplasmal diseases. These include (1) cultural isolation, (2) detection of mycoplasmas in infected tissue by fluorescence- or peroxidase-labeled specific antibody, (3) histopathology, and (4) serology.

1. Culture

Ganaway *et al.* (1973) and Kappel *et al.* (1974) recently demonstrated the effectiveness of culture in monitoring the mycoplasmal status of rat colonies. It is possible to use oropharyngeal swabs and/or nasal washings collected from anesthetized animals. Both *M. pulmonis* and *M. arthritidis* are most frequently isolated from these sites, even in the absence of overt disease. The conjunctiva seems to be the best site for *M. neurolyticum* (Hill, 1974a). Killing the animal is not necessary; therefore all the animals at risk may be evaluated. Even when animals are killed for *M. pulmonis* isolation, culture of tracheobronchial lavages is superior to the use of infected tissue (Taylor-Robinson *et al.*, 1972). However, negative results from only a few animals, regardless of the method, do not demonstrate that a colony is mycoplasma-free. Unfortunately, we do not know how frequently *M. pulmonis* genital infection occurs in the absence of respiratory infection; therefore one cannot use culture of the respiratory tract alone as an indication of the mycoplasmal status of a colony. The uterus, oviduct, and vas deferens can be cultured by gentle washings with 0.3 ml of sterile broth.

Culture of the synovial membrane, as well as other infected tissues, deserves special consideration. Mycoplasmas sometimes grow less well from concentrated tissue suspensions than from dilute ones, because of the presence of a nonspecific inhibitor (Tully and Rask-Nielsen, 1967), probably lysolecithin (Kaklamanis *et al.*, 1969; Mårdh and Taylor-Robinson, 1973). The addition of lysophospholipase appears to abolish the mycoplasmacidal activity.

All pathogenic mycoplasmas require a complex medium, such as Hayflick's (1965). The problems in recovery of mycoplasmas by culture have been well described (Whittlestone, 1974). In general, *M. pulmonis*, *M. arthritidis*, and *M. neurolyticum* grow well aerobically at 37°C. Some strains are easier to isolate on agar than in broth; for others, the reverse is true. Blind restreaking of plates and/or several rapid passes in broth every 48 hr improve the isolation rate. Cultures should not be reported as negative until at least 3 weeks have lapsed.

Once a positive culture is obtained, the organism must be identified as a mycoplasma by the minimal standards proposed by the Subcommittee on the Taxonomy of Mycoplasmatales (1972). Preferably the species should also be established.

2. Detection of Organisms in Infected Tissue

Isolation, cultivation, and positive identification of mycoplasmas may take as long as 3 weeks and can be very laborious. Indirect identification of organisms in infected tissues by immunofluorescence is faster and often more reliable. We have found this method very useful in the diagnosis of MRM and genital mycoplasmosis (Cassell *et al.*, 1979). However, the need for special equipment limits general acceptance of this method. This can be circumvented by replacing the fluorescein label with peroxidase which can be examined by regular light microscopy (Nakane and Kawaoi, 1974; Polak-Vogelzang and Hagenaars, 1976; Hill, 1978). The sensitivity of either of these methods has not been compared with that of cultural detection.

3. Histopathological Character

Because of the difficulties encountered with the above methods, diagnosis of mycoplasmal diseases is often made on the basis of clinical and pathological features and by the process of eliminating other likely infectious agents. The insidious nature of most mycoplasmal diseases often means that there is an active disease process but no apparent gross lesions. For this reason, presumptive diagnosis should be made only on the basis of microscopic evaluation of the entire genital and respiratory tracts and joints. Final diagnosis should be made only on the basis of microscopic examination and positive isolation or detection of organisms.

4. Serology

The indirect detection of mycoplasmal infection by conventional serology is limited. Because most of the infections are restricted to mucosal or serosal surfaces, serum antibodies are usually low. In the early stages of disease when the number of organisms is small and, more particularly, when the infections are latent and the organisms are confined to the oropharynx, diagnosis by serology is particularly difficult. Perhaps the newly developed, more sensitive enzyme-linked immunosorbent (Horowitz and Cassell, 1978) or radioimmunoadsorbent (Brunner *et al.*, 1977) assays will prove to be more suitable for screening purposes.

B. Control

A few investigators have claimed success in eliminating MRM from breeding stocks of rats or mice through programs involving either rigid selection (Nelson and Gowen, 1931; Berg and Harmison, 1957) coupled with the administration of antibacterial drugs (Haberman *et al.*, 1963; Ganaway and Allen, 1969), or principles of cesarean derivation combined with strict isolation procedures (Nelson and Collins, 1961; Ganaway and Allen, 1969; Kappel *et al.*, 1974). In the past decade, much emphasis was placed on the latter techniques with the creation of a large family of terms, such as *specific-pathogen-free* and *pathogen-free*, to describe these stocks for commercial purposes. In actual practice, maintenance of these stocks for significant periods of time has, with rare exceptions, resulted in bitter disappointment. Although these disappointments have generally been attributed to a break in strict isolation procedures, the animals used for hysterectomy or cesarean derivation may have harbored *M. pulmonis* in the genital tract.

Recent studies suggest that rats (Cassell and Davis, 1978) and mice (Cassell *et al.*, 1973b; Taylor *et al.*, 1977; Atobe and Ogata, 1977) can be protected from MRM by immunization and give hope that an effective vaccine will soon be available. It must be kept in mind, however, that the precise relationship between the respiratory and the genital diseases is not known. An effective vaccine may well be required to protect both. Also, before the optimal vaccine can be developed, more information is needed concerning host–parasite interactions at the cellular and subcellular levels, since it appears that subtle details of these interactions determine the outcome of infection. Definition of molecular mechanisms involved in cell surface attachment is of major importance in this regard. *Mycoplasma pulmonis* survival in the presence of antibody suggests that much of the specific antibody may be directed against serotypes of the organism present earlier in the infection or against various metabolites and degradation products irrelevant to immune destruction. Therefore it appears that artificially induced immunity may be more promising in preventing initial colonization than in eliminating the organism after it has established an infection. Definition of the specific antigens, antibodies, and cell types involved in the immune response to *M. pulmonis* then becomes necessary.

In addition, the complexity of MRM makes it necessary not only to understand the mycoplasma–host interrelationships but to have a precise appreciation of the extrinsic factors involved in disease production. This is essential for the application of proper management practices with particular emphasis on prevention.

Disease due to *M. arthritidis* and *M. neurolyticum* is not nearly as common as *M. pulmonis* respiratory or genital disease. Immunoprophylactic methods to control these species therefore do not appear to be necessary at this time. However, investigators should be aware of their presence and the possible influence they have upon scientific research. With regard to detection and control of mycoplasmas in other small animals, much more basic information is needed concerning their incidence and ability to produce disease.

ACKNOWLEDGMENTS

The authors gratefully acknowledge W. H. Wilborn, Department of Anatomy, University of South Alabama, Mobile, Alabama, for the electron micrographs, and J. K. Davis, R. Thorp, and P. Hull for their excellent assistance in preparation of the manuscript. This work was supported by Public Health Service grants RR 00959, HD-11447-01 and HLAI 19741. G.H.C. is recipient of Public Health Service Research Career Development Award 1K04 HL 00387-01 PTHA from the National Heart and Lung Institute.

REFERENCES

Adler, H., and Shifrine, M. (1963). *J. Bacteriol.* **87,** 1245.

Aldridge, K. E., Cole, B. C., and Ward, J. R. (1977a). *Infect. Immun.* **18,** 377–385.

Aldridge, K. E., Cole, B. C., and Ward, J. R. (1977b). *Infect. Immun.* **18,** 386–392.

Andrewes, C. H., and Niven, J. S. F. (1950). *Br. J. Exp. Pathol.* **31,** 773–778.

Andrewes, C. H., and Welch, F. V. (1946). *J. Pathol. Bacteriol.* **58,** 578–580.

Atobe, H., and Ogata, M. (1974). *Jpn. J. Vet. Sci.* **36,** 495–503.

Atobe, H., and Ogata, M. (1977). *Jpn. J. Vet. Sci.* **39,** 39–46.

Barden, J. A., and Tully, J. G. (1969). *J. Bacteriol.* **100,** 5–10.

Barile, M. F., and Leventhal, B. G. (1968). *Nature (London)* **219,** 750–752.

Bartholomew, L. E. (1967). *Ann. N.Y. Acad. Sci.* **143,** 522–534.

Battigelli, M. C., Fraser, D. A., and Cole, H. (1971). *Arch. Intern. Med.* **127,** 1103–1104.

Bemis, D. A., Greisen, H. A., and Appel, M. J. G. (1977). *J. Infect. Dis.* **135,** 753–762.

Berg, B. N., and Harmison, C. R. (1957). *J. Gerontol.* **12,** 370–377.

Biberfeld, G., and Norberg, R. (1974). *J. Immunol.* **112,** 413–415.

Bilder, G. E. (1975). *J. Gerontol.* **30,** 641–646.

Bratthall, D., and Gibbons, R. J. (1975). *Infect. Immun.* **12,** 1231–1236.

Bredt, W. (1973). *Ann. N.Y. Acad. Sci.* **225,** 246–250.

Bredt, W. (1975). *Infect. Immun.* **12,** 694–695.

Bredt, W., and Radestock, U. (1977). *J. Bacteriol.* **130,** 937–938.

Brennan, P. C., and Feinstein, R. N. (1969). *J. Bacteriol.* **98,** 1036–1040.

Brennan, P. C., Fritz, T. E., and Flynn, R. J. (1969) *J. Bacteriol.* **97,** 337–349.

Broderson, J. R., Lindsey, J. R., and Crawford, J. E. (1976). *Am. J. Pathol.* **85,** 115–130.

Brunner, H., Schaeg, W., Schiefer, H. G., and Bruck, U. (1977). *Med. Microbiol. Immunol.* **163,** 25–35.

Cahill, J. F., Cole, B. C., Wiley, B. B., and Ward, J. R. (1971). *Infect. Immun.* **3,** 24–35.

Casillo, S., and Blackmore, D. K. (1972). *J. Comp. Pathol.* **82,** 477–482.

Cassell, G. H., and Davis, J. K. (1978). *Infect. Immun.* **21,** 69–75.

Cassell, G. H., and McGhee, J. R. (1975). *RES, J. Reticuloendothel. Soc.* **18,** B42.

Cassell, G. H., Hiramoto, R. N., Lindsey, J. R., and Baker, H. J. (1971). *Bacteriol. Proc.* p. 78.

Cassell, G. H., Lindsey, J. R., and Broderson, J. R. (1973a). *Abstr. Annu. Meet. Am. Soc. Microbiol., Washington, D. C.* p. 93.

Cassell, G. H., Lindsey, J. R., Overcash, R. G., and Baker, H. J. (1973b). *Ann. N.Y. Acad. Sci.* **225,** 395–412.

Cassell, G. H., Lindsey, J. R., and Baker, H. J. (1974). *J. Immunol.* **115,** 1662–1664.

Cassell, G. H., Carter, P. B., and Silvers, S. H. (1976). *Proc. Soc. Gen. Microbiol.* **3,** 150.

Cassell, G. H., Carter, P. B., and Silvers, S. H. (1978a). Submitted for publication.

Cassell, G. H., Davis, J. K., and McGhee, J. R. (1978b). Submitted for publication.

Cassell, G. H., Davis, J. K., Wilborn, W. M., and Wise, K. S. (1978c). *In* "Microbiology—1978" (D. Schlessinger, ed.). pp. 399–403. Am. Soc. Microbiol., Washington, D. C.

Cassell, G. H., Lindsey, J. R., and Baker, H. J. (1979). *In* "The Laboratory Rat" (H. J. Baker, J. R. Lindsey, and S. H. Weisbroth, eds.), Vol. I. Academic Press, New York. In press.

Cole, B. C., and Ward, J. R. (1973a). *Infect. Immun.* **7,** 416–425.

Cole, B. C., and Ward, J. R. (1973b). *Infect. Immun.* **7,** 691–699.

Cole, B. C., and Ward, J. R. (1973c). *Infect. Immun.* **8,** 199–207.

Cole, B. C., Miller, M. L., and Ward, J. R. (1967). *Proc. Soc. Exp. Biol. Med.* **124,** 103–107.

Cole, B. C., Ward, J. R., and Martin, C. H. (1968). *J. Bacteriol.* **95**, 2022–2030.

Cole, B. C., Cahill, J. F., Wiley, B. B., and Ward, J. R. (1969). *J. Bacteriol.* **98**, 930–937.

Cole, B. C., Golightly-Rowland, L., Ward, J. R., and Wiley, B. B. (1970). *Infect. Immun.* **2**, 419–425.

Cole, B. C., Ward, J. R., Golightly-Rowland, L., and Trapp, G. A. (1971a). *Infect. Immun.* **4**, 431–440.

Cole, B. C., Ward, J. R., Jones, R. S., and Cahill, J. F. (1971b). *Infect. Immun.* **4**, 344–355.

Cole, B. C., Ward, J. R., and Golightly-Rowland, L. (1973). *Infect. Immun.* **7**, 218–255.

Cole, B. C., Golightly-Rowland, L., and Ward, J. R. (1975a). *Infect. Immun.* **11**, 1159–1161.

Cole, B. C., Golightly-Rowland, L., and Ward, J. R. (1975b). *Infect. Immun.* **12**, 1083–1092.

Cole, B. C., Overhall, J. C., Lombardi, P. S., and Glasgow, L. A. (1975c). *Infect. Immun.* **12**, 1349–1354.

Cole, B. C., Overall, J. C., Lombardi, P. S., and Glasgow, L. A. (1976). *Infect. Immun.* **14**, 88–94.

Cole, B. C., Griffiths, M. M., Eichwald, E. J., and Ward, J. R. (1977). *Infect. Immun.* **16**, 382–396.

Collier, A. M., and Clyde, W. A. (1971). *Infect. Immun.* **3**, 694–701.

Collier, W. A. (1939). *J. Pathol. Bacteriol.* **48**, 579–589.

Copperman, R., and Morton, H. E. (1966). *Proc. Soc. Exp. Biol. Med.* **123**, 790–795.

Cotchin, E., and Roe, F. J. (eds.) (1967). "Pathology of Laboratory Rats and Mice," pp. 373–383. Davis, Philadelphia, Pennsylvania.

Davis, J. K., and Cassell, G. H. (1978). In preparation.

Deeb, B. J., and Kenny, G. E. (1967a). *J. Bacteriol.* **93**, 1416–1424.

Deeb, B. J., and Kenny, G. E. (1967b). *J. Bacteriol.* **93**, 1425–1429.

Denny, F. W., Taylor-Robinson, D., and Allison, A. C. (1972). *J. Med. Microbiol.* **5**, 327–336.

Domermuth, C. H., Nielsen, M. H., Freundt, E. A., and Birch-Anderson, A. (1964). *J. Bacteriol.* **88**, 727–744.

Edward, D. G. ff. (1950). *J. Gen. Microbiol.* **4**, 4–15.

Edward, D. G. ff., and Freundt, E. A. (1956). *J. Gen. Microbiol.* **14**, 197–207.

Edward, D. G. ff., and Freundt, E. A. (1965). *J. Gen. Microbiol.* **41**, 263–265.

Edwards, G. A., and Fogh, J. (1960). *J. Bacteriol.* **79**, 267–276.

Eng, J. (1971). *Acta Pathol. Microbiol. Scand.* **79**, 759–763.

Fallon, R. J., and Jackson, D. K. (1967). *Lab. Anim.* **1**, 55–64.

Fenner, F., McAuslan, B. R., Mims, C. A., Sambrook, J., and White, D. O. (1974). "The Biology of Animal Viruses," 2nd Ed., pp. 618–640. Academic Press, New York.

Findlay, G. M., Klieneberger, E., MacCallum, F. O., and MacKenzie, R. D. (1938). *Lancet* **ii**, 1511–1513.

Findlay, G. M., MacKenzie, R. D., MacCallum, F. O., and Kleineberger, E. (1939). *Lancet* **ii**, 7–10.

Forshaw, K. A. (1972). *J. Gen. Microbiol.* **72**, 493–499.

Forshaw, K. A., and Fallon, R. J. (1972). *J. Gen. Microbiol.* **72**, 501–510.

Fraser, L. R., and Taylor-Robinson, D. (1977). *Fertil. Steril.* **28**, 488–498.

Freudenberger, C. B. (1932a). *Am. J. Anat.* **50**, 293–349.

Freudenberger, C. B. (1932b). *Anat. Rec.* **54**, 179–184.

Freundt, E. A. (1974). *In* "Bergey's Manual of Determininative Bacteriology," 8th Ed., pp. 350–382. Williams & Wilkins, Baltimore, Maryland.

Gabridge, M. G., Barden-Stahl, Y. D., Polisky, R. B., and Engelhardt, J. A. (1977). *Infect. Immun.* **16**, 766–772

Ganaway, J. R., and Allen, A. M. (1969). *Lab. Anim. Care* **19,** 71–79.
Ganaway, J. R., Allen, A. M., Moore, T. D., and Bohner, H. J. (1973). *J. Infect. Dis.* **127,** 529–537.
Gay, F. W., Maguire, M. E., and Bakerville, A. (1972). *Infect. Immun.* **6,** 83–91.
Giddens, W. E., Whitehair, C. K., and Carter, G. R. (1971a). *Am. J. Vet. Res.* **32,** 99–114.
Giddens, W. E., Whitehair, C. K., and Carter, G. R. (1971b). *Am. J. Vet. Res.* **32,** 115–129.
Ginsburg, H., and Nicolet, J. (1973). *Nature (London), New Biol.* **246,** 143–146.
Goeth, H., and Appel, K. R. (1974). *Zentralbl. Bakteriol., Parasitenkd., Infektionskr. Hyg., Abt. 1: Orig., Reihe A* **228,** 282–289.
Goldstein, E., and Green, G. M. (1967). *J. Bacteriol.* **93,** 1651–1656.
Golightly-Rowland, L., Cole, B. C., Ward, J. R., and Wiley, B. B. (1970). *Infect. Immun.* **1,** 538–545.
Gourlay, R. N., and Wyld, S. (1976). *Proc. Soc. Gen. Microbiol.* **3,** 142.
Gourlay, R. N., Wyld, S. G., and Taylor-Robinson, D. (1976). *Nature (London)* **259,** 120–123.
Gourlay, R. N., Wyld, S. G., and Leach, R. H. (1977). *Int. J. Syst. Bacteriol.* **27,** 86–96.
Graham, W. R. (1963). *Lab. Anim. Care* **13,** 719–724.
Haberman, R. T., Williams, F. P., McPherson, C. W., and Every, R. R. (1963). *Lab. Anim. Care* **13,** 28–40.
Haller, G. J., Boiarski, K. W., and Somerson, N. L. (1973). *J. Infect. Dis.* **127,** Suppl., 38–42.
Hannan, P. C. (1971). *J. Gen. Microbiol.* **67,** 363–365.
Hannan, P. C. (1976). *Proc. Soc. Gen. Microbiol.* **3,** 147.
Harwick, H. J., Kalmanson, G. M., Fox, M. A., and Guze, L. B. (1973a). *J. Infect. Dis.* **128,** 533–540.
Harwick, H. J., Kalmanson, G. M., Fox, M. A., and Guze, L. B. (1973b). *Proc. Soc. Exp. Biol. Med.* **144,** 561–563.
Hershberger, L. G., Hansen, L. M., and Calhoun, P. W. (1960). *Arthritis Rheum.* **3,** 387–394.
Hill, A. (1971). *J. Gen. Microbiol.* **65,** 109–113.
Hill, A. (1973). "Some aspects of Mycoplasma." I.M.L.S. Thesis, pp. 64–68.
Hill, A. (1974a). *Colloq. INSERM, Mycoplasmes Homme, Anim., Veg. Insectes, Congr. Int., Bordeaux* **33,** 311–315.
Hill, A. (1974b). *Lab. Anim.* **8,** 305–310.
Hill, A. (1974c). *Vet. Rec.* **94,** 385.
Hill, A. (1976). *Proc. Soc. Gen. Microbiol.* **3,** 174.
Hill, A. (1978). *J. Infect. Dis.* **137,** 152–154.
Hill, A., and Dagnall, G. J. R. (1975). *J. Comp. Pathol.* **85,** 45–52.
Horowitz, S. A., and Cassell, G. H. (1978). *Infect. Immun.* **22,** 161–70.
Howell, E. V., and Jones, R. S. (1963). *Proc. Soc. Exp. Biol. Med.* **112,** 69–72.
Hu, P. C., Collier, A. M., and Baseman, J. B. (1975). *Infect. Immun.* **11,** 704–710.
Hudson, J. R., Buttery, S. G., and Cottew, G. S. (1967). *J. Pathol. Bacteriol.* **94,** 257–273.
Hummeler, K., Armstrong, D., and Tomassini, N. (1965a). *J. Bacteriol.* **90,** 511–516.
Hummeler, K., Tomassini, N., and Hayflick, L. (1965b). *J. Bacteriol.* **90,** 517–523.
Innes, J. R. M., McAdams, A. J., and Yevich, P. (1956). *Am. J. Pathol.* **32,** 141–160.
Ito, S., Imaizumi, K., Tajima, Y., Endo, M., and Koyama, R. (1957). *Jpn. J. Exp. Med.* **27,** 243–248.
Jansson, E., and Wager, O. (1967). *Ann. N.Y. Acad. Sci.* **143,** 535–543.
Jansson, E., Makisara, P., Vainio, K., Vainio, V., Snellman, O., and Tuuri, S. (1971). *Ann. Rheum. Dis.* **30,** 506–508.
Jersey, G. C., Whitehair, C. K., and Carter, G. R. (1973). *J. Am. Vet. Med. Assoc.* **163,** 599–604.

Jones, T. C., and Hirsch, J. G. (1971). *J. Exp. Med.* **133,** 231–259.

Jones, T. C., and Yang, L. (1977). *Am. J. Pathol.* **87,** 331–346.

Jones, T. C., Yeh, S., and Hirsch, J. G. (1973). *Proc. Soc. Exp. Biol. Med.* **139,** 464–470.

Jouanneau, M., Brouilhet, H., Kahan, A., Charles, A., and Delbarre, F. (1973). *Biomedicine* **19,** 156–159.

Juhr, von N. C. (1971a). *Z. Versuchstierkd.* **13,** S210–216.

Juhr, von N. C. (1971b). *Z. Versuchstierkd.* **13,** S217–223.

Juhr, von N. C. and Obi, S. (1970). *Z. Versuchstierkd.* **12,** 383–387.

Juhr, von N. C., Obi, S., Hiller, H. H., and Eichberg, J. (1970). *Z. Versuchstierkd.* **12,** 318–320.

Kahan, A., Amor, B., and Delbarre, F. (1964). *C. R. Soc. Biol.* **158,** 1470–1473.

Kaklamanis, E., and Pavlatos, M. (1972). *Immunology* **22,** 695–702.

Kaklamanis, E., and Thomas, L. (1970). *In* "Microbial Toxins" (T. C. Montie, S. Kadis, and S. J. Ajl, eds.), Vol. 3, pp. 493–505. Academic Press, New York.

Kaklamanis, E., Thomas, L., Stavropoulos, I., and Boshwitz, C. (1969). *Nature (London)* **221,** 860–862.

Kappel, H. K., Nelson, J. B., and Weisbroth, S. (1974). *Lab. Anim. Sci.* **24,** 768–772.

Katoch, R. C., and Chandiramani, N. K. (1975). *Indian J. Vet. Sci. Anim. Husb.* **52,** 850–852.

Kenny, G. E. (1971). *Infect. Immun.* **4,** 149–151.

Klein, G. (1977). *Fortschr. Med.* **95,** 408–412.

Klein, G., and Wottawa, A. (1975). *Stud. Biophys.* **50,** S27–S31.

Klieneberger, E. (1938). *J. Hyg.* **38,** 458–476.

Klieneberger, E. (1940). *J. Hyg.* **40,** 204–222.

Klieneberger-Nobel, E. (1962). "Mycoplasmataceae," pp. 13–15. Academic Press, New York.

Klieneberger, E., and Steabben, D. B. (1937). *J. Hyg.* **37,** 143–152.

Kohn, D. F. (1971a). *Lab. Anim. Sci.* **21,** 849–855.

Kohn, D. F. (1971b). *Lab. Anim. Sci.* **21,** 856–861.

Kohn, D. F., and Kirk, B. E. (1969). *Lab. Anim. Care* **19,** 321–330.

Kohn, D. F., Kirk, B. E., and Chov. S. M. (1977). *Infect. Immun.* **16,** 680–689.

Kunishi, M. (1974). *Jpn. J. Opthalmol.* **18,** 150–160.

Laber, G., Schütze, E., Teherani, D. K., Tuschl, H., and Altmann, H. (1974). *Stud. Biophys.* **50,** S21–S26.

Lane-Petter, W. (1970). *Lab. Anim.* **4,** 125–134.

Leach, R. H. (1973). *J. Gen. Microbiol.* **75,** 135–153.

Leach, R. H., and Butler, M. (1966). *J. Bacteriol.* **91,** 934–941.

Leader, R. W., Leader, I., and Witschi, E. (1970). *J. Am. Vet. Med. Assoc.* **157,** 1923–1925.

Lemcke, R. M. (1961). *J. Hyg.* **59,** 401–412.

Lemcke, R. M. (1964). *J. Hyg.* **62,** 199–219.

Lindsey, J. R., and Cassell, G. H. (1973). *Am. J. Pathol.* **72,** 63–90.

Lindsey, J. R. and Conner, M. W. (1978). In preparation.

Lindsey, J. R., Baker, H. J., Overcash, R. G., Cassell, G. H., and Hunt, C. E. (1971). *Am. J. Pathol.* **64,** 675–716.

Lindsey, J. R., Cassell, G. H., and Baker, H. J. (1978). *In* "Pathology of Laboratory Animals" (K. Benirschke, F. M. Garner, and T. C. Jones, eds.), Chap. 15. Springer-Verlag, New York. pp. 1481–1550.

Liu, C., Jayanetra, P., and Voth, D. W. (1970). *Ann. N.Y. Acad. Sci.* **174,** 828–834.

Lutsky, I. I., and Organick, A. B. (1966). *J. Bacteriol.* **92,** 1154–1163.

MacLennan, I. C. M. (1972). *Transplant. Rev.* **13,** 67–90.

Manchee, R. J., and Taylor-Robinson, D. (1969). *J. Bacteriol.* **98,** 914–919.

Mårdh, P. A., and Taylor-Robinson, (1973). *Med. Microbiol. Immunol.* **158,** 219–226.

Mardh, P. A., Skude, G., Akerman, M. and Ursing, B. (1974). *Colloq. INSERM, Mycoplasmes Homme Anim., Veg. Insectes, Congr. Inst., Bordeaux* **33**, 403–410.

Mielens, Z. E., and Rozitis, J. (1964). *Proc. Soc. Exp. Biol. Med.* **117**, 751–754.

Miller, C. E., Wong, K. H., Feeley, J. C., and Forbines, M. E. (1972). *Infect. Immun.* **6**, 739–742.

Morton, H. E., Lecce, J. G., Oskay, J. J., and Coy, N. H. (1954). *J. Bacteriol.* **68**, 697–717.

Morton, H. E., Copperman, R., and Lam, G. T. (1968). *J. Bacteriol.* **95**, 2418–2419.

Nakane, P. K., and Kawaoi, A. (1974). *J. Histochem. Cytochem.* **22**, 1084–1091.

Naot, Y., Tully, J. G., and Ginsburg, H. (1977). *Infect. Immun.* **18**, 310–317.

Nelson, J. B. (1937). *J. Exp. Med.* **65**, 833–860.

Nelson, J. B. (1950a). *J. Exp. Med.* **91**, 309–320.

Nelson, J. B. (1950b). *J. Exp. Med.* **92**, 431–439.

Nelson, J. B. (1954). *J. Exp. Med.* **100**, 311–320.

Nelson, J. B. (1960). *Ann. N.Y. Acad. Sci.* **79**, 450–457.

Nelson, J. B., and Collins, G. R. (1961). *Proc. Anim. Care Panel* **11**, 65–72.

Nelson, J. B., and Gowen, J. W. (1931). *J. Exp. Med.* **54**, 629–636.

Ogata, M., Ohta, T., and Atobe, H. (1967). *Nippon Saikingaku Zasshi* **22**, 618–627.

Organick, A. B., and Lutsky, I. I. (1976). *Lab. Anim. Sci.* **26**, 419–429.

Organick, A. B., Siegesmund, K. A., and Lutsky, I. I. (1966). *J. Bacteriol.* **92**, 1164–1176.

Pachas, W. N. (1970). *Ann. N.Y. Acad. Sci.* **174**, 786–793.

Parkes, M. W., and Wrigley, F. (1951). *Ann. Rheum. Dis.* **10**, 177.

Plackett, P. (1957). *Biochim. Biophys. Acta* **26**, 664–665.

Polak-Vogelzang, A. A., and Hagenaars, R. (1976). *Proc. Soc. Gen. Microbiol.* **3**, 151.

Preston, W. S. (1942). *J. Infect. Dis.* **70**, 180–184.

Razin, S., and Rottem, S. (1967). *J. Bacteriol.* **94**, 1807–1810.

Razin, S., Knyszynski, A., and Lifshitz, Y. (1964). *J. Gen. Microbiol.* **36**, 323–332.

Razin, S., Rottem, S., Hasin, M., and Gershfeld, N. (1973). *Ann. N.Y. Acad. Sci.* **225**, 28–37.

Richter, C. B. (1970). *In* "Morphology of Experimental Respiratory Carcinogenesis" (P. Nettesheim, M. G. Hanna, and J. W. Deatherage, eds.), USAEC Symposium Series No. 21, pp. 365–382. USAEC, Oak Ridge, Tennessee.

Rigby, C., and Langford, E. V. (1976). *J. Appl. Bacteriol.* **41**, 215–221.

Rinaldo, C. R., Cole, B. C., Overall, J. C., and Glasgow, L. A. (1974). *Infect. Immun.* **10**, 1296–1301.

Robinet, H. G. (1962). *J. Bacteriol.* **84**, 896–901.

Rosendal, S., and Thomsen, A. C. (1974). *Acta Pathol. Microbiol. Scand.* **82**, 895–898.

Rudzik, O., Clancy, R. L., Perey, D. Y. E., Bienenstock, J., and Singal, D. P. (1975). *J. Immunol.* **114**, 1–4.

Russell, W. C. (1966). *Nature (London)* **212**, 1537–1540.

Sabin, A. B. (1938a). *Science* **88**, 189–191.

Sabin, A. B. (1938b). *Science* **88**, 575–576.

Schiefer, H. G., Gerhardt, U., Brunner, H., and Krüpe, M. (1974). *J. Bacteriol.* **120**, 81–88.

Sherwin, R. P., Yven, T. G. H., and Richters, V. (1973). *Am. J. Clin. Pathol.* **60**, 268–280.

Simberkoff, M. S., Thorbecke, J., and Thomas, L. (1969). *J. Exp. Med.* **129**, 1163–1181.

Sobeslavsky, O., Prescott, B., and Chanock, R. M. (1968). *J. Bacteriol.* **96**, 695–705.

Sokoloff, L. (1965). *In* "The Pathology of Laboratory Animals" (W. E. Ribelin and J. R. McCoy, eds.), pp. 3–20. Thomas, Springfield, Illinois.

Sokoloff, L. (1967). *Adv. Vet. Sci. Comp. Med.* **6**, 197–203.

Somerson, N. L., Reich, P. R., Chanock, R. M., and Weissman, S. M. (1967). *Ann. N.Y. Acad. Sci.* **143**, 9–20.

Stalheim, O. H. V., and Matthews, P. J. (1975). *Lab. Anim. Sci.* **25**, 70–73.

Stewart, D. D., and Buck, G. E. (1975). *Lab. Anim. Sci.* **25**, 769–773.

Stone, S. S., Masiga, G., and Read, W. C. S. (1969). *Res. Vet. Sci.* **10**, 368–372.
Subcommittee on the Taxonomy of Mycoplasmatales (1972). *Int. J. Syst. Bacteriol.* **22**, 184–188.
Tan, R. J. S., Davey, G. P., and Smith, J. M. B. (1971). *Res. Vet. Sci.* **12**, 390–391.
Taylor, G., and Taylor-Robinson, D. (1974). *Colloq. INSERM. Mycoplasmes Homme, Anim., Veg. Insectes, Congr. Int., Bordeaux* **33**, 331–340.
Taylor, G., and Taylor-Robinson, D. (1975). *Dev. Biol. Stand.* **28**, 195–210.
Taylor, G., and Taylor-Robinson, D. (1976). *Immunology* **30**, 611–618.
Taylor, G., and Taylor-Robinson, D. (1977). *Ann. Rheum. Dis.* **36**, 232–238.
Taylor, G., Taylor-Robinson, D., and Slavin, G. (1974). *Ann. Rheum. Dis.* **33**, 376–384.
Taylor, G., Howard, C. J., and Gourlay, R. N. (1977). *Infect. Immun.* **16**, 422–431.
Taylor-Robinson, D., Denny, F. W., Thompson, G. W., Allison, A. C., and Mårdh, P. A. (1972). *Med. Microbiol. Immunol.* **158**, 9–15.
Taylor-Robinson, D., Rassner, C., Furr, P. M., Humber, D. P., and Barnes, R. D. (1975). *J. Reprod. Fertil.* **42**, 483–490.
Thomas, L. (1969). *Harvey Lect.* **63**, 73–98.
Thomas, L., and Bitensky, M. W. (1966). *J. Exp. Med.* **124**, 1089–1098.
Thomsen, A. C., Rosendal, S., and Thomsen, O. F. (1973). *Acta Pathol. Microbiol. Scand.* **81**, 379–380.
Tram, C., and Guillon, J. C. (1970). *C. R. Soc. Biol.* **164**, 2470–2471.
Tully, J. G. (1965). *J. Infect. Dis.* **115**, 171–185.
Tully, J. G. (1969). *In* "The Mycoplasmatales and the L-Phase of Bacteria" (L. Hayflick, ed.), pp. 581–583. North-Holland Publ., Amsterdam.
Tully, J. G. (1974). *Colloq. INSERM, Mycoplasmes Homme, Anim., Veg. Insectes, Congr. Int., Bordeaux* **33**, 317–324.
Tully, J. G., and Rask-Nielsen, R. (1967). *Ann. N.Y. Acad. Sci.* **143**, 345–352.
Vincze, S., Klein, G., and Altman, H. (1975). *Z. Rheumaforsch.* **34**, 49–54.
Vitullo, B. B., O'Regan, S., Chadarevian, J. P., and Kaplan, B. S. (1977). *Pediatr. Res.* **11**, 559.
Vogelzang, A. A. (1975). *Z. Versuchstierkd.* **17**, 240–246.
Ward, J. R., and Cole, B. C. (1970). *In* "The Role of Mycoplasmas and L Forms of Bacteria in Disease" (J. T. Sharp, ed.), pp 212–239. Thomas, Springfield, Illinois.
Ward, J. R., and Jones, R. S. (1962). *Arthritis Rheum.* **5**, 163–175.
Warren, J. (1942). *J. Bacteriol.* **43**, 211–228.
Westerberg, S. C., Smith, C. B., Wiley, B. B., and Jensen, C. (1972). *Infect. Immun.* **5**, 840–846.
Whittlestone, P. (1974). *Colloq. INSERM, Mycoplasmes Homme, Anim., Veg. Insectes, Congr. Int., Bordeaux* **33**, 143–151.
Whittlestone, P. (1976). *Adv. Vet. Sci. Comp. Med.* **20**, 277–304.
Whittlestone, P., Lemcke, R. M., and Olds, R. J. (1972). *J. Hyg.* **70**, 387–407.
Wilborn, W. H., and Cassell, G. H. In preparation.
Wise, K. S., Cassell, G. H., and Acton, R. T. (1978). *Proc. Natl. Acad. Sci. U.S.A.* **75**, 4479–4483.
Woglom, W. H., and Warren, J. (1938a). *Science* **87**, 370–371.
Woglom, W. H., and Warren, J. (1938b). *J. Exp. Med.* **68**, 513–528.
Woglom, W. H., and Warren, J. (1939). *J. Hyg.* **39**, 266–267.
Woolcock, P. R., Czekalowski, J. W., and Hall, D. A. (1973). *J. Gen. Microbiol.* **78**, 23–32.
Wright, O. N. (1967). *J. Bacteriol.* **93**, 185–190.
Young, C., and Hill, A. (1974). *Lab. Anim.* **8**, 301–304.
Zucker-Franklin, D., Davidson, M., and Thomas, L. (1966). *J. Exp. Med.* **124**, 533–542.

9 / *Mycoplasma pneumoniae* INFECTIONS OF MAN

Wallace A. Clyde, Jr.

I. INTRODUCTION

Most of the more than 60 named *Mycoplasma* species are pathogenic, producing natural diseases in a variety of mammalian, avian, insect, and

THE MYCOPLASMAS, VOL. II

plant hosts. The mycoplasmas indigenous to humans include eight species belonging to two genera (*Mycoplasma pneumoniae, M. orale, M. buccale, M. faucium, M. salivarium, M. fermentans, M. hominis*, and *Ureaplasma urealyticum*); others isolated rarely are *M. lipophilum, M. primatum*, and *Acholeplasma laidlawii*. In contrast to the situation in nonhuman hosts, most of the species isolated from humans appear to be members of the autochthonous microflora colonizing mucous membranes. While pathogenic relationships have been demonstrated for *M. hominis, M. primatum*, and *U. urealyticum*, Koch's postulates have been fulfilled only in the case of *M. pneumoniae* at the present time. It is appropriate, therefore, within the context of this volume that specific attention be given to the features of *M. pneumoniae* disease of humans. Included is information concerning epidemiology, disease characteristics, diagnosis, therapy, and prevention.

History

1. The Disease

The type of pneumonia produced by *M. pneumoniae* was recognized as a clinical entity long before the etiology and nature of the causative organism were established (Reimann, 1938; Gallagher, 1941). When therapy with the sulfonamide group of antimicrobial agents was introduced over four decades ago, and later penicillin, it became apparent that certain cases of pneumonia did not respond dramatically to this treatment as did infections caused by *Streptococcus pneumoniae*. These infections were thus atypical and, having no known exogenous etiological factor, were considered a primary form of lung disease. While the phrase "primary atypical pneumonia" (PAP) was a misnomer in terms of information to be developed subsequently, it provided a basis for classification of pneumonia cases and denoted the recognition of a new clinical syndrome. Generally victims of PAP were healthy children and young adults who experienced a relatively mild form of pneumonitis which was self-limited and rarely fatal. Further definition of this syndrome was made possible by discovery of the cold hemagglutination serological reaction in 1943 (Peterson *et al.*, 1943) and by the advances in diagnosis of viral and rickettsial diseases which have occurred in more recent years.

The fact that PAP had an infectious etiology was established by the pioneering work of Eaton in the early 1940s (Eaton *et al.*, 1944). It was demonstrated that the intranasal inoculation of cotton rats and hamsters with sputum samples from patients produced a form of nonsuppurative pneumonia in these animals. This property of sputum samples could be neutralized by mixing the specimens with patients' convalescent sera before animal inoculation. The additional features of filterability and resistance to certain antimicrobial agents suggested that Eaton's agent of PAP was a virus. An ironic historical note is provided by recovery of a mycoplasma in the course of efforts to propagate the agent in the amniotic cavity of embryonated hens' eggs (van Herick and Eaton, 1945). The mycoplasma was detected by its ability to agglutinate erythrocytes; it was recognized as being dissimilar to Eaton's agent and a contaminant of the eggs themselves, now known to be *Mycoplasma gallisepticum*. Meanwhile clinical studies using human volunteers were being conducted by the Commission on Acute Respiratory Diseases of the Armed Forces Epidemiological Board (1946). These experiments indicated that PAP associated with the development of cold hemagglutinins could be produced in men inoculated via the respiratory route with whole or filtered sputum from patients, but not with an autoclaved portion of the inoculum. Further developments were required before these volunteer experiments and findings of Eaton could be related to each other.

The first practical serological test for Eaton's agent was reported by Liu and co-workers (1959), and this provided an important tool for the rapid development of much new information. The technique was an application of indirect immunofluorescence in which frozen sections from the lungs of infected chicken embryos served as antigen. Upon reacting the lung sections with patients' convalescent sera followed by fluorescein-conjugated anti-human globulin, specific fluorescence could be found in the area of the chick bronchial epithelium. Dilution of the patients' sera to the point of fluorescence extinction provided an expression of antibody titer. Early use of this procedure in seroepidemiological surveys indicated the common nature of Eaton's agent infections in humans (Cook *et al.*, 1960). In addition, by retrospective study of sera preserved from the human volunteer experiments mentioned above it was possible to show that the agent was involved in this demonstration of the transmissibility of PAP (Clyde *et al.*, 1961).

2. The Organism

Further efforts to understand the nature of Eaton's agent began with electron microscopy of infected chick embryo lungs, but these studies were unsuccessful (Donald and Liu, 1959). In 1961, Marmion and Goodburn (1961) first suggested that the agent could be a mycoplasma by demonstrating extracellular, minute coccobacilli in chick bronchial epithelium using intensified Giemsa staining and by showing that this organism was susceptible to treatment with organic gold salts. Further support for this concept was developed by Clyde (1961), who applied indirect immunofluorescence and Giemsa staining to rhesus monkey kidney cell cultures inoculated with chick embryo-derived material. Granular extracellular clusters of minute coccal forms were demonstrated to develop on the cell monolayers, suggesting the appearance of microcolonies of a mycoplasma. Conclusive proof that Eaton's agent was a new *Mycoplasma* species was developed by Chanock *et al.* (1962a) when they succeeded in growing the organisms on artificial media for the first time. The indirect immunofluorescence technique of Liu was used again to show that the mycoplasma colonies seen were identical to Eaton's agent. Shortly thereafter experimental disease was produced in human volunteers inoculated with organisms isolated in the laboratory, thus fulfilling Koch's postulates (Chanock *et al.*, 1961b; Rifkind *et al.*, 1962). Subsequently the name *M. pneumoniae* was proposed for the organism, the nomenclature providing a parallel to that of the common bacterial cause of pneumonia, *S. pneumoniae* (Chanock *et al.*, 1963).

Ability to propagate *M. pneumoniae* in artificial media has greatly facilitated further study of its pathogenicity, to be detailed in Section III, and of its biological properties. It was demonstrated that the organism was hemolytic, an unusual feature among *Mycoplasma* species indigenous to humans (Clyde, 1963a; Somerson *et al.*, 1963); this property was shown to be due to peroxide formation by the mycoplasma (Somerson *et al.*, 1965). Many studies on the antigenicity of *M. pneumoniae* have followed the initial report that a major antigenic determinant was a lipid hapten (Kenny and Grayston, 1965). The fact that the organisms growing in broth fermented a variety of carbohydrates formed the basis for a new serological procedure (Taylor-Robinson *et al.*, 1966). An observation that the mycoplasma attached to and grew on culture vessel surfaces (Somerson *et al.*, 1967) facilitated concentration and purification of organisms for a variety of purposes. Observations of the mycoplasma on glass using phase microscopy and time-lapse cinephotomicrography have indicated that individual organisms are motile, and that they divide by binary fission (Bredt, 1968). It was found further that glass-attached organisms revealed an unusual ultrastructure in possessing a filamentous morphology and a differentiated organelle at one pole (Biberfeld and Biberfeld, 1970). This specialized organelle mediates attachment to host cell surfaces (Collier and Clyde, 1971), a process which involves neuraminic acid moieties on the cell surface (Sobeslavsky *et al.*, 1968). A recent detailed study comparing a fully virulent strain of *M. pneumoniae* with its avirulent derivative—which does not cytoadsorb—provided evidence that the attachment phenomenon was mediated by an actively produced surface protein (Hu *et al.*, 1977).

II. EPIDEMIOLOGY

A. Incidence

Mycoplasma pneumoniae appears to represent one of the more common etiological agents causing lower respiratory tract disease in humans. However, several longitudinal studies suggest that the incidence varies markedly from year to year. Data from a 5-year period of surveillance in Seattle, Washington, revealed that 20% of all pneumonia observed in a general population sample could be associated with *M. pneumoniae* infection (Foy *et al.*, 1970); actual attack rates during this interval varied from 1.2 to 3.0 per 1000 population per year. In a more rural setting represented by Chapel Hill, North Carolina, the rate of infections ranged from 1 to 5 per 1000 population per year, these studies being limited to subjects younger than 16 years of age (Glezen *et al.*, 1971). Serological data accumulated in the Netherlands over a 12-year period revealed that epidemic waves of infection tended to occur at approximately 4.5-year intervals; attack rates are not available for this population (Lind, 1971).

Restricted population groups demonstrating a high incidence of *M. pneumoniae* infections include young adults in university and military settings. At the University of North Carolina, Tulane University, and the University of Wisconsin, approximately half of pneumonia cases could be associated with *M. pneumoniae* infections. During years when *M. pneumoniae* was less prevalent a lower number of pneumonia cases was observed than during years of higher activity (Denny *et al.*, 1971). Studies conducted among the U.S. Armed Forces provide evidence that between 20 and 45% of pneumonia cases are related to mycoplasma infection (summarized in Denny *et al.*, 1971). These figures suggest that the morbidity due to *M. pneumoniae* infections in military populations approaches the magnitude of the recognized problem associated with adenovirus infections.

1. Geographic Factors

Mycoplasma pneumoniae infections probably occur throughout the world, as indicated by reports from countries in Europe, Asia, and North America. However, these studies concern settings in the temperate climate zones, and less information is available on the occurrence of disease in the extremes represented by the tropical and polar areas. A seroepidemiological study involving residents of Alaska and Brazil (Suhs and Feldman, 1966) revealed an incidence of antibodies against *M. pneumoniae* which equaled or exceeded that seen in Montgomery County,

Maryland (Cook *et al.*, 1960). These observations suggest that climate is not an important determinant in the occurrence of *M. pneumoniae* infections.

2. Seasonal Patterns

Reference to the longitudinal studies cited in Section II,A suggests that *M. pneumoniae* disease occurs throughout the year. As with most respiratory diseases there is a tendency for more cases to be seen during the colder months, which probably reflects greater opportunity for transmission among people in more restricted environments. Relative to other common causes of respiratory infections, *M. pneumoniae* has been noted to occur somewhat more frequently in the fall months, as reflected by observations particularly of students and of military personnel (Denny *et al.*, 1971).

3. Age and Sex Factors

One of the more puzzling determinants of *M. pneumoniae* disease is subject age. When a population base of sufficient size and normal distribution is examined, it can be seen that the peak occurrence of mycoplasma pneumonia is about age 10 years; clinical disease is uncommon below age 4 years and after age 50 years (Foy *et al.*, 1970). Despite this peculiar age restriction in the incidence of pneumonia, it has been established that infections occur in infants and young children, the implication being that subclinical disease is more characteristic of these age groups (Fernald *et al.*, 1975). This phenomenon provides a basis for speculations about the pathogenesis of *M. pneumoniae* disease which are presented in Section III,D. Available studies all show that the occurrence of *M. pneumoniae* disease is equal in both sexes.

B. Communicability

Epidemics of *M. pneumoniae* tend to follow a protracted course, which suggests that the degree of communicability is less than with the common respiratory viruses. Transmission from infected individuals to susceptible contacts is thought to occur by the airborne route, and disease has been produced experimentally by aerosol inoculation (Commission on Acute Respiratory Diseases, 1946; Chanock *et al.*, 1961b; Rifkind *et al.*, 1962). The mycoplasma can be isolated from the nose, throat, trachea, and sputum of patients, indicating diffuse involvement of the respiratory mucosa. This extensive parasitism coupled with the persistent cough characteristic of the disease implies that infected secretions are the vehicle of spread. Organisms are present in sputum in large numbers but tend to associate with desquamated cells or cell fragments (Collier and Clyde, 1974); thus, relatively large droplets may be required for transmission. This concept is supported by evidence that epidemic settings generally involve the type of close personal contact present in families, schools, and institutions.

In one study of military personnel, the proximity of bunks was directly proportional to the degree of spread (Steinberg *et al.*, 1969a). During a 12 to 14-week period of basic training, over 40% of recruits showed evidence of seroconversion to *M. pneumoniae*; included were about one-fourth of men who had preexisting antibody, suggesting that reinfections are not uncommon. Steinberg and co-workers also note that the barracks area nearest the shower facilities was the site of the highest level of transmission. It has been demonstrated experimentally that survival of airborne *M. pneumoniae* is a function of both temperature and relative humidity (Wright *et al.*, 1969), optimal conditions being 15°C and 75–85%, respectively.

Several studies conducted in families suggest that the presence of susceptible children is an important element in the transmission of *M. pneumoniae*. When an index case occurred in the home, 84% of children and 41% of adults became infected, according to a survey conducted in Seattle (Foy *et al.*, 1966); similarly high levels of spread were demonstrated in a study in Stockholm (Biberfeld and Sterner, 1969). The manifestations of infection varied widely among household contacts, a factor which should be appreciated in interpreting epidemiological studies based only on clinical classification of illnesses. Foy's data reveal that among 59 infected family members, 42 had lower respiratory tract symptoms, 6 had only pharyngitis, and 9 were entirely asymptomatic. Of interest relative to the age-related incidence cited in Section II,A,3, all the asymptomatic individuals were children. Most of the subjects evaluated in this prospective study were not sufficiently ill to seek medical attention, thus the attack rate of frank pneumonia cannot be determined. In a study of Marine recruits, it was estimated that only 1 infection in 30 presented as clinically apparent pneumonia (Chanock *et al.*, 1961a). However, it has been documented that radiographically demonstrable infiltrates can occur in asymptomatic subjects as well as in those with lower respiratory tract symptoms and signs (Foy *et al.*, 1966; Clyde and Denny, 1967).

III. DISEASE CHARACTERISTICS

The development of culture techniques and specific serological measures for *M. pneumoniae* has allowed much progress in recent years toward a complete understanding of the disease spectrum produced by this organism. Availability of simple diagnostic methods has permitted the large-scale prospective clinical and epidemiological studies necessary to detect inapparent infections and document patterns of transmission. The following section provides a summary of information which has accrued, relates this to data concerning the biology of the causative organism, and highlights areas where unresolved questions remain.

A. Clinical Features

Disease produced by *M. pneumoniae* is generally mild, self-limited, and not accompanied by frequent complications or known long-term sequelae. Based on evidence cited in Section II,B, it can be estimated that approximately half of the infections occurring in adults are completely asymptomatic, probably reflecting some degree of protective immunity. If children also are considered, however, the rate of symptomatic disease following infection climbs to 80% (Foy *et al.*, 1966). The onset of symptoms is usually insidious, following a relatively long incubation period. From studies using human volunteers, initial symptoms began approximately 2 weeks following inoculation (Commission on Acute Respiratory Diseases, 1946; Chanock *et al.*, 1961b). The more natural situation created by the spread of infection within families was characterized by case-to-case intervals averaging between 3 and 4 weeks (Foy *et al.*, 1966). From this point, the clinical expression of disease may follow several patterns.

The most common manifestation of *M. pneumoniae* disease is cough, which can vary from a mild degree to a severe pertussis-like syndrome. Low-grade fever is usually present and together with the cough frequently leads to a clinical diagnosis of nonspecific respiratory illness or acute tracheobronchitis. General symptoms include malaise and headache which often is aggravated by the persistent coughing. Headache may be ascribed in part to the occurrence of sinusitis which has been reported to accompany two-thirds of pneumonia cases (Griffin and Klein, 1971). Many patients complain of having a dry or scratchy throat; at times, only pharyngitis is noted as the clinical evidence of infection (Foy *et al.*, 1966); Glezen *et al.*, 1967).

Many clinical studies report the occurrence of pneumonic infiltrates demonstrable by chest x-ray, which are accompanied by minimal or no physical findings. It is thus difficult to define the frequency with which pneumonia follows *M. pneumoniae* infection, since few studies have included serial x-rays taken on a prospective basis. When pneumonia is present, it is most often unilateral, involving one of the lower lobes. Physical findings include rhonchi, coarse rales, and at times expiratory wheezing. Since the alveoli are usually spared, fine rales and frank consolidation are uncommon; however, variable degrees of atelectasis are present frequently and if extensive produce typical signs of consolidation. Involvement of the pleura, manifested by pleuritic chest pain and signs of effusion, have been reported at times.

The changes described in chest examination are reflected in radiographic findings. Although it should be emphasized that x-ray changes are extremely variable and can mimic a wide variety of lung diseases, there are patterns which typify *M. pneumoniae* disease (George *et al.*, 1966; Foy *et al.*, 1973a). General features include unilateral involvement, perihilar infiltrates that are more dense centrally, and subsegmental areas of atelectasis. As indicated above, pleural effusions have been reported with variable frequency but are not commonly found in larger clinical series. When present, effusions tend to be small and transient.

The duration of clinical *M. pneumoniae* disease is variable and dependent upon the manner of presentation. In untreated patients with tracheobronchitis or pneumonia, the acute febrile phase lasts about 1 week, while cough, malaise, or lassitude may persist an average of two additional weeks. In appropriately treated patients it can be demonstrated that the duration of symptoms and signs is significantly shortened (Kingston *et al.*, 1961); there is a reduction in the progression of disease, as well as accelerated resolution of x-ray abnormalities (see Section V).

B. Complications and Sequelae

A wide range of unusual manifestations of *M. pneumoniae* disease has been described, generally in the form of single case reports or small selected clinical series. These complications involve portions of the respiratory tract and its extensions, in addition to several other organ systems. Sinusitis has been mentioned above, since the reported frequency of this pararespiratory tract involvement precludes consideration of it as a complication. Less common is the occurrence of otitis media in children (Sobeslavsky *et al.*, 1965). Another ear complication, bullous myringitis, was observed in volunteers experimentally infected with *M. pneumoniae* (Rifkind *et al.*, 1962) and has been described in natural disease as well.

Ludlam and co-workers (1964) were the first to suggest an association between *M. pneumoniae* infection and erythema multiforme exudativum (Stevens-Johnson syndrome), and subsequently many similar case studies have been published. It is of historical interest to note that one of the two children originally described by Stevens and Johnson (1922) had pneumonitis at the time of their skin and mucous membrane involvement. Since many other infectious diseases, medications, and the like have been implicated in erythema multiforme, it seems realistic to conclude that *M.*

pneumoniae is only one of many factors related to this syndrome. Less severe, nondescript skin rashes are reported in some studies (Foy *et al.*, 1966), which may pose diagnostic confusion for the clinician.

Central nervous system complications of several types have been reported to accompany some cases of proven *M. pneumoniae* infections, beginning with a publication by Skoldenberg (1965). Syndromes which have been described include psychosis, meningitis, meningoencephalitis, cerebellar ataxia, transverse myelitis, and Guillain-Barre polyradiculopathy. As in the case of skin disease associated with *M. pneumoniae* infections, these conditions are known to have many other causative factors, which leaves unanswered the question of the relative role the mycoplasma may play in this instance. Hemolytic anemia, which can be of subclinical degree, is the most frequently reported hematological complication of *M. pneumoniae* disease; other problems include coagulopathies and thromboembolic phenomena (reviewed in Purcell and Chanock, 1967). The heart is occasionally involved, as indicated by electrocardiographic changes and evidence of myocarditis and pericarditis (Grayston *et al.*, 1965); areas of focal necrosis of the myocardium and liver have been seen in autopsy material (see Section III,C). The occurrence of polyarthritis is another infrequent complication in some patients (Lambert, 1968).

The importance which can be attached to any of the complications that have been listed is difficult to assess with available data. In one large metropolitan study of pneumonia that included 462 cases of *M. pneumoniae* disease, the only complications noted were two instances of bullous myringitis (Foy *et al.*, 1970). It appears that, as in the uncomplicated disease, the various unusual manifestations are generally mild and self-limited. Similarly, the incidence of significant sequelae following *M. pneumoniae* disease remains to be clarified. While one would assume that sequelae are rare in relation to what has been reported about the natural history of the disease, one study has revealed that there may be long-term deficiencies in the pulmonary clearance mechanism following clinical recovery (Jarstrand *et al.*, 1974). Residual pleural abnormalities also have been described (Mufson *et al.*, 1963). The reports cited indicate that both physiological and anatomical disturbances can be produced by *M. pneumoniae* infections.

C. Pathology

In view of the benign course most *M. pneumoniae* cases follow, it is not surprising that limited information is available concerning pathological changes in the infected host. Since postmortem findings represent end-stage disease, it is difficult also to reconstruct sequential changes; further, several fatal cases which have been reported include features of complicating conditions unrelated to *M. pneumoniae* disease. The following discussion summarizes available knowledge in this area, but some information obtained using experimental models is included to supplement the human data.

The literature contains several reports of fatal *M. pneumoniae* disease, beginning with the series of Parker and co-workers (1947). The eight cases reported were collected on the basis of a cold hemagglutinin-positive atypical pneumonia syndrome, although specific etiological information could not be obtained at the time. Later, as discussed by Jordan and Dingle (1965), it was possible to show that an isolate obtained from preserved lung tissue from one case was identical to the original Mac strain of *M. pneumoniae,* also isolated from a fatal case by Eaton and co-workers (1944). Thus there is presumptive evidence that the other similar cases also were mycoplasma pneumonia. The lungs grossly were heavier than normal, showing areas of hemorrhage, congestion, and nodular focal lesions. Small amounts of straw-colored pleural fluid were seen occasionally. Thick exudates were seen within bronchi and bronchioles whose linings were inflamed and ulcerated. The microscopic picture included features of both interstitial pneumonitis and desquamative bronchitis and bronchiolitis. Infiltration of mononuclear cells was prominent in the peribronchial tissues, while the airways were filled with necrotic epithelial cells, mononuclear and polymorphonuclear cells, and fibrin. The involvement of alveoli was irregular and variable, with evidence suggesting this could be due to secondary bacterial invasion. Findings in other organ systems included hemorrhagic encephalitis, acute myocarditis, and focal hepatic necrosis; these changes are of some interest relative to the discussion of complications in Section III,B. The first report of a fatal case from which *M. pneumoniae* was isolated directly from the lung in artificial media is that of Maisel and co-workers (1967). The similarity of features in this case to those reported by Parker supports the relationship of the earlier series to *M. pneumoniae* infection. A report of three other cases, in which serological evidence of mycoplasma infection is provided, again stresses the occurrence of desquamative interstitial pneumonitis; encephalitis was the main clinical and pathological diagnosis in one case (Meyers and Hirschman, 1972). Another report concerns an elderly man who suffered a fatal illness resembling acute rheumatic fever accompanied by pericarditis and pleuropneumonia (Naftalin *et al.*, 1974). Postmortem findings included an endocardial vegetation, a mononuclear myocardial infiltrate, and patchy diaphragmatic necrosis adjacent to the pleural effusions; a thorough microbiological study revealed only *M. pneumoniae* from the heart blood and pericardial fluid.

Several experimental models of *M. pneumoniae* disease have been described, and some information is included in this discussion since it permits reconstruction of events which could produce the pathological changes in humans. The fact that the organism was first isolated in cotton rats, hamsters, and chicken embryos (Eaton *et al.*, 1944) suggested several model systems which could be exploited. Eaton described grossly evident patchy bronchopneumonia in the cotton rat inoculated with sputum or lung tissue from patients. This rat model served as an assay system for organism quantitation and serum neutralization studies. Infected chick embryos, while replicating *M. pneumoniae* on the bronchial mucosa, showed no pathological alterations and hatched normally if undisturbed (Liu, 1957). Use of the Syrian hamster as an experimental model was studied in detail by Dajani and co-workers (1965). Intranasal inoculation of the hamster leads to a sequence of events which closely parallels natural human *M. pneumoniae* pneumonia; there is no mortality nor evident clinical illness. Organisms replicate throughout the respiratory tract of the animal, reaching peak levels about 10–14 days after inoculation and persisting for 4–6 weeks. Pulmonary histopathological changes appear during the first week of infection, become maximal at 2 weeks, and disappear after the third week. Animals develop patchy bronchopneumonia which consists of peribronchial and peribronchiolar infiltration of lymphocytes and plasma cells. There is an exudate in involved airways, which includes a mixture of macrophages and polymorphonuclear leukocytes. Evidence has been developed that the pulmonary changes are the histological expression of the host immune response (see Fernald, this volume, Chapter 12). Young guinea pigs are susceptible also to *M. pneumoniae* infection (Brunner *et al.*, 1973a) and demonstrate a similar disease picture; in contrast to the hamster, guinea pigs have a longer period of respiratory tract colonization and experience some mortality.

D. Pathogenesis

Because of the limited information available on the pathology of natural disease, comments concerning the pathogenesis of *M. pneumoniae* disease are in part speculative or extrapolations from information developed using experimental models. The organism appears to be capable of establishing infection in a susceptible host because of its ability to attach to the surface membrane of ciliated epithelial cells. This has been demonstrated in human fetal trachea infected in organ culture (Collier and Clyde, 1971), as well as in inoculated hamsters and exfoliated cells from human sputum (Collier and Clyde, 1974). In this relationship to host cells the organisms are protected from the normal mucociliary clearance mechanism. There also is experimental evidence that—in the absence of opsonic antibody—

the mycoplasma can evade phagocytosis by alveolar macrophages (Powell and Clyde, 1975). From the position of an obligate extracellular parasite on the respiratory mucosa, it is not clearly understood how *M. pneumoniae* mediates the ensuing disease manifestations. Studies using organ cultures performed by Hu and co-workers (1975) indicate that parasitized epithelial cells show a reduction in glucose utilization, amino acid uptake, and macromolecular synthesis. Oxygen consumption by infected tracheal explants is reduced (Gabridge, 1975). These biochemical alterations are followed by reduction and loss of ciliary activity, histopathological changes, and finally exfoliation of all or part of the infected cell (Collier *et al.*, 1969; Collier and Clyde, 1971; Collier and Baseman, 1973). The mechanism of cell injury has not been defined. One suggestion is that it results from the action of peroxide generated by the mycoplasma (Cohen and Somerson, 1967). It has been reported that isolated *M. pneumoniae* membranes have a cytotoxic activity (Gabridge *et al.*, 1974), but this lacks confirmation by other workers (Hu *et al.*, 1977).

The success of *M. pneumoniae* as a pathogenic microorganism may be due in part to antigenic similarity between its glycerophospholipids and those of host tissues. Thus the related cold hemagglutinin response involves the host's erythrocyte I antigen (Feizi and Taylor-Robinson, 1967); many patients develop antibodies to normal lung tissue (Thomas *et al.*, 1943); and antibodies reactive with human brain and liver have been described (Biberfeld, 1970). This "biological mimicry" of *M. pneumoniae* could limit host immune responsiveness, and the possibility of suppressed antibody formation (Kaklamanis and Pavlatos, 1972) as well as nonspecific blastogenesis (Biberfeld and Gronowicz, 1976) might augment further evasion of host defenses by the parasite. Additional evidence of an immunosuppressive effect of infection is provided by the observation that patients with mycoplasma pneumonia have tuberculin anergy for weeks or months during and following the illness (Biberfeld and Sterner, 1976). Eventually of course an immune response is mounted; this event may be a substantial contribution to the expression of disease in humans, as hypothesized by Fernald and Clyde (1976).

Information of several kinds suggests the involvement of immunopathological phenomena as components of *M. pneumoniae* disease. In humans, the development of antibodies against various tissues has been cited above, and there is evidence that there are circulating immune complexes in serum during acute phases of the disease (Biberfeld and Norberg, 1974). The various complications of the disease described in Section III,B appear to be indirect effects of the organism. The rare reports of isolation of *M. pneumoniae* from nonrespiratory sites is counterbalanced by many attempts with negative results. Epidemiological data can be interpreted to show that repeated infections are required before symptomatic disease occurs, a possible explanation for the age-related incidence of illness (Fernald *et al.*, 1975). The possibility that prior experience with the organism may somehow "sensitize" the host for future infections is suggested by two experiences with inactivated *M. pneumoniae* vaccines. Smith and co-workers (1967) challenged human volunteers who had received prior injections of a vaccine preparation. Volunteers who had developed serum antibodies were protected from challenge infection, while those who had not appeared to have more severe disease than expected. Administration of a similar vaccine to a group of children resulted in the stimulation of circulating lymphocytes but no antibody formation, a type of immunological imbalance which may be detrimental rather than protective (Fernald and Glezen, 1973).

Experimentally, the pneumonic infiltrates of hamsters which mimic the human pathology have been shown to consist of immunoglobulin-producing mononuclear cells (Fernald *et al.*, 1972). This implies that a major component of the pathological picture in the lungs is the histological expression of host immune response. If animals are allowed to recover and are then reinfected, an exaggerated and accelerated pneumonic process is produced (Clyde, 1971a). Further evidence of an immunological basis for the pulmonary pathology is the observation that hamsters pretreated with antithymocyte sera show ablation of pneumonia (Taylor *et al.*, 1974); this is accompanied by no untoward effects of infection other than a slight increase in the numbers of organisms present in the lungs. While this suggests that the organisms per se are not injurious to the host, but rather the host's response to the mycoplasma, a somewhat different pattern is revealed by natural experiments. Four patients with immunodeficiency syndromes characterized by B-cell dysfunction were observed during *M. pneumoniae* infection (Foy *et al.*, 1973b). These patients failed to develop any radiographic evidence of pulmonary infiltration but were more severely ill than expected in regard to systemic symptomatology and persistence of cough. Patients with sickle cell disease (Schulman *et al.*, 1972) and possibly those with Down's syndrome (Baernstein *et al.*, 1965), who are known to have difficulty handling certain kinds of infections, appear to be more severely afflicted on contracting *M. pneumoniae* disease than the general population.

From the foregoing it can be concluded that both organism-related and host-related factors are involved in the pathogenesis of *M. pneumoniae* disease and its attendant complications. Pathogenic properties of the mycoplasma include its ability to attach to and injure respiratory mucosal cells, while evading phagocytosis and modulating the immune response. The host may be responsible in large measure for the appearance of pneumonia by mounting a local immunocyte and phagocytic response to the parasite. Immunopathological phenomena may be responsible for certain clinical manifestations, including the presence of circulating immune complexes (rashes, arthritis) and the formation of tissue-specific antibodies (hemolytic anemia, thrombopenia, myocarditis, hepatic necrosis, neuropathology). Clearly there is marked variability in host reaction, since only about half of patients develop cold hemagglutinins and complications are rare, even among individuals with antitissue globulins (Biberfeld, 1970). The clinical expression of disease may rest with contributing genetic, historical, or environmental factors yet to be defined.

IV. DIAGNOSIS

The presence of *M. pneumoniae* disease can be suspected when the epidemiological and clinical criteria described in Sections II and III are satisfied. Because of the frequency of this disease it should be considered in any case of pneumonia, particularly if older children, adolescents, and young adults are involved. The knowledge of coexisting cases of cold hemagglutinin-positive pneumonia in the community, institution, or family is contributory. Suggestive clinical features include a relatively mild disease in which symptomatology appears disproportionate to the paucity of physical findings. The diagnosis may be inappropriate in certain situations. These include pneumonia of infants and the elderly, and patients who present with isolated manifestations that are unusual features—such as pharyngitis, bullous myringitis, encephalitis, erythema multiforme, or arthritis—more commonly related to other etiological factors.

Both direct and indirect diagnostic methods are discussed in this section. These include consideration of isolation, serological, and rapid methods, as well as exclusion methods involved in differential diagnosis.

A. Isolation Methods

The use of cotton rats, hamsters, guinea pigs, cell cultures, and embryonated hens' eggs for the isolation of *M. pneumoniae* is feasible but largely of historic interest since the advent of suitable artificial media (Chanock *et al.*, 1962a). The formula originally described is still the mainstay of cultural methods, although several variations have been reported. A base of 7 parts beef heart infusion was supplemented with 2 parts horse serum and 1 part yeast extract. The essential ingredient was the yeast extract, the preparation of which was detailed by Hayflick (1965). Rather than a dehydrated enzymic digest of yeast, which is the usual commercial preparation, an aqueous extract of active dry baker's yeast was employed. The needed supplement in this product is heat-stable and dialyzable. Serum provides other constituents necessary for growth, including the cholesterol needed by all members of the genus *Mycoplasma*. Some analysis has been made of a protein-containing substance in serum, which facilitates attachment of *M. pneumoniae* to glass (Hughes *et al.*, 1974). The same basic formula may be used in liquid form or solidified by adding purified agar for isolation attempts. Since manufactured lots of the ingredients vary in ability to support growth of *M. pneumoniae* (and some are frankly inhibitory), rigid quality control practices are required. Another successful medium formulation which has been evaluated extensively uses a papaic digest of soy meal base (Kenny, 1974).

Since *M. pneumoniae* parasitizes the entire respiratory tract mucosa, suitable specimens for isolation attempts include nasopharyngeal or oropharyngeal throat swabs, sputum, tracheal aspirates, or lung tissue samples. Inoculated solid media should be incubated in a humidified atmosphere to prevent drying of the agar, in view of the organism's slow growth rate. Aerobic conditions are satisfactory, but growth is improved in the presence of 5% carbon dioxide. Colonies are not evident before 5 days, and 7–10 days incubation is optimal. Fresh isolates appear as granular, spherical colonies which lack the peripheral zone common to many mycoplasmas. Usually colonies vary between 10 and 100 μm in diameter, but growth often occurs along the edges of mucus streaks or cells from the inoculum which may be difficult to discern. Examination of plates using microscopic magnification of $20\times$ and $60\times$ is recommended.

For the identification of isolates, advantage can be taken of the fact that only *M. pneumoniae* among the human ororespiratory mycoplasmas demonstrates the properties of hemadsorption (Del Giudice and Pavia, 1964) and hemolysis (Clyde, 1963a). Suspect plate cultures may be flooded with a dilute erythrocyte suspension, incubated briefly, washed gently, and examined for hemadsorption. Hemolysis is demonstrated by adding a thin layer of melted 5% blood agar to the plates with reincubation for 24–48 hr. The recovery from a human respiratory specimen of slow-growing mycoplasma colonies having appropriate morphology and demonstrating either hemadsorption or hemolysis is adequate for clinical diagnosis in most cases. This assumes appropriate controls and attention to artifacts which may provide false positive reactions. Direct serological identification of the colonies on agar can be accomplished with the method of Del Giudice and co-workers (1967), if suitable reagents and equipment for immunofluorescence with epi-illumination are available. Lacking these resources, colonies may be subcultured for other identification steps, such as inhibition of growth by specific antiserum (Clyde, 1964).

It has been reported that the use of diphasic (broth over agar) medium for the primary isolation of *M. pneumoniae* roughly doubles the recovery rate obtained with agar alone (Craven *et al.*, 1976). After inoculation, tubes of medium are incubated at 36°C and subcultured at intervals (e.g., 1, 2, 3, and 6 weeks) for demonstration of mycoplasma growth. Incorporation of 1% dextrose and 0.002% phenol red with the broth provides a color change from the pH decrease caused by growth of *M. pneumoniae;* this change is relatively unreliable and should not supplant regular subcultivation as an index of growth. Recovered mycoplasmas are identified as described above. Liquid primary media have advantages over agar plates in being convenient to handle and capable of supporting a small number of organisms. Disadvantages of liquid media are that they preclude direct quantitation, mixed mycoplasma species are difficult to speciate, and processing time and effort are increased significantly. Choice of medium type must be made in consideration of the study purposes and available laboratory resources.

B. Serology

A wide variety of methods for serodiagnosis of *M. pneumoniae* infections has been described. These procedures make use of various biological features of the organism which can be modulated by antibody, e.g., the capacity to hemadsorb, hemagglutinate, attach to inert particles, ferment carbohydrates, reduce tetrazolium salts, be lysed by complement, and produce characteristic glycerophospholipids recognized in several antigen detection systems. All the available methods cannot be described in detail in the context of this section, but they are mentioned for comparative purposes and historical interest. For convenience of presentation, details of serum collection are considered first, followed by a discussion of agglutination methods, inhibition techniques, and direct antigen or antibody detection procedures.

1. Collection of Sera

As with any serological procedure, information obtained using two or more properly timed sera is more meaningful than a single value. This is particularly true in the case of *M. pneumoniae* disease, because of the common nature of the infections and the high prevalence of antibodies in most populations. The acute phase serum sample should be obtained as early as possible in the course of illness. Because of the insidious development of the disease, many patients do not present for medical attention until symptoms have been present for several days; by this time antibodies already may be rising or at high titer. Optimal time for collection of the convalescent-phase sample varies with the serological test to be used (Fernald *et al.*, 1967a). Early samples (1–2 weeks after the acute specimen) are useful for tests in which antibodies of the IgM class are most efficient, as in the case of the agglutination procedures. Later samples (3–8 weeks after the acute specimen) contain a predominance of IgG antibodies which are more effective in the growth inhibition methods. In processing blood samples care should be taken to avoid hemolysis, as hemoglobin interferes with some reactions (tetrazolium reduction). If it is anticipated that cold hemagglutinins will be sought on the same sera, the blood should be clotted and separated at room temperature to avoid loss of antibody by erythrocyte adsorption.

2. Agglutination Methods

Serological tests for *M. pneumoniae* involving agglutination include direct reaction between the mycoplasmas and antibody, and both direct and indirect assays involving organisms attached to larger carrier particles. Kerr and co-workers (1964) described a procedure for *M. pneumoniae* antibody detection, which involved visual agglutination of a heavy organism suspension stained with basic fuchsin. This method has not been thoroughly evaluated in terms of specificity and sensitivity, or with critical clinical trials. Mycoplasmas attached to latex particles have been used to assay animal antisera (Kende, 1969), but again systematic clinical experience with this test has not been recorded. Methods which have been evaluated more fully are hemagglutination techniques. The procedure of Feldman and Suhs (1966) involves direct agglutination of erythrocytes by *M. pneumoniae* suspensions which can be inhibited by the presence of antibody. Critical control of the organism growth phase is required, possibly to provide a sufficient number of dividing organisms or small clusters having multiple attachment organelles to bridge between erythrocytes. Another version of the same phenomenon is the hemadsorption inhibition technique of Del Giudice and Pavia (1964), in which the attachment of erythrocytes to *M. pneumoniae* colonies on agar is prevented by the presence of antibody. A method with greater sensitivity was described by Dowdle and Robinson (1964), who attached the mycoplasma to tanned erythrocytes which then agglutinated in the presence of antibody. This indirect hemagglutination test was later perfected for large-scale applications by using glutaraldehyde-fixed erythrocytes coated with *M. pneumoniae* and stored in liquid nitrogen until needed (Dowdle and Heyward, 1967).

3. Inhibition Methods

Included in this category are techniques that involve the effects of antibody on some biological function of living *M. pneumoniae*. The end results concern restriction of replication measured directly by enumerating organisms or through observation of some metabolic process which reflects growth indirectly. Edward and Fitzgerald (1954) observed that mycoplasmas were inhibited in their growth by the presence of antibody, using a technique of incorporating antisera in agar media. Adaptations of this idea were described subsequently by Huijsmans-Evers and Ruys (1956) and by Clyde (1964), who placed antiserum-saturated filter paper on inoculated plates. While such methods remain useful for species or type identification of isolated mycoplasmas, they are very insensitive and variable measures of antibody and should not be used for quantitative serology.

A sensitive and specific serological procedure for *M. pneumoniae* infections, based on inhibition of the metabolic processes leading to acid production in broth, was described by Taylor-Robinson and co-workers (1966). Antibody titers are expressed as serum dilutions inhibiting a specified number of color change units produced by a standardized inoculum. A more sensitive variation of this test employs serial organism dilutions against a constant amount of serum, in which case the result is given as the quantity of organisms inhibited (Fernald *et al.*, 1967b). Careful control of variables in these tests is required for reproducible results, including the use of accessory factors supplied by fresh normal serum (Fernald *et al.*, 1967b). Since the tests require the presence of live organisms, a potential problem arises when sera of patients on antibiotic therapy are to be examined (Smith and Herrmann, 1971). Tetracycline has a relatively short half-life in sera stored at room temperature or 4°C, but erythromycin is very stable under these conditions. A clever solution described by Niitu and associates (1974a) is the use of an erythromycin-resistant strain of *M. pneumoniae* as the assay organism.

Another type of growth inhibition test which has been applied extensively is the tetrazolium reduction inhibition procedure of Senterfit and Jensen (1966). As the organisms grow in broth containing colorless triphenyltetrazolium solution, they reduce the compound to red formazan, providing a visible color change; this process is inhibited by antibody. Generally, the variables described for the glucose fermentation version apply also to the tetrazolium test. In addition, the presence of hemoglobin interferes with the reaction, which precludes the use of hemolyzed sera or samples from patients having the hemolytic anemia component mentioned in Section III,B.

The basis of a different kind of serological test involving live *M. pneu-*

moniae is the observation that organisms are killed by lysis in the presence of antibody and complement (Gale and Kenny, 1970; Brunner *et al.*, 1971, 1972). This reaction is estimated to be more sensitive in detecting antibody than the complement fixation procedure described below by a factor of 10, although technically it is more difficult to perform.

4. Antigen or Antibody Detection Methods

Procedures grouped in this category do not necessarily require living *M. pneumoniae* organisms, and in general can be used either to detect antibody as serological tests or for the identification of antigen using known antisera. The indirect immunofluorescence procedure of Liu (1957) and Liu and co-workers (1959) was described in Section I,A. Shortly after *M. pneumoniae* was first propagated in artificial media the preparation of antigen for a complement fixation test was reported (Chanock *et al.*, 1962b). Variations in antigen production have appeared in the literature subsequently, the most important being the definition of the reactive component as a lipid hapten (Kenny and Grayston, 1965); extraction of crude organism suspensions with organic solvents yields a product with increased specificity and decreased anticomplementary properties. Since complement fixation tests of various types are widely used in serodiagnosis, this method has been popular for *M. pneumoniae* serology. The only additional reagents required are a mycoplasma antigen preparation and reference antiserum.

In recent years newer technical innovations in antigen or antibody detection systems have been applied to *M. pneumoniae,* although experience with the use of these methods is not yet extensive. The very sensitive technique of radioimmunoprecipitation (RIP) has been evaluated by Brunner and Chanock (1973). In this adaptation ^{14}C-labeled mycoplasmas in suspension are allowed to react with serum dilutions followed by precipitation using anti-human globulin. Radioactivity remaining in the supernatant fluid is measured, and decreases indicate that mycoplasma immune complexes have formed. With this method it can be shown that there is low antibody activity in subjects aged 7–12 months, but rapid acquisition occurs thereafter. These findings may indicate that *M. pneumoniae* infections are more common in early life than previously suspected, or the extreme sensitivity of the test may reflect antibody to some other organism or substance having shared glycolipid antigens (Kenny and Newton, 1973). The RIP test offers the advantage that immunoglobulin class-specific antibodies can be detected. Secretory IgA against *M. pneumoniae* has been measured in respiratory tract secretions; this appears to be the best correlate of protective immunity revealed at present (Brunner *et al.*, 1973b). Use of a newer method, the enzyme-linked immunosorbent assay (ELISA), has the potential for retaining all the advantages offered by the RIP test while being much simpler to perform (Voller *et al.*, 1976).

From the foregoing summary of serological methods for *M. pneumoniae* it can be surmised in view of the extensive list that no single technique has answered all needs. There is a wide variation among the many tests in terms of sensitivity, specificity, cost, and complexity. Choices for a particular application should be made in relation to the study purpose and technical resources available.

C. Rapid Diagnostic Methods

Diagnosis of *M. pneumoniae* infections either by isolation or serological methods offers little help to the clinician dealing with acutely ill patients. Recovery and identification of the mycoplasma cannot be done in less than 1–2 weeks with available methods, and serodiagnosis depends on a comparison of acute- and convalescent-phase samples. The cold hemagglutination method is of some use, since the titers rise early in illness; unfortunately many patients do not develop these agglutinins or have sufficiently high titers ($\geqslant 128$) in single sera to suggest the diagnosis. For the reasons cited there is a genuine need for dependable and specific rapid diagnostic methods.

Immunofluorescence methods have been used for the rapid diagnosis of several infectious diseases. Although this technique has been reported in relation to *M. pneumoniae* disease (Hers, 1963), there is little evidence of wide experience with it. The organisms can be demonstrated in sputum samples by electron microscopy, but this would be impractical and of questionable sensitivity for clinical use; the sputum cytology can be of some value, although this is relatively nonspecific (Collier and Clyde, 1974). It is conceivable that a sensitive antigen detection method, such as the RIP or ELISA procedure mentioned above, could be useful for rapid diagnosis, but this remains to be tested.

D. Differential Diagnosis

A classic presentation of *M. pneumoniae* pneumonia suggests the correct diagnosis in most cases, but the protean manifestations of the disease may be confused with a variety of other conditions. The variable chest x-ray findings can mimic both infectious and noninfectious pulmonary diseases of almost every type. The atypical pneumonia syndrome can be caused by bacteria, mycobacteria, viruses, rickettsia, chlamydiae, fungi, and protozoa; hypersensitivity diseases, chemical pneumonitis, and neoplasia can be added to the list (Clyde and Denny, 1963). The greatest problem is in differentiation of viral and mycoplasmal pneumonias, since very similar epidemiological, clinical, roentgenographic, and laboratory features may be seen in these instances. With attention to all of the factors listed and by a process of excluding diagnoses that can be confirmed rapidly in the clinical laboratory, sufficient information usually can be generated to formulate the therapeutic regimen.

V. THERAPY

Before the identification of *M. pneumoniae* as one of the principal causes of the atypical pneumonia syndrome, clinical trials using various antibiotics were undertaken (summarized in Clyde and Denny, 1963). There was a great deal of controversy concerning clinical efficacy, some of which can be resolved in retrospect by examining case selection factors, antibiotics used, and criteria of clinical response. Studies which indicated a good result of therapy included patients with disease of average severity, most of whom developed cold hemagglutinins; antibiotics in the tetracycline group were used, and response was measured by the proportion of cases that became afebrile within 48 hr. Eaton (1950) demonstrated the sensitivity of his atypical pneumonia agent to chlortetracycline and chloramphenicol, using the culture systems he had described earlier. The development of artificial media for the growth of *M. pneumoniae* and later diagnostic methods made possible definitive studies *in vitro* and *in vivo*.

A. Sensitivity of *Mycoplasma pneumoniae* to Antibiotics

As culture systems for *M. pneumoniae* developed, one of the early applications in each case was study of the effects of antimicrobial agents. The work of Eaton (1950) and of Marmion and Goodburn (1961) used embryonated eggs; Clyde (1963b) employed infected tissue cultures. These reports generally reflected the patterns characteristic of most mycoplasmas, i.e., insensitivity to penicillins and variable sensitivity to tetracyclines, chloramphenicol, and streptomycin. The demonstration of a high degree of effective killing by oleandomycin (Clyde, 1963b) suggested that related macrolide compounds could be useful. With the advent of artificial media several subsequent studies have documented that *M. pneumoniae* is sensitive to erythromycins, a feature not widely shared among mycoplasmas (Slotkin *et al.*, 1967; Jao and Finland, 1967; Niitu *et al.*, 1974b). Development of this information provided a basis for the design of several controlled clinical trials involving documented cases of *M. pneumoniae* disease.

B. Effects of Antibiotics on *Mycoplasma pneumoniae* in Vivo

The efficacy of antibiotic therapy in proven *M. pneumoniae* disease was demonstrated first by Kingston and associates in 1961 (Kingston *et al.*, 1961). A double-blind study was designed using the compound demethyl-chlortetracycline in a disease epidemic observed among Marine recruits. Compared to a group receiving placebo capsules, the treated men showed a significant reduction in duration of cough, fatigue, fever, and rales. Serial chest x-rays demonstrated that therapy interrupted progression and hastened resolution of pulmonary infiltration. Other trials indicated that erythromycin was efficacious in a manner similar to demethylchlortet-racycline (Rasch and Mogabgab, 1965). In later studies other antibiotics were shown to have comparably favorable therapeutic effects, including doxycycline, tetracycline, oxytetracycline, demeclocycline, erythromycin stearate and ethyl succinate, methacycline, and trolean-domycin (Gooch and Mogabgab, 1971; Shames *et al.*, 1970). In contrast, a study employing clindamycin failed to demonstrate the efficacy of this therapeutic agent (Smilack *et al.*, 1974). Of some interest is the observation that antibiotic treatment giving a beneficial clinical response does not produce a microbiological cure (Smith *et al.*, 1967; Gooch and Mogabgab, 1971). Thus the mechanism of action of these antimicrobial agents is not clear.

Slotkin and associates (1967) explored the effects of tetracycline and erythromycin on experimental *M. pneumoniae* disease in the Syrian hamster. The course of pulmonary histopathology was considerably shortened when antibiotic was administered between postinoculation days 15 and 20; in parallel to the human experience, the course of the mycoplasma infection was the same as in untreated control animals. When treatment was given during the first 5 days after inoculation, there was no effect on the expected course of pneumonia or infection, except that onset was delayed for the period of therapy. This experience suggests that antibiotic prophylaxis of *M. pneumoniae* disease would be ineffective (see Section VI,B). These experiments indicate that the mechanism of antimicrobial action is much more subtle than simple microbial eradication, possibly relating to decreased production of an injurious product by the mycoplasma. Further study should be made of this curious phenomenon.

VI. PREVENTION

A. Rationale

Because of the relatively mild nature of most *M. pneumoniae* infections, infrequent complications, lack of known sequelae, and the exceedingly low mortality, the need for development of effective preventive measures can be questioned (Clyde, 1969). The impact of the disease is measured mainly in terms of morbidity, however, and the burden is heavy if consideration is given to the segment of the population involved. The prevalence of the disease among older children, adolescents, and young adults means that the relevant effects are seen in days lost from school and decreased productivity from an important part of the work force, particularly the armed forces. Special problems are presented by institutional settings. In view of these concerns, it seems reasonable to conclude that there is a need for means to prevent *M. pneumoniae* disease, at least in certain population groups.

The incomplete state of knowledge about the pathogenesis of mycoplasma pneumonia and the basis of protective immunity fails to provide clear directives for the development of optimal preventive measures. This section summarizes current experience and insights that have been gained, together with speculations about future directions in this area. Both chemoprophylaxis and immunoprophylaxis are discussed.

B. Chemoprophylaxis

The extreme sensitivity of *M. pneumoniae* to various antibiotics—especially macrolides—suggests that chemoprophylaxis could be an effective tool in disease prevention. However, the observations summarized involving therapy both of natural and experimental disease showing lack of microbiological cure cast some doubt on the feasibility of this approach. Epidemiological considerations add further complexity to the issue. Thus the frequency of asymptomatic infections, age-specific attack rates of disease, lengthy incubation period, and variable case-to-case spread make difficult the selection of subjects for prophylaxis and the timing of administration.

One study has been reported whose goal was the systematic evaluation of oxytetracycline on the epidemiology of *M. pneumoniae* disease in families (Jensen *et al.*, 1965). After identification of an index case in a family unit remaining members were placed on the antibiotic or on a placebo. In an analysis of 242 individuals representing 76 families, it was found that approximately equal numbers of proven infections occurred in the treated and control groups. The difference was that about one-third of the infected patients in the antibiotic group experienced clinical illness, whereas two-thirds in the infected control group were ill. Oxytetracycline did not decrease the number of mycoplasma infections, but the morbidity from infection was significantly lowered. While the data do not indicate true prophylaxis in the sense of epidemiological control of infection, the modification of secondary cases to subclinical disease could be of some benefit in selected situations. The question of chemoprophylaxis needs further evaluation to resolve some of the issues which have been raised.

C. Immunization

The prospects for development of an effective vaccine against *M. pneumoniae* disease are indicated by several studies in the literature but are tempered by consideration of present knowledge concerning disease characteristics and protective immunity. An early experience using an injected vaccine product in human volunteers appeared to produce an adverse effect (Smith *et al.*, 1967). Volunteers who developed serum antibodies following the immunization were protected when challenged with virulent *M. pneumoniae*. However, individuals who failed to generate measurable antibody had more severe illnesses after challenge than unvaccinated control subjects. These results have been interpreted to show that nonresponding vaccinees were somehow sensitized to the mycoplasma, thereby showing greater reaction to experimental infection. Another possible explanation is that the volunteers who developed serum antibodies responded anamnestically to prior experience with the organisms, which was not detected by the preimmunization serology employed; men whose antibodies were not stimulated may have been truly nonimmune and accordingly less protected from challenge infection. This reasoning gains support from a vaccine trial with university students in which antibody-negative subjects failed to respond, while those with preexisting antibody showed a booster effect (Brown *et al.*, 1972). Similarly, administration of vaccine to antibody-negative children resulted in no serological response, but in this case it was shown that T-lymphocyte stimulation had occurred (Fernald and Glezen, 1973). The implications of lymphocyte sensitization in the absence of antibody production by an *M. pneumoniae* vaccine preparation are not clear at the present time.

Other studies using injected *M. pneumoniae* vaccines have provided more promising results than those described above (Mogabgab, 1973). A large field trial was conducted among Air Force personnel using an alum-adsorbed mycoplasma preparation. Most recipients developed serum antibodies equivalent to those seen after natural *M. pneumoniae* infection in terms of titer and persistence. Protective efficacy of the product was 87% for tracheobronchitis and 66% for pneumonia due to *M. pneumoniae*, resulting in a 37–48% reduction in such illnesses due to all causes in the study population. In addition to the demonstration of a significant respiratory disease morbidity decrease in consequence of the vaccine, the data underscore the impact *M. pneumoniae* disease has on a military population. In another large field trial of a different killed raccine, Wenzel *et al.* (1976) achieved protective effects similar to those cited.

Another approach to immunization against *M. pneumoniae* was suggested by a study in which human volunteers were inoculated with live organisms that had been propagated in cell-free media (Couch *et al.*, 1964). These subjects developed less frequent and severe clinical disease than volunteers inoculated with mycoplasmas propagated in a cell culture system. The findings implied that the passage of organisms in cell-free media had resulted in decreased virulence, and that development of a live attenuated vaccine was feasible. Furthermore, experimental data using several vaccine preparations in hamsters revealed that greater resistance to challenge inoculation with *M. pneumoniae* was produced by prior respiratory tract infection than by a parenterally administered vaccine (Fernald and Clyde, 1970). The results in animals suggested that stimulation of local immune mechanisms in the respiratory tract was more consequential for protection than the development of systemic parameters reflected by serum antibody. The local response of importance may be the stimulation of secretory IgA; *M. pneumoniae*-specific antibody of this immunoglobulin class has been measured in respiratory secretions of human subjects and appears to be a better correlate of protective immunity than serum antibody (Brunner *et al.*, 1973b). The logic of the importance attached to local immunity is in keeping with the superficial nature of the infection which involves attachment of the mycoplasma to the respiratory epithelium.

While subcultivation of *M. pneumoniae* produced a strain of decreased virulence for humans, the degree of attenuation was insufficient for vaccine use, since nasal inoculation resulted in a significant amount of illness among recipients. A novel approach to circumvent this problem has been the development of temperature-sensitive mutants of *M. pneumoniae* (Steinberg *et al.*, 1969b, 1971; Brunner *et al.*, 1973c). Strains were sought which could grow at the temperature characteristic of the upper respiratory tract but which would be restricted by the higher core temperature of the lung. A series of mycoplasma mutants induced by treatment with nitrosoguanadine *in vitro* were produced and tested in hamsters and in human volunteers. The animals were infected without showing histopathological changes in the lung; one mutant tested in volunteers resulted in a low incidence of tracheobronchitis. Work has continued on the production of a sufficiently attenuated, genetically stable temperature-sensitive mutant as a vaccine candidate for use in humans (Greenberg *et al.*, 1974), although there have been no recent reports of the successful development of such a vaccine.

Lipman and Clyde (1969) reported the derivation of a strain of *M. pneumoniae* by serial subcultivation in artificial media, which infected hamsters but produced no pneumonia. Comparison of the avirulent strain with its virulent parent showed no change in the properties examined, except for loss of cytoadsorptive ability. This suggests that the ability of *M. pneumoniae* to attach to host cells is a prime determinant of virulence. A relationship between loss of cytoadsorptive ability and deletion of a surface protein of the mycoplasma has been demonstrated by Hu and co-workers (1977). The potential of the avirulent organism as another live vaccine candidate has been explored using the hamster experimental model (Clyde, 1971b). Animals previously infected with the avirulent strain required 1000-fold more virulent challenge organisms to produce pneumonia expected 14 days later than did normal animals; however, further study of the mechanisms involved produced curious results. When hamsters were infected with virulent *M. pneumoniae* and allowed to recover, challenge infection resulted in an exaggerated, accelerated pulmonary histopathological picture relative to the primary infection (Clyde, 1971a). Pneumonic infiltrates were seen between 1 and 3 days after inoculation, rather than at 14 days as in the initial exposure to the organisms. When animals were infected with avirulent organisms no disease was produced; however, challenge inoculation with virulent organisms then produced the same accelerated pneumonia characteristic of two virulent infections. The early pneumonia cleared by 14 days, when changes in unprepared animals were maximal, giving the appearance of protection against challenge when only this time period was examined. The possibility of exaggerated pneumonia following a short incubation period on exposure to natural disease has precluded study of the effects of avirulent organism infection in humans.

Future work on immunoprophylaxis of *M. pneumoniae* disease will depend upon progress in the development of vaccine candidates and comparative studies of their efficacy. It is possible that new innovations will provide materials of better immunogenicity than those described above. For example, one novel idea is the incorporation of purified lipid hapten of *M. pneumoniae* into a heterologous membrane to serve as carrier (Razin *et al.*, 1970). If indeed the prime virulence determinant of *M. pneumoniae* is cytoadsorptive ability, immunization using the protein related to this property might offer a highly selective form of protective immunity (Hu *et al.*, 1977). The use of inactivated preparations applied directly to the respiratory mucosa offers another strategy worth investigation. However, all these prospects must remain in proper perspective relative to natural immunity. It has been shown in a prospective study that infants and children can experience natural reinfections with *M. pneumoniae* within 1- to 3-year periods (Fernald *et al.*, 1975). It has been documented that symptomatic disease can recur in adults within 5 years (Foy *et al.*, 1971), and there is evidence that asymptomatic reinfection also is common (Chanock *et al.*, 1961a; Steinberg *et al.*, 1969). These observations suggest that the protective immunity following natural *M. pneumoniae* disease may be limited in degree and duration; it may be unrealistic to expect more or even the same of artificially induced immunity.

REFERENCES

Baernstein, H. D., Jr., Trevisani, E., Axtell, S., and Quilligan, J. J., Jr. (1965). *J. Pediat.* **66,** 829–837.
Biberfeld, G. (1970). *Clin. Exp. Immunol.* **8,** 319–333.
Biberfeld, G., and Biberfeld, P. (1970). *J. Bacteriol.* **102,** 855–861.
Biberfeld, G., and Gronowicz, E. (1976). *Nature (London)* **261,** 238–239.
Biberfeld, G., and Norberg, R. (1974). *J. Immunol.* **112,** 413–415.
Biberfeld, G., and Sterner, G. (1969). *Scand. J. Infect. Dis.* **1,** 39–46.
Biberfeld, G., and Sterner, G. (1976). *Scand. J. Infect. Dis.* **8,** 71–73.
Bredt, W. (1968). *Pathol. Microbiol.* **32,** 321–326.
Brown, R. C., Hendley, J. O., and Gwaltney, J. M., Jr. (1972). *Infect. Immun.* **5,** 657–661.
Brunner, H., and Chanock, R. M. (1973). *Proc. Soc. Exp. Biol. Med.* **143,** 97–105.
Brunner, H., Razin, S., Kalica, A. R., and Chanock, R. M. (1971). *J. Immunol.* **106,** 907–916.
Brunner, H., James, W. D., Horswood, R. L., and Chanock, R. M. (1972). *J. Immunol.* **108,** 1491–1498.
Brunner, H., James, W. D., Horswood, R. L., and Chanock, R. M. (1973a). *J. Infect. Dis.* **127,** 315–318.
Brunner, H., Greenberg, H. B., James, W. D., Horswood, R. L., Couch, R. B., and Chanock, R. M. (1973b). *Infect. Immun.* **9,** 612–620.
Brunner, H., Greenberg, H., James, W. D., Horswood, R. L,, and Chanock, R. M. (1973c). *Ann. N.Y. Acad. Sci.* **225,** 436–452.
Chanock, R. M., Mufson, M. A., Bloom, H. H., James, W. D., Fox, H. H., and Kingston, J. R. (1961a). *J. Am. Med. Assoc.* **175,** 213–220.
Chanock, R. M., Rifkind, D., Kravetz, H. M., Knight, V., and Johnson, K. M. (1961b). *Proc. Natl. Acad. Sci. U.S.A.* **47,** 887–890.
Chanock, R. M., Hayflick, L., and Barile, M. F. (1962a). *Proc. Natl. Acad. Sci. U.S.A.* **48,** 41–49.
Chanock, R. M., James, W. D., Fox, H. H., Turner, H. C., Mufson, M. A., and Hayflick, L. (1962b). *Proc. Soc. Exp. Biol. Med.* **110,** 884–889.
Chanock, R. M., Dienes, L., Eaton, M. D., Edward, D. G. ff., Freundt, E. A., Hayflick, L., Hers, J. F. P., Jensen, K. E., Liu, C., Marmion, B. P., Morton, H. E., Mufson, M. A., Smith, P. F., Somerson, N. L., and Taylor-Robinson, D. (1963). *Science* **140,** 662.
Clyde, W. A., Jr. (1961). *Proc. Soc. Exp. Biol. Med.* **107,** 716–719.

Clyde, W. A., Jr. (1963a). *Science* **139,** 55.

Clyde, W. A., Jr. (1963b). *Proc. Soc. Exp. Biol. Med.* **112,** 905–909.

Clyde, W. A., Jr. (1964). *J. Immunol.* **92,** 958–965.

Clyde, W. A., Jr. (1969). *J. Infect. Dis.* **120,** 255–257.

Clyde, W. A., Jr. (1971a). *Infect. Immun.* **4,** 757–763.

Clyde, W. A., Jr. (1971b). *Bacteriol. Proc.* p. 78.

Clyde, W. A., Jr., and Denny, F. W. (1963). *Med. Clin. North Am.* **47,** 1201–1218.

Clyde, W. A., Jr., and Denny, F. W. (1967). *Pediatrics* **40,** 669–684.

Clyde, W. A., Jr., Denny, F. W., and Dingle, J. H. (1961). *J. Clin. Invest.* **40,** 1638–1647.

Cohen, G., and Somerson, N. L. (1967). *Ann. N.Y. Acad. Sci.* **143,** 85–87.

Collier, A. M., and Baseman, J. B. (1973). *Ann. N.Y. Acad. Sci.* **225,** 277–289.

Collier, A. M., and Clyde, W. A., Jr. (1971). *Infect. Immun.* **3,** 694–701.

Collier, A. M., and Clyde, W. A., Jr. (1974). *Am. Rev. Respir. Dis.* **110,** 765–773.

Collier, A. M., Clyde, W. A., Jr., and Denny, F. W. (1969). *Proc. Soc. Exp. Biol. Med.* **132,** 1153–1158.

Commission on Acute Respiratory Diseases of the Armed Forces Epidemiological Board (1946). *Bull. Johns Hopkins Hosp.* **79,** 96–167.

Cook, M. K., Chanock, R. M., Fox, H. H., Huebner, R. J., Buescher, E. L., and Johnson, R. T. (1960). *Brit. Med. J.* **1,** 905–911.

Couch, R. B., Cate, T. R., and Chanock, R. M. (1964). *J. Am. Med. Assoc.* **187,** 442–447.

Craven, R. B., Wenzel, R. P., Calhoun, A. M., Hendley, J. O., Hamory, B. H., and Gwaltney, J. M., Jr. (1976). *J. Clin. Microbiol.* **4,** 225–226.

Dajani, A. S., Clyde, W. A., Jr., and Denny, F. W. (1965). *J. Exp. Med.* **121,** 1071–1086.

Del Giudice, R. A., and Pavia, R. (1964). *Bacteriol. Proc.* p. 71.

Del Giudice, R. A., Robillard, N. F., and Carski, T. R. (1967). *J. Bacteriol.* **93,** 1205–1209.

Denny, F. W., Clyde, W. A., Jr., and Glezen, W. P. (1971). *J. Infect. Dis.* **123,** 74–92.

Donald, H. B., and Liu, C. (1959). *Virology* **9,** 20–29.

Dowdle, W. R., and Heyward, J. T. (1967). *Am. J. Clin. Pathol.* **49,** 132–134.

Dowdle, W. R., and Robinson, R. Q. (1964). *Proc. Soc. Exp. Biol. Med.* **116,** 947–950.

Eaton, M. D. (1950). *Proc. Soc. Exp. Biol. Med.* **73,** 24–26.

Eaton, M. D., Meiklejohn, G., and van Herick, W. (1944). *J. Exp. Med.* **79,** 649–668.

Edward, D. G. ff., and Fitzgerald, W. A. (1954). *J. Pathol. Bacteriol.* **68,** 23–30.

Feizi, T., and Taylor-Robinson, D. (1967). *Immunology* **13,** 405–409.

Feldman, H. A., and Suhs, R. H. (1966). *Am. J. Epidemiol.* **83,** 345–356.

Fernald, G. W., and Clyde, W. A., Jr. (1970). *Infect. Immun.* **1,** 559–565.

Fernald, G. W., and Clyde, W. A., Jr. (1976). *In* "Immunologic and Infectious Reactions in the Lung" (C. H. Kirkpatrick and H. Y. Reynolds, eds.), pp. 101–130. Dekker, New York.

Fernald, G. W., and Glezen, W. P. (1973). *J. Infect. Dis.* **128,** 498–504.

Fernald, G. W., Clyde, W. A., Jr., and Denny, F. W. (1967a). *J. Immunol.* **98,** 1028–1038.

Fernald, G. W., Clyde, W. A., Jr., and Denny, F. W. (1967b). *Proc. Soc. Exp. Biol. Med.* **126,** 161–166.

Fernald, G. W., Clyde, W. A., Jr., and Bienenstock, J. (1972). *J. Immunol.* **108,** 1400–1408.

Fernald, G. W., Collier, A. M., and Clyde, W. A., Jr. (1975). *Pediatrics* **55,** 327–335.

Foy, H. M., Grayston, J. T., Kenny, G. E., Alexander, E. R., and McMahan, R. (1966). *J. Am. Med. Assoc.* **197,** 859–866.

Foy, H. M., Kenny, G. E., McMahan, R., Mansy, A. M., and Grayston, J. T. (1970). *J. Am. Med. Assoc.* **214,** 1666–1672.

Foy, H. M., Nugent, C. G., Kenny, G. E., McMahan, R., and Grayston, J. T. (1971). *J. Am. Med. Assoc.* **216,** 671–672.

Foy, H. M., Loop, J., Clarke, E. R., Mansy, A. W., Spence, W. F., Feigl, P., and Grayston, J. T. (1973a). *Am. Rev. Respir. Dis.* **108**, 469–474.

Foy, H. M., Ochs, H., Davis, S. D., Kenny, G. E., and Luce, R. R. (1973b). *J. Infect. Dis.* **127**, 388–393.

Gabridge, M. G. (1975). *Infect. Immun.* **12**, 544–549.

Gabridge, M. G., Johnson, C. K., and Cameron, A. M. (1974). *Infect. Immun.* **10**, 1127–1134.

Gale, J. L., and Kenny, G. E. (1970). *J. Immunol.* **104**, 1175–1183.

Gallagher, J. R. (1941). *Yale J. Biol. Med.* **13**, 663–678.

George, R. B., Ziskind, M. M., Rasch, J. R., and Mogabgab, W. J. (1966). *Ann. Intern. Med.* **65**, 931–942.

Glezen, W. P., Clyde, W. A., Jr., Senior, R. J., Sheaffer, C. I., and Denny, F. W. (1967). *J. Am. Med. Assoc.* **202**, 455–460.

Glezen, W. P., Loda, F. A., Clyde, W. A., Jr., Senior, R. J., Sheaffer, C. I., Conley, W. G., and Denny, F. W. (1971). *J. Pediat.* **78**, 397–406.

Gooch, W. M., III, and Mogabgab, W. J. (1971). *In* "Antimicrobial Agents and Chemotherapy—1970" (G. L. Hobby, ed.), pp. 291–295. *Am. Soc. Microbiol.*, Washington, D.C.

Grayston, J. T., Alexander, E. R., Kenny, G. E., Clarke, E. R., Fremont, J. C., and MacColl, W. A. (1965). *J. Am. Med. Assoc.* **191**, 369–374.

Greenberg, H., Helms, C. M., Brunner, H., and Chanock, R. M. (1974). *Proc. Natl. Acad. Sci. U.S.A.* **71**, 4015–4019.

Griffin, J. P., and Klein, E. W. (1971). *Clin. Med.* **78**, 23–27.

Hayflick, L. (1965). *Tex. Rep. Biol. Med.* **23**, 285–303.

Hers, J. F. P. (1963). *Am. Rev. Respir. Dis.* **88**, 316–333.

Hu, P. C., Collier, A. M., and Baseman, J. B. (1975). *Infect. Immun.* **11**, 704–710.

Hu, P. C., Collier, A. M., and Baseman, J. B. (1977). *J. Exp. Med.* **145**, 1328–1343.

Hughes, J. H., Thomas, D. C., Hamparian, V. V., and Somerson, N. L. (1974). *J. Med. Microbiol.* **7**, 35–40.

Huijsmans-Evers, A. G. M., and Ruys, A. C. (1956) *Antonie van Leeuwenhoek; J. Microbiol. Serol.* **22**, 375–384.

Jao, R. L., and Finland, M. (1967). *Am. J. Med. Sci.* **253**, 639–650.

Jarstrand, C., Camner, P., and Philipson, K. (1974). *Am. Rev. Respir. Dis.* **110**, 415–419.

Jensen, K. E., Senterfit, L. B., Scully, W. E., Conway, T. J., West, R. F., and Drummy, W. W. (1965). *Am. J. Epidemiol.* **86**, 419–432.

Jordan, W. S., Jr., and Dingle, J. H. (1965). *In* "Bacterial and Mycotic Infections of Man" (R. J. Dubos and J. G. Hirsch, eds.), pp. 810–822. Lippincott, Philadelphia, Pennsylvania.

Kaklamanis, E., and Pavlatos, M. (1972). *Immunology* **22**, 695–702.

Kende, M. (1969). *Appl. Microbiol.* **17**, 275–279.

Kenny, G. E. (1974). *In* "Manual of Clinical Microbiology" (E. H. Lennette, E. H. Spaulding, and J. P. Truant, eds.), 2nd Ed., pp. 333–337. Am. Soc. Microbiol., Washington, D.C.

Kenny, G. E., and Grayston, J. T. (1965). *J. Immunol.* **95**, 19–25.

Kenny, G. E., and Newton, R. M. (1973). *Ann. N.Y. Acad. Sci.* **225**, 54–61.

Kerr, K. M., Mascoli, C. C., Olson, N. O., and Campbell, A. (1964). *J. Bacteriol.* **87**, 478–479.

Kingston, J. R., Chanock, R. M., Mufson, M. A., Hellman, L. P., James, W. D., Fox, H. H., Manko, M. A., and Boyers, J. (1961). *J. Am. Med. Assoc.* **176**, 118–123.

Lambert, H. P. (1968). *Brit. Med. J.* **iii**, 156–157.

Lind, K. (1971). *Acta Pathol. Microbiol. Scand. Sect. B* **79**, 239–247.

Lipman, R. P., and Clyde, W. A., Jr. (1969). *Proc. Soc. Exp. Biol. Med.* **131**, 1163–1167.

Liu, C. (1957). *J. Exp. Med.* **106**, 455–466.
Liu, C., Eaton, M. D., and Heyl, J. T. (1959). *J. Exp. Med.* **109**, 545–556.
Ludlam, G. B., Bridges, J. B., and Benn, B. C. (1964). *Lancet* **1**, 958–959.
Maisel, J. C., Babbitt, L. H., and John, T. J. (1967). *J. Am. Med. Assoc.* **202**, 287–290.
Marmion, B. P., and Goodburn, G. M. (1961). *Nature (London)* **189**, 247–248.
Meyers, B. R., and Hirschman, S. Z. (1972). *Mt. Sinai J. Med., N.Y.* **39**, 258–264.
Mogabgab, W. J. (1973). *Ann. N.Y. Acad. Sci.* **225**, 453–461.
Mufson, M. A., Sanders, V., Wood, S. C., and Chanock, R. M. (1963). *N. Engl. J. Med.* **268**, 1109–1111.
Naftalin, J. M., Wellisch, G., Kahana, Z., and Diengott, D. (1974). *J. Am. Med. Assoc.* **228**, 65.
Niitu, Y., Hasegawa, S., and Kubota, H. (1974a). *Antimicrob. Agents Chemother.* **5**, 111–113.
Niitu, Y., Kubota, H., Hasegawa, S., Komatsu, S., Horikawa, M., and Suetake, T. (1974b). *Jpn. J. Microbiol.* **18**, 149–155.
Parker, F., Jr., Jolliffe, L. S., and Finland, M. (1947). *Arch. Pathol.* **44**, 587–608.
Peterson, O. L., Ham, T. H., and Finland, M. (1943). *Science* **97**, 167.
Powell, D. A., and Clyde, W. A., Jr. (1975). *Infect. Immun.* **11**, 540–550.
Purcell, R. H., and Chanock, R. M. (1967). *Med. Clin. North Am.* **51**, 791–802.
Rasch, J. R., and Mogabgab, W. J. (1966). *In* "Antimicrobial Agents and Chemotherapy—1965" (G. L. Hobby, ed.), pp. 693–699. Am. Soc. Microbiol., Washington, D.C.
Razin, S., Prescott, B., and Chanock, R. M. (1970). *Proc. Natl. Acad. Sci. U.S.A.* **67**, 590–597.
Reimann, H. A. (1938). *J. Am. Med. Assoc.* **111**, 2377–2384.
Rifkind, D., Chanock, R., Kravetz, H., Johnson, K., and Knight, V. (1962). *Am. Rev. Respir. Dis.* **85**, 479–489.
Schulman, S. T., Bartlett, J., Clyde, W. A., Jr., and Ayoub, E. M. (1972). *N. Engl. J. Med.* **287**, 164–167.
Senterfit, L. B., and Jensen, K. E. (1966). *Proc. Soc. Exp. Biol. Med.* **122**, 786–790.
Shames, J. M., George, R. B., Holliday, W. B., Rasch, J. R., and Mogabgab, W. J. (1970). *Arch. Intern. Med.* **125**, 680–684.
Skoldenberg, N. (1965). *Brit. Med. J.* **1**, 100–102.
Slotkin, R. I., Clyde, W. A., Jr., and Denny, F. W. (1967). *Am. J. Epidemiol.* **86**, 225–237.
Smilack, J. D., Burgin, W. W., Jr., Moore, W. L., Jr., and Sanford, J. P. (1974). *J. Am. Med. Assoc.* **228**, 729–731.
Smith, C. B., Friedewald, W. T., and Chanock, R. M. (1967). *J. Am. Med. Assoc.* **199**, 353–358.
Smith, T. F., and Herrmann, E. C., Jr. (1971). *Appl. Microbiol.* **21**, 160–161.
Sobeslavsky, O., Syrucek, L., Bruckova, M., and Abrahamovic, M. (1965). *Pediatrics* **35**, 652–657,
Sobeslavsky, O., Prescott, B., and Chanock, R. M. (1968). *J. Bacteriol.* **96**, 695–705.
Somerson, N. L., Taylor-Robinson, D., and Chanock, R. M. (1963). *Am. J. Hyg.* **77**, 122–128.
Somerson, N. L., Walls, B. E., and Chanock, R. M. (1965). *Science* **150**, 226–228.
Somerson, N. L., James, W. D., Walls, B. E., and Chanock, R. M. (1967). *Ann. N.Y. Acad. Sci.* **143**, 384–389.
Steinberg, P., White, R. J., Fuld, S. L., Gutekunst, R. P., Chanock, R. M., and Senterfit, L. B. (1969a). *Am. J. Epidemiol.* **89**, 62–73.
Steinberg, P., Horswood, R. L., and Chanock, R. M. (1969b). *J. Infect. Dis.* **120**, 217–224.
Steinberg, P., Horswood, R. L., Brunner, H., and Chanock, R. M. (1971). *J. Infect. Dis.* **124**, 179–187.
Stevens, A. M., and Johnson, F. C. (1922). *Am. J. Dis. Child.* **24**, 526–533.

Suhs, R. H., and Feldman, H. A. (1966). *Am. J. Epidemiol.* **83,** 357–365.

Taylor, G., Taylor-Robinson, D., and Fernald, G. W. (1974). *J. Med. Microbiol.* **7,** 343–348.

Taylor-Robinson, D., Purcell, R. H., Wong, D. C., and Chanock, R. M. (1966). *J. Hyg.* **64,** 91–104.

Thomas, L., Curnen, E. C., Mirick, G. S., Ziegler, J. E., and Horsfall, F. L., Jr. (1943). *Proc. Soc. Exp. Biol. Med.* **52,** 121–125.

van Herick, W., and Eaton, M. D. (1945). *J. Bacteriol.* **50,** 47–55.

Voller, A., Bidwell, D., and Bartlett, A. (1976). *In* "Manual of Clinical Immunology" (N. R. Rose and H. Friedman, eds.), pp. 506–512. Am. Soc. Microbiol., Washington, D.C.

Wenzel, R. P., Craven, R. B., Davies, J. A., Hendley, J. O., Hamory, B. H., and Gwaltney, J. M., Jr. (1976). *J. Infect. Dis.* **134,** 571–576.

Wright, D. N., Bailey, G. D., and Goldberg, L. J. (1969). *J. Bacteriol.* **99,** 491–495.

10 / MYCOPLASMAS IN HUMAN GENITOURINARY INFECTIONS

David Taylor-Robinson and William M. McCormack[1]

[1] Supported by Research Grant HD 03693 from the National Institute of Child Health and Human Development.

I. MYCOPLASMAS IN THE HUMAN GENITOURINARY TRACT

The first reported isolation of a mycoplasma from humans was by Dienes and Edsall (1937), who recovered organisms in pure culture from a Bartholin's gland abscess. In retrospect, these probably belonged to the species *Mycoplasma hominis*. To date, 11 different *Mycoplasma* species have been isolated. As shown in Table I, at least four of these are found predominantly in the genitourinary tract.

As indicated above, it seems likely that *M. hominis* was the first mycoplasma to be isolated from the genitourinary tract. Several serological subtypes exist (Razin, 1968; Lin and Kass, 1974). It is found commonly in the genitourinary tract but infrequently in the oropharynx or elsewhere. T-strain mycoplasmas, or T mycoplasmas, were first described by Shepard (1954). Since these organisms have the unique ability to metabolize urea, those of human origin were placed in a new genus and species, *Ureaplasma urealyticum* (Shepard *et al.*, 1974), comprising at least eight serotypes (Black, 1973). Ureaplasmas, as these organisms are termed trivially, are also found commonly in the genitourinary tract but infrequently in the oropharynx or elsewhere.

Mycoplasma fermentans, originally referred to as strain G and first isolated by Ruiter and Wentholt (1952), is rarely recovered from the genitourinary tract, perhaps only 1% or less of isolates belonging to this species (Mårdh and Weström, 1970c). *Mycoplasma primatum* (Del Giudice *et al.*, 1971), at one time referred to as the Navel strain, is also rarely isolated (Thomsen, 1974). Infrequent detection of both these mycoplasmas may be a reflection of the technique of isolation and identification. The identification of every colony on a solid medium by the epi-immunofluorescence technique described by Del Giudice *et al.* (1967) might reveal a greater incidence, although so far this has not been found to

TABLE I. Mycoplasmas Isolated from Humans and Their Anatomical Sites

Mycoplasma	Specimen or anatomical site from which isolated											
	Kidney	Bladder urine	Voided urine	Urethral swab	Seminal fluid	Fallopian tube	Cervix and vagina	Rectum	Conjunctiva	Mouth	Lung	Blood
M. hominis	+[a]	+	+	+	+	+[a]	+	+	+	+		+[a]
U. urealyticum (T mycoplasmas)		+	+	+	+	+[a]	+	+	+	+		+[a]
M. fermentans			+	+			+					
M. primatum										+	+[a]	
M. salivarium	+?						+[b]			+		
M. orale										+		
M. buccale										+		
M. faucium										+		
M. lipophilum										+		
A. laidlawii							+[b]			+[a]		
M. pneumoniae											+[a]	

[a] Usually in disease only.
[b] Very rarely found.

be so (D. Taylor-Robinson and P. M. Furr, unpublished observations). *Mycoplasma pneumoniae*, normally isolated from the respiratory tract of persons with disease, has been recovered from a tuboovarian abscess (Thomas *et al.*, 1975) and also from the lower genital tract (Csütörtöki *et al.*, 1975), presumably as a result of orogenital contact. It is not surprising therefore that other mycoplasmas such as *M. salivarium,* normally resident in the oropharynx, are recovered very occasionally from the genital tract (Foy *et al.*, 1975; Gump *et al.*, 1975). Isolation of *M. salivarium* from the kidney has been reported, and this is considered further in Section VII. However, unless otherwise stated, only *M. hominis* and *U. urealyticum* are discussed.

II. COLLECTION AND HANDLING OF SPECIMENS FOR THE ISOLATION OF GENITAL MYCOPLASMAS

A. Specimens from Male Subjects

The manner of obtaining specimens from the male genital tract in order to isolate mycoplasmas has been studied by several groups of workers. Csonka *et al.* (1966, 1967), Sueltmann *et al.* (1971), and Mukhija *et al.* (1973a) isolated ureaplasmas as frequently from the urine of men suffering from urethritis as from urethral swabs. The same claim was made by Klieneberger-Nobel (1959a), Csonka *et al.* (1966, 1967), and Gregory and Cundy (1970) in the case of *M. hominis.* However, Black and Rasmussen (1968) and Sepetjian *et al.* (1969) presented evidence that swabs from men without urethritis more frequently yielded ureaplasma and *M. hominis* organisms, respectively, than voided urines. Subsequently, in a more detailed study of men with and without urethritis, Tarr *et al.* (1976) came to the same conclusion. In view of the known close association of genital mycoplasmas with epithelial cells (Shepard and Calvy, 1965; Manchee and Taylor-Robinson, 1969a), urine specimens from men with and without urethritis may not be comparable. For such comparative purposes, it seems preferable to use a swabbing technique that ensures the presence of urethral epithelial cells. On theoretical grounds, swabbing is likely to remove more cells than the voiding of urine and so provide the most sensitive technique. Tarr *et al.* (1976) suggest that two urethral swabs should be used for optimal ureaplasmal isolation and one urethral and one coronal swab for optimal isolation of *M. hominis.* In addition, experiments in animals, including chimpanzees (Taylor-Robinson *et al.*, 1978), have shown that a swabbing technique can provide consistent data on the numbers of viable organisms present in the lower genital tract. Quantitative information can of course also be provided by examination of urine (Bowie *et al.*, 1977a; Taylor-Robinson *et al.*, 1977), although the time of voiding and the quantity voided may influence the results. Furthermore, examination of early-, mid-, and late-stream specimens of urine is a means of determining the location of mycoplasmas within the genitourinary tract, something which cannot be achieved by swabbing.

B. Specimens from Female Subjects

It seems obvious that urine specimens from female subjects cannot replace swab specimens for the isolation of mycoplasmas from the genital tract. Several workers found clean-voided specimens of urine to be somewhat less sensitive than direct genital specimens for the isolation of ureaplasmas from infants (Foy *et al.*, 1970a) and adults (Braun *et al.*, 1970a; Mårdh and Weström, 1970a; Lee *et al.*, 1972a), although both techniques were comparable for the isolation of *M. hominis* in two studies (Csonka *et al.*, 1966; Braun *et al.*, 1970a). In adults, apart from the cervix and vagina, the urethra is often infected or may be "contaminated" by secretions from the former sites. It would be surprising therefore if the results of examining urine specimens did not sometimes parallel those of genital swabs. Indeed, Csonka *et al.* (1966) and Archer (1968) found urine equivalent to cervical or vaginal swabs for the isolation of ureaplasmas, and Kundsin (1976) reported a slightly higher recovery from urines than from cervical swabs. Failure to clean the perineum before the collection of urine samples and centrifugation of urine before culture increase the mycoplasmal yield. Despite the increased yield from "dirty" urine specimens, W. M. McCormack (unpublished observations) has evidence to indicate clearly that this does not justify the use of a urine specimen as a substitute for a vaginal swab.

C. Handling of Specimens

For optimal isolation, swabs should be expressed immediately into mycoplasma medium, and they should certainly not be allowed to dry, even though drying does not rapidly kill all ureaplasmas as might be expected of cell wall-deficient organisms (Taylor-Robinson *et al.*, 1969a). Blood samples should also be inoculated into medium soon after taking, since the recovery of genital mycoplasmas has been shown to decline appreciably over an hour (Lee *et al.*, 1972b). Once in medium, there is no great urgency for transportation to the laboratory. However, this should be done as soon as possible, preferably within 24 hr, and in the meantime the medium containing organisms should be kept at 4°C. This is particularly important if an estimation of the number of organisms in a specimen is to be made, since the mean generation time of ureaplasmas at 37°C is not more than 1–2 hr (Furness, 1975). Urine samples should also be kept cool and, for greater isolation sensitivity, centrifuged at a minimum of 600 g to remove epithelial and other cells from fluids to be cultured.

III. METHODS USED FOR THE LABORATORY DIAGNOSIS OF GENITAL MYCOPLASMAL INFECTION

A. Isolation and Identification

Mycoplasmas are Gram-negative and do not take up the counterstain sufficiently well for the small individual organisms to be recognized on microscopic examination of Gram-stained clinical specimens. Although there is a correlation between vaginal smears which appear "dirty" and the isolation of *M. hominis* (Jones and Davson, 1967; Mårdh *et al.*, 1971), a definitive diagnosis cannot be made on the basis of cytology but depends on culturing specimens on appropriate media with identification of isolates. The basic medium is a beef heart infusion broth, available commercially as PPLO broth, supplemented with 10% (vol/vol) fresh yeast extract (25% wt/vol) and 20% (vol/vol) horse serum. The latter supplies cholesterol or related sterols which are required by all genital mycoplasmas (Razin and Tully, 1970), including ureaplasmas (Rottem *et al.*, 1971), for growth. In broth, all genital mycoplasmas grow well under atmospheric conditions, but on agar, colonies develop best in an atmosphere of nitrogen–5% carbon dioxide. An atmosphere of 100% carbon dioxide is conducive to the development of large ureaplasma colonies (Razin *et al.*, 1977).

In order to detect mycoplasma growth in broth medium, advantage is taken of the metabolic activity of mycoplasmas. Clinical material is added to separate vials of broth containing phenol red (0.002%) and 0.1% glucose, arginine, or urea. *Mycoplasma fermentans* catabolizes glucose to lactic acid by a glycolytic pathway, thus lowering the pH of the medium from an initial 7.5 and producing a color change from pink to yellow. *Mycoplasma hominis* metabolizes arginine using a three-enzyme system to convert it via ornithine to ammonia, thus raising the pH of the medium from an initial 7.0 and producing a color change from yellow to pink. Ureaplasmas grow best at pH 6.0 or less, and they possess a urease which breaks down urea to ammonia, and therefore a similar color change is produced. Aliquots of medium from cultures showing these color changes are subcultured into fresh broth media and onto agar medium for the development of colonies. On agar medium which contains added urea and a sensitive indicator of ammonia, manganous sulfate, ureaplasma colonies are identified as dark-brown colonies (Shepard and Lunceford, 1976). Use of the "liquid to agar medium" technique provides the most sensitive method for the isolation of both ureaplasmas (Taylor-Robinson *et al.*, 1969b; Shepard and Lunceford, 1970) and *M. hominis* (Braun *et al.*, 1970a). Moreover, for ureaplasmas it is the simplest and most rapid diagnostic method. Dilution of the original specimens in liquid medium also allows a rapid estimation to be made of the number of organisms (Taylor-Robinson and Purcell, 1966) and provides assurance that the color changes observed are not spurious, which might be the case with a single vial of inoculated medium.

Colonies of *M. hominis*, *M. fermentans*, and *M. primatum* are about 200–300 μm in diameter and have a characteristic "fried egg" appearance due to a dense center of growth in the agar and a more translucent peripheral growth on the surface. Ureaplasmas were originally termed T strain or T mycoplasmas (T for tiny) because of the very small colonies they produce (15–30 μm in diameter). These colonies usually lack surface peripheral growth, hence do not have the "fried egg" morphology. However, colony size and appearance are hazardous criteria for identification. The volume of agar has been shown to affect the size and appearance of ureaplasma colonies, larger colonies forming on deep agar (Lee *et al.*, 1974a). Furthermore, on buffered medium ureaplasmas may develop typical colonies up to 300 μm (Manchee and Taylor-Robinson, 1969b), and ureaplasma colonies and, indeed, those of *M. hominis* and other mycoplasmas may be small and lack peripheral zones when crowded together.

On conventional blood agar, *M. hominis* strains, but not ureaplasmas, produce nonhemolytic pinpoint colonies, the organisms of which do not of course Gram-stain. *Mycoplasma hominis* also grows in most routine blood culture media, without changing their appearance, and blind subculture onto blood agar can be used by a routine laboratory to diagnose bloodstream invasion (Wallace *et al.*, 1978).

Mycoplasma medium is usually supplemented with penicillin G or with a broader-acting synthetic penicillin, such as ampicillin, which has no effect on the multiplication of mycoplasmas. Thallium acetate is also added as a bacterial inhibitor. However, ureaplasmas are much more sensitive to thallium than other mycoplasmas (Lee *et al.*, 1972a) and, although some investigators report that they have used it successfully at a low concentration, many are adamant that it has no place in the medium and choose to omit it. Lincomycin and erythromycin have differential effects on genital mycoplasmas (Braun *et al.*, 1970b). Lincomycin is active *in vitro* against *M. hominis* (minimal inhibitory concentration

(MIC) of 3.1 μg/ml) and *M. fermentans* (MIC of 0.16 μg/ml) but not against ureaplasmas (MIC of 500 μg/ml). Erythromycin has the reverse effect, inhibiting the multiplication of ureaplasmas (MIC of 12.5 μg/ml) but being far less active against *M. hominis* (MIC of 1000 μg/ml) and *M. fermentans* (MIC of 125 μg/ml). These differences in susceptibility have been used to separate genital mycoplasmas in culture (Braun *et al.*, 1970b; Csonka and Corse, 1970). However, definitive identification of genital mycoplasmas is made by means of the serological techniques described in the following section.

B. Serological Techniques

Numerous serological tests have been used for detecting antibody to mycoplasmas (Purcell *et al.*, 1969; Brunner *et al.*, 1973). Some methods are not very sensitive but are specific and therefore useful for identifying mycoplasmas. Thus growth inhibition on agar, in which specific antisera inhibit the development of colonies, falls into this category. The specific antisera are usually incorporated in disks which are then placed on the agar (Clyde, 1964), although placing the antisera in wells in the agar and other modifications increase the sensitivity of the technique (Black, 1973). *Mycoplasma hominis* and the other large-colony-forming mycoplasmas found in the genital tract are usually identified by the agar growth inhibition technique, although more than one antiserum to *M. hominis* may be required (Lin *et al.*, 1975). The same technique has been used to identify the serotypes of *U. urealyticum* (Black, 1973; Piot, 1976, 1977), although the metabolism inhibition test (Purcell *et al.*, 1966) and the complement-dependent mycoplasmacidal test (Lin *et al.*, 1972; Lin and Kass, 1973) have been more frequently employed. There is no doubt that the epi-immunofluorescence technique (Del Giudice *et al.*, 1967; Barile and Del Giudice, 1972), in which colonies on agar are identified directly with specific fluorescent antibody, holds a distinct advantage over other methods in that it affords the opportunity to detect a mixture of different mycoplasma species or ureaplasma serotypes. Mixtures are far less easily detected by other methods, the mycoplasma which grows best being the one most likely to be identified. Piot (1977) has demonstrated the existence of mixtures of ureaplasma serotypes in specimens from the male genital tract by means of the epi-immunofluorescence technique, and there is clearly a need for its more extensive use.

Several serological methods, such as radioimmunoprecipitation, mycoplasmacidal, metabolism inhibition, and indirect hemagglutination tests are both sensitive and specific and therefore useful for detecting low levels of antibody developed by a host as a result of mycoplasmal infection. The first method has not, so far, been used to study genital mycoplasmas. Indirect hemagglutination with sensitized erythrocytes has been used in studies of both *M. hominis* (Taylor-Robinson *et al.*, 1965) and ureaplasmas (Jansson *et al.*, 1971), but the method is difficult to standardize. In the metabolism inhibition test, specific metabolites (arginine for *M. hominis*, urea for ureaplasmas, etc.) are incorporated into broth containing phenol red, organisms, and antibody. The last-mentioned inhibits multiplication and metabolism of homologous organisms, thus preventing a change in color of the pH indicator (Purcell *et al.*, 1966). Complement in fresh guinea pig serum augments inhibitory activity (Taylor-Robinson *et al.*, 1966). The results of the test must be recorded when a color change commences, continued incubation often causing a decrease in antibody titers. Reading tests at the appropriate time is not always easy to achieve and failure to do so is a major cause of nonreproducibility of results. Lin and Kass (1970, 1975) showed that arginine and urea interfered with the killing of *M. hominis* and ureaplasma organisms, respectively, probably because of the release of ammonia and inactivation of ammonia-labile components of complement. They therefore devised a two-stage mycoplasmacidal test, antibody and complement being allowed to react with the organisms and kill them in the absence of arginine or urea, killing of the mycoplasmas then being demonstrated by addition of the appropriate substrate. The method is sensitive, but doubts have been raised (Ford and Henderson, 1976a; D. Taylor-Robinson, unpublished observations) about its alleged increased sensitivity as compared to the conventional metabolism inhibition technique. However, familiarity with a method is an important factor in its successful use.

IV. EPIDEMIOLOGY

A. Colonization of Infants

Infants become colonized with genital mycoplasmas usually during passage through the birth canal, since infants delivered by cesarean section are colonized less often than those delivered vaginally (Klein *et al.*, 1969). Ureaplasmas have been isolated from the vulval region of about one-quarter to one-third of infant girls, and *M. hominis* from a smaller proportion (Klein *et al.*, 1969; Foy *et al.*, 1970a; Braun *et al.*, 1971). The mucosa of the male genital tract is probably less exposed, and this is reflected in the less frequent recovery of mycoplasmas from the genital tracts of infant boys; Foy *et al.* (1970a) found that 6% of them were colonized by ureaplasmas. Mycoplasmas, mainly ureaplasmas, have been isolated from the nose and throat of up to about 15% of infants of both sexes (Klein *et al.*, 1969) and also from the umbilicus and conjunctivae. In one study (Prentice *et al.*, 1977), conjunctival colonization with ureaplasmas was detected in only about 2% of newborn infants, possibly because the eyes are closed before birth. The figures presented above are an estimate of the incidence of infant colonization by genital mycoplasmas. It is reasonable to suppose, however, that such figures may vary from one study to another, depending upon the proportion of pregnant women who are vaginally infected. As indicated in Section IV,C, this proportion depends on several factors and varies from one group of women to another.

Neonatal colonization by mycoplasmas does not persist. Those on the conjunctivae disappear rapidly, often within a week (M. J. Prentice, G. R. Hutchinson, and D. Taylor-Robinson, unpublished observations). There is also a progressive decrease in the proportion of infants who are colonized in the nose, throat, and genital tract. At the last-mentioned site, female infants have been found to harbor the organisms for a longer time than male infants, but Foy *et al.* (1970a) found that less than 5% of 1-year-olds were still colonized. This isolation rate may depend, however, on the population studied. Female infants who are still colonized at this time may carry the organisms into adult life (Hammerschlag *et al.*, 1978).

B. Colonization of Children

Genital mycoplasmas are rarely, if ever, isolated from prepubertal boys (Klieneberger-Nobel, 1959a,b; Lee *et al.*, 1974b; Foy *et al.*, 1975). Most investigators (Csonka *et al.*, 1966; Mårdh and Weström, 1970a; Lee *et al.*, 1974b) have found ureaplasmas in about 10% of prepubertal girls, and *M. hominis* usually in a smaller proportion, although Hammerschlag *et al.* (1978) recorded a somewhat higher ureaplasmal isolation rate. After puberty the isolation rate rises with increasing age, colonization to some extent probably reflecting sexual experience (see Section IV,C). Foy *et al.* (1975) found genital mycoplasmas in urine from girls of an earlier age (13 years) than boys (16 years), and the isolation rate among girls was eightfold higher than among boys of the same age.

C. Colonization of Adults

1. Role of Sexual Experience

After puberty, there is an increase in the proportion of men and women who are colonized by *M. hominis* and ureaplasmas, primarily through sexual contact. As shown in Table II, the frequency of infection, in both sexes, appears to be related to sexual activity. Thus, about 14% of men

TABLE II. Relationship of Sexual Experience to Male Urethral or Vaginal Colonization with Genital Mycoplasmas

Sexual experience	Normal male college students[a]			Female students and graduate nurses[b]		
	Number studied	With U. urealyticum (%)	With M. hominis (%)	Number studied	With U. urealyticum (%)	With M. hominis (%)
No genital contact	21	0	0	71	5.6	1.4
Genital contact without vaginal penetration	15	6.7	0	30	26.7	0
Sexual intercourse						
One partner	32	18.8	0	32	37.5	9.4
Two partners	23	26.1	4.3	11	54.5	9.1
Three or more partners	87	44.8	13.8	12	75.0	16.7

[a] Data of McCormack et al. (1973c).
[b] Data of McCormack et al. (1972b).

without overt disease who had considerable sexual experience were found to be infected with *M. hominis* and about 45% of them with ureaplasmas. Likewise, genital mycoplasmas were infrequently recovered from the vagina of sexually mature young women without a history of sexual contact, whereas *M. hominis* was recovered from about 17% and ureaplasmas from 75% of those who had had intercourse with three or more partners. It is interesting to note that colonization increases more rapidly with increasing sexual experience in women than in men, suggesting that women are more susceptible to colonization with these organisms. The above observations are in line with the infrequent occurrence of genital mycoplasmas in the urine of nuns (Archer, 1968; Kundsin *et al.*, 1971a, 1973), compared to the very frequent occurrence of the organisms in women with obvious sexual experience attending venereal disease clinics (Dunlop *et al.*, 1969; Gregory and Payne, 1970).

Infection of the adult male genitourinary tract by ureaplasmas may be transient (Coufalik *et al.*, 1979), the organisms disappearing spontaneously, or it may be persistent. As a result of repeated sexual contact, persistence may be more apparent than real. However, this is not always the case, as some strains have been shown to persist for a year in the absence of sexual contact (Holmes *et al.*, 1974; MacLeod *et al.*, 1976).

2. Other Factors Associated with Colonization

a. Race. Shepard (1954) and Holt *et al.* (1967) isolated genital mycoplasmas more frequently from black than from white men, although the comparability of sexual activity within the two groups was not assessed. The colonization rates among nonpregnant black women are also higher (McCormack *et al.*, 1973a,d). Furthermore, *M. hominis* and ureaplasmas have been isolated more frequently from black than from white pregnant women (Foy *et al.*, 1970b; Steytler, 1970; Braun *et al.*, 1971). The extent to which these differences are due to differences in sexual activity, the usual reason proposed, rather than to a real racial predisposition to colonization is not clear. However, recent evidence indicates that, when the sexual experience factor is carefully controlled, black women are still more often colonized by *M. hominis* and ureaplasmas than are other women (W. M. McCormack, unpublished observations).

b. Disadvantaged groups. In addition to the observations mentioned in Section IV,C,2,a, Ford (1967) reported that large-colony-forming mycoplasmas were twice as common among women in jail as among patients of private gynecologists. Furthermore, McCormack *et al.* (1973d) found *M. hominis* in 53.6% and ureaplasmas in 76.3% of patients attending prenatal and gynecology clinics at Boston City Hospital compared with 21.3 and

52.9%, respectively, of patients visiting private obstetricians and gynecologists in the same area. Whether this apparent socioeconomic difference is a reflection of a difference in sexual activity or whether other environmental factors are involved is unknown. Foy *et al.* (1975) found that colonization of adolescent girls by genital mycoplasmas was associated with certain sociological determinants such as dating and cigarette smoking, but this more advanced life-style is very likely to encompass sexual experimentation.

  c. **Contraception.** The evidence for different means of contraception influencing mycoplasmal colonization of the female genital tract is conflicting. McCormack (1974) found significantly higher rates of colonization by *M. hominis* in women with intrauterine devices than in those without, in agreement with the observations of Gregory and Payne (1970). However, the latter workers reported that oral contraceptives had no influence, whereas other workers (Mårdh and Weström, 1970a; McCormack *et al.*, 1973d) found *M. hominis* and ureaplasmas more frequently in women using oral contraceptives. Recently, Gump *et al.* (1975) reported that neither intrauterine devices nor oral contraceptives had any significant effect on genital colonization by *M. hominis* or ureaplasmas.

  d. **Menstrual cycle.** There are very few data on whether isolation is affected by acquiring specimens at different times in the menstrual cycle. Singer and Ivler (1975) reported that they had isolated genital mycoplasmas from women attending a family planning clinic more frequently after midcycle (75%) than at midcycle (56.5%).

  e. **Pregnancy.** In some studies (Freundt, 1958; Sachdev and Flamm, 1969) genital mycoplasmas were recovered about equally from pregnant and nonpregnant women. Although there are no studies in which sexual experience has been matched in the two groups, the weight of evidence suggests that both *M. hominis* and ureaplasmas are recoverable more frequently from pregnant women (Csonka *et al.*, 1966; Jones, 1967a; Archer, 1968; Mårdh and Weström, 1970a,b). Harwick *et al.* (1970) and de Louvois *et al.* (1975) found that the incidence of *M. hominis* increased between the first and third trimesters of pregnancy. Although not proven, the increased frequency of recovery during pregnancy may be due to changes in the local environment of the vagina, providing conditions conducive to mycoplasmal growth.

  f. **Menopause.** Comparisons of women in different age groups suggest that a decrease in the incidence of genital mycoplasmas occurs after the menopause (Csonka *et al.*, 1966; Archer, 1968; Mårdh and Weström, 1970a,b), although there has not always been control of the factors, already mentioned, that influence the results of comparing different groups of women.

g. Anatomical site. There is evidence that *M. hominis* exists more frequently in the prepuce than in the urethral canal, being isolated more often from uncircumcised men, particularly from the coronal sulcus, than from circumcised men. The rate of isolation of ureaplasmas, however, does not seem to be influenced by circumcision (Hare *et al.*, 1969; Taylor-Robinson and Furr, 1973; Tarr *et al.*, 1976), suggesting that they are more associated with the urethral canal than the glans or prepuce (Davis *et al.*, 1973).

In women, the organisms seem to be vaginal, since swabs from the vagina, the posterior fornix, or even the periurethral area are more likely to contain mycoplasmas than swabs obtained from the endocervical canal (Dunlop *et al.*, 1969; McCormack *et al.*, 1972a). This is worth emphasizing for two reasons. First, studies of gonorrhea have made the endocervix the site most likely to be sampled, not only for gonococci but also for mycoplasmas; and second, some studies may be facilitated by using self-obtained vaginal specimens.

The proximal urethra, bladder, uterus, and fallopian tubes are usually free of mycoplasmas, and the circumstances under which they become infected are discussed.

D. Serological Observations

Newborn infants, some of which are colonized by genital mycoplasmas, frequently possess serum antibodies to genital and other mycoplasmas (D. Taylor-Robinson and T. Feizi, unpublished observations) (Table III). These antibodies, however, appear to be of maternal origin and not due to a response of the infants to infection, since the antibody titers parallel the maternal serum antibody titers and antibody disappears by 6 months of age. Thereafter an increase is seen in the frequency of antibody to large-colony-forming mycoplasmas (Taylor-Robinson *et al.*, 1965; Jones and Sequeira, 1966; Purcell *et al.*, 1969; Mårdh and Weström, 1970b) and to ureaplasmas (Purcell *et al.*, 1966) at or soon after puberty. These results are consistent with the acquisition of genital mycoplasmas at this time. Correlation between the presence of mycoplasmas and the development of antibody was also seen in the study of Kundsin *et al.* (1973), in which the infrequent finding of metabolism-inhibiting antibody to ureaplasmas in the sera of nuns and its much more common occurrence in the sera of other groups of women correlated with the rate of isolation of ureaplasmas from women in the various groups.

In addition, Lin *et al.* (1978) showed that postpartum rises in the titers of *M. hominis* antibody are correlated with the presence of mycoplasmas in the genital tract and that almost 90% of women colonized with *M.*

TABLE III.   Mycoplasma Metabolism-Inhibiting Antibody in the Sera of Mothers and Their Infants at Birth and Subsequently[a]

Subject	Time at which serum was taken	Titer of antibody to:		
		M. hominis	*M. salivarium*	*M. pneumoniae*
Mother	Delivery and 6 months later	<2	16	4
Infant	Delivery	<2	2	4
	6 months later	<2	<2	<2
Mother	Delivery and 6 months later	<2	2	32
Infant	Delivery	2	4	64
	6 months later	<2	<2	<2
Mother	Delivery and 6 months later	<2	32	16
Infant	Delivery	<2	16	8
	6 months later	<2	<2	<2
Mother	Delivery and 6 months later	8[b]	4	<2
Infant	Delivery	8	4	<2
	6 months later	<2	<2	<2
Mother	Delivery and 6 months later	16	4	<2
Infant	Delivery	16	4	<2
	6 months later	<2	<2	<2

[a] Data of D. Taylor-Robinson and T. Feizi (unpublished observations).
[b] Titer rose to 64 at 6 months.

hominis and 40% colonized with *U. urealyticum* have significant changes in the titer of antibodies to these mycoplasmas throughout an apparently normal pregnancy. Furthermore, the possession of antibody is associated with the number of pregnancies, the lowest antibody titers being found in women experiencing their first pregnancy.

V. ROLE OF GENITAL MYCOPLASMAS IN DISEASES OF MEN

A. Nongonococcal Urethritis

1. Role of Large-Colony-Forming Mycoplasmas

a. Isolation studies. Soon after mycoplasmas were first isolated from the male urethra, attempts were made to determine whether they were a cause of nongonococcal urethritis (NGU) (Smith, 1942; Beveridge *et al.*, 1946), and many studies on large-colony-forming mycoplasmas have since been reported. Studies in which the findings in men with disease have been compared with those on men who were apparently healthy have been summarized previously (Taylor-Robinson *et al.*, 1969a), and several studies were analyzed in detail by King (1964). Because *M. fermentans* and *M. primatum* are rarely isolated from the genital tract in health or disease, they cannot be considered significant causes of NGU. Even though most of the mycoplasmas, particularly in the earlier studies, were not identified, it is reasonable to suppose that the majority of them were *M. hominis*. If this is so, when the studies are viewed as a whole, the frequency of isolation of this mycoplasma from men with disease and from apparently healthy men is not different. However, when the studies are considered separately (King, 1964), there are remarkable differences in results, probably because the criteria for selection of cases differed widely. Some of the earlier workers compared men suffering from NGU, 50% or more of whom were found to be infected, with medical personnel and even with boys in whom colonization rates were negligible (Beveridge *et al.*, 1946; Harkness and Henderson-Begg, 1948; Klieneberger-Nobel, 1959a,b). These differences were supported by differences in the prevalence of complement-fixing antibody in the various groups (Card, 1959). This disparity in isolation rate and antibody prevalence between one group and another led to the belief that *M. hominis* was of etiological importance. However, when control groups more comparable to the patients were studied, the differences in isolation rates were less apparent (Salaman, 1946; Melén and Linnros, 1952; Shepard, 1954; Freundt, 1956; Ford, 1960; Ford *et al.*, 1962; Ford and DuVernet, 1963; Csonka *et al.*, 1966; Ruys *et al.*, 1967; Hare *et al.*, 1969; Piot, 1976). Indeed, some workers (Osoba, 1972; Holmes *et al.*, 1975) have isolated *M. hominis* more frequently from persons without urethritis than from patients suffering from NGU. Recently, Bowie *et al.* (1977b,c) examined patients without urethritis and those suffering from NGU, dividing the latter into chlamydia-positive and chlamydia-negative groups. *Mycoplasma hominis* was isolated from the first voided urine of 19–22% of men in all the groups, and these investigators did not consider it a cause of disease.

   b. Studies based on differential antibiotics. Although, as mentioned previously, *M. hominis* is resistant to erythromycin *in vitro*, this antibiotic has been found to be effective in the treatment of NGU (Willcox, 1954, 1968). Conversely, lincomycin, which inhibits *M. hominis in vitro*, was found to be no more effective in treating the disease than a placebo (Csonka and Spitzer, 1969). Thus the effect of antibiotics on *M. hominis in vitro*, which does not correspond with their effect on the disease, has not lent support to the idea that this mycoplasma is pathogenic in the male urethra. In a recent study, Coufalik *et al.* (1978) used rifampicin, which is active against chlamydiae but ineffective against both *M. hominis* and ureaplasmas, to treat patients with NGU. Although the study was not designed to examine the pathogenic role of *M. hominis*, the results were not consistent with this mycoplasma being important. However, to further exclude this possibility it seems best to treat NGU patients infected by *M. hominis* and ureaplasmas but not by chlamydiae with lincomycin, which inhibits *M. hominis* but not ureaplasmas, and a similar group of patients with erythromycin, which has the reverse effect.

2. Role of *Ureaplasma urealyticum*

Numerous efforts have been made, since ureaplasmas were first isolated from the urethral discharge of men suffering from NGU (Shepard, 1954), to determine whether these organisms are a cause of the disease. Some of the studies have been commented upon previously (Taylor-Robinson *et al.*, 1969a; McCormack *et al.*, 1973a; Taylor-Robinson, 1976, 1977a).

a. Isolation studies. As shown in Table IV, in about half the investigations, ureaplasmas have been isolated significantly more frequently from patients suffering from NGU than from control subjects apparently free of disease, whereas in the other studies the rate of isolation in the two groups has been about the same. The factor which has probably contributed most to the difference between the results of one study and another is the selection of inappropriate controls. It seems desirable that subjects in the control group should be free from NGU and have sexual habits similar to those of patients suffering from the disease because, as mentioned before, the mycoplasmal isolation rate increases with increased sexual experience (McCormack *et al.*, 1973c). The overall equivocal results of the various studies certainly do not provide any incentive to continue this comparative approach. It is particularly difficult to obtain groups of persons of comparable sexual experience, although when this was achieved (Lee *et al.*, 1976), the rate of isolation in the groups with and without disease was about the same, again providing no evidence that ureaplasmas caused disease. One of the failures of the various studies is that they have been qualitative rather than quantitative, the numbers of organisms isolated from individual patients not having been documented. If ureaplasmas are involved in the pathogenic process, it is reasonable to expect them to be present in larger numbers than if they had a commensal role only. Hare *et al.* (1969), who studied postgonococcal, nonspecific urethritis, did not recover larger numbers of organisms from patients with disease, but Bowie *et al.* (1977a) and Weidner *et al.* (1978) have quantitative data to support the hypothesis. It is necessary, however, to be aware of the possibility that a larger number of organisms might be isolated from a patient who has a discharge than from one who has not, as a mere consequence of culturing a larger volume of material.

Wong *et al.* (1977) found that there was an association between ureaplasmas and NGU only when chlamydia-positive patients were excluded

TABLE IV. *Ureaplasma urealyticum* Isolated from the Genitourinary Tract of Men in Controlled Studies

Reference	Patients with NGU		Normal controls	
	Number studied	Percent positive	Number studied	Percent positive
Ford et al. (1962)	45	60	55	22
Ford and DuVernet (1963)	100	79	200	34
Csonka et al. (1966)	101	70	95	13
Shepard (1966)	1500	70–80	600	26
Ingham et al. (1966)	45	66	54	48
Ruys et al. (1967)	39	51	7	29
Holmes et al. (1967)	104	21	75	9
Black and Rasmussen (1968)	56	46	46	54
Catalano et al. (1968)	29	31	20	45
Shipley et al. (1968)	24	70	13	23
Fowler and Leeming (1969)	179	53	123	41
Hare et al. (1969)[a]	35	60	85	69
Haas et al. (1971)	52	65	27	47
Jansson et al. (1971)	157	58	36	53
Sueltmann et al. (1971)	193	68	36	25
Markham et al. (1972)	115	85	29	52
Osoba (1972)	93	19	65	20
Waldman (1972)	52	50	58	43
Bennett et al. (1973)	121	64	85	19
Davis et al. (1973)	34	64	15	20
Furness et al. (1973)	36	31	35	30
Hofstetter (1973)	93[b]	68	60	0
McChesney et al. (1973)	57	76	70	27
Mukhija et al. (1973b)	40	60	45	11
Sepetjian et al. (1973)	122	43	40	13
Sompolinsky et al. (1973)	78	63	28	7
Douboyas and Papapanagiotou (1975)	165	58	70	21
Holmes et al. (1975)	112	63	62	58
Lee et al. (1976)	57	44	43	63
Piot (1976)	47	57	66	50
Vaughan-Jackson et al. (1977)[a]	49	45	17	71

[a] A study of postgonococcal nonspecific urethritis.
[b] This group contained some patients with chronic prostatourethritis.

from their analysis. In addition, Bowie *et al.* (1976, 1977a,b,c) isolated ureaplasmas significantly more frequently and in larger numbers (Bowie *et al.*, 1977a) from patients with chlamydia-negative NGU than from those with chlamydia-positive urethritis. However, Taylor-Robinson *et al.* (1979) did not find this to be the case, so at the present time it seems unwise to believe that ureaplasmas are especially associated with chlamydia-negative disease.

b. Studies based on antibiotic therapy. *(1) Suboptimal therapy.* Shepard (1974) used suboptimal doses of doxycycline to treat patients with NGU. There was a temporary disappearance of both symptoms and ureaplasmas from the urine, and the return of symptoms was associated with a reappearance of the organisms in numbers similar to those found before treatment. A similar phenomenon was also noted in a man who was given a short course of tetracycline therapy for NGU which he had developed while enroute to an Antarctic base (MacLeod *et al.*, 1976). Because of the seclusion, the recurrence of symptoms and ureaplasmas about 3 weeks after therapy could not have been due to sexual reexposure. Although it is tempting to consider the concomitant return of symptoms and ureaplasmas as being indicative of a causative role for these organisms in NGU, this cannot be inferred because in neither of the studies mentioned were other tetracycline-sensitive organisms, such as chlamydiae, excluded.

(2) Placebo-controlled trial of tetracycline. Although there have been many trials of tetracycline in the treatment of NGU (Csonka, 1965; Grimble and Amarasuriya, 1975), few have been placebo-controlled or carried out with a comprehensive microbiological investigation. However, in such a placebo-controlled trial of minocycline, Prentice *et al.* (1976) not only obtained clear evidence that chlamydiae were etiologically involved in some cases but also noted a significant association between minocycline therapy and the resolution of symptoms and signs in patients from whom only ureaplasmas had been isolated. This provided some evidence for the pathogenicity of these organisms.

(3) Use of differential antibiotics. Another valuable approach to understanding the role of ureaplasmas in NGU is to treat patients with antibiotics which differentiate between ureaplasmas and other potentially pathogenic microorganisms.

Bowie *et al.* (1976, 1977a,b) found that urethritis persisted in men not only after treatment with aminocyclitols (streptomycin and spectinomycin), which eradicated ureaplasmas but not chlamydiae, but also after treatment with sulfafurazole which eliminated chlamydiae but not ureaplasmas. The results suggested therefore that both chlamydiae and ureaplasmas were important as a cause of NGU. Coufalik *et al.* (1979) treated patients suffering from NGU with minocycline or rifampicin, the latter being active *in vitro* against chlamydiae but inactive against ureaplasmas (Shepard *et al.*, 1974). This was borne out *in vivo*, because of 123 patients given rifampicin, chlamydiae were isolated after treatment from only 1 of 53 who were initially chlamydia-positive, whereas ureaplasmas were isolated from 55 of 68 men who were initially ureaplasma-positive. Clinically, rifampicin was less effective than minocycline, and patients infected with ureaplasmas failed to respond to rifampicin treatment significantly more often than those who were not infected. Furthermore, 44% of men whose ureaplasmas persisted failed to recover, whereas only about 8% of men whose ureaplasmas disappeared did not respond to treatment. These workers thought that their results suggested that ureaplasmas were a cause of urethritis in some of the men, an estimated 10% at least.

The occurrence of tetracycline-resistant ureaplasmas also provides a differential antibiotic situation. Ford and Smith (1974) were the first to isolate such an organism from a patient whose urethritis did not respond to this antibiotic. However, there was a clinical response to erythromycin, to which the ureaplasma was sensitive, which suggested that the organism caused the disease. Unfortunately, chlamydiae were not sought. The opportunity to repeat this observation in conjunction with more extensive microbiological investigations is likely to arise, since other workers have observed tetracycline-resistant ureaplasmas (Hofstetter *et al.*, 1976a; Spaepen *et al.*, 1976), such strains comprising about 10% of those isolated in different areas of London (Evans and Taylor-Robinson, 1978).

c. Serological studies. Jansson *et al.* (1971) found a rise or fall in antibody titer measured by indirect hemagglutination in 13 (24%) of 54 patients. In tests on the same sera, D. Taylor-Robinson (unpublished observations) could not reproduce these findings nor detect responses by the metabolism-inhibition technique. Indeed, nearly all attempts to detect antibody by the latter method have been unsuccessful (Purcell *et al.*, 1966, 1967; Ruys *et al.*, 1967; Catalano *et al.*, 1968; Fowler and Leeming, 1969; Hill *et al.*, 1973; Le Quan Sang and D. Taylor-Robinson, unpublished observations). However, Ford (1967) detected a small rise in antibody titer in 2 of 11 paired sera, and Black and Krogsgaard-Jensen (1974) found a few responses by both metabolism inhibition and immunofluorescence. To detect the maximum number of responses, the latter workers used a large number of ureaplasma serotypes in the metabolism inhibition test, a procedure also advocated by Lin (1977) for the complement-dependent mycoplasmacidal test. By means of this test, however, Bowie *et al.* (1977a) detected a fourfold rise or fall in titer of antibody in only 6 of 59 NGU patients. The persistence of ureaplasmas in the genitourinary tract and the existence of several serotypes at one time may culminate in failure to select the strain that has infected recently. This, in addition to a poor response of the host to infection of the genital mucosa, may explain the infrequent detection of antibody responses.

The available serological tests (Black and Krogsgaard-Jensen, 1974; Lin *et al.*, 1972) make it possible to serotype isolates and so determine whether a particular serotype is associated with NGU. Those who have done this (Lin *et al.*, 1972; Black, 1973; Piot, 1976; Lin, 1977) have not found any serotype to predominate, although the total number of isolates examined was relatively small. Piot (1977) found by using the epi-immunofluorescence technique that 36% of the isolates in his study consisted of more than one serotype. Clearly greater use of this method is to be recommended.

d. Studies in animal models and in human volunteers. Animal models may be of considerable value for studying NGU (Taylor-Robinson, 1977a; Taylor-Robinson *et al.*, 1978), and, indeed, the importance of the chimpanzee as a model of ureaplasmal infection has now been established (D. Taylor-Robinson, unpublished observations). It seems to be much more difficult to produce a persistent ureaplasmal infection reproducibly in lower primates (Bowie *et al.*, 1978). The use of ureaplasma-infected and, also, *M. hominis*-infected subcutaneous chambers in mice and guinea pigs (Kraus *et al.*, 1977) may be more applicable to the study of mycoplasmal infections which do not involve a mucosal surface.

It seems that the most certain way of determining whether ureaplasmas cause human urethritis is to infect humans deliberately. Volunteers have been used in many studies concerned with the etiology of infectious respiratory disease, but clearly there are greater problems with any study in which infection of the genitourinary tract is proposed. It does not seem reasonable or ethical to ask volunteers to be inoculated. However, Jänsch (1972) developed a polymorphonuclear cell discharge after inoculating himself intraurethrally with ureaplasmas. Unfortunately, their origin, purity of culture, and number inoculated have not been published, and it is difficult to assess whether the discharge was attributable to the ureaplasmas. In a study by Taylor-Robinson *et al.* (1977) two of the investigators inoculated themselves intraurethrally. Each subject received a different ureaplasma strain, although both strains were identified subsequently as Black's serotype 5. These strains had been isolated from patients with NGU from whom no other potentially pathogenic organisms could be recovered. Because it was necessary to make certain that the inocula contained ureaplasmas only, the strains to be inoculated were cloned three times during the course of nine passages on artificial media. Both subjects, free of ureaplasmas and other potentially pathogenic microorganisms, received about 5×10^4 ureaplasma organisms. The first subject (Fig. 1) developed urethritis characterized by dysuria, frequency, and urethral discomfort; early morning specimens of urine contained threads and had a hazy appearance, and there were polymorphonuclear leukocytes in the centrifuged deposits. Ureaplasmas were isolated consistently from the urine samples, but these and the associated symptoms and signs

Month (1975)		May	June		July		August	
Date		28 30 1 3 5 7 9 11 13 15 17 19 21 23 25 27 29		1 3 5 7 9		28 30 1 3 5 7 9 11 13 15		
Day postinoculation		1 3 5 7 9 11 13 15 17 19 21 23 25 27 29 31 33 35 37 39 41 43				62 64 2 4 6 8 10 12 14 16		
Event	Inoc. ureaplasmas 38α●	●—Minocycline therapy—●		Alcohol test●		Inoc. of medium●		
Symptoms	Urinary							
	Pyrexia							
	Arthralgia							
Appearance of urine	Thread							
	Bits							
	Haze							
Urine leukocyte count mm⁻³	40– 30– 20– 10–							
Polymorphs in centrifuged urine		+++ ++++	+	+ +	− − + − − −	− +		−
Titer of ureaplasmas in urine Orgs.ml⁻¹	10³– 10–							

● Urine IgG above normal

FIGURE 1. Observations on a human male subject before and after intraurethral inoculation of ureaplasmas. · or − indicates negative test. (From Taylor-Robinson et al., 1977.)

disappeared on institution of minocycline therapy and did not recur subsequently. The second subject also developed evidence of mild urethritis and, like the first, a transient metabolism-inhibiting antibody response. The predominant feature of disease in the second subject, however, was the appearance of urinary threads in which polymorphonuclear leukocytes were regularly observed. The threads persisted for at least 6 months after minocycline therapy, which eliminated the organisms from meatal, urine, and semen samples. The analysis of fractionated semen samples indicated that the ureaplasmas had infected the prostate, and therefore it is possible that the threads were of prostatic origin. However, their persistence following treatment, which was apparently effective in eliminating viable organisms, was mysterious. There was no evidence for the production of autoantibodies against prostatic tissue, but the results of immunofluorescence tests, performed with antiserum against the ureaplasmas that had originally been inoculated, suggested, but did not unequivocally prove, that the continued production of threads might be due to the persistence of ureaplasma antigen in a nonviable form. These results indicated that some ureaplasmas are likely to be pathogenic under natural conditions and that they may be capable of initiating chronic disease.

The report by Ford and Henderson (1976b), although not concerning a volunteer experiment, describes a similar situation in the sense that it was known that a man would come in contact, through intercourse, with ureaplasmas but not chlamydiae. He became infected, developed urethritis, and was cured only when his partner, in addition to himself, was treated with tetracycline.

B. Other Conditions

1. Balanitis and Paraurethral Abscess

Mycoplasma fermentans has been isolated from patients with balanitis (Ruiter and Wentholt, 1952), and unidentified large-colony-forming mycoplasmas from paraurethral abscesses (Dienes *et al.*, 1948; Krücken, 1959). In neither of these conditions, however, is there sufficient evidence to associate the organisms with the disease.

2. Acute and Nonacute Prostatitis

Some of the early workers (Dienes and Smith, 1942, 1946; Morton *et al.*, 1951) noted that many of the men from whom they isolated large-colony-forming mycoplasmas had prostatitis. Other investigators (Salaman, 1946; Röckl and Nasemann, 1959) isolated mycoplasmas about as frequently from patients with prostatitis as from healthy men. Some of these patients had urethroprostatitis and, although this must have been true of many subsequent studies of alleged NGU, the element of acute prostatitis has not usually been dissociated from urethritis. Hofstetter and colleagues (Marx and Hofstetter, 1975; Hofstetter, 1976, 1977) have investigated more than 4000 patients suffering from urethroprostatitis and, in recent years, patients attending a prostatitis clinic. Mycoplasmas, mainly ureaplasmas, were found significantly more often and in greater numbers (10^6 organisms/ml prostatic secretion) in the secretions of patients with disease than in those of healthy persons ($<10^3$ organisms/ml). However, the problems, discussed previously, of assessing the role of mycoplasmas, including ureaplasmas, in NGU must be relevant to acute urethroprostatitis and prostatitis. Furthermore, microorganisms found in expressed prostatic secretion may merely reflect those present in the urethra (Mårdh and Colleen, 1975). In this regard, it is interesting that Hofstetter (1977) isolated mycoplasmas from prostatic tissue biopsied by perineal punch. Although this procedure has its antagonists, it should obviously be exploited from a microbiological point of view whenever the opportunity arises.

Meares (1973) could not find ureaplasmas in the genital tracts of patients suffering from nonbacterial chronic prostatitis (prostatosis). However, Swedish investigators (Mårdh and Colleen, 1975; Colleen and Mårdh, 1975) found *M. hominis* in 10% of 79 patients with nonacute prostatitis but in none of 20 aged-matched controls with no history or signs of genital infection. Only one patient, mycoplasma-positive, possessed mycoplasmacidal serum antibodies to *M. hominis* (Mårdh *et al.*, 1975). To what extent these results can be regarded as indicating a real association between *M. hominis* and nonacute prostatitis is difficult to assess, but the difference in frequency of isolation is emphasized by the fact that the occurrence of ureaplasmas in the patients (47%) was not significantly different from that in the controls (35%). However, the possibility of ureaplasmas initiating chronic disease has been mentioned previously (Section V,A, 2d).

3. Reiter's Disease

a. Isolation studies. Mycoplasmas cause arthritis in animals, but numerous attempts to implicate them in rheumatoid arthritis have failed (Taylor-Robinson and Taylor, 1976). Several investigators have considered the possibility that arthritis and conjunctivitis following or concomitant with sexually transmissible NGU (Reiter's disease) might be due to mycoplasmal infection. However, when considering Reiter's disease, it is clear that the problems encountered in defining the role of mycoplasmas in NGU are no less apparent. In particular, whether the proportion of Reiter's patients who carry urethral organisms is greater than in a control group depends entirely on how the latter is selected, a point discussed previously. Several workers (Ford and Rasmussen, 1964; Csonka *et al.*, 1966; Ford, 1967, 1968) have isolated *M. hominis* and/or ureaplasmas from the genital tracts of Reiter's patients as frequently as from those suffering from NGU, and the strains seem serologically similar in both conditions (Ford, 1966). As expected, organisms are more likely to be isolated from patients with active than with inactive treated disease (Oates *et al.*, 1959). Indeed, a major difficulty in investigating Reiter's disease is that patients have often been treated with antibiotics before microbiological investigations can be attempted. An added problem is the part played by chlamydiae. Coufalik *et al.* (1979) saw two untreated NGU patients from whom ureaplasmas, but not chlamydiae, were isolated from the urethra and who subsequently developed arthritis. Clearly, ureaplasmas should not be ignored, and the best approach to the problem is to examine cases of NGU for both chlamydiae and mycoplasmas before Reiter's disease develops (Taylor-Robinson, 1979).

Attempts to isolate mycoplasmas from diseased joints have not met with much success. Dienes *et al.* (1948), using solid medium, isolated mycoplasmas from joint fluid in two cases of Reiter's disease. Bartholomew (1965) reported that he had isolated mycoplasmas from the synovial fluids taken from five of six patients with Reiter's disease or systemic lupus erythematosus. However, he used a cell culture technique, and it seems that the "isolates" came from mycoplasma-contaminated cells and not from the fluids. Jansson *et al.* (1972) isolated a mycoplasma, "related to *M. arthritidis*," from joint fluid, but the diagnosis of Reiter's disease was only tentative. The diagnosis was not in doubt, however, in a series of cases investigated by Ford (1967, 1968). He failed to isolate ureaplasmas from 15 synovial fluids, and other investigators have also been unsuccessful (see McCormack *et al.*, 1973a). Confirmation of the scanty evidence for the existence of mycoplasmas in the joints would help to establish the relationship between mycoplasmas and Reiter's disease beyond reasonable doubt. Failure to do so should not necessarily be regarded as an indication of a lack of association between mycoplasmas and disease, because it may be an immunopathological process triggered by organisms in the genital tract in individuals who are genetically predisposed to the development of Reiter's disease.

b. Serological studies. Ford and Henderson (1976a) and Ford (1977) detected low levels of metabolism-inhibiting antibodies to ureaplasmas in a somewhat higher proportion of patients with Reiter's disease than in patients attending a venereal disease clinic for a variety of reasons. The difference, however, was insufficiently striking to suggest an etiological association between the organisms and the disease. However, the data provided no evidence against such an hypothesis.

VI. ROLE OF GENITAL MYCOPLASMAS IN DISEASES OF WOMEN

A. Bartholin's Gland Abscess

A Bartholin's gland abscess was the site from which a human mycoplasma was first isolated (Dienes and Edsall, 1937). Unidentified mycoplasmas (Dienes and Smith, 1942; Dienes *et al.*, 1948), *M. hominis* (Russell and Fallon, 1970), and ureaplasmas (Solomon *et al.*, 1970) have been isolated subsequently. The possibility that these isolations were due to the gland being superficially contaminated by mycoplasma-containing secretions from the cervix and vagina rather than to infection of the gland was not excluded. Furthermore, the data did not indicate the proportion of abscesses that might have a mycoplasmal etiology. However, Lee *et al.* (1977) have probably answered these questions by examining percutaneous aspirates from 34 intact Bartholin's gland abscesses and 12 cysts for genital mycoplasmas and other microorganisms. Most of the isolates were gonococci, Gram-negative bacilli and mixed aerobic and anaerobic organisms that are part of the vaginal flora. Although genital mycoplasmas were isolated from the vagina of most of the patients, *M. hominis* was isolated from only one and ureaplasmas from none of the aspirates.

B. Vaginitis and Cervicitis

1. Isolation Studies

a. *Mycoplasma hominis*. As in the studies of NGU in men, a majority of the large-colony-forming mycoplasmas isolated in early studies were not identified specifically, although it is likely that most of them were *M. hominis*. The results of studies up to about 1963, summarized previously (Taylor-Robinson *et al.*, 1969a), indicated that the isolation rate in persons with disease was more than twice that in persons considered to be free of disease. However, interpretation of this is difficult, because most investigators do not provide a precise clinical definition of the disease and selection of control groups may not always have been appropriate. It is particularly difficult to ensure that women in control groups are disease-free. Furthermore, the possibility cannot be excluded in many cases that another microorganism caused the disease and at the same time provided conditions favorable for the growth of mycoplasmas. Indeed, it has been shown in several studies that *M. hominis* is more frequently isolated when there is infection by another microorganism. Thus there has been an increased rate of isolation of *M. hominis* from patients with vaginitis associated with *Trichomonas vaginalis* (Freundt, 1953; Nicol and Edward, 1953; Bercovici *et al.*, 1962; Holt *et al.*, 1967; Müller *et al.*, 1967; Romano and Romano, 1968; Mendel *et al.*, 1970). Furthermore, an increase in the rate of isolation of large-colony-forming mycoplasmas or *M. hominis* has been found in women infected by gonococci (Salaman, 1946; Nicol and Edward, 1953; Somerson *et al.*, 1955; Klieneberger-Nobel, 1959a,b), in women infected by *Haemophilus vaginalis* (Edmunds, 1958; Spitzbart, 1967; Mendel *et al.*, 1970), and in women with monilial vaginitis (Bercovici *et al.*, 1962; Romano and Romano, 1968; Mendel *et al.*, 1970). The increased mycoplasmal isolation rate is often associated with a rise in vaginal pH (Freundt, 1953; Huijsmans-Evers and Ruys, 1956; Bercovici *et al.*, 1962; Romano and Romano, 1968; Mårdh *et al.*, 1975), which occurs when the normal flora, consisting mainly of lactobacilli, is replaced by a mixed flora. Furthermore, de Louvois *et al.* (1975) noted that the isolation rate of *M. hominis* in early pregnancy was increased when lactobacilli were adjudged to be absent.

Mycoplasma hominis has been isolated from one-third (Bercovici *et al.*, 1962; Mendel *et al.*, 1970) to 50% or more (Csonka *et al.*, 1966; Mårdh and Weström, 1970b,c; Mårdh, 1972) of women with nongonococcal or nonspecific vaginitis and cervicitis, the latter being a disease from which other organisms were not isolated. The high isolation rate noted by the Swedish workers was in women who had clinical and cytological signs of lower genital tract infections which may not have been entirely confined to the cervix and vagina. In women in whom such signs were absent, the isolation rate was about 5%. This may suggest an etiological relationship, but there are no data concerning the sexual activity of the women in the two groups. Furthermore, the complicating factor of the role of chlamydiae was not considered, although these organisms are far more likely to be related to cervicitis than to vaginitis. de Louvois *et al.* (1975) observed that the isolation rate of *M. hominis* was increased in women suspected of having vulvovaginitis in pregnancy, a finding they thought was worth further investigation.

b. *Ureaplasma urealyticum.* In contrast to the isolation results for *M. hominis*, Romano and Romano (1968) did not isolate ureaplasmas more frequently from patients with nonspecific vaginitis, or trichomonal or monilial vaginitis, than from women in a control group. Nor could Mårdh and Weström (1970a) demonstrate any significant difference in the isolation rate for ureaplasmas from the lower genital tract of women with signs of infection than from a carefully matched control group without signs. Kundsin *et al.* (1973) isolated ureaplasmas from 80% of women with genitourinary tract infections, including cervicitis and vaginitis, and from 51% of women with reproductive problems who were otherwise asymptomatic and who visited private practitioners. The difference in isolation rates probably reflects the difference in sexual attitudes of the women in the two groups, those in the latter group being more selective in their sexual contacts.

2. Studies Based on Antibiotic Therapy

Some of these studies have given conflicting results. Thus in a study of patients with positive cultures for both *T. vaginalis* and *M. hominis* (Bercovici *et al.*, 1962), treatment that eliminated only *T. vaginalis* led to clinical improvement, whereas treatment that eliminated only *M. hominis* did not. However, in a study of 12 patients who had positive cultures for both microorganisms, treatment with metronidazole, which eradicated *T. vaginalis* but not *M. hominis*, did not result in clinical cure (Weström and Mårdh, 1971). Pheifer *et al.* (1978) also used metronidazole to treat patients suffering from nonspecific vaginitis. The drug had no effect on *M. hominis*, but it eliminated *H. vaginalis*, and this was associated with clinical improvement. Less confusing are the results of studies in which antibiotics which inhibit *M. hominis in vitro,* such as tetracyclines, have been given to women harboring this mycoplasma (Leberman *et al.*, 1952; Bercovici *et al.*, 1962; Weström and Mårdh, 1971). Treatment has usually produced a clinical cure, with disappearance of the abnormal cytological picture and eradication of the organisms. It may of course be argued that clinical improvement is due to eradication of some other tetracycline-sensitive organisms and, on the whole, the results of all these various studies do not suggest an important role for *M. hominis* in vaginitis.

3. Serological Studies

Mårdh and Weström (1970b) and Mårdh *et al.* (1975) detected indirect hemagglutinating antibodies to *M. hominis* in the sera of 27.1% of women with lower genital tract infections and in those of 10.5% of noninfected healthy controls. Moreover, Kundsin *et al.* (1973) found that the incidence of metabolism-inhibiting antibody to several ureaplasmas was greatest in a group of women with lower genital tract infections than in other groups of women. However, the reservations mentioned previously about regarding differences in isolation rates as being indicative of an etiological relationship also apply to antibody studies.

C. Pelvic Inflammatory Diseases

1. Isolation Studies

a. *Mycoplasma hominis.* There have been numerous reports of the isolation of large-colony-forming mycoplasmas (Dienes and Smith, 1942; Dienes *et al.*, 1948; Randall *et al.*, 1950; Hirsch, 1952; Gotthardson and Melén, 1953; Stokes, 1955; Klieneberger-Nobel, 1959a; Zeltzer and Palti, 1963), including *M. hominis* (Russell and Fallon, 1970; Solomon *et al.*, 1970, 1973; Eschenbach *et al.*, 1975) and *M. fermentans* (Freundt, 1953), from inflamed fallopian tubes, tuboovarian abscesses, and pelvic abscesses or fluid. However, the most illuminating observations have been made by Swedish investigators (Mårdh and Weström, 1970c; Mårdh *et al.*, 1975; Weström and Mårdh, 1975). They studied 50 women with salpingitis diagnosed by direct vision through a laparoscope, 50 women with lower genital tract infections, and 50 carefully matched noninfected women who served as controls. Specimens were obtained directly from the fallopian tubes, and *M. hominis* was isolated from the tubes of 4 (8%) women with salpingitis. In no case did tubal specimens from women without signs of salpingitis yield *M. hominis*. In addition, there were more isolations of *M. hominis* from cervical and urethral cultures of patients with salpingitis than from the control patients. Although *Neisseria gonorrhoeae* was isolated from the cervix or urethra of 17 of the 50 patients with salpingitis and from the tubes of 2 of them, the latter isolations were not concurrent with those of *M. hominis*. Eschenbach *et al.* (1975) also found *M. hominis,* but not ureaplasmas, more often in endocervical swabs from women with acute pelvic inflammatory disease than in those from women in a comparison group without inflammatory disease; in one instance, *M.*

hominis was isolated from a culdocentesis specimen taken from a patient with inflammatory disease. However, for persons without gonococcal disease the mycoplasmal isolation rates in the two groups were little different, being 64 and 54%, respectively.

b. *Ureaplasma urealyticum.* Ureaplasmas have been less extensively studied, but they were isolated directly from the fallopian tubes of 2 of 50 patients with acute salpingitis (Mårdh and Weström, 1970c) and from pelvic fluid (Solomon *et al.*, 1973; Eschenbach *et al.*, 1975) and from a tuboovarian abscess (Braun and Besdine, 1973).

2. Organ Culture Studies

Tissues can be maintained in an organ culture system more or less in the same physiological condition as they occur *in vivo*. Organ cultures of genital mucosa provide a valuable tool for looking at the relationship that exists between a microorganism and the epithelial cell surface. Fallopian tube organ cultures are particularly useful, because ciliary activity may be assessed and used as an index of cell viability. In such cultures, *N. gonorrhoeae* has been shown to produce profound damage to the epithelium (Carney and Taylor-Robinson, 1973; Taylor-Robinson *et al.*, 1975a). In contrast, *M. hominis* organisms multiplied and persisted in the cultures, but they did not cause damage (Taylor-Robinson and Carney, 1974). However, Mårdh *et al.* (1976) observed by scanning electron microscopy that the organisms induced pathological changes in the ciliated cells in the form of ciliary swelling. This may be due to the effect of ammonia produced by mycoplasmal metabolism. The reason for believing this is that ciliary swelling has been observed in bovine oviduct cultures infected by bovine ureaplasmas (Stalheim *et al.*, 1976) and has been attributed to ammonia production (Stalheim and Gallagher, 1977).

Ureaplasmas of human origin have been inoculated into fallopian tube organ cultures without obvious damage ensuing (Taylor-Robinson and Carney, 1974). It may be worthwhile, however, to look at their effect again by means of the quantitative technique of assessing ciliary activity described by McGee *et al.* (1976). Failure to demonstrate loss of activity cannot necessarily be taken as meaning avirulence of the ureaplasmas, since the organ culture system is divorced from the immunological mechanisms of the host which may play an integral part in pathogenesis.

3. Serological Studies

Complement-fixing antibodies to large-colony-forming mycoplasmas, presumably *M. hominis,* were found by Melén and Gotthardson (1955), and to *M. hominis* by Lemcke and Csonka (1962), in some patients with salpingitis. The antibody titers were greater than in sera from other groups of women serving as controls. In addition, indirect hemagglutinating antibodies to *M. hominis* were demonstrated in the sera of 53.8% of patients with salpingitis, compared to 10.5% of healthy women (Mårdh and Weström, 1970b). Furthermore, significant rises or falls in antibody titer were detected during the course of disease in the sera of 9 of 16 women who had *M. hominis* in the lower genital tract, 3 of them also having the organisms in their fallopian tubes (Mårdh and Weström, 1970b). Mårdh (1970) also found an increased level of IgM in 34% of patients with acute salpingitis. This was associated with the isolation of *M. hominis* and with the presence of indirect hemagglutinating antibody to the mycoplasma. A rise in titer of metabolism-inhibiting antibody to ureaplasmas was demonstrated in only 1 of 50 patients with salpingitis (Mårdh and Weström, 1970a). Eschenbach *et al.* (1975), who used the mycoplasmacidal test, also detected a greater number of antibody responses to *M. hominis* in paired sera from patients with acute pelvic inflammatory disease than in a selected control group.

These various data, in particular those concerning *M. hominis,* suggest that mycoplasmas may have a primary pathogenic role in some cases of acute pelvic inflammatory disease. This suggestion is not unreasonable when an organism has been isolated from a site where it does not normally occur and has stimulated an antibody response. Furthermore, it is supported by the finding that *M. hominis* inoculated into the oviducts of grivet monkeys produced salpingitis and an antibody response (Møller *et al.*, 1978). However, although mycoplasmas were isolated apparently in pure culture from human fallopian tubes, chlamydiae were not sought in the studies mentioned. The subsequent isolation of chlamydiae from fallopian tubes of persons suffering from salpingitis (Eilard *et al.*, 1976; Mårdh *et al.*, 1977), and therefore their possible occurrence in the tubes of patients from whom *M. hominis* and ureaplasmas have been isolated, means that the role of these mycoplasmas in pelvic inflammatory disease needs to be reassessed.

D. Postabortal Fever

Isolation and Serological Studies

Mycoplasma hominis has been isolated from the blood of two patients with septic abortion, each of whom developed an antibody response (Tully *et al.*, 1965; Harwick *et al.*, 1967), and from the blood of another patient (Solomon *et al.*, 1973). In addition, Jones (1967b) isolated *M. hominis* from the vagina of 36 women who aborted. Three of them had been febrile at the time of abortion, and they developed a rise in the titer of *M. hominis* complement-fixing antibody after abortion. In another study (Harwick *et al.*, 1969) (Table V), amniotic fluid taken from 50 patients yielded *M. hominis* on 4 occasions, 3 of the 4 patients being febrile.

The most striking evidence for the role of *M. hominis* in postabortal fever comes from a prospective study by Harwick *et al.* (1970). They isolated *M. hominis* from the blood of 4 (7.8%) of 51 women who had febrile abortions but not from 53 women who had afebrile abortions or from 102 normal pregnant women. *Mycoplasma hominis* occurred also more frequently in the cervix of women who had febrile abortions. Furthermore, antibody responses to *M. hominis* were detected in 50% of women who had febrile abortions but in only 2 (14%) of 14 women who had afebrile abortions.

A suggestion that ureaplasmas might cause postabortal fever is seen in the results of a study by Stray-Pedersen *et al.* (1978). Retrospective examination of gynecological histories revealed that 6 of 13 habitual abortion patients with ureaplasma-positive endometria had suffered from postabortal fever, whereas only 1 of 33 patients with negative cultures had done so. However, the evidence was inconclusive, because bacteria were significantly associated with the ureaplasma-positive cultures.

E. Postpartum Fever

Isolation and Serological Studies

The relation between vaginal colonization with *M. hominis* or ureaplasmas and puerperal fever is not absolutely clear. McCormack *et al.* (1973b) detected no association between the isolation of these organisms from vaginal cultures and postpartum fever in a study of over 300 women examined consecutively. However, in another study (Jones, 1967a), 6 of 13 women harboring *M. hominis* developed postpartum fever and 5 developed an antibody response, whereas only 2 of 12 women from whom *M. hominis* was not isolated developed fever, and there were no antibody responses. In addition, Harwick *et al.* (1971) isolated *M. hominis* from the cervix of 12 (32%) of 37 patients with postpartum fever but from only 4 (11%) of 37 afebrile patients serving as controls. They also found more serological responses to *M. hominis* among the febrile patients than among the controls. The association between vaginal colonization and postpartum fever is likely to be best seen where there is uterine invasion before or after delivery. Such invasion undoubtedly occurs, as shown in Table V, ureaplasmas having been isolated more frequently than *M. hominis*. There is a greater chance of isolation being made following previous vaginal examination and prolonged labor (Caspi *et al.*, 1976) but, as shown in Table V, both sorts of microorganisms are most likely to be isolated after rupture of the membranes (Caspi *et al.*, 1976); according to Jones and Tobin (1969), the longer the interval between membrane rupture and delivery, the greater the chance of placental or amniotic fluid contamination by mycoplasmas. These investigators cultured the amniotic surface of placentas obtained at cesarean section. They found that patients who had placental cultures positive for *M. hominis* or ureaplasmas were more likely to be febrile after delivery than those who had negative cultures, and that there had been prolonged rupture of the membranes in most of the febrile women. A similar finding was reported by Caspi *et al.* (1976), but it does not necessarily mean that mycoplasmas cause the fever, because other vaginal microorganisms can be isolated following prolonged rupture of the membranes.

Since mycoplasmas within the vagina can invade the uterus, it is perhaps not surprising that, after delivery, as after abortion, a proportion of them are capable of entering the blood. Indeed, McCormack *et al.* (1975) detected a transient invasion by *M. hominis* for a few minutes after delivery. This was probably not associated with fever because, although 5 (50%) of 10 women with *M. hominis* in the blood developed fever, 93 (31%) of 301 women from whom the mycoplasma was not isolated also developed fever. However, more persistent invasion after delivery has been noted for large-colony-forming mycoplasmas (Slingerland and Morgan, 1952) including *M. hominis* (Stokes, 1955; Tully and Smith, 1968; Sharp, 1970; Russell and Fallon, 1970; Solomon *et al.*, 1973; Wallace *et al.*, 1978) and ureaplasmas (Caspi *et al.*, 1971; Sompolinsky *et al.*, 1971; Solomon *et al.*, 1973; R. Platt, unpublished observations). The various results indicate that *M. hominis* strains can be isolated from the blood of about 8% of febrile women after delivery (McCormack *et al.*, 1973b) and that no particular serotype predominates (Lin *et al.*, 1976). Furthermore, an antibody response is detectable in nearly all cases (McCormack *et al.*, 1975; Lin, 1977; Wallace *et al.*, 1978). Thus the isolation of *M. hominis* from the blood of febrile patients long after delivery, an antibody response, and the apparent absence of the mycoplasma from the blood of patients who are well (Wallace *et al.*, 1978) are points strongly in favor of *M. hominis* causing some cases of postpartum fever. The patients develop a low-grade fever for a day or two after delivery, are not severely ill, and recover uneventfully even without antibiotic therapy (Wallace *et al.*, 1978). How often *M. hominis*-endometritis occurs without bloodstream invasion and its contribution to postpartum fever are outstanding questions. Some information on these points is provided by a study of R. Platt and W. M. McCormack (unpublished) in which antibody responses to *M.*

hominis were found in about 50% of women with unexplained mild postpartum fever.

Although ureaplasmas may be found in the blood of women after delivery, bloodstream invasion is far less frequently associated with an antibody response (Harwick *et al.*, 1971; McCormack *et al.*, 1975; Lin, 1977), and it is much less certain that they are responsible for postpartum fever.

Mycoplasmas have also been isolated from the blood of men (see Section VII).

VII. ROLE OF GENITAL MYCOPLASMAS IN DISORDERS OF THE URINARY TRACT

The role of genital mycoplasmas in extragenital disease has been reviewed by McCormack (1977), and it is particularly appropriate that disorders of the urinary tract should be considered in a discussion of genital mycoplasmas.

In a study of infants, a few days to 2 months old, 250 urine specimens obtained by suprapubic bladder puncture were cultured for genital mycoplasmas (Lee *et al.*, 1974b). Only one specimen, from a patient who had an *Escherichia coli* urinary tract infection, contained *M. hominis*. There is therefore no evidence to implicate genital mycoplasmas as a cause of urinary tract infection in infants. In older children, particularly after puberty, there is evidence that the urinary tract occasionally becomes invaded by genital mycoplasmas. Thus Foy *et al.* (1975) found genital mycoplasmas more frequently in the urine of adolescent girls who had abnormal urine analyses or in postpubertal girls attending a renal clinic than in other girls of comparable age. However, they had insufficient evidence to incriminate the organisms as a cause of renal disease, believing that more sophisticated clinical studies were necessary.

A. Cystitis

There are early reports (Dienes and Smith, 1946; Dienes *et al.*, 1948; Harkness and Henderson-Begg, 1948) of the isolation of mycoplasmas from the urine of adult patients of both sexes with abacterial pyuria and/or acute hemorrhagic cystitis. Berg *et al.* (1957) described a series of 15 men suffering from acute hemorrhagic cystitis in whom mycoplasmas were recovered from urine during the active phase of the disease. These workers also observed remission of symptoms and a simultaneous disappearance of the organisms after treatment with streptomycin. Pachas (1970) described a similar case, *M. hominis* being isolated from the urine of a woman who improved symptomatically following tetracycline therapy. However, whether the mycoplasmas in these cases were present in the bladder or whether isolation from urine only represents their presence in the urethra or prepuce is not known. Observation of the existence of mycoplasmas in suprapubic cystostomy specimens from such patients and not from those who are disease-free would be a valuable finding, but even so, evidence that the organisms were associated with the bladder mucosal lesions and that they were not just free in the urine would need to be considered. The fact that mycoplasmas have been found above the urethra (see Section VII, B and C) means that there is a possibility of their causing cystitis, but other potential pathogenic microorganisms, such as chlamydiae, have also to be taken into account.

B. Urinary Calculi

Friedlander and Braude (1974) produced magnesium-ammonium phosphate stones in the bladders of male, but not female, rats by inoculating ureaplasmas directly into the bladder or renal pelvis. The production of calculi is thought to be related, *inter alia,* to the urease activity of the organisms and can be prevented by treating the animals with acetohydroxamic acid (Lamm *et al.*, 1977). Mårdh *et al.* (1975) wondered whether ureaplasmas could be associated with the production of calculi in humans too, and they have searched for such organisms in the urinary tract and kidney tissue of patients with calculi in the ureter and/or renal pelvis who were subjected to nephrectomy or pyelolithotomy. In the case of two such patients, ureaplasmas were isolated, not only from urine collected from the ureter and renal pelvis, but also from the renal cortex and medulla. Further investigations of this kind are obviously needed.

C. Nephritis

The isolation of *M. salivarium,* but not bacteria, from the renal cortex of a man who had focal glomerulonephritis and chronic focal pyelonephritis was described by Pachas (1970). Cultures of a renal biopsy obtained 2 years later were sterile, and a serological response to the mycoplasma was not demonstrated. It was postulated that there had been hematogenous spread of the mycoplasma from the oropharynx of the patient but, in view of its identification as an oropharyngeal commensal, accidental contamination of the kidney tissue by organisms in the mouths of the investigators is another possibility. The significance of the finding is unclear, and no conclusions can be drawn on the basis of a single report.

The ascent of mycoplasmas from the lower genitourinary tract is probably a more likely means by which they might infect the kidney. Witzleb et al. (1968) found more than 10^5 genital mycoplasma organisms per milliliter of urine in 12 (16%) of 75 patients with infections of the urinary tract, including chronic pyelonephritis, such numbers of organisms not being found in a disease-free group of 71 persons. No distinction was made between M. hominis and ureaplasmas and, even though midstream urine specimens were examined, it is not possible to say in which part of the urinary tract the organisms were present. However, the same workers (Witzleb et al., 1969) examined urines taken by suprapubic cystostomy. They found mycoplasmas not only in the urines of 3 of 30 patients suffering from urinary tract infections, mostly chronic pyelonephritis, but also in those of 3 of 30 patients with other diseases of the urinary tract. In view of the latter finding, it is difficult to know the relationship, if any, of the organisms to pyelonephritis, even though they were not recovered from 21 persons without disease. Mårdh et al. (1972) also examined suprapubic aspiration specimens, as well as voided urines, from 87 patients, all of whom had findings suggestive of urinary tract infection and 42 of whom had a diagnosis of chronic pyelonephritis. Mycoplasma hominis was isolated by cystostomy from 2.3% of the cases, and ureaplasmas were isolated from 11.5%. Because patients without signs of inflammatory disease were not included in the study and because the mycoplasmas were isolated from bacteria-positive cases as frequently as from bacteria-negative ones, it is not surprising that these investigators came to no conclusion about the significance of the organisms in causing disease. It is worth noting that only seven of the patients in the series were men, so that, although the frequency with which mycoplasmas occur in the bladder and upper urinary tract of men in health and disease is not clear, one might surmise that it is less than in women. Bredt et al. (1974) isolated ureaplasmas from 13.6% and M. hominis from about 1% of 257 urine specimens collected by suprapubic cystostomy. They thought that preexisting damage favored infection of the kidneys and/or upper urinary tract.

Thomsen (1974) isolated ureaplasmas from the cortex of a kidney showing nonspecific inflammation at autopsy. Later, he isolated M. hominis from the upper urinary tract of 3 women and ureaplasmas from the renal pelvis of 2 women in a group of 40 patients with chronic pyelonephritis, but not from the upper urinary tract of 40 patients with noninfectious urinary tract diseases (Thomsen, 1975). Only 1 of the 3 patients who harbored M. hominis had associated bacteriuria, and all had signs of acute exacerbation of pyelonephritis, 2 of them developing an antibody response to the mycoplasma. More recently, Thomsen (1978a) also isolated

M. hominis from the upper urinary tract of 7 of 80 patients with acute pyelonephritis; in 4 of these cases, the mycoplasma was isolated apparently in pure culture. Antibodies to *M. hominis,* measured by indirect hemagglutination, were demonstrable in serum and in ureteric and bladder urine from some of these patients (Thomsen, 1978b). In contrast, the mycoplasma was not recovered from the upper urinary tract of 60 patients with noninfectious urinary diseases, and antibody was not detected. *Ureaplasma urealyticum* strains were isolated from the upper urinary tract of 5 patients, one of whom was also infected by *M. hominis,* but the ureaplasmal isolation rate was not significantly different from that in the control group. The data suggest that *M. hominis* causes some cases of acute pyelonephritis, that it is associated with acute exacerbations of chronic pyelonephritis, but that ureaplasmas are unlikely to be involved. The same group of investigators (Thomsen *et al.*, 1973; Rosendal and Thomsen, 1974) also produced focal suppurative pyelonephritis in rats with a strain of *Mycoplasma arthritidis,* obstruction of the ureter being an important factor in the development of disease. This model may have a useful function in further investigations in this area.

Mycoplasmemia. The occurrence of *M. hominis* in the blood is not entirely confined to women. Simberkoff and Toharsky (1976) found this mycoplasma to be present transiently in the blood of five men who had had obstruction, manipulation, or surgery of the genitourinary tract. One man developed a metabolism-inhibiting antibody response, and all were pyrexial. Two of the men became afebrile after tetracycline therapy, one did so without treatment, and the other two died of their underlying disease.

VIII. ROLE OF GENITAL MYCOPLASMAS IN DISORDERS OF REPRODUCTION

The association of genital mycoplasmas with various aspects of reproductive disorders was reviewed by McCormack (1976).

A. Involuntary Infertility

Mycoplasmas could reduce male fertility by inhibiting spermatogenesis, causing the formation of abnormal spermatozoa, reducing sperm motility, and impairing the passage of spermatozoa as a consequence of damaging the genital tract. In the female genital tract, mycoplasmas might directly interfere with the transmission of spermatozoa and with the fertilization of ova. Inflammatory changes within the genital tract caused by mycoplasmas could also produce these effects and, in addition, interfere with the movement and implantation of ova and so reduce female fertility. The influence of mycoplasmas on male fertility is considered separately but, because the fertility of a union is the sum of the fertilities of the two partners, particular attention is given to the "infertile couple."

1. Male Infertility

Taylor-Robinson and Manchee (1967, 1969) demonstrated that spermatozoa adsorbed to colonies and suspensions of certain mycoplasmas, including some strains of ureaplasmas. This raised the question, considered by several investigators, of whether mycoplasmas, in particular ureaplasmas, might cause male infertility. Thus semen samples from men who accompanied their wives to an infertility clinic, and samples from a few men seeking advice from their general practitioners, were examined for volume, sperm number, motility, and aberrant forms (Taylor-Robinson and Furr, 1973); on the basis of these factors, the men were graded into normal or low-fertility categories. Ureaplasmas were isolated from 47% of the specimens from men of normal fertility and from 57% of those from men of low fertility. Further, Vogt (1973) found about an equal distribution of ureaplasmas among normal and abnormal seminal fluids, although the frequency of isolation in this study was low. In another study, Schoub et al. (1976) found M. hominis and ureaplasmas in seminal fluids which had normal cytology as frequently as in those in which the cytology was regarded as pathological. O'Leary and Frick (1975) found that samples in which there were no spermatozoa contained ureaplasmas even less frequently than samples in which there were more than 20×10^6 spermatozoa per milliliter. However, the presence of ureaplasmas was associated with decreased sperm motility. In another investigation, but one in which the results were subjected to a more detailed analysis, Fowlkes et al. (1975a) concluded that semen samples containing ureaplasmas also had poorer motility, in addition to fewer spermatozoa and more aberrant forms, than samples without ureaplasmas. S. Yoshida, Y. Saito, and M. Yoshioka (unpublished observations) have also noted abnormally shaped spermatozoa in semen samples containing ureaplasmas but not in ureaplasma-free samples. Recently, Jurmanova and Sterbova (1977) reported that spermatozoa in bovine semen samples containing mycoplasmas, including ureaplasmas, were less motile than those in samples not containing them, but it was not made clear which species of mycoplasma was responsible. Furthermore, a small reduction in sperm motility has been observed in experiments in which bovine spermatozoa have been mixed with M. bovis (E. V. Langford, personal communication) and in those in which human spermatozoa have been mixed with large numbers of suspended *M. hominis,* ureaplasmas, or other mycoplasma organisms (Hofstetter *et al.*, 1976b). Decreased motility could be brought about by the adherence of ureaplasmas (Gnarpe and Friberg, 1972, 1973b; Fowlkes *et al.*, 1975b) and *M. hominis* (Busolo *et al.*, 1975; D. Taylor-Robinson and P. M. Furr, unpublished observations) to spermatozoa.

Attempts to isolate genital mycoplasmas from the vas deferens taken at vasectomy from men who had *M. hominis* and/or ureaplasmas in urine or seminal samples have been unsuccessful (Traub *et al.*, 1973; D. Taylor-Robinson and P. M. Furr, unpublished observations). There is of course no information of the same kind for infertile men, but it is unlikely that all of them have mycoplasmas in the vas deferens. It seems more likely that semen is contaminated at the time of ejaculation by ureaplasmas residing in the urethra, and it would be surprising therefore if the organisms could affect spermatogenesis. Furthermore, because of the probable time of mycoplasma access to semen, and in view of the small number of mycoplasma organisms relative to the number of spermatozoa (usually at least 1:10) even in an infertile semen sample, it seems remarkable that these organisms could appreciably affect motility in a freshly collected specimen. Nevertheless, spermatozoa again come in contact with ureaplasmas in the female genital tract, perhaps for a sufficient length of time to reduce their motility. Whether mycoplasmal infection in the male genital tract could cause sufficient damage to the tract to impair the passage of sperm is of course an open question.

2. Female Infertility and the Infertile Couple

a. Isolation studies. Several workers have considered the infertile couple. Gnarpe and Friberg (1972, 1973a) investigated primary sterility of at least 5 years' duration in 52 couples. Ureaplasmas were isolated from the cervix of 90% of the women and from the semen of 86% of their husbands, but only from 23% of cervices of 40 pregnant women and from 26% of seminal fluids from 23 men married to pregnant or recently delivered women. In a further study, Friberg and Gnarpe (1974) found ureaplasmas in 76% of ejaculates from 50 men of couples with unexplained infertility; the semen samples were otherwise normal. In contrast, ureaplasmas were isolated from 47% of ejaculates from 32 men with high titers of sperm-agglutinating antibodies, the ejaculates having various degrees of sperm motility, but from only 19% of ejaculates from 32 men who had recently proven their fertility. On the basis of these differences in the isolation of ureaplasmas these investigators suggested that there was an association between ureaplasmal infection and infertility.

Love *et al.* (1973) studied the relationship between *M. hominis* and subfertility. They found this mycoplasma to be present more frequently in the cervical secretions of infertile women who had an associated discharge or pelvic abnormality than in those of normal healthy pregnant or nonpregnant women. Later, more women who were not infected by *M. hominis* were found to have conceived than those who were infected by this microorganism. It is possible that the presence of discharge or pelvic abnormality provided a suitable situation for the multiplication of *M. hominis* and that its disappearance and improved frequency of conception were unrelated except as an index of improved genital health.

Taylor-Robinson (1974) questioned some of the above findings, and de Louvois *et al.* (1974) refuted them. They isolated *M. hominis* from 13.2% of one or both partners of 38 fertile couples and from 14.7% of 109 infertile couples; ureaplasmas were isolated from 52.6% of one or both partners of fertile couples and from 57.2% of infertile couples, differences which were not significant. During the next 12 months, 22.5% of the couples conceived (Harrison *et al.*, 1975). Ureaplasmas were isolated from 63% of these couples, and *M. hominis* from 18%, compared with 56 and 13%, respectively, from those who did not conceive. The ureaplasmal isolation results of de Louvois *et al.* (1974) were confirmed by Mårdh *et al.* (1975) and by Matthews *et al.* (1974, 1975), although the findings of the latter workers for *M. hominis* were similar to those of Love *et al.* (1973). W. M. McCormack (unpublished observations) also found genital mycoplasmas as often in fertile as in infertile women, *M. hominis* being isolated from about 20% of the women and ureaplasmas from about 50% of them. The most recent published data are those of Stray-Pedersen *et al.* (1978). They isolated ureaplasmas from the cervix of infertile women (83%) more frequently than from fertile women (49%), but this difference was less striking than when endometrial specimens were examined. In this instance, 50% of specimens from infertile women were positive, but only 7% of those from fertile women. However, bacteria were also significantly associated with ureaplasma-positive endometrial cultures. Most of the endometrial specimens from the infertile women were taken by curettage, so that cervical contamination is a factor which needs to be taken into consideration when assessing the significance of the findings. C. D. Graber, P. Creticos, and S. Phansey (unpublished observations) have also mentioned recently that their data suggest that ureaplasmas are recovered more frequently and in larger numbers from infertile than from fertile women, and that this seems to be so only if the endocervical canal is sampled and not if the vagina is tested.

b. Observations based on antibiotic therapy. Horne and Rock (1952) treated 43 infertile women with oxytetracycline during the week before ovulation, and 10 of them became pregnant. Although specimens were not taken for culture, these workers postulated that the antibiotic acted on cervical microorganisms that were interfering with the migration of sperm. Later, Kundsin (1970a) suggested that mycoplasmas might cause some cases of infertility, because an infertile woman who harbored them became pregnant after tetracycline treatment. Furthermore, on the basis of their ureaplasmal isolation results, Swedish workers (Gnarpe and Friberg, 1973a; Friberg and Gnarpe, 1973) treated infertile couples with doxycycline during the first half of the menstrual cycle for up to five consecutive months. Twenty-nine percent of the women conceived within a few months of eradication of the ureaplasmas. Friberg and Gnarpe (1974) later reported that the treatment of 40 infertile couples with doxycycline was followed by 9 (22%) pregnancies. Hofstetter (1973) commented in a similar vein: Two patients with primary female sterility and adnexitis, from whom mycoplasmas had been isolated, conceived 3 or 4 weeks after antimycoplasmal therapy to both partners. Horne *et al.* (1973, 1974) described their regime for treating patients with Declomycin in some detail without giving a clear indication of its effect. However, Kundsin (1976) mentioned that the antibiotic had been given to 36 women and their husbands in whom infection by ureaplasmas seemed to be the only explanation for infertility. Fifteen (43%) of the women became pregnant within 3 months and 29 (84%) within a year. It is well known, however, that a proportion of women of infertile couples eventually become pregnant without antibiotic treatment. Thus, Taylor-Robinson and G. T. Smedley (Taylor-Robinson, 1974) studied 32 infertile couples, 69% of whom were infected by ureaplasmas. Nine (28%) of the women, 5 (56%) of whom carried ureaplasmas, became pregnant within 1 year. As mentioned previously, Harrison *et al.* (1975) recorded a similar pregnancy rate for untreated women. In view of these observations and because none of the aforementioned antibiotic studies were controlled in any way, the double-blind controlled prophylactic trial carried out by Harrison *et al.* (1975) was much required and timely. They treated 88 couples who had primary infertility of unknown cause with doxycycline. Although a 28-day course of the antibiotic eradicated *M. hominis* and ureaplasmas, the rate of conception (16%) was no higher in those treated with the drug than in those given a placebo. These investigators concluded that doxycycline, although it eradicates mycoplasmas, is of no use in the treatment of primary infertility of unknown cause, and that mycoplasmas are not associated with the condition. However, it is worth mentioning that in all these studies, except that of Stray-Pedersen *et al.* (1978), only myco-plasmas occurring in the vagina and cervix were considered, and it is known that they can infect the fallopian tubes, where it is possible that they may cause damage. Chronic inflammatory changes could result in infertility similar to that produced by gonococcal pelvic inflammatory disease. Indeed, in Sweden, nongonococcal salpingitis, of whatever cause, has been associated with a worse prognosis in terms of infertility than gonococcal salpingitis (Weström, 1975; Weström and Mårdh, 1975). Furthermore, although antibiotic therapy can eliminate mycoplasmas, it may not reverse changes they have produced. If infertility is a consequence of remote mycoplasmal infection, it may be very difficult to establish an etiological association. It is necessary therefore to take a cautious attitude in interpreting the results of studies which have so far been designed to evaluate the role of mycoplasmas in infertility. There are, however, no data to support the notion that infertile couples should be examined for *M. hominis* and ureaplasmas and treated with antibiotics if they are found to be colonized.

B. Chorioamnionitis

The fact that mycoplasmas gain access to the amniotic cavity (Table V) means that potentially they may be able to cause certain pregnancy-related conditions, including chorioamnionitis. Shurin *et al.* (1975) isolated ureaplasmas, but not *M. hominis,* from newborn infants twice as frequently where there was an associated histologically severe chorioamnionitis than where there was less severe disease or no disease at all, and they and others (Caspi *et al.*, 1971; Tafari *et al.*, 1976) have suggested that chorioamnionitis might be due to ureaplasmal infection. It is known that the inflammation is related to rupture of the membranes (Fox, 1977) and that ureaplasmas are most likely to gain entry to the amniotic cavity and colonize the fetus when this happens (Table V). In this circumstance the association between chorioamnionitis and colonization of the infant might be spurious, chorioamnionitis being due in fact to several other factors or to any one of a number of other microorganisms that could gain entry to the amniotic cavity at the same time. The findings of Shurin *et al.* (1975) are provocative, however, because they took into account the duration of membrane rupture in their analysis and still found a significant association between chorioamnionitis and ureaplasmal infection.

C. Habitual Spontaneous Abortion and Stillbirth

1. Isolation Studies

Many studies of this subject have been based on the isolation of mycoplasmas from the vagina, cervix, or urine. Jones (1967b) and Harwick *et al.* (1970) found that women who had uncomplicated spontaneous abor-

TABLE V. Isolation of Mycoplasmas from the Uterus and Amniotic Fluid during and Immediately after Pregnancy[a]

Reference	Gestation	Site tested	Membranes ruptured	Number of cases	Number of isolations	Mycoplasma
Jones (1967a)	Term	Uterine cavity	Yes	1	1	*M. hominis*
Brunell et al. (1969)	Term	Amniotic fluid	Yes	1	1	*M. hominis*
Harwick et al. (1969)	Term	Amniocentesis	Yes	6	1	*M. hominis*
	14–20 weeks	Amniocentesis	No	44	3	*M. hominis*
Jones and Tobin (1969)	Term	Amniotic side of placenta	Yes	7	7	*M. hominis* (2) and ureaplasmas (5)
	Term	Amniotic side of placenta	?	113	0	—
Caspi et al. (1971)	4 weeks premature	Amniotic fluid	No	1	1	Ureaplasmas
Solomon et al. (1973)	Term	Placental membranes	Yes	2	2	Ureaplasmas
Lamey et al. (1974)	Term	Endometrium	Yes	39	21	Mainly ureaplasmas
	Term	Endometrium	No	40	8	Mainly ureaplasmas
Schneider et al. (1974)	14–20 weeks	Amniocentesis	No	10	0	—
Caspi et al. (1976)	Term	Placenta	Yes	79	24	Mainly ureaplasmas
	Term	Placenta	No	44	4	Mainly ureaplasmas
Weissenbacher et al. (1976)	Term	Amniocentesis	?	185	0	—

[a] The data presented concern specimens collected at cesarean section or by amniocentesis, so that isolations are not the result of contamination from the lower genital tract.

tions were colonized by *M. hominis* no more frequently than women who had normal pregnancies. Moreover, Foy *et al.* (1970b) found that colonization with *M. hominis* or ureaplasmas did not correlate either with a history of prior abortion or stillbirth or with abortion itself. Nevertheless, the idea that genital mycoplasmas might be responsible for some cases was stimulated by the results of two prospective studies (Kundsin and Driscoll, 1970a; Braun *et al.*, 1971) in which there was a trend, albeit not statistically significant, for early maternal colonization to occur more frequently among women who had spontaneous abortions and stillbirths than among those who did not.

Mycoplasmal colonization of fetal membranes and fallopian tubes may be more relevant to fetal wastage, as suggested by Kundsin (1970b). It is clear (Table V) that genital mycoplasmas are sometimes found in amniotic fluid even when the membranes are intact, and the presence of mycoplasmas early in pregnancy would increase their chance of causing fetal damage. Although they are present probably less frequently in early than in late pregnancy (Table V), there being insufficient data to be dogmatic, their occurrence early in pregnancy in some cases seems inevitable in view of the known ability of ureaplasmas to infect the upper genital tract (see Section VI,C). To emphasize this, Kundsin (1970b) reported a patient who had suffered repeated spontaneous abortions; cervical cultures for mycoplasmas were negative, but ureaplasmas were isolated from a fallopian tube at hysterectomy. The data in Table V are based on studies of amniocentesis or cesarean-derived material, so that mycoplasmal isolations which have been made from the products of conception are not due to vaginal contamination. This point is relevant to several studies. Kundsin *et al.* (1967) isolated ureaplasmas, but no other microorganisms, from the chorion, amnion, and decidua of a spontaneous abortus, a predictable result when the products of conception passed through an infected vagina. In further studies, Kundsin and Driscoll (1970b) isolated mycoplasmas, in particular ureaplasmas, more frequently from fetal membranes of aborted fetuses or premature babies than from those of therapeutic abortions or normal full-term babies. In addition, genital mycoplasmas have been isolated from the products of early abortions (Caspi *et al.*, 1972) and midtrimester fetal losses (Sompolinsky *et al.*, 1975) more often than from the products of conception of induced abortions. Recently, Stray-Pedersen *et al.* (1978) reported a study which is relevant to mycoplasmal infection beyond the cervix. They isolated ureaplasmas more often from the endometrium of women who had habitual abortions (28%) than from the same site in women comprising a control group (7%); most of the specimens in the two groups were taken by aspiration, which may be less likely to lead to contamination from the cervix than curettage. Clearly, therefore, the results of these various studies suggest that there is an association between maternal infection and/or infection of the products of conception by genital mycoplasmas and spontaneous abortion. However, whether the association is more apparent than real is problematical, since it is difficult to evaluate the comparability of the various groups of women. Furthermore, the possible role of other microorganisms, such as chlamydiae, is a complicating factor which has not been assessed.

The ability to isolate mycoplasmas from aborted fetuses and stillborn infants is not entirely due to superficial contamination, because they have been isolated from the lungs (Jones, 1967b; Pease *et al.*, 1967; Romano *et al.*, 1968, 1971; Sompolinsky *et al.*, 1975; Tafari *et al.*, 1976) and from the brain, heart, and viscera (Harwick *et al.*, 1967; Jones, 1967b; Hayflick and Stanbridge, 1967; Romano *et al.*, 1968; Bashmakova and Soldatova, 1969; Sompolinsky *et al.*, 1975). Isolation from the respiratory tract is probably due to aspiration of infected amniotic fluid, whereas isolation from the heart and viscera may be indicative of hematogenous spread, possibly due to invasion of the fetus via the umbilical vessels. In considering the relationship of mycoplasmal infection to fetal death, it is interesting to note that there is a report of the isolation of *M. hominis* from the cord blood of 5.5% of infants alive at birth (Steytler, 1970) and of the isolation of ureaplasmas also (Klein *et al.*, 1969). However, the possibility of contamination by vaginal organisms has to be kept in mind, particularly in this situation. In relation to mycoplasmemia, it is also pertinent to note the observations of McCormack *et al.* (1975). They found that 2 of 10 women who had *M. hominis* in the blood immediately after delivery had produced stillborn infants, whereas only 1 of 301 women from whom the mycoplasma was not isolated had a stillbirth. Although the difference was significant, these workers were reluctant to place too much emphasis on the finding until it had been confirmed. Unfortunately, none of these observations provide an answer to the major problem, recognized by Caspi *et al.* (1972), of whether abortion of the fetus occurs because mycoplasmas invade it and cause its death or whether the fetus dies for some other reason and is then invaded by the organisms.

2. Studies Based on Antibiotic Therapy

Since mycoplasmas are sensitive to tetracyclines and other broad-spectrum antibiotics *in vitro*, fetal loss, if due to these organisms, could conceivably be prevented by appropriate antimicrobial therapy. In a study by Driscoll *et al.* (1969), 6 women who had had a total of 29 unsuccessful pregnancies, most of which had ended in spontaneous abortion during the first trimester, were given demethylchlortetracycline each day beginning before or shortly after conception and continuing for 28 weeks. Before treatment, 5 of the women were tested for genital myco- plasmas and 4 were found to be infected. Although 1 woman had an early abortion and another a stillbirth, 3 of the other women carried to term, and the fourth had a premature infant. Other reports by the same group of workers (Kundsin *et al.*, 1969; Kundsin, 1970a) are along similar lines, describing successful pregnancies after antibiotic treatment of women who were colonized by ureaplasmas and who had had frequent abortions previously. These observations have led these investigators to postulate that subclinical mycoplasmal infection is an important cause of reproduc- tive failure (Horne *et al.*, 1974). They have also suggested that ureaplas- mas cause endometritis (Horne *et al.*, 1973) and have used their evidence for this to support the hypothesis. However, to do so seems inadvisable, because other microorganisms, such as chlamydiae, which might cause endometritis, were not sought. Stray-Pedersen *et al.* (1978) have also used a tetracycline (doxycycline) to treat women who had previously experi- enced habitual spontaneous abortion and reported that a large proportion of the women had normal pregnancies. Despite these various observa- tions, the effectiveness of antibiotics in preventing spontaneous abortion remains controversial, largely because all the antibiotic trials have been uncontrolled. Nevertheless, the information available at the moment is interesting enough to justify placebo-controlled trials of antibiotics, pref- erably not tetracyclines, in patients with repeated spontaneous abortions.

3. Serological Studies

Jones (1967b) found complement-fixing antibody to *M. hominis* in 29% of sera from 70 women after abortion but in only 15% of sera from 171 normal pregnant women before delivery, although the occurrence of this mycoplasma in the cervix of the women in the two groups was not different. Entry of mycoplasmas into the circulation (McCormack *et al.*, 1975) and stimulation of an antibody response may occur quite frequently during or after a normal pregnancy (Jones, 1967a; Foy *et al.*, 1970b; Lin *et al.*, 1978), so that this finding in itself is not supportive evidence for *M. hominis* causing the abortions.

4. Chromosomal Aberrations

Chromosomal damage, including open breaks, gaps, and rearrange- ments, has been observed in cultures of various cells infected with myco- plasmas *in vitro*. Such changes have been seen in cell cultures infected by genital mycoplasmas, namely, *M. fermentans* (Fogh and Fogh, 1965), *M. hominis* (Allison and Paton, 1966), and *U. urealyticum* (Kundsin *et al.*, 1971b), as well as by other mycoplasmas of human and animal origin

(Taylor-Robinson, 1978). The reason for the changes brought about by ureaplasmas is unknown. However, some of the defects noted *in vitro* are known to be due to depletion of arginine by mycoplasmal metabolism in the closed cell culture system. It seems unlikely that such a mechanism would operate in an "open" *in vivo* situation. Although chromosome changes in WI-38 cell cultures infected by *M. hominis* are similar to those noted in patients with Down's syndrome (Allison and Paton, 1966), mycoplasmal infection has not been directly associated with chromosomal abnormalities in the human fetus. Therefore whether the observations of damage in cell cultures have any relevance to the *in vivo* situation is entirely speculative. Conceivably, if mycoplasmal infections caused chromosomal abnormalities in the fetus, they could produce abortion or developmental anomalies.

5. Animal Models

a. Experimental infections. There have been few experimental observations concerning the ability of mycoplasmas to cause abortion in animals (Taylor-Robinson, 1977b). However, Hartman *et al.* (1964) found that *M. bovis* (*M. agalactiae* subsp. *bovis*) inoculated into the uterus of heifers produced varying degrees of endometritis, endosalpingitis, and salpingoperitonitis, and Stalheim and Proctor (1976) noted that intraamniotic inoculation resulted in abortion. Further, Tan and Miles (1974) inoculated pregnant cats intravaginally with feline ureaplasmas and attributed an ensuing abortion and early neonatal deaths to the ureaplasmal infection. Not surprisingly, perhaps, rodents have been used most as models for mycoplasma-induced abortion. Cole *et al.* (1973) noted that *M. arthritidis* caused fetal death when injected intravenously into pregnant mice, and Gabridge and Cohen (1976) observed fetal resorptions following intraperitoneal inoculations of *M. hominis* and *M. fermentans*. Taylor-Robinson *et al.* (1975b) inoculated mice intravenously with *M. pulmonis* before or after mating and examined them just before parturition. Significantly more dead fetuses were found than in uninoculated controls, although the deaths were probably due to maternal infection and disturbance rather than fetal infection per se. Furthermore, Naot *et al.* (1978) inoculated gravid rats intravenously with *M. arthritidis* and found that the newborn offspring were significantly reduced in number compared with those of uninoculated rats and that half the offspring of the inoculated rats died within the first 10 days of birth, whereas almost all those of the uninoculated rats survived. These various results indicate that mycoplasmas are able to produce abortions in animals and presumably have the potential for doing so in humans. It would be unwise, however, to use such observations to strengthen what is, at the moment, inadequate evidence for mycoplasmas causing human abortion.

b. Naturally occurring infections. Although mycoplasmas occur in the genital tracts of many animal species and cause disease in some, their association with reproductive failure is sufficiently obscure (Taylor-Robinson, 1977b) to be unhelpful in elucidating the problem in humans. As an example, Kundsin *et al.* (1975) isolated ureaplasmas from the genital tracts of talapoin and patas monkeys which had evidence of reproductive failure in the form of infertility, spontaneous abortions, or stillbirths. In view, however, of the numerous factors known to influence breeding and the fact that only ureaplasmas were sought, it is not possible to associate them with the reproductive problems. However, it must be admitted that nonhuman primates may serve as useful models for investigating the possible role of mycoplasmas, including ureaplasmas, in human reproductive failure.

D. Prematurity and Low-Birth-Weight Infants

1. Antibiotic Studies

In two studies conducted before it was recognized that there was an association between prenatal tetracycline administration and staining of the primary teeth, this antibiotic was administered to pregnant women (Elder *et al.*, 1968, 1971). In each study, carried out on a controlled, double-blind basis, women who were treated with tetracycline for 6 weeks during pregnancy gave birth to significantly fewer infants weighing 2500 gm or less than women who were given a placebo. Although no microbiological investigations were conducted, it was postulated that tetracycline-sensitive microorganisms might be responsible, and mycoplasmas were considered among these.

2. Isolation Studies

a. *Ureaplasma urealyticum.* The first direct evidence for an association between mycoplasmas and birth weight was seen in a study of unselected newborn infants at the Boston City Hospital (Klein *et al.*, 1969). About 15% of them were found to be colonized in the nose or throat or at both sites with genital mycoplasmas, mainly ureaplasmas, and colonized infants had a significantly lower mean birth weight (2605 gm) than those who were not colonized (2952 gm). In a further study by Braun *et al.* (1971), 28% of infants with a birth weight of 2500 gm or less were colonized by ureaplasmas, whereas only 5% of those weighing more than 2500 gm were colonized.

TABLE VI. Summary of the Association of Mycoplasmas with Genitourinary Disease[a]

Disease	Association of indicated mycoplasma with disease		Comments
	M. hominis	U. urealyticum	
Nongonococcal urethritis	−	+	The weight of evidence indicates that ureaplasmas cause some cases of NGU, but the proportion is unknown
Balanitis and paraurethral abscess	−	−	No evidence to associate either microorganism with disease
Acute and chronic prostatitis	±	−	An association with chronic disease has been reported, but an etiological relationship has not been proved
Reiter's disease	−	−	So far no evidence for an association, but the possible role of ureaplasmas should not be ignored
Bartholin's gland abscess	−	−	Recent work provides no evidence to associate either microorganism with the disease
Vaginitis and cervicitis	−	−	Mycoplasma hominis, in particular, often isolated more frequently from women with disease than from those without, but inadequate evidence for an etiological relationship
Pelvic inflammatory diseases	+	−	Isolations from fallopian tubes and antibody responses indicate that M. hominis causes some cases of acute salpingitis, but its role in nonchlamydial disease needs to be assessed
Postabortal fever	+	−	Isolations from blood and antibody responses strongly indicate an etiological relationship in some cases of fever

			Comments
Postpartum fever	+		Comments as for postabortal fever
Cystitis	−	−	Genital mycoplasmas found in the bladder, but so far no evidence for an association with disease
Urinary calculi	−	±	Ureaplasmas produce calculi in rats experimentally, but no evidence that they produce natural disease in humans
Nephritis	+	−	Increasing evidence that *M. hominis* causes some cases of acute pyelonephritis and acute exacerbations of chronic disease
Involuntary infertility	−	−	Some reports that ureaplasmas cause decreased motility of spermatozoa, but no data to support the notion that infertile couples possessing genital mycoplasmas should be treated with tetracyclines
Chorioamnionitis	±	±	An undoubted association between ureaplasmal isolation and inflammation, provocative enough to stimulate further work
Spontaneous abortion and stillbirth	−	±	An association between abortion and the presence of ureaplasmas in the mother or in the abortus is undeniable, but evidence that the organisms cause abortion is lacking
Prematurity and low-birth-weight infants	−	+	An association between low birth weight, but not decreased gestational age, and ureaplasmas in the mother or in the infant is undoubted, but it is unknown whether the organisms are directly responsible

a +, ±, or −, strong, weak, or no association with disease. Whether or not there is an etiological relationship is considered under "Comments."

Since colonization of the newborn infant is obviously related to the presence of mycoplasmas in the genital tract of the mother, a prospective study was carried out by the Boston workers (Braun *et al.*, 1971) on 484 prenatal women. Urine and cervical specimens obtained at the first prenatal clinic visit were examined for mycoplasmas. Women who were colonized with ureaplasmas gave birth to infants with a significantly lower mean birth weight (3099 ± 595 gm) than those who were not colonized (3297 ± 510 gm). Foy *et al.* (1970b) studied a much smaller group of women, which may explain why there was only a trend, and not a significant association, between maternal colonization with ureaplasmas and lower mean birth weight; ureaplasma-positive mothers gave birth to infants weighing 3172 gm, whereas ureaplasma-negative mothers produced infants weighing 3304 gm.

b. *Mycoplasma hominis.* The association between infant or maternal colonization with this mycoplasma and low birth weight is less striking than in the case of *U. urealyticum*. Braun *et al.* (1971) found that few infants were colonized with *M. hominis* and that it was not associated with low birth weight. Furthermore, Foy *et al.* (1970b) could not detect a relationship between maternal colonization with *M. hominis* and low birth weight. While Braun *et al.* (1971) failed to find any striking association, they noted that the combined effect of *M. hominis* and ureaplasmas on birth weight was greater than the effect of ureaplasmas alone. A more positive finding was reported by di Musto *et al.* (1973), who noted that *M. hominis* culture-positive mothers gave birth to infants of mean weight 2799 gm, while culture-negative mothers produced infants of 3103 gm. Isolates from mothers who produced babies of low birth weight were found to be serologically diverse (Lin *et al.*, 1976).

The results of the various studies have not indicated that genital mycoplasmal infection of either infant or mother is associated with a decreased gestational age. There seems no doubt, however, that the association between infection, particularly with ureaplasmas, and low birth weight is a real phenomenon, because it is independent of other factors which contribute to low birth weight, such as maternal age and weight, race, parity, history of previous abortion and prematurity, cigarette smoking, and bacteriuria (Braun *et al.*, 1971). Despite this, it cannot be concluded at the present time that genital mycoplasmas are directly responsible for low birth weight, because it is possible that women who have a predisposition to smaller babies are selectively colonized. Clearly, however, in view of the importance of low birth weight in perinatal morbidity and mortality, the phenomenon warrants further investigation.

IX. CONCLUSIONS

The major conclusions concerning the role of mycoplasmas in human genitourinary diseases are summarized in Table VI.

REFERENCES

Allison, A. C., and Paton, G. R. (1966). *Lancet* **ii**, 1229–1230.

Archer, J. F. (1968). *Br. J. Vener. Dis.* **44**, 232–234.

Barile, M. F., and Del Giudice, R. A. (1972). *Ciba Found. Symp. Pathogen. Mycoplasmas*, pp. 165–185. Elsevier, Amsterdam.

Bartholomew, L. E. (1965). *Arthritis Rheum.* **8**, 376–388.

Bashmakova, M. A., and Soldatova, V. M. (1969). *Vopr. Okhr. Materin. Det.* **14**, 69–73.

Bennett, A. H., Kundsin, R. B., and Shapiro, S. R. (1973). *J. Urol.* **109**, 427–429.

Bercovici, B., Persky, S., Rozansky, R., and Razin, S. (1962). *Am. J. Obstet. Gynecol.* **84**, 687–691.

Berg, R. L., Weinberger, H., and Dienes, L. (1957). *Am. J. Med.* **22**, 848–864.

Beveridge, W. I. B., Campbell, A. D., and Lind, P. E. (1946). *Med. J. Aust.* **1**, 179–180.

Black, F. T. (1973). *Appl. Microbiol.* **25**, 528–533.

Black, F. T., and Krogsgaard-Jensen, A. (1974). *Acta Pathol. Microbiol. Scand., Sect. B* **82**, 345–353.

Black, F. T., and Rasmussen, O. G. (1968). *Br. J. Vener. Dis.* **44**, 324–330.

Bowie, W. R., Alexander, E. R., Floyd, J. F., Holmes, J., Miller, Y., and Holmes, K. E. (1976). *Lancet* **ii**, 1276–1278.

Bowie, W. R., Wang, S.-P., Alexander, E. R., Floyd, J., Forsyth, P. S., Pollock, H. M., Lin, J.-S., Buchanan, T. M., and Holmes, K. K. (1977a). *J. Clin. Invest.* **59**, 735–742.

Bowie, W. R., Wang, S.-P., Alexander, E. R., and Holmes, K. K. (1977b). *In* "Nongonococcal Urethritis and Related Infections" (D. Hobson and K. K. Holmes, eds.), pp. 19–29. Am. Soc. Microbiol., Washington, D.C.

Bowie, W. R., Pollock, H. M., Forsyth, P. S., Floyd, J. F., Alexander, E. R., Wang, S.-P., and Holmes, K. K. (1977c). *J. Clin. Microbiol.* **6**, 482–488.

Bowie, W. R., Digiacomo, R. F., Holmes, K. K., and Gale, J. L. (1978). *Br. J. Vener. Dis.* **54**, 235–238.

Braun, P., and Besdine, R. (1973). *Am. J. Obstet. Gynecol.* **117**, 861–862.

Braun, P., Klein, J. O., Lee, Y. H., and Kass, E. H. (1970a). *J. Infect. Dis.* **121**, 391–400.

Braun, P., Klein, J. O., and Kass, E. H. (1970b). *Appl. Microbiol.* **19**, 62–70.

Braun, P., Lee, Y.-H., Klein, J. O., Marcy, S. M., Klein, T. A., Charles, D., Levy, P., and Kass, E. H. (1971). *N. Engl. J. Med.* **284**, 167–171.

Bredt, W., Lam, P. S., Fiegel, P., and Höffler, D. (1974). *Dtsch. Med. Wochenschr.* **99**, 1553–1556.

Brunell, P. A., Dische, R. M., and Walker, M. B. (1969). *J. Am. Med. Assoc.* **207**, 2097–2099.

Brunner, H., Horswood, R. L., and Chanock, R. M. (1973). *J. Infect. Dis.* **127**, Suppl., 52–55.

Busolo, F., Conventi, L., Bertoloni, G., and Meloni, G. A. (1975). *Atti Congr. Naz. Soc. Ital. Microbiol., 17th, Padua*, pp. 1111–1115.

Card, D. H. (1959). *Br. J. Vener. Dis.* **35**, 27–34.

Carney, F., E., and Taylor-Robinson, D. (1973). *Br. J. Vener. Dis.* **49**, 435–440.

Caspi, E., Herczeg, E., Solomon, F., and Sompolinsky, D. (1971). *Am. J. Obstet. Gynecol.* **111**, 1102–1106.

Caspi, E., Solomon, F., and Sompolinsky, D. (1972). *Isr. J. Med. Sci.* **8**, 122–127.

Caspi, E., Solomon, F., Langer, R., and Sompolinsky, D. (1976). *Obstet. Gynecol.* **48**, 682–684.

Catalano, G., Varone, G. L., and Argenziano, G. (1968). *G. Mal. Infett. Parassit.* **20**, 1009–1013.

Clyde, W. A., Jr. (1964). *J. Immunol.* **92**, 958–965.

Cole, B. C., Ward, J. R., and Golightly-Rowland, L. (1973). *Infect. Immun.* **7**, 218–225.

Colleen, S., and Mårdh, P.-A. (1975). *In* "Genital Infections and Their Complications" (D. Danielsson, L. Juhlin, and P.-A. Mårdh, eds.), pp. 121–131. Almqvist & Wiksell, Stockholm.

Coufalik, E. D., Taylor-Robinson, D., and Csonka, G. W. (1979). *Br. J. Vener. Dis.* **55**, 36–43.

Csonka, G. W. (1965). *Br. J. Vener. Dis.* **41**, 1–8.

Csonka, G. W., and Corse, J. (1970). *Br. J. Vener. Dis.* **46**, 203–204.

Csonka, G. W., and Spitzer, R. J. (1969). *Br. J. Vener. Dis.* **45**, 52–54.

Csonka, G. W., Williams, R. E. O., and Corse, J. (1966). *Lancet* **i**, 1292–1296.

Csonka, G. W., Williams, R. E. O., and Corse, J. (1967). *Ann. N.Y. Acad. Sci.* **143**, 794–798.

Csütörtöki, V., Stipkovits, L., and Varga, L. (1975). *Acta Microbiol. Acad. Sci. Hung.* **22**, 353.

Davis, G., Smithurst, B., Talbot, A., Townsend, E., and Parry, A. (1973). *Med. J. Aust.* **2**, 268–271.

Del Giudice, R. A., Robillard, N. F., and Carski, T. R. (1967). *J. Bacteriol.* **93**, 1205–1209.

Del Giudice, R. A., Carski, T. R., Barile, M. F., Lemcke, R. M., and Tully, J. G. (1971). *J. Bacteriol.* **108**, 439–445.

de Louvois, J., Blades, M., Harrison, R. F., Hurley, R., and Stanley, V. C. (1974). *Lancet* **i**, 1073–1075.

de Louvois, J., Hurley, R., and Stanley, V. C. (1975). *J. Clin. Pathol.* **28**, 731–735.

Dienes, L., and Edsall, G. (1937). *Proc. Soc. Exp. Biol. Med.* **36**, 740–744.

Dienes, L., and Smith, W. E. (1942). *Proc. Soc. Exp. Biol. Med.* **50**, 99–101.

Dienes, L., and Smith, W. E. (1946). *J. Clin. Invest.* **25**, 911–912.

Dienes, L., Ropes, M. W., Smith, W. E., Madoff, S., and Bauer, W. (1948). *N. Engl. J. Med.* **238**, 509–515.

di Musto, J. C., Bohjalian, O., and Millar, M. (1973). *Obstet. Gynecol.* **41**, 33–37.

Douboyas, J., and Papapanagiotou, J. (1975). *Zentralbl. Bakteriol., Parasitenkd. Infektionskr. Hyg., Abt. 1: Orig., Reihe A* **233**, 575–579.

Driscoll, S. G., Kundsin, R. B., Horne, H. W., Jr., and Scott, J. M. (1969). *Fertil. Steril.* **20**, 1017–1019.

Dunlop, E. M. C., Hare, M. J., Jones, B. R., and Taylor-Robinson, D. (1969). *Br. J. Vener. Dis.* **45**, 274–281.

Edmunds, P. N. (1958). *J. Obstet. Gynaecol. Br. Emp.* **66**, 917–926.

Eilard, T., Brorsson, J.-E., and Hamark, B. (1976). *Scand. J. Infect. Dis., Suppl.* **9**, 82–84.

Elder, H. A., Smith, R., and Kass, E. H. (1968). *Intersci. Conf. Antimicrob. Agents Chemother., 8th, New York.*

Elder, H. A., Santamarina, B. A. G., Smith, S., and Kass, E. H. (1971). *Am. J. Obstet. Gynecol.* **111**, 441–462.

Eschenbach, D. A., Buchanan, T. M., Pollock, H. M., Forsyth, P. S., Alexander, E. R.,

Lin, J.-S., Wang, S.-P., Wentworth, B. B., McCormack, W. M., and Holmes, K. K. (1975). *N. Engl. J. Med.* **293,** 166–171.

Evans, R. T., and Taylor-Robinson, D. (1978). *J. Antimicrob. Chemother.* **4,** 57–63.

Fogh, J., and Fogh, H. (1965). *Proc. Soc. Exp. Biol. Med.* **119,** 233–238.

Ford, D. K. (1960). *Arthritis Rheum.* **3,** 395–402.

Ford, D. K. (1966). *Arthritis Rheum.* **9,** 503–504.

Ford, D. K. (1967). *Ann. N.Y. Acad. Sci.* **143,** 501–504.

Ford, D. K. (1968). *Can. Med. Assoc. J.* **99,** 900–910.

Ford, D. K. (1977). *In* "Nongonococcal Urethritis and Related Infections" (D. Hobson and K. K. Holmes, eds.), pp. 64–66. Am. Soc. Microbiol., Washington, D.C.

Ford, D. K., and DuVernet, M. (1963). *Br. J. Vener. Dis.* **39,** 18–20.

Ford, D. K., and Henderson, E. (1976a). *Arthritis Rheum.* **19,** 1328–1332.

Ford, D. K., and Henderson, E. (1976b). *Br. J. Vener. Dis.* **52,** 341–342.

Ford, D. K., and Rasmussen, G. (1964). *Arthritis Rheum.* **7,** 220–227.

Ford, D. K., and Smith, J. R. (1974). *Br. J. Vener. Dis.* **50,** 373–374.

Ford, D. K., Rasmussen, G., and Minken, J. (1962). *Br. J. Vener. Dis.* **38,** 22–25.

Fowler, W., and Leeming, R. J. (1969). *Br. J. Vener. Dis.* **45,** 287–293.

Fowlkes, D. M., MacLeod, J., and O'Leary, W. M. (1975a). *Fertil. Steril.* **26,** 1212–1218.

Fowlkes, D. M., Dooher, G. B., and O'Leary, W. M. (1975b). *Fertil. Steril.* **26,** 1203–1211.

Fox, H. (1977). *In* "Infections and Pregnancy" (C. R. Coid, ed.), pp. 251–288. Academic Press, New York.

Foy, H., Kenny, G. E., Levinsohn, E. M., and Grayston, J. T. (1970a). *J. Infect. Dis.* **121,** 579–587.

Foy, H., Kenny, G. E., Wentworth, B. B., Johnson, W. L., and Grayston, J. T. (1970b). *Am. J. Obstet. Gynecol.* **106,** 635–643.

Foy, H., Kenny, G. E., Bor, E., Hammar, S., and Hickman, R. (1975). *J. Clin. Microbiol.* **2,** 226–230.

Freundt, E. A. (1953). *Acta Pathol. Microbiol. Scand.* **32,** 468–480.

Freundt, E. A. (1956). *Br. J. Vener. Dis.* **32,** 188–194.

Freundt, E. A. (1958). "The Mycoplasmataceae (The Pleuropneumonia Group of Organisms): Morphology, Biology and Taxonomy." Aarhus Stiftsbogtrykkerie, Copenhagen.

Friberg, J., and Gnarpe, H. (1973). *Am. J. Obstet. Gynecol.* **116,** 23–26.

Friberg, J., and Gnarpe, H. (1974). *Andrologia* **6,** 45–52.

Friedlander, A. M., and Braude, A. I. (1974). *Nature (London)* **247,** 67–69.

Furness, G. (1975). *J. Infect. Dis.* **132,** 592–596.

Furness, G., Kamat, M. H., Kaminski, Z., and Seebode, J. J. (1973). *Invest. Urol.* **10,** 387–391.

Gabridge, M. G., and Cohen, L. J. (1976). *Lab. Anim. Sci.* **26,** 206–210.

Gnarpe, H., and Friberg, J. (1972). *Am. J. Obstet. Gynecol.* **114,** 727–731.

Gnarpe, H., and Friberg, J. (1973a). *Nature (London)* **242,** 120–121.

Gnarpe, H., and Friberg, J. (1973b). Nature (*London*) **245,** 97–98.

Gotthardson, A., and Melén, B. (1953). *Acta Pathol. Microbiol. Scand.* **33,** 291–293.

Gregory, J. E., and Cundy, K. R. (1970). *Appl. Microbiol.* **19,** 268–270.

Gregory, J. E., and Payne, F. E. (1970). *Am. J. Obstet. Gynecol.* **107,** 220–226.

Grimble, A. S., and Amarasuriya, K. L. (1975). *Br. J. Vener. Dis.* **51,** 198–205.

Gump, D. W., Horton, E., Phillips, C. A., Mead, P. B., and Forsyth, B. R. (1975) *Fertil. Steril.* **26,** 1135–1139.

Haas, H., Dorfman, M. L., and Sacks, T. G. (1971). *Br. J. Vener. Dis.* **47,** 131–134.

Hammerschlag, M. R., Alpert, S., Rosner, I., Thurston, P., McComb, D., Semine, D. Z., and McCormack, W. M. (1978). *Pediatrics* **62,** 57–62.

Hare, M. J., Dunlop, E. M. C., and Taylor-Robinson, D. (1969). *Br. J. Vener. Dis.* **45,** 282–286.

Harkness, A. H., and Henderson-Begg, A. (1948). *Br. J. Vener. Dis.* **24,** 50–58.

Harrison, R. F., de Louvois, J., Blades, M., and Hurley, R. (1975). *Lancet* **i,** 605–607.

Hartman, H. A., Tourtellotte, M. E., Nielsen, S. W., and Plastridge, W. N. (1964). *Res. Vet. Sci.* **5,** 303–310.

Harwick, H. J., Iuppa, J. B., Purcell, R. H., and Fekety, F. R. (1967). *Am. J. Obstet. Gynecol.* **99,** 725–727.

Harwick, H. J., Iuppa, J. B., and Fekety, F. R. (1969). *Obstet. Gynecol.* **33,** 256–259.

Harwick, H. J., Purcell, R. H., Iuppa, J. B., and Fekety, F. R. (1970). *J. Infect. Dis.* **121,** 260–268.

Harwick, H. J., Purcell, R. H., Iuppa, J. B., and Fekety, F. R. (1971). *Obstet. Gynecol.* **37,** 765–768.

Hayflick, L., and Stanbridge, E. (1967). *Ann. N.Y. Acad. Sci.* **143,** 608–621.

Hill, D. A., Philip, R. N., Greaves, A. B., and Purcell, R. H. (1973). *Br. J. Vener. Dis.* **49,** 524–530.

Hirsch, W. (1952). *Bull. Res. Counc. Isr.* **2,** 207.

Hofstetter, A. (1973). *Infection* **1,** 247–249.

Hofstetter, A. (1976). *Fortschr. Prakt. Dermatol. Venerol.* **8,** 389–394.

Hofstetter, A. (1977). *Hautarzt* **28,** 295–298.

Hofstetter, A., Blenk, H., and Rangoonwala, R. (1976a). *Muench. Med. Wochenschr.* **118,** 49–50.

Hofstetter, A., Schill, W.-B., Hoppe, W., and David, R. (1976b). *Ges. Urol.* **28,** 447–450.

Holmes, K. K., Johnson, D. W., Floyd, T. M., and Kvale, P. A. (1967). *J. Am. Med. Assoc.* **202,** 467–473.

Holmes, K. K., Handsfield, H. H., Wang, S. P., Wentworth, B. B., Turck, M., Anderson, J. B., and Alexander, E. R. (1975). *N. Engl. J. Med.* **292,** 1199–1205.

Holmes, M. J., Furr, P. M., and Taylor-Robinson, D. (1974). *J. Hyg.* **72,** 355–363.

Holt, S., Pederson, A. H. B., Wang, S. P., Kenny, G. E., Foy, H. M., and Grayston, J. T. (1967). *Am. J. Ophthalmol.* **63,** 1057–1064.

Horne, H. W., Jr., and Rock, J. (1952). *Fertil. Steril.* **3,** 321–327.

Horne, H. W., Jr., Hertig, A. T., Kundsin, R. B., and Kosasa, T. S. (1973). *Int. J. Fertil.* **18,** 226–231.

Horne, H. W., Jr., Kundsin, R. B., and Kosasa, T. S. (1974). *Fertil. Steril.* **25,** 380–389.

Huijsmans-Evers, A. G. M., and Ruys, A. C. (1956). *Antonie van Leeuwenhoek* **22,** 371–376.

Ingham, H. R., MacFarlane, W. V., Hale, J. H., Selkon, J. B., and Codd, A. A. (1966). *Br. J. Vener. Dis.* **42,** 269–271.

Jänsch, H. H. (1972). *Hautarzt* **23,** 558.

Jansson, E., Lassus, A., Stubbs, S., and Tuuri, S. (1971). *Br. J. Vener. Dis.* **47,** 122–125.

Jansson, E., Vaino, U., Lassus, A., and Tuuri, S. (1972). *Br. J. Vener. Dis.* **48,** 304–305.

Jones, D. M. (1967a). *J. Clin. Pathol.* **20,** 633–635.

Jones, D. M. (1967b). *Br. Med. J.* **i,** 338–340.

Jones, D. M., and Davson, J. (1967). *Nature (London)* **213,** 828.

Jones, D. M., and Sequeira, P. L. J. (1966). *J. Hyg.* **64,** 441–449.

Jones, D. M., and Tobin, B. M. (1969). *J. Med. Microbiol.* **2,** 347–352.

Jurmanova, K., and Sterbova, J. (1977). *Vet. Rec.* **100,** 157–158.

King, A. (1964). "Recent Advances in Venereology," pp. 352–394. Churchill, London.

Klein, J. O., Buckland, D., and Finland, M. (1969). *N. Engl. J. Med.* **280,** 1025–1030.

Klieneberger-Nobel, E. (1959a). *Br. Med. J.* **i,** 19–23.

Klieneberger-Nobel, E. (1959b). *Br. J. Vener. Dis.* **35**, 20–23.

Kraus, S. J., Jacobs, N. F., Chandler, F. W., and Arum, E. A. (1977). *Infect. Immun.* **16**, 302–309.

Krücken, H. (1959). *Dermatol. Wochenschr.* **140**, 1342–1346.

Kundsin, R. B. (1970a). *Prog. Gynecol.* **5**, 275–282.

Kundsin, R. B. (1970b). *N. Engl. J. Med.* **282**, 928–929.

Kundsin, R. B. (1976). *Health Lab. Sci.* **13**, 144–151.

Kundsin, R. B., and Driscoll, S. G. (1970a). *Surg., Gynecol. Obstet.* **131**, 89–92.

Kundsin, R. B., and Driscoll, S. G. (1970b). *Ann. N.Y. Acad. Sci.* **174**, 794–797.

Kundsin, R. B., Driscoll, S. G., and Ming, P.-M. L. (1967). *Science* **157**, 1573–1574.

Kundsin, R. B., Driscoll, S. G., and Praznik, J. (1969). *In* "Mycoplasma Diseases of Man" (M. Sprössig and W. Witzleb, eds.), pp. 141–148. Fischer, Jena.

Kundsin, R. B., Kirsch, A., and Parreno, A. (1971a). *Bacteriol. Proc.* p. 77.

Kundsin, R. B., Ampola, M., Streeter, S., and Neurath, P. (1971b). *J. Med. Genet.* **8**, 181–187.

Kundsin, R. B., Parreno, A., and Kirsch, A. (1973). *Br. J. Vener. Dis.* **49**, 381–384.

Kundsin, R. B., Rowell, T., Shepard, M. C., Parreno, A., and Lunceford, C. D. (1975). *Lab. Anim. Sci.* **25**, 221–224.

Lamey, J. R., Foy, H. M., and Kenny, G. E. (1974). *Obstet. Gynecol.* **44**, 703–708.

Lamm, D. L., Johnson, S. A., Friedlander, A. M., and Gittes, R. F. (1977). *Urology* **10**, 418–421.

Leberman, P. R., Smith, P. F., and Morton, H. E. (1952). *J. Urol.* **68**, 399–402.

Lee, Y.-H., Bailey, P. E., and McCormack, W. M. (1972a). *J. Infect. Dis.* **125**, 318–321.

Lee, Y.-H., Bailey, P. E., and McCormack, W. M. (1972b). *Appl. Microbiol.* **23**, 824–825.

Lee, Y.-H., Donner, A., Bailey, P. E., Alpert, S., and McCormack, W. M. (1974a). *J. Lab. Clin. Med.* **84**, 766–770.

Lee, Y.-H., McCormack, W. M., Marcy, S. M., and Klein, J. O. (1974b). *Pediatr. Clin. North Am.* **21**, 457–466.

Lee, Y.-H., Tarr, P. I., Schumacher, J. R., Rosner, B., Alpert, S., and McCormack, W. M. (1976). *Sex. Transm. Dis.* **3**, 25–28.

Lee, Y.-H., Rankin, J. S., Alpert, S., Daly, A. K., and McCormack, W. M. (1977). *Am. J. Obstet. Gynecol.* **129**, 150–153.

Lemcke, R., and Csonka, G. W. (1962). *Br. J. Vener. Dis.* **38**, 212–217.

Lin, J.-S. L. (1977). *In* "Nongonococcal Urethritis and Related Infections" (D. Hobson and K. K. Holmes, eds.), pp. 370–375. Am. Soc. Microbiol., Washington, D.C.

Lin, J.-S., and Kass, E. H. (1970). *J. Infect. Dis.* **122**, 93–95.

Lin, J.-S., and Kass, E. H. (1973). *Infect. Immun.* **7**, 499–500.

Lin, J.-S. L., and Kass, E. H. (1974). *Infect. Immun.* **10**, 535–540.

Lin, J.-S., and Kass, E. H. (1975). *J. Med. Microbiol.* **8**, 397–404.

Lin, J.-S. L., Kendrick, M. I., and Kass, E. H. (1972). *J. Infect. Dis.* **126**, 658–663.

Lin, J.-S. L., Alpert, S., and Radnay, K. M. (1975). *J. Infect. Dis.* **131**, 727–730.

Lin, J.-S. L., Radnay, K., Kendrick, M. I., and Kass, E. H. (1976). *Scand. J. Infect. Dis.* **8**, 45–48.

Lin, J.-S. L., Radnay, K., Kendrick, M. I., Rosner, B., and Kass, E. H. (1978). *J. Infect. Dis.* **137**, 266–273.

Love, W., Jones, M., Andrews, B., and Thomas, M. (1973). *Lancet* **i**, 1130–1131.

McChesney, J. A., Zedd, A., King, H., Russell, C. M., and Hendley, J. O. (1973). *J. Am. Med. Assoc.* **226**, 37–39.

McCormack, W. M. (1974). *Intersci. Conf. Antimicrob. Agents Chemother., 14th, San Francisco, Calif.,* p. 385.

McCormack, W. M. (1976). *J. Clin. Pathol.* **29,** Suppl. 10, 95–98.
McCormack, W. M. (1977). *In* "Nongonococcal Urethritis and Related Infections" (D. Hobson and K. K. Holmes, eds.), pp. 98–105. Am. Soc. Microbiol., Washington, D.C.
McCormack, W. M., Rankin, J. S., and Lee, Y.-H. (1972a). *Am. J. Obstet. Gynecol.* **112,** 920–923.
McCormack, W. M., Almeida, P. C., Bailey, P. E., Grady, E. M., and Lee, Y.-H. (1972b). *J. Am. Med. Assoc.* **221,** 1375–1377.
McCormack, W. M., Braun, P., Lee, Y.-H., Klein, J. O., and Kass, E. H. (1973a). *N. Engl. J. Med.* **288,** 78–89.
McCormack, W. M., Lee, Y.-H., Lin. J.-S., and Rankin, J. S. (1973b). *J. Infect. Dis.* **127,** 193–196.
McCormack, W. M., Lee, Y.-H., and Zinner, S. H. (1973c). *Ann. Intern. Med.* **78,** 696–698.
McCormack, W. M., Rosner, B., and Lee, Y.-H. (1973d). *Am. J. Epidemiol.* **97,** 240–245.
McCormack, W. M., Rosner, B., Lee, Y.-H., Rankin, J. S., and Lin, J.-S. (1975). *Lancet* **i,** 596–599.
McGee, Z. A., Johnson, A. P., and Taylor-Robinson, D. (1976). *Infect. Immun.* **13,** 608–618.
MacLeod, A. D., Furr, P. M., and Taylor-Robinson, D. (1976). *Br. J. Vener. Dis.* **52,** 337–340.
Manchee, R. J., and Taylor-Robinson, D. (1969a). *Br. J. Exp. Pathol.* **50,** 66–75.
Manchee, R. J., and Taylor-Robinson, D. (1969b). *J. Bacteriol.* **100,** 78–85.
Mårdh, P.-A. (1970). *Acta Pathol. Microbiol. Scand., Sect. B* **78,** 726–732.
Mårdh, P.-A. (1972). "Mycoplasmas in Acute Salpingitis and in Colpitis and Their Occurrence in Urine." Staffanstorps Tryckeri A.B., Lund.
Mårdh, P.-A., and Colleen, S. (1975). *Scand. J. Urol. Nephrol.* **9,** 8–16.
Mårdh, P.-A., and Weström, L. (1970a). *Acta Pathol. Microbiol. Scand., Sect. B* **78,** 367–374.
Mårdh, P.-A., and Weström, L. (1970b). *Br. J. Vener. Dis.* **46,** 390–397.
Mårdh, P.-A., and Weström, L. (1970c). *Br. J. Vener. Dis.* **46,** 179–186.
Mårdh, P.-A., Stormby, N., and Weström, L. (1971). *Acta Cytol.* **15,** 310–315.
Mårdh, P.-A., Lohi, A., and Fritz, H. (1972). *Acta Med. Scand.* **191,** 91–95.
Mårdh, P.-A., Weström, L., and Colleen, S. (1975). *In* "Genital Infections and Their Complications" (D. Danielsson, L. Juhlin, and P.-A. Mårdh, eds.), pp. 53–62. Almqvist & Wiksell, Stockholm.
Mårdh, P.-A., Weström, L., von Mecklenburg, C., and Hammar, E. (1976). *Br. J. Vener. Dis.* **52,** 52–57.
Mårdh, P.-A., Ripa, K. T., Wang, S.-P., and Weström, L. (1977). *In* "Nongonococcal Urethritis and Related Infections" (D. Hobson and K. K. Holmes, eds.), pp. 77–83. Am. Soc. Microbiol., Washington, D.C.
Markham, N. P., Markham, J. G., and Smith, E. R. (1972). *Br. J. Vener. Dis.* **48,** 200–204.
Marx, F. J., and Hofstetter, A. (1975). *Muench. Med. Wochenschr.* **117,** 1023–1028.
Matthews, C. D., Elmslie, R. G., Clapp, K. H., and Svigos, J. M. (1974). *Lancet* **ii,** 108.
Matthews, C. D., Elmslie, R. G., Clapp, K. H., and Svigos, J. M. (1975). *Fertil. Steril.* **26,** 988–990.
Meares, E. M. (1973). *J. Am. Med. Assoc.* **224,** 1372–1375.
Melén, B., and Gotthardson, A. (1955). *Acta Pathol. Microbiol. Scand.* **37,** 196–200.
Melén, B., and Linnros, B. (1952). *Acta Derm.-Venerol.* **32,** 77–85.
Mendel, E. B., Rowan, D. F., Graham, J. H. M., and Dellinger, D. (1970). *Obstet. Gynecol.* **35,** 104–108.
Møller, B. R., Freundt, E. A., Black, F. T., and Frederiksen, P. (1978). *Infect. Immun.* **20,** 248–257.
Morton, H. E., Smith, P. F., and Leberman, P. R. (1951). *Am. J. Syph., Gonorrhea, Vener. Dis.* **35,** 14–17.

Mukhija, R. D., Gupta, U., Bhujwala, R. A., Bhutani, L. K., and Kandhari, K. C. (1973a). *Indian J. Med. Res.* **61,** 1771–1774.

Mukhija, R. D., Gupta, U., Bhujwala, R. A., Mahajan, V. M., Bhutani, L. K., and Kandhari, K. C. (1973b). *Indian J. Med. Res.* **61,** 1766–1770.

Müller, W. A., Holtorff, J., and Blaschke-Hellmessen, E. (1967). *Arch. Hyg. Bakteriol.* **151,** 609–621.

Naot, Y., Sharf, M., and Klein, A. (1978). *J. Med. Microbiol.* **11,** 261–267.

Nicol, C. S., and Edward, D. G. ff. (1953). *Br. J. Vener. Dis.* **29,** 141–150.

Oates, J. K., Whittington, M. J., and Wilkinson, A. E. (1959). *Br. J. Vener. Dis.* **35,** 184–186.

O'Leary, W. M., and Frick, J. (1975). *Andrologia* **7,** 309–316.

Osoba, A. O. (1972). *Br. J. Vener. Dis.* **48,** 116–120.

Pachas, W. N. (1970). *Ann. N.Y. Acad. Sci.* **174,** 786–793.

Pease, P., Rogers, K. B., and Cole, B. C. (1967). *J. Pathol. Bacteriol.* **94,** 460–462.

Pheifer, T. A., Forsyth, P. S., Durfee, M. A., Pollock, H. M., and Holmes, K. K. (1978). *N. Engl. J. Med.* **298,** 1429–1434.

Piot, P. (1976). *Br. J. Vener. Dis.* **52,** 266–268.

Piot, P. (1977). *Br. J. Vener. Dis.* **53,** 186–189.

Prentice, M. J., Taylor-Robinson, D., and Csonka, G. W. (1976). *Br. J. Vener. Dis.* **52,** 269–275.

Prentice, M. J., Hutchinson, G. R., and Taylor-Robinson, D. (1977). *Br. J. Ophthalmol.* **61,** 601–607.

Purcell, R. H., Taylor-Robinson, D., Wong, D., and Chanock, R. M. (1966). *J. Bacteriol.* **92,** 6–12.

Purcell, R. H., Wong, D., Chanock, R. M., Taylor-Robinson, D., Canchola, J., and Valdesuso, J. (1967). *Ann. N.Y. Acad. Sci.* **143,** 664–675.

Purcell, R. H., Chanock, R. M., and Taylor-Robinson, D. (1969). *In* "The Mycoplasmatales and the L-phase of Bacteria" (L. Hayflick, ed.), pp. 221–264. Appleton, New York.

Randall, J. H., Stein, R. J., and Ayres, J.-C. (1950). *Am. J. Obstet. Gynecol.* **59,** 404–413.

Razin, S. (1968). *J. Bacteriol.* **96,** 687–694.

Razin, S., and Tully, J. G. (1970). *J. Bacteriol.* **102,** 306–310.

Razin, S., Masover, G. K., Palant, M., and Hayflick, L. (1977). *J. Bacteriol.* **130,** 464–471.

Röckl, H., and Nasemann, T. (1959). *Urol. Int.* **9,** 266–274.

Romano, N., and Romano, F. (1968). *G. Mal. Infett. Parassit.* **20,** 585–591.

Romano, N., Carollo, F., and Romano, F. (1968). *Riv. Ist. Sieroter. Ital.* **43,** 217–224.

Romano, N., Romano, F., and Carollo, F. (1971). *N. Engl. J. Med.* **285,** 950–952.

Rosendal, S., and Thomsen, A. C. (1974). *Acta Pathol. Microbiol. Scand., Sect. B* **82,** 895–898.

Rottem, S., Pfendt, E. A., and Hayflick, L. (1971). *J. Bacteriol.* **105,** 323–330.

Ruiter, M., and Wentholt, H. M. M. (1952). *J. Invest. Dermatol.* **18,** 313–325.

Russell, F. E., and Fallon, R. J. (1970). *Lancet* **i,** 1295.

Ruys, A. C., Herderscheê, D., and Waldman, J. (1967). *Ann. N.Y. Acad. Sci.* **143,** 390–393.

Sachdev, K. S., and Flamm, H. (1969). *Ger. Med. Mon.* **14,** 512–516.

Salaman, M. H. (1946). *J. Pathol. Bacteriol.* **58,** 31–35.

Schneider, E. L., Stanbridge, E. J., Epstein, C. J., Golbus, M., Abbo-Halbasch, G., and Rodgers, G. (1974). *Science* **184,** 477–480.

Schoub, B. D., Jacobs, Y. R., Hylén, E., and Freedman, R. (1976). *S. Afr. Med. J.* **50,** 445–447.

Sepetjian, M., Thivolet, J., Monier, J.-C., and Salussola, D. (1969). *Pathol. Biol.* **17,** 953–959.

Sepetjian, M., Thivolet, J., Monier, J.-C., and Salussola, D. (1973). *Pathol. Biol.* **21,** 949–954.

Sharp, J. T. (1970). *Arthritis Rheum.* **13**, 263–271.

Shepard, M. C. (1954). *Am. J. Syph., Gonorrhea, Vener. Dis.* **38**, 113–124.

Shepard, M. C. (1966). *Health Lab. Sci.* **3**, 163–169.

Shepard, M. C. (1974). *In* "Les Mycoplasmes de l'Homme, des Animaux, des Vegetaux et des Insectes" (J. M. Bové and J. F. Duplan, eds.), Colloques INSERM, No. 33, pp. 375–379. INSERM, Paris.

Shepard, M. C., and Calvy, G. L. (1965). *N. Engl. J. Med.* **272**, 848–851.

Shepard, M. C., and Lunceford, C. D. (1970). *Appl. Microbiol.* **20**, 539–543.

Shepard, M. C., and Lunceford, C. D. (1976). *J. Clin. Microbiol.* **3**, 613–625.

Shepard, M. C., Lunceford, C. D., Ford, D. K., Purcell, R. H., Taylor-Robinson, D., Razin, S., and Black, F. T. (1974). *Int. J. Syst. Bacteriol.* **24**, 160–171.

Shipley, A., Bowman, S. J., and O'Connor, J. J. (1968). *Med. J. Aust.* **1**, 794–796.

Shurin, P. A., Alpert, S., Rosner, B., Driscoll, S. G., Lee, Y.-H., McCormack, W. M., Santamarina, B. A. G., and Kass, E. H. (1975). *N. Engl. J. Med.* **293**, 5–8.

Simberkoff, M. S., and Toharsky, B. (1976). *J. Am. Med. Assoc.* **236**, 2522–2524.

Singer, G. R., and Ivler, D. (1975). *N. Engl. J. Med.* **293**, 780.

Slingerland, D. W., and Morgan, H. R. (1952). *J. Am. Med. Assoc.* **150**, 1309–1310.

Smith, W. E. (1942). *J. Bacteriol.* **43**, 83.

Solomon, F., Sompolinsky, D., Caspi, E., and Alkan, W. J. (1970). *Isr. J. Med. Sci.* **6**, 605–610.

Solomon, F., Caspi, E., Bukovsky, I., and Sompolinsky, D. (1973). *Am. J. Obstet. Gynecol.* **116**, 785–792.

Somerson, N. L., Rubin, A., Smith, P. F., and Morton, H. E. (1955). *Am. J. Obstet. Gynecol.* **69**, 848–853.

Sompolinsky, D., Solomon, F., Leiba, H., Caspi, E., Lewinsohn, G., and Almog, C. (1971). *Isr. J. Med. Sci.* **7**, 745–748.

Sompolinsky, D., Harari, Z., Solomon, F., Caspi, E., Krakowski, D., and Henig, E. (1973). *Isr. J. Med. Sci,* **9**, 438–446.

Sompolinsky, D., Solomon, F., Elkina, L., Weinraub, Z., Bukovsky, I., and Caspi, E. (1975). *Am. J. Obstet. Gynecol.* **121**, 610–616.

Spaepen, M. S., Kundsin, R. B., and Horne, H. W. (1976). *Antimicrob. Agents Chemother.* **9**, 1012–1018.

Spitzbart, H. (1967). *Geburtshilfe Frauenheilkd.* **27**, 889–894.

Stalheim, O. H. V., and Gallagher, J. E. (1977). *Infect. Immun.* **15**, 995–996.

Stalheim, O. H. V., and Proctor, S. J. (1976). *Am. J. Vet. Res.* **37**, 879–883.

Stalheim, O. H. V., Proctor, S. J., and Gallagher, J. E. (1976). *Infect. Immun.* **13**, 915–925.

Steytler, J. G. (1970). *S. Afr. J. Obstet. Gynaecol.* **8**, 10–13.

Stokes, E. J. (1955). *Lancet* **i**, 276–279.

Stray-Pedersen, B., Eng, J., and Reikvam, T. M. (1978). *Am. J. Obstet. Gynecol.* **130**, 307–311.

Sueltmann, S., Allen, V., Inhorn, S. L., and Benforado, J. M. (1971). *Health Lab. Sci.* **8**, 62–66.

Tafari, N., Ross, S., Naeye, R. L., Judge, D. M., and Marboe, C. (1976). *Lancet* **i**, 108–109.

Tan, R. J. S., and Miles, J. A. R. (1974). *Aust. Vet. J.* **50**, 142–145.

Tarr, P. I., Lee, Y.-H., Alpert, S., Schumacher, J. R., Zinner, S. H., and McCormack, W. M. (1976). *J. Infect. Dis.* **133**, 419–423.

Taylor-Robinson, D. (1974). *Nature (London)* **248**, 267.

Taylor-Robinson, D. (1976). *In* "Scientific Foundations of Urology" (D. I. Williams and G. D. Chisholm, eds.), pp. 258–262. Heinemann, London.

Taylor-Robinson, D. (1977a). *In* "Nongonococcal Urethritis and Related Infections" (D. Hobson and K. K. Holmes, eds.), pp. 30–37. Am. Soc. Microbiol., Washington, D.C.

Taylor-Robinson, D. (1977b). *In* "Infections and Pregnancy" (C. R. Coid, ed.), pp. 141–206. Academic Press, New York.

Taylor-Robinson, D. (1978). *In* "Mycoplasma Infection of Cell Cultures" (G. J. McGarrity, D. G. Murphy, and W. W. Nichols, eds.), pp. 47–56. Plenum, New York.

Taylor-Robinson, D. (1979). *In* "Current Research in Rheumatoid Arthritis and Allied Diseases" (D. C. Dumonde and R. N. Maini, eds.) Medical and Technical Publications Press, Lancaster. (In press.)

Taylor-Robinson, D., and Carney, F. E. (1974). *Br. J. Vener. Dis.* **50**, 212–216.

Taylor-Robinson, D., and Furr, P. M. (1973). *Ann. N.Y. Acad. Sci.* **225**, 108–117.

Taylor-Robinson, D., and Manchee, R. J. (1967). *Nature (London)* **215**, 484–487.

Taylor-Robinson, D., and Manchee, R. J. (1969). *In* "Mycoplasma Diseases of Man" (M. Sprössig and W. Witzleb, eds.), pp. 113–129. Fischer, Jena.

Taylor-Robinson, D., and Purcell, R. H. (1966). *Proc. R. Soc. Med.* **59**, 1112–1116.

Taylor-Robinson, D., and Taylor, G. (1976). *In* "Infection and Immunology in the Rheumatic Diseases" (D. C. Dumonde, ed.), pp. 177–186. Blackwell, Oxford.

Taylor-Robinson, D., Ludwig, M. W., Purcell, R. H., Mufson, M. A., and Chanock, R. M. (1965). *Proc. Soc. Exp. Biol. Med.* **118**, 1073–1083.

Taylor-Robinson, D., Purcell, R. H., Wong, D. C., and Chanock, R. M. (1966). *J. Hyg.* **64**, 91–104.

Taylor-Robinson, D., Addey, J. P., Hare, M. J., and Dunlop, E. M. C. (1969a). *Br. J. Vener. Dis.* **45**, 265–273.

Taylor-Robinson, D., Addey, J. P., and Goodwin, C. S. (1969b). *Nature (London)* **222**, 274–275.

Taylor-Robinson, D., Johnson, A. P., and McGee, Z. A. (1975a). *In* "Genital Infections and Their Complications" (D. Danielsson, L. Juhlin, and P.-A. Mårdh, eds.), pp. 243–252. Almqvist & Wiksell, Stockholm.

Taylor-Robinson, D., Rassner, C., Furr, P. M., Humber, D. P., and Barnes, R. D. (1975b). *J. Reprod. Fertil.* **42**, 483–490.

Taylor-Robinson, D., Csonka, G. W., and Prentice, M. J. (1977). *Q. J. Med., New Ser.* **46**, 309–326.

Taylor-Robinson, D., Purcell, R. H., London, W. T., and Sly, D. L. (1978). *J. Med. Microbiol.* **11**, 197–201.

Taylor-Robinson, D., Evans, R. T., Coufalik, E. D., Prentice, M. J., Munday, P. E., Csonka, G. W., and Oates, J. K. (1979). *Br. J. Vener. Dis.* **55**, 30–35.

Thomas, M., Jones, M., Ray, S., and Andrews, B. (1975). *Lancet* **ii**, 774–775.

Thomsen, A. C. (1974). *Acta Pathol. Microbiol. Scand., Sect. B* **82**, 653–656.

Thomsen, A. C. (1975). *Acta Pathol. Microbiol. Scand., Sect. B* **83**, 10–16.

Thomsen, A. C. (1978a). *J. Clin. Microbiol.* **1**, 84–88.

Thomsen, A. C. (1978b). *J. Clin. Microbiol.* **2**, 197–202.

Thomsen, A. C., Rosendal, S., and Thomsen, O. F. (1973). *Acta Pathol. Microbiol. Scand., Sect. A* **81**, 379–380.

Traub, R. G., Madden, D. L., Fuccillo, D. A., and McLean, T. W. (1973). *N. Engl. J. Med.* **289**, 697–698.

Tully, J. G., and Smith, L. G. (1968). *J. Am. Med. Assoc.* **204**, 827–828.

Tully, J. G., Brown, M. S., Sheagren, J. N., Young, V. M., and Wolff, S. M. (1965). *N. Engl. J. Med.* **273**, 648–650.

Vaughan-Jackson, J. D., Dunlop, E. M. C., Darougar, S., Treharne, J. D., and Taylor-Robinson, D. (1977). *Br. J. Vener. Dis.* **53**, 180–183.

Vogt, H. J. (1973). *Infection* **1**, 250–252.

Waldman, J. (1972). "De Isolate von T-stam Mycoplasmas bij Mannen," Thesis. Van Steijn's Drukkerji N.V., Amsterdam.

Wallace, R. J., Jr., Alpert, S., Brown, K., Lin, J.-S. L., and McCormack, W. M. (1978). *Obstet. Gynecol.* **51,** 181–185.

Weidner, W., Brunner, H., Krause, W., and Rothauge, C. F. (1978). *Dtsch. Med. Wochenschr.* **103,** 465–470.

Weissenbacher, E.-R., Bredt, W., Jonatha, W., and Zahn, V. (1976). *Proc. Soc. Gen. Microbiol.* **iii**(4), 145.

Weström, L. (1975). *Am. J. Obstet. Gynecol.* **121,** 707–713.

Weström, L., and Mårdh, P.-A. (1971). *Acta Obstet. Gynecol. Scand.* **50,** 25–31.

Weström, L., and Mårdh, P.-A. (1975). *In* "Genital Infections and Their Complications" (D. Danielsson, L. Juhlin, and P.-A. Mårdh, eds.), pp. 157–167. Almqvist & Wiksell, Stockholm.

Willcox, R. R. (1954). *Lancet* **ii,** 684–685.

Willcox, R. R. (1968). *Br. J. Vener. Dis.* **44,** 157–159.

Witzleb, W., Färber, I., Thieler, H., and Blumöhr, T. (1968). *Zentralbl. Bakteriol., Parasitenkd., Infektionskr. Hyg., Abt. 1: Orig.* **208,** 427–430.

Witzleb, W., Färber, I., Blumöhr, T., and Thieler, H. (1969). *In* "Mycoplasma Diseases of Man" (M. Sprössig and W. Witzleb, eds.), pp. 149–154. Fischer, Jena.

Wong, J. L., Hines, P. A., Brasher, M. D., Rogers, G. T., Smith, R. F., and Schachter, J. (1977). *Sex. Transm. Dis.* **4,** 4–8.

Zeltzer, H., and Palti, Z. (1963). *Harefuah* **65,** 156–158.

11 / MYCOPLASMAS AS ARTHRITOGENIC AGENTS

Barry C. Cole and John R. Ward

I. INTRODUCTION

Members of the Mycoplasmatales are the causative agents of a wide variety of animal diseases which most commonly result in respiratory and joint infections as well as systemic involvement including brain, liver, kidney, and heart. The genitourinary tract may also become infected. Many of these infections are chronic in nature, suggesting an intimate host–parasite interaction. Although some species are primarily arthritogenic agents, others including the respiratory pathogens can also exhibit associated joint complications.

In this chapter we compare the main features of the various animal arthritides induced by mycoplasmas and summarize current thoughts on the mechanisms of invasion of the host, the immune responses to the agents, and the mechanisms of the inflammatory process. The general

THE MYCOPLASMAS, VOL. II

physiological and biological properties of these organisms are dealt with elsewhere in this volume and are mentioned here only as they relate to arthritogenicity. Finally we consider attempts to implicate mycoplasmas directly in the pathogenesis of human rheumatoid arthritis (RA).

II. MYCOPLASMA-INDUCED ARTHRITIS IN ANIMALS

A. Clinical, Pathological, and Microbiological Features

1. Murine Arthritis

One of the earliest mycoplasma infections to be studied was rat arthritis induced by *Mycoplasma arthritidis*. The disease occurs naturally in rat colonies and may also be produced by the injection of mycoplasma cultures (Ward and Cole, 1970). Onset of the experimental disease induced by intravenous (IV) injection of organisms varies from 2 to 9 days depending upon inoculum size and virulence of the organisms (Ward and Jones, 1962). The arthritis can affect all four extremities and the vertebral articulations. The joints exhibit pronounced swelling, redness, and tenderness, and the synovial cavity contains a thick, purulent exudate. Histologically the infection is markedly suppurative and progresses from intense polymorphonuclear leukocyte (PMN) infiltration of the synovial membrane and adjacent tissues to abscess production and periostial osteoneogenesis and destruction of articular cartilage. Rats frequently develop associated urethritis, rhinitis, conjunctivitis, and corneal opacity. Arthritis of interspinal articulations produces paralysis of the hind limbs. The disease appears to be self-limited and usually resolves by 50 days. Increases in peripheral blood PMNs and lymphocytes are seen during the infection, and the erythrocyte sedimentation rate (ESR), hemolytic serum complement level, and serum lysozyme level are also elevated (Eisen and Loveday, 1973).

Organisms are readily cultured from involved joints during the peak of arthritis but cannot be recovered 6–8 weeks after infection (Ward and Jones, 1962; Hill and Dagnall, 1975). Immunofluorescence studies have shown that antigen persists in the joint for a further 2 weeks after cultivable organisms have been eliminated (Hill and Dagnall, 1975). Although *M. arthritidis* can be harbored in the oropharynx, middle ear, and lung of normal rats (Ward and Cole, 1970; Stewart and Buck, 1975), no overt pulmonary disease has been described. This organism has also been reportedly isolated from humans and other nonhuman primates, but its capacity to induce disease in these hosts has not been established (Chapter 6).

In contrast with the limited arthritis seen in rats, experimental arthritis induced by the IV injection of *M. arthritidis* into mice is capable of progressing to a migratory chronic phase which can persist for the life of the animal (Cole *et al.*, 1971a, and unpublished observations). Whereas the disease often subsides 70–150 days after inoculation, a spontaneous pronounced resurgence of arthritis can occur after this time. Although the onset of this disease is similar to that seen in rats, less virulent cultures often do not exhibit an early acute phase of arthritis, and sometimes clinical disease is delayed for 72 days after injection (Cahill *et al.*, 1971). It is not known whether arthritis occurs spontaneously, and there have been no published reports on the isolation of *M. arthritidis* from normal mice.

With virulent organisms, the histological lesions at 3 days consist of edema and scattered periarticular infiltration with PMNs and a mild proliferation of synoviocytes. The disease rapidly progresses to an intense infiltration of synovial membrane and adjacent tissues, with abscess formation. Late lesions are characterized by massive proliferation of the synovial membrane, with villus hypertrophy and a predominantly lymphocytic and plasma cell infiltrate (Fig. 1). Articular cartilage is gradually

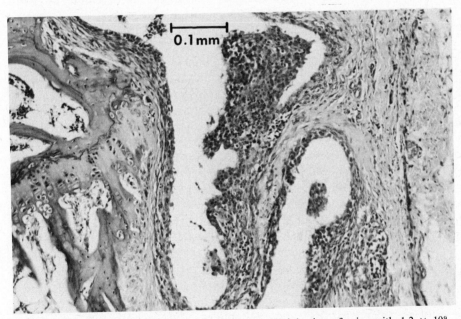

FIGURE 1. Joint lesions obtained 76 days after IV injection of mice with 1.2×10^9 colony-forming units (CFU) of *M. arthritidis*. Pronounced villus hypertrophy with mononuclear cell and PMN infiltration is seen. Cartilage destruction and collagen deposition are also apparent. (Reproduced from Cole *et al.*, 1971a.)

eroded, and pannus formation leads to extensive invasion of bone. Although evidence of repair is also seen late in the disease, active areas of destructive inflammation persist. Peripheral blood neutrophilia (Cole *et al.*, 1976) and sometimes lymphopenia are seen during the first 3 weeks of infection, and mild anemia is apparent through 60 days (Edwards *et al.*, 1975). An important feature of the mouse disease induced by *M. arthritidis* is that organisms can be isolated from involved joints at all stages of the arthritis, although the number of positive isolations decreases in the chronic stage of the disease. The organism can also induce a spreading necrotizing abscess in mice and results in abortion or resorption of fetuses following IV injection of the organisms into pregnant mice (Cole *et al.*, 1973a; Kaklamanis and Thomas, 1970).

Mycoplasma pulmonis can also induce arthritis in mice. Mycoplasmas have been known to be associated with mouse arthritis for many years (Sabin, 1939), although in some cases, because of the inadequate taxonomy at the time, definitive identification of all the isolates was not possible. At least one of Sabin's arthritogenic mouse isolates has now been identified as *M. pulmonis* (Tully and Ruchman, 1964), a known respiratory pathogen of mice and rats. This species is a common inhabitant of the respiratory tract of rodents and can also localize and produce inflammation of the genital tract (this volume, Chapter 8; Goeth and Appel, 1974).

Barden and Tully (1969) described spontaneously occurring nonsuppurative chronic polyarthritis in mice which had received tumor material. Subsequent experiments showed that *M. pulmonis* was the etiological agent and that chronic migratory arthritis could be induced experimentally by the IV injection of this species into normal mice. The disease was characterized in more detail by Harwick *et al.* (1973b, 1976). After the initial acute phase of infection, which was much less suppurative than that seen with *M. arthritidis,* the changes observed bore a close similarity to those seen in the chronic phase of *M. arthritidis*-induced arthritis of mice. The *M. pulmonis*-induced disease also exhibited periods of varying severity and persisted for the 46 weeks' duration of the experiments. Studies by Cassell (personal communication) suggest that other strains of *M. pulmonis* can induce a more suppurative type of infection in mice (Fig. 2) and that rats can also develop mild transient arthritis when injected with this organism. As with *M. arthritidis*, *M. pulmonis* can be recovered from arthritic joints even in the late chronic phase of the disease. In contrast with *M. arthritidis*, *M. pulmonis* induces pronounced peripheral blood lymphocytosis but only a mild neutrophilia in mice 7–14 days after IV inoculation (Cole *et al.*, 1975b).

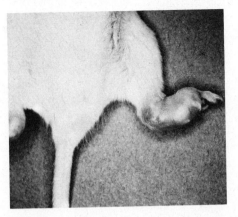

FIGURE 2.   Joint of mouse 96 days after IV injection with 1.2×10^8 CFU *M. pulmonis*. (Reproduced courtesy of G. H. Cassell, University of Alabama, Birmingham.)

2. Rabbit Arthritis

Recently, Cole *et al.* (1977b) reported that both *M. arthritidis* and *M. pulmonis* induced arthritis in rabbits following injection of the organisms into knee joints. The arthritis progresses from acute to chronic inflammation, as seen in mouse arthritis (Figs. 3–6). There is preliminary evidence that the arthritis, which is restricted to the injected joints, can persist for at least 14 months in some animals. In striking contrast to the mouse arthritides, mycoplasmas cannot be cultured from rabbit joints later than 4 weeks after inoculation despite the continuation of active disease. Preliminary studies using immunofluoresence indicate that the organisms do not localize on the surface of the synovial membrane, but that within a few days they move into the deeper layers of the synovium where they rapidly become undetectable (Washburn *et al.*, 1978). Thus, these observations contrast quite significantly with those seen in murine respiratory and genital infections caused by *M. pulmonis,* in which epithelial surfaces are extensively colonized (this volume, Chapter 8).

Although *M. pulmonis* has been isolated from the nasopharynx of rabbits suffering from respiratory disease (Deeb and Kenny, 1967), its etiological role in this condition remains to be established, as does its frequency of isolation from normal rabbits. *Mycoplasma arthritidis* has not been isolated from rabbits.

3. Swine Arthritis

Two distinct species of mycoplasma are known to produce spontaneous arthritis in swine, and both can result in considerable economic loss.

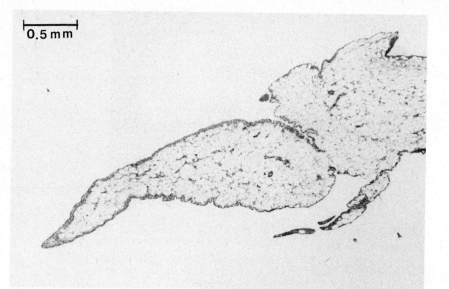

FIGURE 3.   Normal rabbit synovium. Note the simple outline, even surface layer, and acellular stroma. (Reproduced from Cole *et al.*, 1977b.)

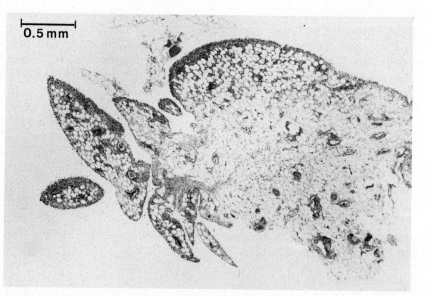

FIGURE 4.   Rabbit synovium 7 days after intra-articular injection of 10^6 CFU of *M. arthritidis*. Note proliferation of villi, infiltration of surface layer with inflammatory cells, increased vascularity, and desquamation. (Reproduced from Cole *et al.*, 1977b.)

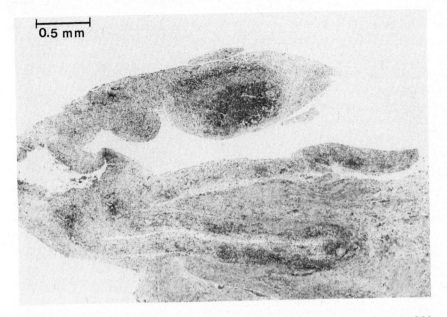

0.5 mm

FIGURE 5. Rabbit synovium 30 days after intra-articular injection with 10^9 CFU of *M. arthritidis*. Villus hypertrophy, massive cellular infiltration, and formation of lymphoid follicles are apparent. (Reproduced from Cole *et al.*, 1977b.)

Mycoplasma hyorhinis predominantly affects swine less than 8 weeks of age (Duncan and Ross, 1973). Fever and lameness usually occur by 4–10 days following the intraperitoneal (IP) injection of *M. hyorhinis*. The early histological lesions are characterized by hyperemia, edema, and infiltration of the synovium with PMNs, macrophages, and some lymphocytes. By 6–9 weeks there is chronic synovitis with cartilage and bone destruction. Clinical arthritis has been observed to persist for 18 months (Decker and Barden, 1975). As well as synovitis, polyserositis is also evident in a high proportion of swine naturally or experimentally infected with *M. hyorhinis*, and lymphoid accumulations are evident in liver, lung, brain, and myocardium (Roberts *et al.*, 1963a,b; Ennis *et al.*, 1971). The erythrocyte sedimentation rate (ESR) is increased in the early stages of the disease, and lymphocytosis is present through 20 weeks.

Although *M. hyorhinis* is readily recovered through 57 days, the organisms are only rarely found in the joints after this time (Barden and Decker, 1971; Duncan and Ross, 1973; Roberts *et al.*, 1963b). The finding by immunofluorescence that *M. hyorhinis* antigen can be detected in the synovial membrane many months after viable organisms can no longer be isolated suggests that nonviable or noncultivable organisms may be re-

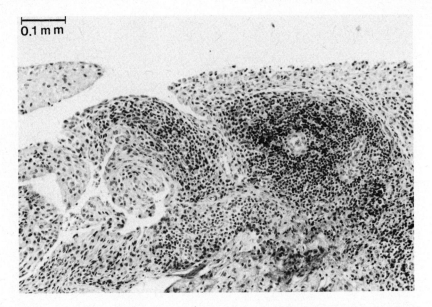

0.1 m m

FIGURE 6.   Rabbit synovium 90 days after injection of 10^6 CFU of *M. arthritidis*. Note the perivascular lymphoid follicle and hyperplasia of vascular epithelium. The thickened synovial surface layer contains macrophages, lymphocytes, plasma cells, and fibroblasts. (Reproduced from Cole *et al.*, 1977b.)

sponsible for the continued inflammation (Decker and Barden, 1975). Electron microscope examination of acutely inflamed synovium has failed to demonstrate the presence of mycoplasma cells (Duncan and Ross, 1969). This organism can be harbored in the nasopharynx of adult swine but does not regularly induce respiratory disease. It is frequently isolated from the lungs of pneumonic swine, and pure cultures of the organism induce pneumonia and pericarditis in gnotobiotic piglets after intranasal administration (Goiš *et al.*, 1971).

Swine arthritis induced by *M. hyosynoviae* is generally less severe than that seen with *M. hyorhinis*, is nonsuppurative, and predominantly affects older animals (Ross and Duncan, 1970; Ross *et al.*, 1971). Experimental induction of the arthritis has been inconsistent. The onset of disease occurs with sudden lameness 4–8 days after IV injection of the organisms. In many animals the arthritis resolves after a short, acute phase, but in others the disease persists. The pathological lesions appear to be restricted to hyperemia, edema, and mild hypertrophy of the synovial membrane, with increased serofibrinous synovial fluid. Detailed studies over a long period of time have not been undertaken. It appears that viable organisms are fairly rapidly eliminated from the joints, although they can persist for a longer time on the tonsils. In fact, *M. hyosynoviae* is harbored naturally on the tonsils and respiratory mucosa of adult sows, and the infection can be passed to suckling piglets after 6 weeks of age (Ross and Spear, 1973). There is no evidence at this time that *M. hyosynoviae* causes respiratory disease.

4. Avian Arthritis

Mycoplasma gallisepticum is a versatile natural pathogen of turkeys and chickens causing severe respiratory disease, polyarteritis affecting the brain and heart, and less commonly arthritis. Early work has been reviewed by Adler (1970). Following IV or foot pad inoculation of chickens (Kerr and Olson, 1967; DaSilva and Adler, 1969) polyarteritis of periarticular tissues and synovitis are seen as early as 3 days. Suppurative arthritis develops which leads to chronic synovial changes with erosion of cartilage. In some birds, evidence of arthritis persisted for 206 days, and successful isolations of *M. gallisepticum* were reported at this time (Kerr and Olson, 1967). It is interesting that, in animals injected in one foot pad, the arthritis progressed only to the joints of the injected limb. Contact-infected chickens only rarely developed arthritis but did develop respiratory disease. The organisms are harbored naturally in the respiratory tract, and egg transmission of the agent is a common and troublesome occurrence (Adler, 1970).

In contrast to *M. gallisepticum, Mycoplasma synoviae* is primarily an arthritogenic avian mycoplasma, but there can be associated systemic involvement affecting the lungs, liver, heart, kidneys, and spleen (Sevoian *et al.*, 1958). *Mycoplasma synoviae* disease can be acquired by the respiratory route and by egg transmission. Kerr and Olson (1970) reported a comparison of 2-week-old chickens injected in the foot pad with *M. synoviae* with uninoculated contact-infected chickens. Arthritis began after 5 days in the joints of the inoculated limb and after 14 days had spread to the joints of other limbs. Arthritis was not seen in contact-infected birds before 30 days, and the infection was less severe and involved fewer joints. Histologically the arthritis progressed through an acute suppurative stage to a more chronic phase in which erosion of articular cartilage and destruction of tendons was prominent. After 175 days there was complete destruction of tarsal joints in 5% of the birds. A striking feature of the *M. synoviae*-induced disease was the marked infiltration of the heart, liver, spleen, and other organs with mononuclear cells and heterophils. During the first 40–50 days of infection there was an increase in peripheral blood heterophils and monocytes but a marked decrease in lymphocytes. Pronounced anemia was apparent for the first 30 days. Viable organisms sometimes persisted in the joints as long as 189 days after inoculation and were regularly isolated from the trachea for the 206 days' duration of the experiment.

Recently *M. synoviae* was shown to induce air sacculitis in chickens in which epithelial hyperplasia and predominantly lymphocytic infiltration of connective tissue were seen (Fletcher *et al.*, 1976). Turkey poults also develop air sacculitis following inoculation of *M. synoviae* into the air sac and arthritis when the organisms are given IV (Ghazikhanian *et al.*, 1973). However, the joint lesions and inflammatory involvement of other organs is generally much less severe than that seen in chickens. Organisms persisted in involved joints for the 28 days' duration of the experiments.

Mycoplasma meleagridis infects a high proportion of turkey flocks and is primarily egg-transmitted. Although the organism is of low pathogenicity, it induces mild air sacculitis and synovitis in turkeys (Adler, 1970). Recent studies suggest that experimental *M. meleagridis* may result in more severe synovitis with pronounced bone deformity (Bigland and Jordan, personal communication). The joint lesions induced by this organism have not been studied in detail.

5. Bovine, Caprine, and Ovine Arthritis

Arthritis is a complicating feature of bovine pleuropneumonia and has been commonly seen during attempts to vaccinate cattle against the etiological agent, *Mycoplasma mycoides* subsp. *mycoides*. However, the strict eradication of infected herds has largely precluded more detailed studies of the ability of this organism to cause joint disease (Meyer, 1909; Trethewie and Turner, 1961; Sharp and Riggs, 1967). Only in comparatively recent years has it been realized that mycoplasma species other than *M. mycoides* are capable of causing spontaneous bovine arthritis (Moulton *et al.*, 1956; Simmons and Johnston, 1963). The best studied of these is *Mycoplasma bovis*, formerly classified as *M. agalactiae* subsp. *bovis* or *M. bovimastitidis,* the most common causative agent of bovine mastitis (Gourlay, 1973). This mycoplasma has recently been isolated from cases of spontaneous arthritis in calves and feedlot cattle (Hjerpe and Knight, 1972; Stalheim and Stone, 1975). Stalheim and Page (1975) demonstrated that intra-articular or IV injection of *M. bovis* resulted in a severe arthritis. Animals receiving intramammary injections developed severe mastitis and arthritis. The organisms persisted in the joints for the 28 days of observation. Preliminary pathological studies revealed severe fibrinopurulent synovitis with synovial cell proliferation and villus hypertrophy. Using gnotobiotic calves, Gourlay *et al.* (1976) showed that 2 weeks following inoculation of *M. bovis* into the respiratory tract mild subclinical pneumonia and arthritis resulted, with positive isolations of mycoplasma from lungs and joints.

As reviewed by Cottew (1970) and elsewhere in this volume (Chapter 3), it is clear that mycoplasmas can induce joint disease in goats and sheep. Although in some cases the organisms were not identified, in others *M. agalactiae* (the causative agent of agalactia) appeared to be responsible. More work is clearly required to define the arthritogenic potential of mycoplasmas for these hosts.

6. Arthritis in Nonhuman Primates

Whereas mycoplasmas have been claimed to be associated with arthritis in gorillas and rhesus monkeys, conclusive evidence on their role in these conditions remains to be presented (see this volume, Chapter 6).

7. Summary

Although many of the arthritic diseases caused by mycoplasmas have been incompletely studied, especially with regard to chronic symptoms, some trends are apparent. Thus, while some mycoplasmas are primarily arthritogenic agents, most of the respiratory pathogens can also induce varying degrees of joint involvement. In general the histopathological characteristics of the lesions induced by these organisms bear a close similarity to each other, and an acute suppurative phase of arthritis is usually followed by a chronic disease characterized by synovial proliferation, mononuclear cell infiltration, and cartilage destruction. In many cases the organisms can persist within the synovial tissues. The ability of some species to survive within the respiratory tract provides a potential reservoir for continued infection.

B. Chemotherapy of Animal Arthritis

In general, antibiotic therapy of mycoplasma-induced arthritis has not been successful, especially in the case of established disease. This has been particularly true with spontaneous arthritis of cattle induced by *M. bovis* (Stalheim, 1976). Thus, intramuscular injections of dihydro-streptomycin and tylosin followed by oral tetracycline administered in water or milk failed to produce remission of the arthritis. Similarly, neither intramuscular injections of tylosin nor intra-articular administration of tylosin, lincomycin, or clindamycin suppressed the experimentally induced disease, and mycoplasmas were still recoverable from the arthritic joints at autopsy. Tylosin only delayed the onset of disease when given at the time of inoculation of organisms.

The inoculation of eggs with antibiotics appears to control infection with *M. gallisepticum* and *M. synoviae,* but considerably less success has been obtained in controlling adult disease. Although tetracyclines can suppress arthritis, cessation of treatment may lead to a recurrence of the disease (Adler, 1970). Swine arthritis and polyserositis appear to be similarly resistant to antibiotic therapy, and the successful elimination of nasal carriers of *M. hyorhinis* has not been accomplished. Tylosin and lincomycin given in conjunction with corticosteroids can suppress swine arthritis induced by *M. hyosynoviae* when given during the onset of the disease (Ross and Duncan, 1970).

As previously reviewed (Ward and Cole, 1970), murine models of arthritis have been used extensively to test the chemotherapeutic effectiveness of antibiotics and organic gold compounds. Although it was originally thought that the ability of the latter compounds to suppress arthritis was due to their mycoplasmacidal properties, recent work suggests that they may also act nonspecifically on the inflammatory process. Tetracyclines are also known to suppress arthritis when given prior to infection or during the onset of the disease. Hannan (1976) showed that large doses of intramuscularly-administered tetracycline were required to suppress established (21 days) *M. pulmonis*-induced disease. Orally administered drug had no effect. The levels of tetracycline used to suppress arthritis in these studies were greater than those which could be tolerated by humans.

Additional experiments in our laboratory have shown that tetracycline treatment of the early phase of mouse arthritis induced by *M. arthritidis* is effective but that cessation of treatment results in exacerbation of the disease (unpublished). Furthermore, when treatment is initiated 6 months after infection, no decrease in clinical disease is seen, and a few mycoplasmas are still recoverable from arthritic joints. Other studies by G. Taylor (personal communication) are interesting, since they showed that lymecycline treatment of established (5 months) *M. pulmonis* arthritis reduced the incidence of mycoplasmas and resulted in a decrease in the inflammatory cells from the synovium. Gross pathology as evidenced by joint swelling was unaffected by the treatment. Studies by Hannan and Dixon (1978) on arthritic mice injected over 1 year previously with *M. pulmonis* indicate that gentamicin is more effective than tetracycline in reducing the numbers of organisms in the joints.

We might conclude from these studies that mycoplasma-induced arthritis does not in general respond well to the usual antimicrobial doses of antibiotics but that continually applied high doses may exhibit a beneficial effect. Since disease often returns after cessation of treatment, it is also apparent that the organisms must be sequestered at a protected site. We therefore suggest that murine arthritis induced by mycoplasmas may serve as a model to develop more effective chemotherapeutic approaches to the problem of chronic infection.

C. Immune Responses and Resistance to Reinfection

In mycoplasmal diseases of economic importance, the development of diagnostic serological tests and vaccines has received much attention and is described in detail elsewhere in this volume. The precise roles of humoral and cellular immune responses in protection of the host have been more difficult to define. Although the immune phenomena associated with arthritis of laboratory animals has been studied in somewhat more detail, many important questions remain unresolved. Comparisons of studies conducted in different laboratories should be made with caution because of differences in host and mycoplasma strains utilized (see also this volume, Chapter 12).

1. Humoral Immune Responses

In this section we use the *M. arthritidis* models of arthritis to illustrate the diversity of host-immune responses and will only briefly summarize pertinent observations from other mycoplasma-induced arthritides.

The self-limited arthritis of rats induced by *M. arthritidis* is associated with the elimination of organisms from involved joints and the development of a complete immunity to reinfection (Ward and Jones, 1962; Cole *et al.*, 1969). Protection is also observed by the SC administration of viable organisms or by IV administration of formalin-killed cells. There is evidence that a humoral factor plays a major role in resistance, since serum from convalescent rats protects normal rats against disease (Cole and Ward, 1973a). The nature of the factor responsible is not known. Convalescent rat serum is incapable of neutralizing actively growing organisms and is without metabolism-inhibiting (MI) antibody activity (Cole *et al.*, 1969). Furthermore, convalescent serum apparently does not contain opsonizing antibodies, as evidenced by its failure to promote phagocytosis of *M. arthritidis* by immune peritoneal macrophages (Cole *et al.*, 1973b). In contrast, rabbit hyperimmune serum against *M. arthritidis* promotes active phagocytosis. However, it should be noted that other phagocytic cells were not examined and that opsonin activity may have been masked by the reported ability of *M. arthritidis* to suppress phagocytic action (Simberkoff and Elsbach, 1971). Interestingly, the adsorption of convalescent rat serum with *M. arthritidis* antigen did not diminish the protective effect, although the CF antibody titer of the serum was drastically reduced (Cole *et al.*, 1969). These results suggest that the protective property of the serum might be directed against a soluble mycoplasma product.

The chronic nature of mouse arthritis induced by *M. arthritidis* and the ability of the organisms to persist in joints indicate that these animals are less able to control the infection than are rats. These observations correlate with the lesser effectiveness of active or passive vaccination procedures in protecting mice against arthritis and with the inability of convalescent serum to promote clearance of IV injected organisms (Cole *et al.*, 1976; Cole and Ward, 1973a). It is clear, however, that some immune processes are in effect, since a decrease in severity of disease or even spontaneous resolution can occur. Furthermore, convalescent mice fail to develop major disease when the organisms are reinjected either IV or intraarticularly (Cole *et al.*, 1976). As with rats, mice readily produce CF antibodies in response to infection with *M. arthritidis*. The MI antibody response of mice is variable and only low titers have been detected (Cole *et al.*, 1971b and 1976). There is preliminary evidence that the strain of mouse affects the MI antibody response as does also the strain of *M. arthritidis* utilized (B. C. Cole *et al.*, unpublished observations).

Rabbits respond quite differently to *M. arthritidis* in that the organisms are very rapidly eliminated from the injected joints although disease persists. The disappearance of viable organisms is not surprising in view of the strong immune responses which they evoke in this host. High levels of MI antibody can be detected in serum and even higher titers have been found in joint fluids. This latter observation, combined with the demonstration of IgG and IgA producing plasma cells in infected synovial tissue, suggests that antibody is synthesized locally (Cole *et al.*, 1977b; L. R. Washburn, B. C. Cole, and J. R. Ward, unpublished observations). Swine infected with *M. hyorhinis* or *M. hyosynoviae* also produce high levels of MI antibody (Decker and Barden, 1975; Ross *et al.*, 1973; Zimmerman and Ross, 1977), which may also correlate with the failure to isolate viable organisms during the chronic phase of these diseases. Although the resistance of rabbits to reinfection has not been studied, it is known that the serum of rabbits hyperimmunized against *M. arthritidis* can very effectively protect both mice and rats against arthritis and that it will enhance clearance of injected organisms and promote phagocytosis.

There is now evidence that the three different arthritic disease syndromes induced by *M. arthritidis* in rats, mice, and rabbits also occur in these same hosts after injection with *M. pulmonis*. Certain similarities are also apparent in the immune responses of these hosts to the latter organism. Thus, whereas CF antibody can readily be detected in all animals, MI antibody has been less consistently found except in rabbits (Taylor *et al.*, 1974; Cole *et al.*, 1975b, 1977b; Harwick *et al.*, 1976). Humoral antibody is believed to play a major role in protection of mice against *M. pulmonis* arthritis, because the serum from convalescent animals is highly effective when passively administered to normal mice. Interestingly, the protective properties of the serum could not be removed by adsorption with *M. pulmonis* antigen (Taylor and Taylor-Robinson, 1977). Other studies have shown that convalescent mouse serum does contain opsonizing antibodies (G. Taylor, personal communication).

As reviewed by Adler (1970), chickens infected with both *M. gallisepticum* and *M. synoviae* appear to develop resistance to reinfection and antibodies persist in serum for many months. It appears that a humoral antibody response also plays a major role in the protection of these hosts, since bursectomized birds develop a more severe infection with both *M. synoviae* and *M. gallisepticum* in comparison with that seen in control chickens (Vardaman *et al.*, 1973; Bryant *et al.*, 1973). However, growth inhibiting antibodies have not been detected in the sera of arthritic birds (Jordan, 1975), and this may explain the ability of the organisms to persist in diseased tissues.

2. Cell-Mediated Immune Responses

In the arthritic diseases which have been studied, a cell-mediated immune response also develops against the invading organisms. Thus active infection of mice with either *M. arthritidis* or *M. pulmonis* results in an increase in the uptake of [³H]thymidine by immune lymphocytes *in vitro* in the presence of homologous antigen, as compared with that seen with normal lymphocytes in the presence of antigen (Cole *et al.*, 1975a,b, 1976). This reaction was detected at all stages of the disease process, but the degree of the response did not appear to correlate with the severity of the arthritis. A similar response has been detected in rabbits injected intraarticularly with *M. arthritis* or *M. pulmonis* (Cole *et al.*, 1977b). A lymphocyte transformation reaction, as well as positive leukocyte migration inhibition and skin tests have also been demonstrated in cattle infected with *M. mycoides* (Roberts *et al.*, 1973). Decker and Barden (1975) showed that a single swine chronically infected with *M. hyorhinis* exhibited a delayed hypersensitivity skin reaction when given homologous antigen, and this procedure was associated with a flare in arthritis.

The role played by cell-mediated immune phenomena in protection of the host against arthritogenic mycoplasmas has been much more difficult to evaluate. Immune spleen cells passively administered to normal mice protect against arthritis induced with *M. pulmonis* and result in fewer positive isolations of the organisms from the tissues (Taylor and Taylor-Robinson, 1977). Although it remains to be determined whether immune spleen cells from *M. arthritidis*-infected mice exhibit a similar effect, it is known that these cells do not promote clearance of *M. arthritidis* from the blood stream of recipient mice. In contrast, spleen and lymph node cells taken from rats infected with *M. arthritidis* promoted the clearance of circulating mycoplasmas in recipient animals, but the latter are not protected against the subsequent development of arthritis (Cole and Ward, 1973a). Preliminary experiments with athymic nude mice indicate that more severe arthritis is produced in response to infection with *M. arthritidis* than occurs with normal litter mates (B. C. Cole, unpublished observations). However, the ability of the animals to survive the 21 days of the experiment suggests the presence of other protective components.

Possible evidence of a role for cell-mediated immunity was reported by Taylor *et al.* (1974), who showed that thymectomized and x-irradiated mice developed more severe arthritis when injected with *M. pulmonis*. However, treatment with cyclophosphamide, a suppressor of B-cell functions, also resulted in more severe infection often leading to death. Additional studies indicated that immune serum was much more effective in overcoming the cyclophosphamide-enhanced infection than immune spleen cells.

In conclusion, although there is some evidence that cell-mediated immune phenomena contribute to resistance to reinfection, on the basis of present data humoral mechanisms appear to play the major role in protection of the host against arthritogenic mycoplasmas.

3. Autoimmunity

Rheumatoid factors (anti-gamma-globulin antibodies) have been identified in the sera of chickens with spontaneous synovitis (Porter and Gooderham, 1966) and in the sera of chickens experimentally infected with *M. synoviae* and *M. gallisepticum* (Roberts and Olesiuk, 1967). Swine infected with *M. hyorhinis* also produce rheumatoid factors, although these antibodies were only detected in synovial fluids (Ross *et al.*, 1973), thus suggesting local synthesis.

Agglutinins against red blood cells have been detected in the sera of arthritic swine infected with *M. hyorhinis* (Ross *et al.*, 1973), but it is not yet known whether they are the result of a shared antigen or due to a mycoplasma-mediated change in the antigenicity of host antigens. The cold agglutinins induced by *M. pneumoniae* against human blood group I could be due to the latter mechanism (Feizi *et al.*, 1969). Although preliminary studies to detect the presence of rheumatoid factors in murine models of arthritis have failed, Harwick *et al.* claimed to have detected a humoral (Harwick *et al.*, 1976) and cell-mediated immune response (Harwick *et al.*, 1973a) to normal synovial tissue in mice infected with *M. pulmonis*, although the precise source of the antigen was not clear. Cross-reactivity between *M. arthritidis* and rat tissues was previously described by Cahill *et al.* (1971).

D. Mechanisms of Invasion of the Host

The large dose of organisms required to induce experimental arthritis raises the question as to how these diseases are initiated naturally. It is apparent that certain environmental conditions render the host more susceptible to infection. Inadequate sanitation, close contact through overcrowding, poor diet, and trauma constitute environments which might increase herd or individual susceptibility to organisms which are usually present as harmless commensals. Mycoplasmas invade damaged tissues, as evidenced by the detection of *M. arthritidis* in the joints of rats with arthritis induced by Freund's adjuvant (Pearson, 1959) or 6-sulfanilamidoindazole (Mielens and Rozitis, 1964). It has been established that the organisms are not responsible for the primary arthritic lesions caused by these compounds. Many of the first accounts of murine mycoplasmal disease were based upon experiments involving injection of the animals with other infectious agents or foreign material. Even concentrated uninoculated broth constituents can dramatically enhance the ability of *M. arthritidis* to induce abscesses following subcutaneous inoculation (Cole *et al.*, 1973a).

Genetic factors appear to play a role in determining host susceptibility to infection with mycoplasmas, although the precise mechanisms are not understood. Thus different mouse strains vary considerably in their arthritic response to infection with *M. arthritidis* (Cole *et al.*, 1973a) and *M. pulmonis* (Hannan, 1971; Taylor *et al.*, 1974). Similar differences in host strain susceptibility have been observed with *M. hyorhinis* (Barden *et al.*, 1973) and *M. hyosynoviae* (Ross, 1973) arthritis of swine.

When the organisms have entered the host, the establishment of a successful infection requires the ability to either bypass or suppress host defense mechanisms. Mycoplasmas appear to bypass host defenses in several ways. Thus *M. pulmonis* possesses a surface protein which protects the organism against phagocytosis by peritoneal macrophages (Jones *et al.*, 1972). Other mycoplasmas appear to produce substances which promote survival of the organisms *in vivo*, for example, the galactan of *M. mycoides* subsp. *mycoides* (Hudson *et al.*, 1967). The ability of some mycoplasmas to adsorb host proteins (Bradbury and Jordan, 1972) could result in decreased immunogenicity and increased resistance to host defenses. Impaired immunogenicity appears to occur with *M. arthritidis* infection of rats. Thus during studies on arthritis of rats induced by *M. arthritidis* it was observed that MI antibodies were not produced against this organism, whereas the animals were capable of producing these antibodies to other mycoplasma species (Cole *et al.*, 1969). Since *M.*

arthritidis induced high levels of MI antibody in other hosts, it was clear
that a specific relationship existed between *M. arthritidis* and the rat.
Preliminary evidence suggested that *M. arthritidis* shared an antigenic
component with rat tissues, thus rendering the organisms less im-
munogenic in their natural host (Cahill *et al.*, 1971).

Virulent strains of *M. arthritidis* can persist in the peripheral circulation
of rats for many days after IV injection (Cole and Ward, 1973a) and can
also resist phagocytosis *in vitro* by peritoneal macrophages (Cole and
Ward, 1973b). These observations, together with the failure to detect
opsonizing antibodies in the serum of convalescent rats, could also be due
to the occurrence of antigens shared with the host. However, the observations of Simberkoff and Elsbach (1971) indicate that *M. arthritidis* not
only resists phagocytosis by rabbit peritoneal cells or human PMNs but
that this organism suppresses the ability of the cells to phagocytize *Escherichia coli*. Whether these observations are related to the ability of *M.
arthritidis* to suppress lymphocyte functions *in vitro* by virtue of arginine
depletion from the medium (Barile and Leventhal, 1968; Kaklamanis and
Pavlatos, 1972) is not known.

The ability of some mycoplasmas to suppress cell functions *in vitro*
raises the question as to whether these organisms can overcome host
defenses *in vivo* by an immunosuppressive effect. In fact it has been
shown that *M. arthritidis* can suppress the neutralizing antibody response
of rats to $\phi 5$ bacteriophage and the hemagglutinating antibody response of
rabbits to common antigens derived from *E. coli* and *Staphylococcus
aureus* (Bergquist *et al.*, 1974). It is not clear whether these responses
were due to antigenic competition. Additionally, Kaklamanis and Pavlatos
(1972) showed that lymphocytes taken from rats infected with *M. arthritidis* exhibited a decreased *in vitro* mitogenic response to phytohemagglutinin. This suppression of lymphocyte functions was not demonstrated by
lymphocytes taken from mice infected with *M. arthritidis* (Cole *et al.*, 1976).

Other recent observations may also have a bearing on the inhibition of
host cell functions *in vivo*. Mice injected intraperitoneally with *M. arthritidis* produce a transient interferon response (Rinaldo *et al.*, 1974).
There is now increasing evidence that interferon can act as an immunoregulatory agent (Chester *et al.*, 1973), although high concentrations
are apparently required for this effect. Of even greater interest is the
finding that when the interferon response of mice to *M. arthritidis* has
subsided, the animals become hyporeactive to further interferon induction by other potent interferon inducers (Cole *et al.*, 1975c, 1978). Furthermore, serum taken from these hyporeactive mice can suppress the
ability of mouse embryo fibroblasts *in vitro* to produce interferon when
challenged with Newcastle disease virus, a potent inducer of interferon. It

is possible that this serum factor can suppress host cell functions other than interferon production.

A further understanding of the mechanisms by which mycoplasmas invade the host might come through studies comparing the biological, biochemical, and serological properties of virulent and avirulent strains. Only very limited studies have thus far been conducted on the arthritogenic mycoplasmas. In the case of *M. arthritidis* it is known that avirulent strains are eliminated from the peripheral circulation of rodents more rapidly than virulent strains (Cole *et al.*, 1973a). Furthermore, avirulent cultures appeared to be less susceptible to the growth-inhibiting properties of hyperimmune rabbit antisera than virulent cultures (Golightly-Rowland *et al.*, 1970). However, the specific property which determines these apparent differences has not been identified.

E. Mechanisms of the Inflammatory Response

We have already discussed the host and agent factors which might permit invading organisms to become established in the host. In this section we deal with the actual inflammatory process, which leads to clinical disease, and present some alternative hypotheses on the mechanisms of acute and chronic inflammation.

1. Acute Inflammation

Microorganisms produce a wide variety of toxic substances which can directly contribute to the inflammatory response, although there is no direct evidence that arthritogenic mycoplasmas synthesize classic exotoxins. However *M. arthritidis* produces a spreading necrotizing abscess in mice following subcutaneous injection and death of mice after large IV doses of the organisms (Cole *et al.*, 1973a; Kaklamanis and Thomas, 1970). Proteolytic enzymes have been detected in cultures of *M. arthritidis* (Czekalowski *et al.*, 1973). Neurotoxic properties have been ascribed to *M. gallisepticum,* and severe arthritis leading to the occlusion of capillaries is believed to be responsible for necrosis of brain tissue (Manuelidis and Thomas, 1973).

As reviewed by Stanbridge (1971) and Barile (this volume, Chapter 13), mycoplasmas exert a wide variety of effects on cultured cells. The ability of many mycoplasmas to adsorb avidly to cells would further potentiate the action of toxic substances. Of the arthritogenic species, *M. synoviae* and *M. gallisepticum* strongly adsorb to cells at a neuraminic acid receptor site (Aldridge, 1975; Gesner and Thomas, 1965). There is evidence that *M. arthritidis* is also capable of a close association with cells. Studies in our laboratory indicate that both *M. arthritidis* and *M. pulmonis* colonize the surface of cultured rabbit synovial cells (L. R. Washburn, B. C. Cole, and J. R. Ward, unpublished observations). The infection of swine synovial cell cultures with *M. hyorhinis* leads to rapid cell death. In contrast, *M. hyosynoviae* appeared to associate with only a small percentage of cells, and cytopathic effects were much less prominent (Potgieter *et al.*, 1972). Whether synovial cells provide a particularly attractive surface for adsorption, thus accounting for the specific localization of the organisms, is not known at this time.

How do the attached organisms mediate cell damage? First, *M. pulmonis*, *M. hyorhinis*, *M. gallisepticum*, and *M. synoviae* (Cole *et al.*, 1968; Kerr and Olson, 1970) are all potent producers of a peroxide hemolysin. Peroxide appears to contribute to cell death in tracheal organ cultures infected with mycoplasmas (Cherry and Taylor-Robinson, 1970). Many mycoplasmas deplete arginine from the medium (Stanbridge, 1971), thus altering cell functions. For example, arginine-deprived cells have been shown to exhibit enhanced susceptibility to lysis by a variety of agents including interferon (Lee and Rozee, 1975). Competitive arginine utilization also appears to be responsible for the *in vitro* suppression of lymphocyte transformation in response to mitogens such as phytohemagglutinin. It has even been postulated that this reaction may contribute to *in vivo* inflammation. However, Ibrahim and Yamomoto (1977) failed to detect a decrease in the plasma levels of arginine in *M. meleagridis*-infected turkey poults, and arginine supplementation of the animals failed to abrogate the inflammatory response. Mycoplasmas also utilize nucleic acid precursors (Stanbridge *et al.*, 1971) which are probably obtained from animal cells by the ability of the organisms to associate closely with cell surfaces and to secrete nucleases (Razin *et al.*, 1964). This reaction might also result in cytotoxic effects.

Mycoplasmas may cause cell damage not only by a direct toxic effect on cells but by activating host mediators of inflammation. Lymphokines such as chemotactic factor, macrophage migration inhibitory factor, mitogenic factor, lymphotoxin, and so on, are receiving increasing attention as mediators of inflammation. These substances can be produced by the interaction of normal lymphocytes with nonspecific mitogens such as phytohemagglutinin, or by the interaction of specifically sensitized lymphocytes with homologous antigen. In 1973, Ginsburg and Nicolet (1973) reported that *M. pulmonis* was mitogenic for unsensitized rat lymphocytes. A similar reaction has been demonstrated for *M. pulmonis* toward mouse lymphocytes (Cole *et al.*, 1975b) and for *M. pneumoniae* toward mouse and hamster lymphocytes (Biberfeld and Gronowicz, 1976). Recent work suggests that mitogenesis may in fact be a general property of the Mycoplasmatales (Cole *et al.*, 1977a; Naot *et al.*, 1977). The ability of mycoplasmas to cap lymphocytes in the absence of added antibody provides a partial explanation for these phenomena (Stanbridge and Weiss, 1978). What is the significance of these observations? Since mycoplasmas appear to be mitogenic for normal unsensitized lymphocytes, an inflammatory reaction would be initiated as soon as the organisms localized in the joint. It is also clear that the later development of a cell-mediated immune response to the invading organisms might enhance this inflammation by the induction of an additional lymphokine release. As discussed earlier, a cell-mediated immune response develops in animal arthritides, and evidence has been presented to suggest that this reaction contributes to inflammatory processes (this volume, Chapter 12).

What is the specific evidence that lymphocyte activitation *by mycoplasmas* constitutes an inflammatory mechanism? During control experiments for studies to determine the role of cell-mediated immunity in tissue damage, mouse fibroblasts labeled with ^{51}Cr were treated with a mixture of viable *M. arthritidis* and normal lymphocytes. Death of the fibroblasts occurred as detected by release of the ^{51}Cr. The presence of both mycoplasmas and lymphocytes was required (Aldridge *et al.*, 1977). This cytotoxic reaction might be due to a soluble lymphotoxin produced in association with the mitogenic effect induced by this mycoplasma species (Cole *et al.*, 1977a), or to direct activation of lymphocytes possessing cytotoxic effector activities. The role of mycoplasma-induced activation of lymphocytes in joint inflammation remains to be defined. However, studies by Andreis *et al.* (1974) indicate that lymphokines produced *in vitro* can exhibit inflammatory effects such as synovial hyperplasia following injection into rabbit joints. It is noteworthy that an intense lymphocytic infiltration of synovial tissue is characteristic of many mycoplasma-induced arthritides. The pronounced lymphocytic infiltration of organs seen in diseases due to *M. synoviae* and *M. gallisepticum* might thus be related to the particularly strong mitogenic potential of these organisms (Cole *et al.*, 1977a).

2. Chronic Inflammation

In cases in which mycoplasmas are known to persist within joint tissues, i.e., arthritis of mice induced by *M. arthritidis* and *M. pulmonis* and chicken synovitis induced by *M. synoviae*, the continued inflammatory response could be mediated by the mechanisms already discussed. The failure to recover cultivable organisms from the arthritic joints of swine and rabbits might require another explanation for the mechanism of these chronic forms of inflammation. However, can we be sure that mycoplasmas have in fact been eliminated from these tissues?

The ability of *M. hyorhinis* to develop an obligate parasitic phase *in vitro*, in which the presence of living cells is required for replication

(Hopps *et al.*, 1973), suggests that in some cases viable organisms might persist within joints yet not be detectable by the usual culture techniques. Failure to culture the organisms could be made more difficult because of the presence of high levels of neutralizing antibody, the mycoplasmacidal properties of tissue extracts (Kaklamanis *et al.*, 1969), or a failure to culture the actual site where the organisms are localized. An alternative explanation is that continued inflammation is due to the retention of nonviable mycoplasma antigen. In this regard, arthritis of rabbits can be induced by the injection of bovine serum albumin into the joints of hyperimmunized animals, and the antigen persists in the articular cartilage and menisci (Cooke and Richer, 1974). Persistence of antigen appears to be dependent on a presensitized host, thus suggesting the selective retention of immune complexes within the cartilage. Consequently it is possible that in some chronic mycoplasma-induced arthritides a strong immune reaction could eliminate viable organisms but lead to the deposition and retention of immune complexes in articular cartilage. Such complexes, by activating the complement sequence and promoting lysosomal release from the phagocytosing cells, might ensure a continued inflammatory response. It should be noted that, in the case of swine arthritis, *M. hyorhinis* antigen can be detected by immunofluorescence in joint tissues long after cultivable organisms have been eliminated (Decker and Barden, 1975).

It is clear that the question of persistence of mycoplasma antigen in chronically inflamed joints must be answered before a complete understanding of these diseases can be obtained. Is it possible, however, that there are pathogenetic mechanisms which are not dependent upon persistence of the initiating antigen? Autoimmune phenomena in the form of rheumatoid factors are characteristic of human RA and, as we have noted, are also present in the sera of chronically arthritic swine and chickens. It is commonly held that these antibodies are directed against immune complexes of host gamma-globulin and an unknown antigen. Other mycoplasma infections exhibit autoimmune sequelae. Thus *M. pneumoniae* infection not only results in the appearance of cold agglutinins directed against red blood cells, but also antibodies against brain, lung, and lymphocytes (Biberfeld *et al.*, 1976). It has also been reported that mice develop an immune reaction against normal mouse synovial tissue following infection with *M. pulmonis*. However, these studies, which utilized the macrophage migration inhibition technique, were complicated by the observation that, in the absence of antigen, macrophages from infected mice migrated further than macrophages from control mice.

Autoimmune phenomena against tissue antigens could arise through extensive cell damage, resulting in the appearance of host antigens with an altered configuration. These antigens might be retained in cartilage in the form of immune complexes. Alternatively, as discussed earlier, the occurrence of antigens shared by parasite and host (Cahill *et al.*, 1971) could initiate an autoimmune response, especially if the heterogenetic antigens differed slightly in antigenic specificity. The observations of Cassell *et al.* (1978) are of interest in this regard, since they indicated that *M. hyorhinis* selectively bound Thy-l and H-2 antigens during infection in mouse lymphoblastoid lines. The close association of these antigens with mycoplasma membranes could initiate an autoimmune response with potential for altered host immunocompetency.

It has been postulated that autoimmunity can arise through immunodeficiency (Fudenberg and Wells, 1976). A key example is in the development of anti-DNA antibodies in NZB mice due to a lack of suppressor T cells (Steinberg, 1974). Anti-DNA antibodies have been reported to occur in the sera of rats infected with *M. arthritidis* (Klien and Wottawa, 1975). The reported immunosuppressive properties of *M. arthritidis* described earlier may be relevant to this, although considerable work is required to define the specific host function which is altered.

III. ROLE OF MYCOPLASMAS IN HUMAN ARTHRITIS

A. Introduction

In humans, arthritis is frequently associated with infection. The infectious agent may directly invade a joint, producing acute or chronic arthritis. In other cases, such as bacterial endocarditis and hepatitis B virus infection, sterile arthritis may occur and yet clear with resolution of the infection. Permanent or chronic inflammatory joint changes are not seen. Furthermore sterile arthritis can also develop after the infectious disease has seemingly resolved. This latter "reactive arthritis," which can be chronic, occurs after *Yersinia, Salmonella,* and *Shigella* infections and is associated with the presence of the H-LA B27 antigen.

In contrast RA is of unknown etiology and is characterized by chronic polyarthritis in which extensive synoviocyte hyperplasia and infiltration of synovial tissues with PMNs, lymphoid cells, and macrophages is seen. Cartilage destruction may also occur. There is frequent systemic involvement including pleuritis, pulmonary nodules, diffuse interstitial pulmonary fibrosis, pericarditis, myocardial and endocardial lesions, lymphadenopathy, splenomegaly, and anemia. The disease may be associated with autoimmune phenomena such as rheumatoid factors, and other immunological aberrations are apparent.

A main hypothesis is that RA is initiated by an infectious agent. Autoimmune phenomena could thus be explained by an agent-mediated alteration of host antigens, i.e., by the production of antibodies against immune complexes of agent and host gamma-globulin, by neoantigen production, or by an abnormal response to cross-reacting antigens similar to the response seen with rheumatic fever.

There appears to be a consensus that the accumulation of inflammatory cells, activation of the complement system by immune complexes, and the release of lymphokines by activated lymphoid cells are important in the pathogenesis of RA. An immune response against a persisting antigen could initiate and perpetuate these reactions. It may not be necessary that antigen persist within the joints, since immune complexes could be generated at a distant site and later trapped in articular cartilage.

Whatever the pathogenetic mechanisms involved, it seems clear that neither the initiating nor the sustaining event(s) have been identified. Despite the recent interest in a viral etiology for RA, most of the features of this disease can be seen in the various chronic animal arthritides induced by mycoplasmas. In the next section we review attempts to implicate mycoplasmas directly in the etiology of human RA.

B. Detection of Mycoplasmas

1. Isolation of Organisms

Sabin's (1939) early work on chronic mouse arthritis induced by mycoplasmas prompted a still continuing search for these agents in the tissues of RA patients. However, many of the reports on the isolation of mycoplasmas from rheumatoid tissues cannot be adequately evaluated, since in some instances the organisms isolated could not be transferred and in others the isolates were not identified or characterized.

With the use of conventional mycoplasma media infrequent isolations of *Mycoplasma arthritidis, M. fermentans,* and *M. hominis* have been reported from the joint tissues of RA patients and sometimes from non-RA patients (Jansson and Wager, 1967; Mårdh *et al.*, 1973). However, a majority of other workers have failed to isolate mycoplasmas (reviewed in Cole *et al.*, 1973b, 1975d; Stewart *et al.*, 1974; Taylor-Robinson and Taylor, 1976). Utilizing more complex media containing egg yolk, Jansson *et al.* (1971) described the isolation of mycoplasmas from each of 27 rheumatoid synovia, whereas 24 nonrheumatoid synovia failed to yield mycoplasmas. The isolates, which were slow-growing, appeared to be related to *M. arthritidis*. The latter species was also claimed to have been isolated from the pleural effusion of a patient exhibiting RA (Brown *et al.*, 1973). Other investigators (Ford and Wort, 1972; Person *et al.*, 1972; B. C. Cole and J. R. Ward, unpublished observations) have failed to confirm Jansson's observations, and the interpretation was that many of the so-called mycoplasma colonies were in fact artifacts derived from the media.

Jansson *et al.* (1971) also injected synovial specimens into yolk sacs of embryonated hens' eggs and reported the isolation of mycoplasma in six instances when recovery was not possible with direct inoculation on conventional media. However, Sharp (1970), who also injected material into yolk sacs, failed to detect mycoplasmas either by transfer to mycoplasma media or by the use of ^{125}I-labeled antisera probes. More recently, Markham and Myers (1976), using a modified Jansson's egg yolk broth medium, reported that a slow-growing microorganism was isolated after 6 weeks incubation from 9 of 11 synovial fluids from patients in an "acute" (not defined) stage of RA. Non-RA fluids were not studied. Replication in broth culture was deduced by the incorporation of $^{32}PO_4$ into RNA extracts for the only isolate tested. On agar, initial colonies resembled T mycoplasmas but could not be transferred. Limited electron microscope examination provided some support for their resemblance to mycoplasmas.

In an entirely different approach, Williams (1968) employed sucrose density gradient centrifugation of synovial fluid to concentrate the organisms and to separate them from synovial fluid inhibitors. Bands corresponding to the density of mycoplasmas were inoculated into conventional mycoplasma medium. By this technique, *M. fermentans* was isolated from 40% of RA synovial fluids and 20% of non-RA fluids. Unfortunately his intriguing observation has not been confirmed by other investigators (Cole *et al.*, 1973b; Mårdh *et al.*, 1973; Windsor *et al.*, 1974).

Cell culture systems have also been used to isolate mycoplasmas from rheumatoid tissues, although the frequent contamination of established cell lines with mycoplasmas poses problems in the interpretation of these studies. By this means Bartholomew (1965) reported the isolation of mycoplasma strains similar to *M. hyorhinis* from rheumatoid synovial fluids. Fraser *et al.* (1971) claimed a higher isolation rate of mycoplasmas from RA as compared with non-RA synovial membrane, but the isolates were not identified. Other workers (Barnett *et al.*, 1966; Middleton and Highton, 1975; Wilkes *et al.*, 1973) using similar methods have failed. In a more sophisticated approach, Person *et al.* (1973) used synovial fluid cells cocultivated with Vero cells, explant synovial cell cultures, or continuous-passage synovial cell cultures to detect mycoplasmal nucleic acids in specimens from 13 RA patients and 7 patients with non-RA joint disease. However, all results were negative.

2. Immunological Studies

The presence of specific antibody in the serum or synovial fluid of RA patients has been used to implicate mycoplasmas in RA. Bartholomew (1967) used a polyvalent antigen composed of four mycoplasmas supposedly isolated from RA and Reiter's disease patients and reported CF antibodies in RA patients. Williams (1968)) reported MI antibodies to *M. fermentans* in RA patients, and Jansson *et al.* (1971) found occasional anti-*M. arthritidis* antibodies in their human RA patients. Conversely, numerous other investigators have failed to demonstrate a unique association with RA (Chanock *et al.*, 1967; Stewart *et al.*, 1974; Mårdh *et al.*, 1973; Chandler *et al.*, 1971; Cole *et al.*, 1975d).

Further evidence for the role of *M. fermentans* was presented by Williams *et al.* (1970), who showed that the migration of leukocytes taken from rhematoid patients, but not from control patients, was inhibited in the presence of *M. fermentans* antigen. However, recent findings suggest that the observed inhibition of migration of leukocytes in the presence of *M. fermentans* antigen also occurs with leukocytes from normal control patients. The inhibition appears to be due to IgG associated with the mycoplasma membranes (Maini *et al.*, 1975), since aggregated IgG alone was shown to exhibit a similar effect (Brostoff *et al.*, 1973). Finally other studies have failed to provide evidence of increased lymphocyte transformation to mycoplasmas by RA lymphocytes (Cole *et al.*, 1975d).

A very recent report suggests that arthritis may be a secondary complication in infection with *M. pneumoniae*, the agent of primary atypical pneumonia of humans (Hernandez *et al.*, 1977). In this study 7 of 45 patients who had recently suffered from *M. pneumoniae* disease developed an arthritic condition which lasted from 1 to 18 months. One of these patients, who exhibited multiple joint involvement with clinical synovial hypertrophy, developed rheumatoid factor which persisted until the symptoms resolved at 10 months. These studies are interesting in view of the observations of Obeck *et al.* (1976), who found that a rhesus monkey with severe chronic polyarthritis developed cold agglutinins and CF antibodies against *M. pneumoniae*. However neither mycoplasmas nor bacteria were isolated from the arthritic joints.

IV. CONCLUSIONS AND FUTURE PROSPECTS

It is apparent that much more work is required to answer some key questions concerning the mechanisms of mycoplasma-induced arthritis. The means by which these organisms resist host defense mechanisms are poorly understood, as are the mechanisms by which disease can continue in the apparent absence of cultivable organisms. The role played by persisting nonviable antigen also requires further examination, as does the precise site of localization of mycoplasmal antigens, be it in the joint or at some site distant from the lesion such as the respiratory or genital tract. Despite the chronic nature of these diseases, the infected hosts neverthe-less exhibit immunity to reinfection, although the mechanisms involved are not clear. This apparent paradox requires further study. Recent work on mycoplasma–lymphocyte interactions suggests a possible inflamma-tory pathway by lymphokine production and also points to potential altera-tion of the host's immunoresponsiveness by the ability of some organisms to bind selectively the H-2 and Thy-l antigens and to induce interferon, an immunoregulatory agent. The role of mycoplasma viruses in these dis-eases might also be considered, especially in view of our observations that the MVL2 virus of *Acholeplasma laidlawii* can induce lymphocytes to produce interferon (Lombardi and Cole, 1977, 1978).

A genetic component clearly plays a role in susceptibility to infection by mycoplasmas. In addition, the observation that varied arthritic syn-dromes develop in rats, mice, and rabbits to the same mycoplasma species (*M. arthritidis*) illustrates the importance of host responses in the expression of disease.

There is a paucity of data on most of the chronic phases of mycoplasma-induced arthritides. This is unfortunate, since a more de-tailed knowledge of the natural history of these models of chronic inflam-mation would have a direct bearing on further understanding the nature of human arthritis. It is hoped that additional work on chronic animal ar-thritis will permit the development of more sensitive techniques for the detection of mycoplasmas and will more precisely identify the *in vivo* sites from which mycoplasmas might be recovered.

Despite numerous investigations, convincing evidence implicating mycoplasmas in the etiology of human RA remains to be presented. Much less attention has been given to the potential role of mycoplasmas in other forms of human arthritis. The recent isolations of *M. pneumoniae* (Taylor-Robinson *et al.*, 1978) and *U. urealyticum* (Quinn *et al.*, 1978) from the arthritic joints of immuno-compromised patients should encour-age additional studies in this area.

The close similarity between chronic arthritis of animals induced by mycoplasmas and human rheumatoid arthritis warrants continued investi-gation with regard to a possible common etiology. We would like to suggest a few guidelines for future work in this area.

1. Sampling of Patients

Since mycoplasmas may be rapidly eliminated from joint tissues, it is essential that individuals be cultured during the onset of arthritis. When possible, synovial fluid, membrane, and articular cartilage should be examined. Respiratory and genital tracts should also be cultured, since mycoplasmas can localize in these sites; comparison with normal flora must be made. Repeated samplings should be performed.

2. Culture Procedures

Both undiluted samples and serial dilutions should be examined to avoid the cidal properties of certain tissue suspensions (Kaklamanis *et al.*, 1969). Artificial media should include those for mycoplasmas, ureaplasmas, and spiroplasmas. "Noncultivable" mycoplasmas should be sought by metabolic probes using synovial fluids or cell cultures derived from rheumatoid patients or using normal mycoplasma-free synovial lines inoculated with clinical samples.

3. Immunological Procedures

Sequential serum and joint fluid samples should be collected throughout the course of disease and examined for a rise in antibody titers against any mycoplasmas isolated. Immunofluorescence studies on joint fluids and tissues should also be undertaken to determine the extent and site of the infection. Cell-mediated immune responses using the lymphocyte transformation technique might also be of value in providing further evidence of a specific infection.

4. Transfer of the Disease to Experimental Animals

All isolates should be tested for pathogenic potential in laboratory animals. If isolates are not obtained, joint fluid and arthritic tissues can be administered intra-articularly into animals, since our experimental studies indicate that very few organisms are required to establish an infection by this method.

5. Handling of Isolates

Isolate(s) should be characterized as belonging to the Mycoplasmatales and identified at the species level using reference reagents. Finally, deposition of the organisms in a culture collection is imperative.

ACKNOWLEDGMENTS

We are indebted to those investigators who kindly supplied us with unpublished material. We thank Dr. Gail H. Cassell for supplying Fig. 2, and the American Society for Microbiology for allowing us to reproduce Figs. 1, 3, 4, 5, and 6.

The authors' work described in this chapter was supported by grant No. AM02255 from the National Institute of Arthritis, Metabolism and Digestive Disease, by grant No. AI12103 from the National Institute of Allergy and Infectious Diseases, and by a grant from the Kroc Foundation.

REFERENCES

Adler, H. E. (1970). *In* "The Role of Mycoplasmas and L-Forms of Bacteria in Disease" (J. T. Sharp, ed.), pp. 240–261. Thomas, Springfield, Illinois.

Aldridge, K. E. (1975). *Infect. Immun.* **12**, 198–204.

Aldridge, K. E., Cole, B. C., and Ward, J. R. (1977). *Infect. Immun.* **18**, 377–385.

Andreis, M., Stastny, P., and Ziff, M. (1974). *Arthritis Rheum.* **17**, 537.

Barden, J. A., and Decker, J. L. (1971). *Arthritis Rheum.* **14**, 193–211.

Barden, J. A., and Tully, J. G. (1969). *J. Bacteriol.* **100**, 5–10.

Barden, J. A., Decker, J. L., Dalgard, D. W., and Aptekar, R. G. (1973). *Infect. Immun.* **8**, 887–890.

Barile, M. F., and Leventhal, B. G. (1968). *Nature (London)* **219**, 751–752.

Barnett, E. V., Balduzzi, P., Vaughan, J. H., and Morgan, H. R. (1966). *Arthritis Rheum.* **9**, 720–724.

Bartholomew, L. E. (1965). *Arthritis Rheum.* **8**, 376–388.

Bartholomew, L. E. (1967). *Ann. N.Y. Acad. Sci.* **143**, 522–534.

Bergquist, L. M., Lau, B. H. S., and Winter, C. E. (1974). *Infect. Immun.* **9**, 410–415.

Biberfeld, G., and Gronowicz, E. (1976). *Nature (London)* **261**, 238–239.

Biberfeld, G., Biberfeld, P., and Wigzell, H. (1976). *Scan. J. Immunol.* **5**, 87–95.

Bradbury, J. M., and Jordan, F. T. W. (1972). *J. Hyg.* **70**, 267–278.

Brostoff, J., Howell, A., and Roitt, I. M. (1973). *Clin. Exp. Immunol.* **15**, 1–7.

Brown, T. McP., Bailey, J. S., and Clark, H. W. (1973). *Int. Congr. Rheumatol., 13th, Excerpta Med.* p. 172.

Bryant, B. J., Adler, H. E., Cordy, D. R., Shifrine, M., and DaMassa, A. J. (1973). *Eur. J. Immunol.* **3**, 9–15.

Cahill, J. R., Cole, B. C., Wiley, B. B., and Ward, J. R. (1971). *Infect. Immun.* **3**, 24–35.

Cassell, G. H., Davis, J. K., Wilbourn, W. H., and Wise, K. S. (1978). "Microbiology" (D. Schlessinger, ed.), pp. 399–403. Amer. Soc. Microbiol., Washington, D.C.

Chandler, R. W., Robinson, H., and Masi, A. T. (1971). *Ann. Rheum. Dis.* **30**, 274–278.

Chanock, R. M., Purcell, R. H., and Decker, J. L. (1967). *In* "Third Nuffield Conference on Rheumatism," pp. 18.1–18.2. Nuffield Found., London.

Cherry, J. D., and Taylor-Robinson, D. (1970). *Infect. Immun.* **2**, 431–438.

Chester, T. J., Paucker, K., and Merigan, T. C. (1973). *Nature (London)* **246**, 92–94.

Cole, B. C., and Ward, J. R. (1973a). *Infect. Immun.* **7**, 416–425.

Cole, B. C., and Ward, J. R. (1973b). *Infect. Immun.* **7**, 691–699.

Cole, B. C., Ward, J. R., and Martin, C. H. (1968). *J. Bacteriol.* **95**, 2022–2030.

Cole, B. C., Cahill, J. F., Wiley, B. B., and Ward, J. R. (1969). *J. Bacteriol.* **98**, 930–937.

Cole, B. C., Ward, J. R., Jones, R. S., and Cahill, J. F. (1971a). *Infect. Immun.* **4**, 344–355.

Cole, B. C., Ward, J. R., Golightly-Rowland, L., and Trapp, G. A. (1971b). *Infect. Immun.* **4**, 431–440.

Cole, B. C., Ward, J. R., and Golightly-Rowland, L. (1973a). *Infect. Immun.* **7**, 218–225.

Cole, B. C., Ward, J. R., and Smith, C. B. (1973b). *Arthritis Rheum.* **16**, 191–198.

Cole, B. C., Golightly-Rowland, L., and Ward, J. R. (1975a). *Infect. Immun.* **11**, 1159–1161.

Cole, B. C., Golightly-Rowland, L., and Ward, J. R. (1975b). *Infect. Immun.* **12**, 1083–1092.

Cole, B. C., Overall, J. C., Jr., Lombardi, P. S., and Glasgow, L. A., (1975c). *Infect. Immun.* **12**, 1349–1354.

Cole, B. C., Taylor, M. B., and Ward, J. R. (1975d). *Arthritis Rheum.* **18,** 435–441.

Cole, B. C., Golightly-Rowland, L., and Ward, J. R. (1976). *Ann. Rheum. Dis.* **35,** 14–22.

Cole, B. C., Aldridge, K. E., and Ward, J. R. (1977a). *Infect. Immun.* **18,** 393–399.

Cole, B. C., Griffiths, M. M., Eichwald, E. J., and Ward, J. R. (1977b). *Infect. Immun.* **16,** 382–396.

Cole, B. C., Lombardi, P. S., Overall, J. C., Jr., and Glasgow, L. A. (1978). *Proc. Soc. Exp. Biol. Med.* **157,** 83–88.

Cooke, T. D., and Richer, S. M. (1974). *J. Rheumatol.* **1,** 143–152.

Cottew, G. S. (1970). *In* "The Role of Mycoplasmas and L-Forms of Bacteria in Disease" (J. T. Sharp, ed.), pp. 198–211. Thomas, Springfield, Illinois.

Czekalowski, J. W., Hall, D. A., and Woolcock, P. R. (1973). *J. Gen. Microbiol.* **75,** 125–133.

DaSilva, J. M. L., and Adler, H. E. (1969). *Pathol. Vet.* **6,** 385.

Decker, J. L., and Barden, J. A. (1975). *In* "Immunological Aspects of Rheumatoid Arthritis," Rheumatology, Vol. 6, pp. 338–345. Karger, Basel.

Deeb, B. J., and Kenny, G. E. (1967). *J. Bacteriol.* **93,** 1416–1424.

Duncan, J. R., and Ross, R. F. (1969). *Am. J. Pathol.* **57,** 171–186.

Duncan, J. R., and Ross, R. F. (1973). *Am. J. Vet. Res.* **34,** 363–366.

Edwards, C. Q., Deiss, A., Cole, B. C., and Ward, J. R. (1975). *Proc. Soc. Exp. Biol. Med.* **150,** 664–668.

Eisen, V., and Loveday, C. (1973). *Br. J. Pharmacol.* **47,** 272–281.

Ennis, R. S., Dalgard, D., Willerson, J. T., Barden, J. A., and Decker, J. L. (1971). *Arthritis Rheum.* **14,** 202–211.

Feizi, T., Taylor-Robinson, D., Shields, M. D., and Carter, R. A. (1969). *Nature (London)* **222,** 1253–1256.

Fletcher, O. J., Anderson, D. P., and Kleven, S. H. (1976). *Vet. Pathol.* **13,** 303–314.

Ford, D. K., and Wort, B. (1972). *Arthritis Rheum.* **15,** 650–651.

Fraser, K. B., Shirodaria, P. V., Haire, H., and Middleton, D. (1971). *J. Hyg.* **69,** 17–25.

Fudenberg, H. H., and Wells, J. V. (1976). *In* "Infection and Immunology in the Rheumatic Diseases" (D. C. Dumonde, ed.), pp. 549–562. Blackwell, Oxford.

Gesner, B., and Thomas, L. (1965). *Science* **151,** 590–591.

Ghazikhanian, G., Yamamoto, R., and Cordy, D. R. (1973). *Avian Dis.* **17,** 122–136.

Ginsburg, H., and Nicolet, J. (1973). *Nature (London), New Biol.* **246,** 143–146.

Goeth, H., and Appel, K. R. (1974). *Zentralbl. Bakteriol., Parasitenkd., Infektionskr. Hyg., Abt. 1: Orig., Reihe A:* **228,** 282–289.

Goiš, M., Pospišil, Z., Černy, M., and Vrva, V. (1971). *J. Comp. Pathol.* **81,** 401–410.

Golightly-Rowland, L., Cole, B. C., Ward, J. R., and Wiley, B. B. (1970). *Infect. Immun.* **1,** 538–545.

Gourlay, R. N. (1973). *J. Am. Vet. Med. Assoc.* **163,** 905–909.

Gourlay, R. N., Thomas, L. H., and Howard, C. J. (1976). *Vet. Rec.* **98,** 506–507.

Hannan, P. C. T. (1971). *J. Gen. Microbiol.* **67,** 363–365.

Hannan, P. C. T. (1976). *J. Med. Microbiol.* **10,** 87–102.

Hannan, P. C. T., and Dixon, R. A. (1978). *Zentralbl. Bakteriol., Parasitenkd., Infektionskr. Hyg., Abt. 1: Orig., Reihe A:* **241,** 277–278.

Harwick, H. J., Kalmanson, G. M., Fox, M. A., and Guze, L. B. (1973a). *Proc. Soc. Exp. Biol. Med.* **144,** 561–563.

Harwick, H. J., Kalmanson, G. M., Fox, M. A., and Guze, L. B. (1973b). *J. Infect. Dis.* **128,** 533–546.

Harwick, H. J., Mahoney, A. D., Kalmanson, G. M., and Guze, L. B. (1976). *J. Infect. Dis.* **133,** 103–112.

Hernandez, L. A., Urquhart, G. E. D., and Dick, W. C. (1977). *Br. Med. J.* **2,** 14–16.

Hill, A., and Dagnall, G. J. R. (1975). *J. Comp. Pathol.* **85,** 45–52.

Hjerpe, C. A., and Knight, H. D. (1972). *J. Am. Vet. Med. Assoc.* **160,** 1414–1418.

Hopps, H. E., Meyer, B. C., and Barile, M. F. (1973). *Ann. N.Y. Acad. Sci.* **225,** 265–276.

Hudson, J. R., Buttery, S. H., and Cottew, G. S. (1967). *J. Pathol. Bacteriol.* **94,** 257–273.

Ibrahim, A. A., and Yamomoto, R. (1977). *Infect. Immun.* **18,** 226–229.

Jansson, E., and Wager, O. (1967). *Ann. N.Y. Acad. Sci.* **143,** 535–543.

Jansson, E., Mäkisara, P., Vainio, K., Vainio, U., Snellman, O., and Turri, S. (1971). *Ann. Rheum. Dis.* **30,** 506–508.

Jones, T. C., Yeh, S., and Hirsch, J. G. (1972). *Proc. Soc. Exp. Biol. Med.* **139,** 464–470.

Jordan, F. T. W. (1975). *Avian Pathol.* **4,** 165–174.

Kaklamanis, E., and Pavlatos, M. (1972). *Immunology* **22,** 695–702.

Kaklamanis, E., and Thomas, L. (1970). *In* "Microbial Toxins" (T. C. Montie, S. Kadis, and S. T. Ajl, eds.), Vol. 3, pp. 493–505. Academic Press, New York.

Kaklamanis, E., Thomas, L., Stavropoulos, K., Borman, I., and Boshwitz, C. (1969). *Nature (London)* **221,** 860–862.

Kerr, K. M., and Olson, N. O. (1967). *Avian. Dis.* **11,** 559–578.

Kerr, K. M., and Olson, N. O. (1970). *Avian Dis.* **14,** 291–320.

Klien, G., and Wottawa, A. (1975). *Stud. Biophys.* **50,** S27–S31.

Lee, S. H. S., and Rozee, K. R. (1975). *Exp. Cell Res.* **93,** 143–151.

Lombardi, P. S., and Cole, B. C. (1977). *Abstr. Annu. Meet., A.S.M.,* p. 134.

Lombardi, P. S., and Cole, B. C. (1978). *Infect. Immun.* **20,** 209–214.

Maini, R. N., Lemcke, R. M., Windsor, G. D., Roffe, L. M., Magrath, I. T., and Dumonde, D. C. (1975). *In* "Immunological Aspects of Rheumatoid Arthritis" (J. Clot and J. Sang, eds.), Rheumatology, Vol. 5, pp. 118–130. Karger, Basel.

Manuelidis, E. E., and Thomas, L. (1973). *Proc. Natl. Acad. Sci. U.S.A.* **70,** 706–709.

Mårdh, P.-A., Nilsson, F. J., and Bjelle, A. (1973). *Ann. Rheum. Dis.* **32,** 319–325.

Markham, J. G., and Myers, D. B. (1976). *Ann. Rheum. Dis.* **35,** 1–7.

Meyer, K. F. (1909). *Transvaal Dep. Agric. Rep. Bov. Vet. Bacteriol.* **135,** 159–163.

Middleton, P. J., and Highton, T. C. (1975). *Ann. Rheum. Dis.* **34,** 369–372.

Mielens, Z. E., and Rozitis, J. (1964). *Proc. Soc. Exp. Biol. Med.* **117,** 751–754.

Moulton, J. E., Bordin, A. G., and Rhode, E. A. (1956). *J. Am. Vet. Med. Assoc.* **129,** 364–367.

Naot, Y., Tully, J. G., and Ginsburg, H. (1977). *Infect. Immun.* **18,** 310–317.

Obeck, D. K., Toft, J. D., II, and Dupuy, H. J. (1976). *Lab. Anim. Sci.* **26,** 613–618.

Pearson, C. M. (1959). *In* "Mechanisms of Hypersensitivity" (J. H. Shaffer, G. A. Logrippo, and M. W. Chase, eds.), pp. 647–671. Little, Brown, Boston, Massachusetts.

Person, D. A., Whitworth, M. E., and Sharp, J. T. (1972). *Arthritis Rheum.* **15,** 649–650.

Person, D. A., Sharp, J. T., and Rawls, W. E. (1973). *Arthritis Rheum.* **16,** 677–687.

Porter, P., and Gooderham, K. R. (1966). *Res. Vet. Sci.* **7,** 25–34.

Potgieter, L. N. D., Frey, M. L., and Ross, R. F. (1972). *Can. J. Comp. Med.* **36,** 145–149.

Quinn, P. A., Stuckey, M., Gelfand, E. W. (1978). *Zentralbl. Bakteriol., Parasitenkd., Infektionskr. Hyg., Abt. 1: Orig., Reihe A:* **241,** 248–249.

Razin, S., Knszynski, A., and Lifshitz, Y. (1964). *J. Gen. Microbiol.* **36,** 323–331.

Rinaldo, C. R., Jr., Cole, B. C., Overall, J. C., Jr., and Glasgow, L. A. (1974). *Infect. Immun.* **10,** 1296–1301.

Roberts, D. H., and Olesiuk, O. M. (1967). *Avian Dis.* **11,** 104–119.

Roberts, D. H., Windsor, R. S., Masiga, W. N., and Kariavu, C. G. (1973). *Infect. Immun.* **8,** 349–354.

Roberts, E. D., Switzer, W. P., and Ramsey, F. K. (1963a). *Am. J. Vet. Res.* **24,** 9–18.

Roberts, E. D., Switzer, W. P., and Ramsey, F. K. (1963b). *Am. J. Vet. Res.* **24,** 19–31.

Ross, R. F. (1973). *J. Infect. Dis.* **127,** Suppl., S84–S86.

Ross, R. F., and Duncan, J. R. (1970). *J. Am. Vet. Med. Assoc.* **157**, 1515–1518.

Ross, R. F., and Spear, M. L. (1973). *Am. J. Vet. Res.* **34**, 373–378.

Ross, R. F., Switzer, W. P., and Duncan, J. R. (1971). *Am. J. Vet. Res.* **32**, 1743–1749.

Ross, R. F., Dale, S. E., and Duncan, J. R. (1973). *Am. J. Vet. Res.* **34**, 367–372.

Sabin, A. B. (1939). *Science* **89**, 228–229.

Sevoian, M., Snoeyenbos, G. H., Basch, H. I., and Reynolds, I. M. (1958). *Avian Dis.* **2**, 499–513.

Sharp, J. T. (1970). *Arthritis Rheum.* **13**, 263–271.

Sharp, J. T., and Riggs, S. (1967). "Rheumatology," Vol. 1, pp 51–106. Karger, Basel.

Simberkoff, M. S., and Elsbach, P. (1971). *J. Exp. Med.* **134**, 1417–1430.

Simmons, G. C., and Johnston, L. A. Y. (1963). *Aust. Vet. J.* **39**, 11–14.

Stalheim, O. H. V. (1976). *J. Am. Vet. Med. Assoc.* **169**, 1096–1097.

Stalheim, O. H. V., and Page, L. A. (1975). *J. Clin. Microbiol.* **2**, 165–168.

Stalheim, O. H. V., and Stone, S. S. (1975). *J. Clin. Microbiol.* **2**, 169–172.

Stanbridge, E. (1971). *Bacteriol. Rev.* **35**, 206–227.

Stanbridge, E. J., and Weiss, R. L. (1978). "Microbiology" (D. Schlessinger, ed.), pp. 394–398. Amer. Soc. Microbiol., Washington, D.C.

Stanbridge, E. J., Hayflick, L., and Perkins, F. T. (1971). *Nature (London), New Biol.* **232**, 242–244.

Steinberg, A. D. (1974). *Arthritis Rheum.* **17**, 11–14.

Stewart, D. D., and Buck, G. E. (1975). *Lab. Anim. Sci.* **25**, 769–773.

Stewart, S. M., Duthie, J. J. R., Mackay, J. M. K., Marmion, B. P., and Alexander, W. R. M. (1974). *Ann. Rheum. Dis.* **33**, 346–352.

Taylor, G., and Taylor-Robinson, D. (1977). *Ann. Rheum. Dis.* **36**, 232–238.

Taylor, G., Taylor-Robinson, D., and Slavin, G. (1974). *Ann. Rheum. Dis.* **33**, 376–384.

Taylor-Robinson, D., and Taylor, G (1976). *In* "Infection and Immunology in the Rheumatic Diseases" (D. C. Dumonde, ed.), pp. 177–186. Blackwell, Oxford.

Taylor-Robinson, D., Gumpel, J. M., Hill, A., and Swannell, A. J. (1978). *Ann. Rheum. Dis.* **37**, 180–182.

Trethewie, E. R., and Turner, A. W. (1961). *Aust. Vet. J.* **37**, 27–36.

Tully, J. G., and Ruchman, I. (1964). *Proc. Soc. Exp. Biol. Med.* **115**, 554–558.

Vardaman, T. H., Landreth, K., Whatley, S., Dreesen, L. J., and Glick, B. (1973). *Infect. Immun.* **8**, 674–676.

Ward, J. R., and Cole, B. C. (1970). *In* "The Role of Mycoplasmas and L-Forms of Bacteria in Disease" (H. T. Sharp, ed.), pp. 212–239. Thomas, Springfield, Illinois.

Ward, J. R., and Jones, R. S. (1962). *Arthritis Rheum.* **5**, 163–175.

Washburn, L. R., Cole, B. C., and Ward, J. R. (1978). *Zentralbl. Bakteriol., Parasitenkd., Infektionskr. Hyg., Abt. I: Orig., Reihe* A: **241**, 238–239.

Wilkes, R. M., Simsarian, J. P., Hopps, H. E., Roth, H., Decker, J. L., Aptekar, R. G., and Meyer, H. M. (1973). *Arthritis Rheum.* **16**, 446–454.

Williams, M. H. (1968). *In* "Recovery of Mycoplasma from Rheumatoid Synovial Fluid" (J. J. R. Duthie and W. R. M. Alexander, eds.), Third Pfizer International Symposium on Rheumatic Diseases, pp. 171–181. Edinburgh Univ. Press, Edinburgh.

Williams, M. H., Brostoff, J., and Roitt, I. M. (1970). *Lancet* **2**, 277–280.

Windsor, G. D., Nicholls, A., Maini, R. N., Edward, D. G. ff., Lemcke, R. M., and Dumonde, D. C. (1974). *Ann. Rheum. Dis.* **33**, 70–74.

Zimmerman, B. J., and Ross, R. F. (1977). *Am. J. Vet. Res.* **38**, 2075–2076.

12 / HUMORAL AND CELLULAR IMMUNE RESPONSES TO MYCOPLASMAS

Gerald W. Fernald

I. INTRODUCTION

Mycoplasmas, a unique group among microorganisms in general, deserve special consideration from immunologists interested in infection and immunity. These organisms, whose individual characteristics are detailed elsewhere in this treatise, are found throughout the animal and plant kingdoms, yet they receive little attention compared to bacteria and viruses. Most of the literature concerning host immune responses to mycoplasmas relates to serological diagnosis and vaccine prophylaxis of disease. A few investigators have addressed themselves to the basic immunology of mycoplasma–host interactions. The purpose of this chap-

THE MYCOPLASMAS, VOL. II

ter is, first, to review their work, particularly in terms of humoral and cellular immune responses in natural or experimental infections. Generalities which characterize mycoplasmas as antigenic entities and distinguish them from bacteria, viruses, and other microorganisms are emphasized. Such information should be of interest to biological scientists and clinicians concerned with immunological reactions to mycoplasmas in animal hosts.

Second, in addition to eliciting an immune response, many mycoplasmas have immunosuppressive properties. In some instances, depletion of arginine accounts for reduced reactivity of lymphocytes *in vitro*, but in others, both *in vivo* and *in vitro*, the mechanism is not clear. These observations are not only curious but have important implications for investigators studying the immunopathology of diseases caused by mycoplasmas, including pneumonia and arthritis. The implications of such experiments for the development and testing of mycoplasma vaccines are alarming, especially in view of reports that, following natural *Mycoplasma pneumoniae* infection, a state of anergy may exist for several weeks (Biberfeld and Sterner, 1976b).

A third component of this chapter addresses briefly the application of immunological principles to vaccine prophylaxis of mycoplasma diseases. Emphasis is given to experiments which demonstrate the elements of the immune response which seem most effective in mediating, moderating, or preventing subsequent infections.

II. ANTIGENIC COMPONENTS OF MYCOPLASMAS

Antigenic characterization of mycoplasmas is addressed extensively in Volume I (see Chapter 13). In this chapter the main points to be considered are antigenic components presented to the infected host, antigen processing (i.e., phagocytosis and degradation of mycoplasmas), and antigenic stimulation of the host immune response, both cellular and humoral.

A. Location of Antigenic Moieties

Lacking cell walls, the surface antigens mycoplasmas present to the infected host are components of the cell membrane. Mycoplasma membranes consist essentially of a phospholipid bilayer with its hydrophilic, polar components presenting externally (Smith *et al.*, 1973). Such membranes appear to behave as a fluid mosaic with proteins floating in the surface layer (Singer and Nicholson, 1972). In keeping with this concept, the major surface antigens of mycoplasmas have been found to be glycolipids and proteins. Additional antigens such as enzyme proteins and nucleic acids are contained intracellularly but may become exposed during death and degradation of the mycoplasma. The surface antigens probably are important in stimulating immune defenses aimed at preventing or modifying infection.

B. Antigenicity and Immunogenicity of Mycoplasma Components

In characterizing mycoplasma antigens, a distinction must be made between antigenicity and immunogenicity. While glycolipids are active in complement fixation (CF) and growth inhibition reactions, they are generally poor immunogens (Kenny and Grayston, 1965; Sobeslavsky et al., 1967). Much of the literature characterizing antibody responses in laboratory animals involves adjuvants which promote the immunogenicity of weak antigens. The response in vivo to the inoculation of organisms without adjuvant may be less spectacular, albeit more representative of the immune response under natural conditions. Depending upon the site of immunization (i.e., respiratory tract infection versus intramuscular injection of killed vaccine) the level of circulating antibody may have no direct relation to the state of immunity (Fernald and Clyde, 1970).

1. Glycolipid Haptens

The glycolipid haptens of mycoplasmas have been studied extensively and are discussed in detail elsewhere (see Volume I, Chapter 13). The purified glycolipids of M. pneumoniae act as antigens in CF, growth inhibition, and other in vitro antigen–antibody reactions. They are, however, poor immunogens in vivo unless attached to proteins (Sobeslavsky et al., 1966). On the surface membrane of M. pneumoniae galactosyl and glycosyl diglycerides appear to be the antigens responsible for stimulation of humoral immunity. Glucose and galactose are detectable, using lectins, on the surface membranes of Mycoplasma pneumoniae, M. mycoides, M. pulmonis, M. gallisepticum, and M. gallinarum. Pronase treatment does not diminish the lectin response, suggesting that there are no glycoproteins present (Schiefer et al., 1974). However, Kahane and Brunner (1977) recently described an immunologically active glycoprotein in M. pneumoniae membranes. In the case of Mycoplasma fermentans and Acholeplasma laidlawii, carbohydrates are detectable only after pronase treatment, suggesting that the glycolipids are masked by proteins (Schiefer *et al.*, 1974).

2. Protein Antigens

A large variety of protein antigens is demonstrable with antisera to whole organisms prepared in rabbits. Most of these proteins are probably intracellular, since membrane proteins seem not to be soluble unless lysed with detergents (Hollingdale and Lemcke, 1969). These mycoplasma protein antigens are revealed to the host immune system through phagocytosis and degradation but, because they are not on the membrane surface, they may not be important in surface immunity.

While protein antigens do not stimulate antibodies detectable by common serological techniques, they apparently are the principal antigens responsible for cell-mediated reactions to mycoplasmas. Mizutani and Mizutani (1975b) reported that the *M. pneumoniae* antigens responsible for eliciting macrophage migration inhibition were contained in a lipid-free protein fraction. Suzuki *et al.* (1976) further characterized these water-soluble antigens as pronase-resistant with a high polysaccharide content, namely, galactose, glucose, and mannose. These glycoprotein antigens inhibited migration of peritoneal macrophages from immune guinea pigs and elicited a delayed cutaneous reaction but did not fix complement. In contrast the acetone-soluble glycolipid fraction of *M. pneumoniae* was active as a CF antigen but not in the macrophage assay or the skin reaction.

During the active growth stage, mycoplasmas present theoretically only surface membrane structures and soluble antigens to the host. Once the organism dies, whether or not it is phagocytosed, internal antigens become exposed. Phagocytosis of the injured or dead mycoplasma results in further breakdown, making more antigenic moieties available. Eventually the immune system may be presented with a large number of antigens derived from the infecting mycoplasmas. Those related to surface receptors on host cells or possessing toxic or antimetabolic properties may stimulate antibodies to each of these functional entities. Antibodies to such surface antigens may block surface receptor sites, neutralize toxic activities, or serve simply as opsonins. Immune responses to internal organism components, chiefly proteins, may produce antigen–antibody complexes which, by fixing complement, attract an inflammatory cellular infiltrate to the area of infection. As mentioned above, protein antigens are probably responsible for stimulating T-lymphocyte reactions which may generate lymphocytic cellular infiltrates, as in the delayed hypersensitivity reaction.

III. HOST RESPONSES TO MYCOPLASMAS

A. Nonimmune Reactions

In gaining entrance to the host organism, mycoplasmas must supervene the natural barriers to noxious substances which protect all living organisms. The initial mode of parasitism of mycoplasmas is to attach to surface epithelia of the respiratory or genital tract (see this volume, Chapter 14). Mucous secretions, ciliary motion, and physical factors such as coughing and sneezing probably prevent large numbers of invading mycoplasmas from achieving this goal. Organisms which remain, like most foreign bodies, are subject to ingestion, digestion, and elimination by phagocytes. As hypothesized in Section II,B, antigenic stimulation of the immune system may arise either from components of phagocytosed mycoplasmas or from factors released by intact organisms which manage to colonize mucosal epithelial surfaces. Certain pathogenic mycoplasmas, as well as commensals, remain in this extracellular position (*M. pneumoniae*). Other pathogens, capable of systemic invasion, localize in joints (*Mycoplasma arthritidis*), brain (*M. gallisepticum*), pleura, and subcutaneous tissues (*M. mycoides*).

1. Polymorphonuclear (PMN) Phagocytosis

Until an immune response is mounted against the invading mycoplasmas, phagocytic cells must work in the absence of specific antibodies. In general it appears that mycoplasmas resist degradation by PMN leukocytes in the absence of specific antiserum. Simberkoff and Elsbach (1971) found that *Mycoplasma hominis* and *M. arthritidis* were not ingested or killed by human or rabbit leukocytes under conditions which permitted rapid killing of *Escherichia coli*. Neither the presence nor the absence of specific antiserum affected this system. Resistance to phagocytosis appeared to relate to the absence of tight adherence to the leukocyte membrane. These workers proposed that the mechanism by which these two mycoplasmas resisted phagocytosis related to injury of the leukocyte membrane. This was based on the observation that *E. coli* ingestion and killing were reduced in the presence of whole mycoplasmas or supernatant fluid from a mycoplasma culture.

Howard *et al.* (1976) reported that *Mycoplasma dispar* and *M. agalactiae* resisted phagocytosis by bovine leukocytes. However, when bovine antimycoplasma antibody was added, phagocytosis and killing were observed. This suggested that failure to use a homologous system of phagocytic cells and antiserum, and a mycoplasma infective for the experimental host, may explain the lack of antibody effect in the Simberkoff study.

2. Mononuclear Phagocytosis

Several investigators have observed that mononuclear phagocytes (macrophages) are unable to ingest mycoplasmas in the absence of specific antibody. The organisms attach to the macrophage membrane, but only with the addition of antibody do endocytosis and killing occur (Jones and Hirsh, 1971; Cole and Ward, 1973; Powell and Clyde, 1975).

3. Complement

In each of the experiments above, sera were heat-inactivated and therefore devoid of complement activity. Under natural conditions *in vivo* complement probably works in concert with antibody to opsonize mycoplasmas. Bredt showed that complement alone, in the absence of specific antibody, was activated by *M. pneumoniae* (Bredt and Bitter-Suermann, 1975). Activated complement alone, presumably C3b, promotes phagocytosis by macrophages (Bredt, 1975). Thus, in the absence of specific antibody, clearance of mycoplasmas by macrophages probably occurs *in vivo* in the early stages of infection. Since cross-reacting antibodies to mycoplasmas are known to be stimulated by antigens in nature, it is likely that "natural antibodies" also act as opsonins to promote phagocytic activity (Gale and Kenny, 1970; Kenny and Newton, 1973).

B. Immune Reactions

In this and subsequent sections of this chapter experimental observations on the various models of mycoplasma lung infections serve as the main theme. This choice is made arbitrarily for the sake of simplicity and because several laboratories have focused on the immunology of mycoplasma pneumonia. Most of the generalities derived from these studies should relate to other organ systems, however. General reviews of immune mechanisms in the lung should be consulted for backgound material (Kaltreider, 1976; Newhouse *et al.*, 1976).

1. Local Proliferation of Immunocytes

The initial site of interaction between the organism and the host's immune system probably occurs at or near the site of infection. In the lower respiratory tract of animals infected intranasally, a peribronchial proliferation of lymphoid cells appears after several days (Dajani *et al.*, 1965; Lindsey *et al.*, 1971; Brunner *et al.*, 1973b). In *M. pulmonis* infection of specific-pathogen-free mice (Cassell *et al.*, 1974) and in *M. pneumoniae*-infected hamsters (Fernald *et al.*, 1972) IgM plasmacytes become apparent in this peribronchial infiltrate by the end of the first week. IgG and IgA cells appear subsequently, giving further evidence of local antibody formation in the submucosal tissues.

Non-immunoglobulin-containing lymphoid cells were seen to cluster around small blood vessels in the lamina propria in the hamster model. These perivascular cellular infiltrates resembled histologically the lesions of cutaneous delayed hypersensitivity, suggesting that they might be T lymphocytes (Fernald *et al.*, 1972).

The histopathology of other mycoplasma infections has been described and varies depending on the species of mycoplasma and host and the site of infection. In pigs, *Mycoplasma suipneumoniae* produces chronic pneumonia characterized by prolonged colonization of the mucous epithelium and a perivascular and peribronchiolar mononuclear infiltrate (Whittlestone, 1972). In rats a similar lesion is produced by *M. pulmonis* infection, but it frequently progresses to bronchiectasis (Lindsey *et al.*, 1971). Mycoplasma pneumonias in other animals, including humans (see this volume, Chapter 9), have a similar histological pattern, suggesting that the accumulation of immunoglobulin-producing lymphoid cells in the submucosa is a characteristic of all mycoplasma infections of the respiratory tract.

2. Regional Lymph Nodes

In the mouse with *M. pulmonis* pneumonia, concurrent enlargement of paratracheal nodes is apparent. These lymphoid tissues also contain large numbers of immunoglobulin-bearing cells (Cassell *et al.* 1974). Lymph node enlargement is also seen in *M. pneumoniae*-infected guinea pigs but rarely in the hamster model (Fernald, unpublished observations). The involvement of regional lymph nodes in these mycoplasma pneumonias suggests traffic of antigen and/or cells from the infected bronchi via afferent lymph channels. In the gut, depending upon the degree of antigenic stimulation, lymphocytes of both B (antibody-producing) and T (thymus-dependent) types may feed into the systemic circulation via the efferent lymphoid system (Heremans, 1969). Sensitive techniques for tracing the course of mycoplasma antigens or antigen-bearing macrophages will be required to establish that this is the route of immune induction against mycoplasma infection in the lung.

3. Local Immunoinflammatory Response

Coincident with the evolution of peribronchial and other cellular infiltrates in mycoplasma pneumonia, an inflammatory exudate develops within the bronchi and bronchioles. This consists of both PMN and mononuclear phagocytes and follows a predictable course (Clyde, 1971; Whittlestone, 1972). Total mononuclear cells remain relatively stable in numbers throughout the course of *M. pneumoniae* infection in the hamster (Clyde, 1971; Fernald and Clyde, 1976). Although the size and morphology of these mononuclear cells varies, over 90% contain acid phosphatase and adhere to glass or plastic; thus functionally they appear to be macrophages (G. W. Fernald, unpublished observations). At the peak of the peribronchial pneumonic reaction, and during its resolution, macrophages in the bronchial lumen appear to enlarge, contain more vacuoles, and are more irregular in shape. This is in contrast to the small, rounded appearance of macrophages seen in antithymocyte serum-suppressed animals (Fernald and Clyde, 1974). Either antibody or lymphokines, secreted locally, could be the factor which activates pulmonary macrophages during mycoplasma pneumonia. It has been shown that pulmonary macrophages exposed to *M. pneumoniae* organisms *in vitro* are not activated until specific antibody is added (Powell and Clyde, 1975). Antibody stimulates increased cellular movement; the mycoplasmas are endocytosed and appear to disintegrate in the cytoplasmic vacuoles of the macrophages.

PMN leukocytes, which are few in number in bronchial washings and tissue sections of normal uninfected lungs, increase manyfold during *M. pneumoniae* infection, reaching a peak at the height of the peribronchial infiltrate (Clyde, 1971). A correlation between the increase in antibody-forming cells in the lamina propria and PMN leukocytes in the adjacent bronchial lumen is suggested by the suppression of both cellular responses when animals are treated with antithymocyte serum (Fernald and Clyde, 1974). PMNs are not seen in hamsters infected intranasally with avirulent *M. pneumoniae* which does not attach to mucosal cells. Although the organisms persist in the lung for several days and evoke a modest increase in intrabronchial mononuclear cells, no peribronchitis is seen (G. W. Fernald, unpublished observations).

Evidence that antibody is present in the bronchial lumen at the peak of the histological response is provided by the observation that leukocytes form rosettes about sloughed, infected epithelial cells in hamsters (Clyde, 1971) and in humans (Collier and Clyde, 1974). These rosettes may be constructed *in vitro* in the presence of antimycoplasma antibody and complement (Clyde, 1971). This phenomenon also appears in immune animals 3 days after intranasal challenge, coincident with an accelerated peribronchial round cell infiltrate. Such observations suggest, but do not prove, that PMN phagocytosis depends upon the generation of antibody locally in response to the infecting mycoplasmas, and that this is a significant component of the immunological defense mechanism.

4. Secretory Antibody System

As immunologists have become aware of the secretory immunological system, a component of most mucosal surfaces in the body, its role in defending against infections has been a focus of investigation. Initial efforts to detect *M. pneumoniae* antibodies in upper respiratory secretions of humans (Smith *et al.*, 1967) and in bronchial washings of the hamster model (Fernald, 1969b) were unsuccessful because of the insensitivity of the serological methods used. Biberfeld and Sterner (1971) utilized an indirect immunofluorescent test to detect *M. pneumoniae* antibody in sputum samples obtained from patients with pneumonia. IgA antibody was present in all 31 samples with detectable antimycoplasma activity. IgG antibodies were present in 24, and IgM was found in 13, all of which contained IgA as well. In 5 sputa, only IgA antibody was found. Both local synthesis of secretory IgA and transudation of serum into bronchial secretions were postulated as the origin of the *M. pneumoniae* antibodies found in respiratory tract secretions.

Holmgren (1974) collected sputa, tracheobronchial washings, and sera from disease-free pigs inoculated intranasally with *Mycoplasma hyopneumoniae*. Indirect hemagglutinating antibodies (IHA) were detectable in bronchial secretions within 2 weeks of inoculation, peaked between 8 and 9 weeks, and persisted through the 13-week period of study. Serum IHA antibodies appeared by the fourth week. Antibody activity in the secretory fluids collected 2 weeks after infection was found in fractions containing only IgA. Secretions collected at 13 weeks contained IHA antibody in both IgA and IgG fractions. IgA antibodies in tracheobronchial secretions separated by gel filtration with higher-molecular-weight proteins (i.e., IgM), while serum IgA antibodies eluted in fractions containing both 19S and 7S molecules. Thus, although secretory IgA was not characterized immunologically, this investigator suggested the antibody detected in tracheobronchial washings was 11S IgA.

Martinez-Tello *et al.* (1968) noted that, while IgA predominates in secretions of the uninfected normal human lung, immunohistological studies of uninfected bronchial mucosa from autopsy cases revealed plasma cell IgA, IgG, and IgM in a ratio of 5:5:1. In patients with chronic infection, such as cystic fibrosis, IgA and IgG cell numbers were increased, with IgA predominating. No such studies have been possible in patients with *M. pneumoniae* pneumonia, but in hamsters which normally have a scant background of IgA plasmacytes, all three cell types are generated by *M. pneumoniae* infection (Fernald *et al.*, 1972).

Cassell *et al.* (1974) also found large numbers of all three Ig-containing plasma cells near bronchi of mice with *M. pulmonis* pneumonia. *Mycoplasma pulmonis* antibodies in tracheobronchial secretions of these mice were detected by the second week after inoculation and persisted through the eighth week. IgG$_1$ and IgG$_2$ appeared first, followed by IgA in the fifth week. IgM was intermittently detected from the fourth week onward. When considered in light of such studies documenting localized production of three major immunoglobulin types in the lamina propria, Biberfeld's results probably reflect local secretion of IgA, IgG, and IgM during the course of *M. pneumoniae* pneumonia in humans (Biberfeld and Sterner, 1971).

While detection of IgA-specific mycoplasma antibody in bronchial secretions established that local antibody was being synthesized and secreted, the biological function of these antibodies remained undefined. In an effort to develop more sensitive methods for detecting the apparently minimal amounts of local antibody generated in the human respiratory tract, Brunner developed both a complement-mediated lysis assay (Brunner *et al.*, 1972) and a radioimmunoprecipitation technique (Brunner and Chanock, 1973). The latter method was used to measure IgA-specific *M. pneumoniae* antibody in nasal washings and sputa in a group of experimentally infected volunteers (Brunner *et al.*, 1973a). Men with preexisting titers of nasal IgA antibody showed the most resistance to the challenge infection. Serum antibody levels statistically were unrelated to resistance. This report confirmed that resistance to *M. pneumoniae* infection was more dependent upon secretory than serum antibodies.

While it is evident that local antibodies correlate with protective immunity, their mechanism of action still remains elusive. Potential opsonic activity has been suggested above, i.e., that IgG fixes complement on the mycoplasma membrane and facilitates attachment and engulfment via Fc and C3b receptors on the macrophage membrane. IgA may activate complement by the alternative pathway and thereby promote phagocytosis. While these activities are predictable from *in vitro* studies, proof that they actually operate *in vivo* is yet to be obtained.

Brunner *et al.* (1973a) has suggested that local IgA may protect the host by blocking adsorption of *M. pneumoniae* to respiratory epithelial cells. This would not only prevent colonization and serve to limit the infection (Williams and Gibbons, 1972) but would also prevent organisms from secreting toxins in direct apposition to the epithelial cells. Preliminary experiments, utilizing radioisotope-labeled *M. pneumoniae* in hamster tracheal organ cultures (Powell *et al.*, 1976), indicate that serum antibodies can block the attachment of mycoplasmas to respiratory epithelium, but the low level of mycoplasma antibody in tracheobronchial secretions requires a more sensitive technique to detect secretory IgA blocking antibody (D. A. Powell, personal communication).

5. Local Cell-Mediated Immune (CMI) Responses

The role of local cell-mediated immunity in mycoplasma infections has been addressed by several investigators (Denny et al., 1972; Fernald, 1973; Taylor et al., 1974; Fernald and Clyde, 1974; Taylor and Taylor-Robinson, 1975). This limb of the immune system appeared to be part of the local response to mycoplasma infection because of the histological similarity of the peribronchial and perivascular lesion to that of delayed hypersensitivity (Fernald, 1969b). However, most of the cells comprising these infiltrates are derived from B lymphocytes (Fernald et al., 1972), and antibody production obviously plays a major role in the local pathogenesis of disease as discussed above. There is ample evidence that CMI reactivity can be detected in the respiratory tract of humans and animals either when exposed experimentally to noninfectious agents (Waldman and Henny, 1971) or infected with viruses (Waldman et al., 1972) or bacteria (Reynolds et al., 1974; Cantey and Hand, 1974). No direct evidence of a local cell-mediated response to mycoplasmas has been reported, but CMI is exhibited in vitro by lymphocytes and macrophages obtained from extrarespiratory sites (see Section III,B,6).

6. Systemic Manifestations of Mycoplasma Immunity

Early studies on the nature of the immune response to mycoplasma infection concerned immunoglobulin characterization of serum antibody in infected patients and experimental animals (Fernald et al., 1967; Biberfeld, 1968; Fernald, 1969a). These experiments established that IgM, IgG, and IgA antibodies appeared sequentially within the first few weeks of infection with M. pneumoniae, as had been observed in many other infections. A large variety of serological reactions has been utilized to characterize the systemic humoral responses to mycoplasma infection, most of which are laboratory phenomena with no direct relation to in vivo function (Sethi, 1973; Whittlestone, 1976; Fernald et al., 1979). Certain in vitro antibody functions do have biological correlates which may be of functional significance in vivo. These are opsonins which promote phagocytosis of mycoplasmas by macrophages (Jones and Hirsch, 1971; Powell and Clyde, 1975; Jones and Yang, 1977), antibodies which fix complement on the mycoplasma membrane and cause lysis (Brunner et al., 1971), and antibodies capable of inhibiting the attachment of M.

pneumoniae to hamster tracheal epithelial cells (D. A. Powell, personal communication). The list might also include antibodies which cross-react with host antigens such as erythrocytes (Costea *et al.*, 1971, 1972) and brain and other tissue (Biberfeld, 1971). (The implications for immunopathogenicity related to cross-reacting antibodies in mycoplasma disease in humans is discussed by Clyde, this volume, Chapter 9.)

Cellular immunity to mycoplasmas has been a subject of study since *in vitro* methods for analysis of lymphocyte reactivity were developed (Leventhal *et al.*, 1969). Lymphocyte responses *in vitro* to *M. pneumoniae* organisms appear early after natural infection in humans and persist for several years (Fernald, 1972; Biberfeld *et al.*, 1974; Mogensen *et al.*, 1976). Similar studies of this phenomenon have been reported in guinea pigs (Brunner, 1974; Fernald and Clyde, 1976), swine (Roberts, 1973), and cattle (Roberts *et al.*, 1973). Human lymphocyte studies have been more successful than those performed on animals, although the reasons for this are unknown (Fernald and Metzgar, 1971; Fernald, 1973).

The relation of circulating antigen-reactive lymphocytes to the local immune response to mycoplasma pneumonia is even less understood than humoral immunity. Since this manifestation of CMI is absent in children experiencing their first episodes of *M. pneumoniae* infection, we have assumed that sensitized lymphocytes do not reach systemic circulation until a sufficient local response has been generated in lung and regional lymph nodes (Fernald *et al.*, 1975, 1979).

In addition to lymphocyte transformation, macrophage migration inhibition has been studied as an *in vitro* parameter of CMI. Arai *et al.* (1971) demonstrated inhibition of the migration of peritoneal macrophages from guinea pigs and hamsters by splenic or peritoneal lymphocytes from *M. pneumoniae*-infected hamsters. Biberfeld (1973) confirmed this finding in hamsters and noted that migration inhibition was present 1 week after intranasal inoculation. CF antibodies did not appear until the end of the second week. This suggests that sensitized lymphocytes are released into the circulation during the early phase of *M. pneumoniae* pneumonia and that this test is more sensitive than lymphocyte transformation. However, studies of leukocyte migration in *M. pneumoniae*-infected patients revealed the opposite; i.e., lymphocyte transformation was more often positive than leukocyte migration inhibition (Biberfeld, 1974).

Mycoplasma pneumoniae infection has been shown to generate delayed cutaneous hypersensitivity in humans (Mizutani *et al.*, 1971; Suzuki *et al.*, 1976) and in guinea pigs (Mizutani and Mizutani, 1975a; Fernald and Clyde, 1976; Suzuki *et al.*, 1976). As with the *in vitro* parameters of CMI discussed above, such reactions reflect that T lymphocytes are sensitized during *M. pneumoniae* infection but shed no light on their role in the local immune response in the lung.

7. Experimental Ablation of the Immune Response as a Means for Study of Its Components

Experimental manipulation of the immune system in animal models has been utilized by several investigators to isolate T- and B-lymphocyte function in mycoplasma pneumonias. These experiments fall into two groups: those in which immunosuppressive drugs or antilymphocyte serum (ALS) was employed on otherwise normal animals and those in which thymectomy or bursectomy was performed to ablate T- or B-cell function. In some instances combinations of both procedures were utilized.

a. Thymus-dependent immunity (T cells). Denny *et al.* (1972) studied the role of thymus-dependent immunity to *M. pulmonis* in thymectomized, x-irradiated, ALS-treated mice. These T-lymphocyte-deficient animals were more readily infected, and systemic spread of mycoplasmas to other organs occurred more frequently than in normal controls. Peribronchiolar and perivascular lymphoid cell infiltrates, characteristic of *M. pulmonis* pneumonia in controls, were much less prominent in the immunosuppressed group. These results were interpreted to indicate (1) that local immunity, under T-cell control, acted to limit infection in the lung as well as systemic spread of organisms, and (2) that much of the "pneumonia" was a manifestation of the local cellular immune response. Similar observations were reported in cyclophosphamide-treated mice by Singer *et al.* (1972). Antibody levels were not determined in these experiments, and therefore the degree of B-lymphocyte function was not known, although presumably it also was depressed, especially in Denny's study since bone marrow cell reconstitution was not employed.

Subsequent studies of *M. pneumoniae*-infected hamsters showed antithymocyte serum treatment slightly increased the numbers of organisms infecting the lung and depleted pneumonic cellular infiltrates, although systemic spread of organisms in this model did not occur (Taylor *et al.*, 1974). These experiments were repeated, using the serological response to sheep erythrocytes (SRBC) and *Brucella* organisms to monitor T-cell-dependent and -independent antibody production (Fernald and Clyde, 1974). While SRBC hemolytic antibody responses were suppressed along with the pneumonia, *Brucella* agglutinins, a manifestation of B-cell function, were produced (Rouse and Warner, 1972). Indeed, specific *M. pneumoniae* antibodies, measured as CF and growth-inhibiting activity, are also suppressed in antithymocyte serum- (ATS) treated hamsters (G.

W. Fernald, unpublished observations). Thus, in both *M. pulmonis* and *M. pneumoniae* infection, the host immune response apparently depends upon intact thymic function (Taylor and Taylor-Robinson, 1975). Nevertheless, the factor which affects organisms directly is antibody which apparently cannot be generated in the absence of T lymphocytes.

b. Bursa-dependent immunity (B lymphocytes). Mycoplasma infections in birds provide a unique immunological model for study of the B-cell system, since the avian bursa of Fabricius functions as the central lymphoid organ in the control of humoral immunity (Cooper *et al.*, 1966). Adler *et al.* (1973) showed that antibodies to *M. gallisepticum* were markedly reduced in chemically bursectomized chickens; the low titers which are detectable are restricted to the IgM class. This may represent a primitive B-cell response originating elsewhere in the central lymphoid organs (Bryant *et al.*, 1973). Resistance to infection in such bursectomized birds was inversely proportional to the amount of lymphoid tissue persisting at autopsy.

Vardaman *et al.* (1973) surgically bursectomized chickens at hatch and challenged them with *Mycoplasma synoviae* at age 3 weeks. Normal controls were similarly infected. Antibodies to *M. synoviae* were delayed in synthesis and reduced in titer in bursectomized chicks. Air sac lesions were markedly increased in the bursaless birds, indicating an enhanced degree of infection. These data also suggested that antibody production was necessary for immune resistance to mycoplasma infection, but a supporting role for thymic dependent lymphocytes was not excluded.

c. Passive transfer of immune serum. The simplest way to isolate the effect of humoral immunity on an infectious process is to transfer immune serum passively. This method reportedly was employed by Nocard and later by Gourlay and Shifrine (1966) in demonstrating a protective effect of convalescent-phase serum against *M. mycoides* in cattle (Taylor and Taylor-Robinson, 1976). Goiš *et al.* (1974) reported that passively transferred immune serum protected gnotobiotic piglets against *M. hyorhinis* infection. The major effect was to prevent systemic spread to organs other than the respiratory tract. However, organism concentrations in the lung were significantly reduced and pneumonic lesions were fewer. IgM and IgG fractions of *M. hyorhinis* immune sera produced the same effect. A similar effect of immune serum on mycoplasma-infected pigs was reported by Lam and Switzer (1971).

In contrast to the above reports, several workers have commented on the failure of serum antibody, whether actively or passively acquired, to influence mycoplasma infections. We and others have noted that serum antibody titers produced by parenteral vaccination do not correlate with protection (Goodwin *et al.*, 1969; Fernald and Clyde, 1970). When compared to nasal antibodies, serum antibody titers are poor predictors of resistance to *M. pneumoniae* in humans (Brunner *et al.*, 1973a).

The relative effects of passively acquired immunity, both cellular and humoral, were studied definitively by Taylor and Taylor-Robinson (1976). Transfer of 10^8 immune spleen cells between syngeneic (C3H) mice failed to prevent typical disease due to *M. pulmonis*. In contrast, convalescent sera from infected mice showed a progressively protective effect when injected intraperitoneally into recipient mice infected with the same organism. Both numbers of organisms colonizing the respiratory tract and degree of lung lesions were reduced by the passively acquired antiserum. The effect of passive antibody on colonization could be overcome by increasing the size of the inoculum, but still lung lesions did not develop. These investigators postulated that specific antibodies blocked the host immune response by competing with mycoplasma receptors on lymphocytes and macrophages. This specificity was not removed by adsorption of CF antibodies with whole mycoplasmas. This discrepancy suggested that common serological methods may not detect antibody specificities responsible for blocking the local immune response in lung to mycoplasmas, thus offering an explanation for the variable effect of serum antibody levels on mycoplasma infections.

8. Summary and Conclusions

While further experiments will be necessary to clarify the relative roles of cellular and humoral immunity in mycoplasma disease, the present data are overwhelming in favor of antibody as the prime mediator of resistance. These antibodies are most likely of local origin but include IgG, and perhaps IgM, as well as IgA. They function as opsonins to promote removal by phagocytosis and prevent reattachment of mycoplasmas to the mucosal epithelium, thereby interfering with progress of the infection. That most mycoplasmas are well adapted to withstand this defense on the part of the host is suggested by the prolonged course of these infections. Thymus-dependent immunity probably plays a supporting role in the generation of mycoplasma antibodies by B lymphocytes, but there is still no evidence that T lymphocytes directly attack mycoplasmas.

Apart from the direct antimycoplasma effect of the immune response, there is also much evidence to suggest that the disease produced in the host is a manifestation of the immune response to foreign antigens proliferating in the target organ. That this immunopathological response is lacking in the absence of all or part of the immune system has been observed in mice (Denny *et al.*, 1972), hamsters (Taylor *et al.*, 1974), and humans (Foy *et al.*, 1973). The presumed selective effect of ALS in suppressing mycoplasma pneumonia (Fernald and Clyde, 1974; Taylor *et al.*, 1974) suggests that the process is mediated by the T lymphocyte. However, the failure of passively transferred immune cells to generate immunity of any sort seems to refute the role of T cells in this process (Taylor and Taylor-Robinson, 1976). Such experiments are notoriously difficult to perform successfully, however, even between syngeneic animals, and much more elaborate and extensive trials will be necessary before the validity of this negative observation can be accepted.

Another line of evidence in support of the host immune response as the source of the pulmonary infiltrates in mycoplasma pneumonia comes from observation of immune animals subjected to rechallenge (Clyde, 1971; Fernald *et al.*, 1972). Within 3 days of infection, peribronchial and vascular lesions, consisting predominantly of small lymphocytes, develop. By the tenth day, when unimmunized controls are developing maximum infection and pneumonia, lesions in the immunized group are diminishing and numbers of organisms in the lung have fallen off markedly (Fernald and Clyde, 1976). Increased numbers of phagocytes and evidence of immune phagocytosis are also seen to peak 3 days after challenge (Clyde, 1971). Thus all the immune phenomena which progress so slowly in the previously uninfected animal are accelerated, as if by anamnesis, upon reinfection. No correlate of this experimental observation in hamsters has been seen clinically. It may occur whenever local immunity has waned to the point where local antibody protection is absent but sufficient cellular immunity persists to evoke an accelerated immune response to the invading mycoplasmas (Fernald *et al.*, 1979).

IV. NONSPECIFIC EFFECTS OF MYCOPLASMAS ON THE IMMUNE RESPONSE

A. *In Vitro* Effects on Cultured Lymphocytes

Both suppression and stimulation of lymphocyte activity have been observed due to mycoplasmas or mycoplasma products.

1. Immunosuppressive Activity *in Vitro*

Toxicity of certain mycoplasmas for lymphocytes *in vitro* was first reported by Copperman and Morton (1966). They described reversible inhibition of mitosis in cultured lymphocytes by nonviable suspensions of *M. hominis.* The inhibitor was shown to be arginine deiminase, and its effect could be countered by adding arginine or by washing the lymphocytes and culturing them in fresh medium (Barile and Leventhal, 1968). The inhibitory effect was found to be common to all arginine-utilizing mycoplasmas, but not to glucose-fermenting species (Simberkoff *et al.*, 1969). The effect of mycoplasmas on cells in culture, including lymphocytes, has been reviewed extensively by Stanbridge (1971).

2. Immunostimulatory Effects *in Vitro*

Since the original reports of the toxicity of arginine deiminase for lymphocyte cultures, descriptions of other effects unrelated to arginine have appeared. Ginsburg and Nicolet (1973) observed an immunostimulatory effect of *M. pulmonis* on rat lymphocytes *in vitro*. Extensive blastogenesis was observed after 2 days in culture, resembling the mitogenic effect of phytohemagglutinin (PHA), but heating to 60°C or filtration removed the effect, suggesting that live organisms were involved. The mitogenicity of *M. pulmonis* has been confirmed by Cole *et al.* (1975) in studies on mouse lymphocytes. In neither study was there evidence of prior sensitization of the lymphocytes; rather, the evidence favors a direct nonspecific effect of the viable mycoplasma on lymphocytes.

In a second paper, Ginsburg's experiments have been reconfirmed in germ-free animals, and the effect of other mycoplasmas on rat lymphocytes has been reported (Naot *et al.*, 1977). In these experiments, *M. pneumoniae*, *M. fermentans*, *M. hominis*, *M. orale*, and *A. laidlawii* did not activate rat lymphocytes, but *M. pulmonis, M. arthritidis*, and *M. neurolyticum* did. In a study of the inhibiting effect of porcine mycoplasmas on PHA-induced lymphocyte transformation Roberts (1972) observed that *M. hyorhinis,* a glucose-fermenting species, produced the same effect as arginine-utilizing organisms. *Mycoplasma hyopneumoniae* and *Acholeplasma granularum* also inhibited transformation, but to a lesser extent than the arginine-utilizing species, *Mycoplasma iners, M. hyosynoviae*, and *M. gallinarum*.

Biberfeld and Gronowicz (1976) reported that *M. pneumoniae* was a polyclonal activator for B lymphocytes in pathogen-free mice. They proposed that such direct stimulation of antibody-forming cells could account for the early production of nonspecific IgM antibodies in natural infection. Further evidence of mycoplasma-mediated activation of lymphocytes *in vitro* was presented by Cole and co-workers who reported that interferon was induced by several mycoplasma species in sheep and human lymphocyte cultures (Cole *et al.*, 1976).

Recently, Cole *et al.* (1977) reported studies on the mitogenic potential of a large number of mycoplasma strains. Both arginine-utilizing and glucose-fermenting species, including *A. laidlawii* and *Spiroplasma citri,* were mitogenic for mouse lymphocytes. In the case of arginine deiminase-containing mycoplasmas, heat inactivation removed the inhibitory effect and allowed expression of a heat-stable mitogenic factor. The mitogenic factor in *M. pneumoniae* reported by Biberfeld and Gronowicz (1976) was also heat-stable, but in Ginsburg and Nicolet's experiments with *M. pulmonis* it was not. Further characterization of this factor (or factors) should be forthcoming now that its existence has been established. Studies presently in progress in the laboratory of Naot and co-workers suggest this factor is a membrane protein (Naot *et al.*, 1979).

B. *In Vivo* Effects of Mycoplasmas on the Immune Response

1. Experimental Animal Models

An immunosuppressive effect on antibody formation to phage $\phi5$ has been reported in *M. arthritidis*-infected rats by Kaklamanis and Pavlatos (1972). Lymphocyte responses to PHA *in vitro* were also suppressed in these animals. *Mycoplasma arthritidis* membranes injected intravenously suppressed the primary and secondary hemagglutinin response to *E. coli* common antigen in rabbits (Bergquist *et al.*, 1974). Suppression of PHA-induced lymphocyte mitogenesis was reported during the course of *M. mycoides* infection in cattle, but the serological response was unaffected (Roberts *et al.*, 1973). Eckner *et al.* (1974) found that thymus cellularity was decreased in mice inoculated with *M. arthritidis* extracts. Histological depletion of T-dependent areas of thymus and lymph nodes and suppression of *in vitro* responses to PHA and concanavalin A was observed, but the antibody response to sheep erythrocytes was preserved, suggesting selective suppression of a T-cell subpopulation. A similar involutionary effect of *M. fermentans* on mouse tissues has been observed by Gabridge and Schneider (1975). These observations, although unexplained as to underlying mechanisms, suggest that mycoplasmas or their products directly influence the function of lymphocytes *in vivo*.

2. Suppression of Delayed Hypersensitivity in Humans

Biberfeld and Sterner (1976a) have documented anergy to tuberculin skin testing in patients with *M. pneumoniae* pneumonia. In light of the universal use of BCG in Sweden, negative purified protein derivative skin tests early after onset of disease were notable in 22 of 36 patients. Repeated skin testing yielded a return of delayed hypersensitivity to tuberculin within 3–6 weeks, but prolonged tuberculin anergy was observed for more than 5 months in two patients. Control skin tests with *Candida* or other frequently positive antigens were not studied.

In a subsequent report, Biberfeld and Sterner (1976b) extended these observations to include 47 recently infected subjects, with the same results. In addition, lymphocyte activation *in vitro* by PPD and *M. pneumoniae* antigens was studied in 13 patients. In eight cases thymidine uptake stimulated by PPD was threefold lower during the *M. pneumoniae* illness than after recovery. This documentation of tuberculin nonreactivity, both *in vivo* and *in vitro*, strongly suggests that mycoplasma infections exert direct effects upon the immune response of the host, as do certain viruses such as measles. The implications of this phenomenon, if confirmed, are far-reaching both for experimental studies on the pathogenesis of mycoplasma diseases and for vaccine immunoprophylaxis.

V. EFFECTS OF VACCINATION ON IMMUNITY TO MYCOPLASMA INFECTIONS

Mycoplasmas cause significant disease in many animal species, and attempts at control by immunoprophylaxis have been equally numerous. The recent and extensive review of this subject by Whittlestone (1976) should be consulted for details.

Certain observations recur in studies of the protective effect of vaccination against mycoplasmas, most of which relate directly to immunological processes discussed in the previous sections of this chapter. They are:

1. Prior natural infection conveys the most effective state of resistance, as expressed by limitation of colonization, degree of pneumonic response in the host, and duration of immunity (Whittlestone, 1976). However, there is now solid evidence that *M. pneumoniae* infections in humans recur at intervals of several years (Foy *et al.*, 1971; Biberfeld *et al.*, 1974; Fernald *et al.*, 1975). These observations suggest that immunity to a single infection is relatively short-term, particularly in early childhood (Fernald *et al.*, 1979).

2. Intranasal inoculation with live, virulent organisms induces a degree of immunity similar to that of natural infection (Fernald and Clyde, 1970; Taylor *et al.*, 1977). However, the usefulness of an unattenuated vaccine is severely limited by its pathogenic effect on the host, as well as possible spread by contagion (Couch *et al.*, 1964).

3. Attenuation of mycoplasma strains tends to reduce both immunogenicity and virulence. In most cases attenuation has not yielded an effective vaccine for commercial production. A unique exception exists for *M. mycoides* vaccination in cattle where subcutaneous inoculation of live organisms into the tail serves to generate effective immunity in a manner analogous to vaccination against smallpox (Gourlay, 1975).

4.   Killed vaccines administered intranasally are relatively ineffective unless boosted by parenteral inoculation of vaccine (Taylor *et al.*, 1977; Howard *et al.*, 1977). This may be because an effective antigenic mass is not retained for a sufficient time in the lung.

5. Parenterally killed vaccines, particularly if combined with adjuvant, produce adequate protection. This is primarily a reduction in pneumonia, with a minimal effect on the numbers of organisms growing in lung (Fernald and Clyde, 1970; Mogabgab, 1973). A similar effect can be achieved briefly by inoculation of hyperimmune serum into mice (Taylor and Taylor-Robinson, 1976), cattle (Masiga and Windsor, 1975), and swine (Lam and Switzer, 1971; Goiš *et al.*, 1974).

Most of these studies indicate that a single dose of vaccine, in a form suitable for clinical use, is unlikely to produce lasting immunity to myco-plasma infection. Stimulation of systemic antibodies may prevent clinical manifestations of pneumonia, but additional local stimulation with live or killed organisms may be necessary to evoke resistance to colonization. In view of Taylor and Taylor-Robinson's (1976) observation of the suppression of colonization by systemic antibody, it may nevertheless be feasible to protect against mycoplasma infection with a vaccine prepared from the components of the organism responsible for epithelial cell attachment, such as the P-1 protein of *M. pneumoniae* characterized by Hu *et al.* (1977).

VI. SUMMARY AND CONCLUSIONS

The immune response to mycoplasmas is stimulated by two main classes of antigens: membrane glycolipids and lipid-free proteins. Glycolipid antigens elicit most of the common serological reactions and also serve as receptors for complement-mediated lysis and growth inhibition by antibody. Protein antigens are reactive in eliciting delayed hypersensitivity and macrophage migration inhibition, both examples of cell-mediated immunity.

The biological functions of antigen–antibody reactions *in vivo* are poorly delineated, but two separate categories of activity are suggested by this chapter. The first is the interaction of antibodies with surface antigens of the mycoplasma. These antibodies appear to be secreted locally. Plasma cells in the lamina propria in the lung are the source of secretory IgA, as well as IgG and IgM. Such antibodies probably protect the host by aiding in the clearance of infecting organisms and blocking their deleterious effects on host cells. Included in this category are opsonins, antibodies which fix complement and lyse cell membranes, antitoxins, and antiattachment antibodies. There is solid evidence in support of the biological importance of the first two antibody reactions; confirmation of the latter two should be forthcoming.

The second category of interactions between mycoplasma antigens and host immune factors involves the local immunoinflammatory response to dying organisms and their degradation products. Both humoral and cellular immunity are involved in promoting phagocytosis of infectious debris which accumulates as part of the disease process. Mycoplasmas generally resist phagocytosis until opsonized. As organisms become coated with antibody and complement, leukocytes are attracted to the infected tissue and constitute the bulk of the inflammatory exudate. Macrophages also accumulate locally and appear to become activated. Both antibody and lymphokines derived from T lymphocytes in local lymphoid cellular infiltrates may contribute to macrophage activation. In the lung this immunoinflammatory response seems to comprise most of what is perceived clinically as pneumonia.

In addition to the local immune response to mycoplasmas, systemic humoral and cellular responses can be detected by various serological tests and by assessment of antigen stimulability of lymphocytes *in vitro*. These systemic reactions are peripheral manifestations of the local immune response to mycoplasmas and appear not to be directly responsible for combating the infecting organisms.

Studies based upon ablation of thymus-dependent components of the immune response suggest that the generation of local plasmacyte infiltrates and leukocyte exudates is T-lymphocyte-dependent. In bursectomized chickens, it is apparent that antibody production is essential for the resolution of infection and resistance to subsequent challenge. However, since antibody production is dependent upon T-lymphocyte helper functions, the assumption must be made that both systems must interact to mount an effective defense against mycoplasmas.

Interaction of mycoplasmas with the host immune system is complicated by potential direct effects of the organisms on lymphocytes. Examples of both stimulation and suppression of lymphocyte function have been reported. Most impressive are the *in vitro* and *in vivo* inhibitory effects of *M. arthritidis*, the *in vitro* mitogenic effects of *M. pulmonis*, and reports of human B-cell stimulation and T-cell suppression by *M. pneumoniae*.

Further research on immunological reactions to mycoplasmas promises to yield important information concerning the pathogenesis of mycoplasma disease in a variety of animal species. To the cellular biochemist, the study of interactions between mycoplasmas and the host cell may eventually reveal how cell injury is mediated. To the immunopathologist the separation of host responses into those which are primarily protective and those which are detrimental to the host may provide insight into the pathogenesis of clinical disease syndromes. To the immunologist, further study of the interactions of organisms and lymphocytes, both specific and nonspecific, will be essential to understanding how the host immune response is mediated. To the clinician interested in prophylaxis of mycoplasma infections, both the beneficial and detrimental effects of mycoplasmas and their products on the immune response will have to be considered in the evaluation of future vaccine programs.

REFERENCES

Adler, H. E., Bryant, B. J., Cordy, D. R., Shifrine, M., and DaMassa, A. J. (1973). *J. Infect. Dis.* **127**, Suppl., S61–S66.
Arai, S., Hinuma, Y., Matsumoto, K., and Nakamura, T. (1971). *Jpn. J. Microbiol.* **15**, 509–514.
Barile, M. F., and Leventhal, B. G. (1968). *Nature (London)* **219**, 751–752.
Bergquist, L. M., Lau, B. H. S., and Winter, C. E. (1974). *Infect. Immun.* **9**, 410–415.
Biberfeld, G. (1968). *J. Immunol.* **100**, 338–347.
Biberfeld, G. (1971). *Clin. Exp. Immunol.* **8**, 319–333.
Biberfeld, G. (1973). *J. Immunol.* **110**, 1146–1150.
Biberfeld, G. (1974). *Clin. Exp. Immunol.* **17**, 43–49.
Biberfeld, G., and Gronowicz, E. (1976). *Nature (London)* **261**, 238–239.
Biberfeld, G., and Sterner, G. (1971). *Acta Pathol. Microbiol. Scand.* **79**, 599–605.
Biberfeld, G., and Sterner, G. (1976a). *Scand. J. Infect. Dis.* **8**, 71–73.
Biberfeld, G., and Sterner, G. (1976b). *Infection* **4**, Suppl., S17–S20.
Biberfeld, G., Biberfeld, P., and Sterner, G. (1974). *Clin. Exp. Immunol.* **17**, 29–41.
Bredt, W. (1975). *Infect. Immun.* **12**, 694–695.
Bredt, W., and Bitter-Suermann, D. (1975). *Infect. Immun.* **11**, 497–504.
Brunner, H. (1974). *In* "Les Mycoplasmes de l'Homme, des Animaux, des Vegetaux et des Insectes" (J. M. Bové and J. F. Duplan, eds.), Colloques INSERM, No. 33, pp. 411–420. INSERM, Paris.
Brunner, H., and Chanock, R. M. (1973). *Proc. Soc. Exp. Biol. Med.* **143**, 97–105.
Brunner, H., Razin, S., Kalica, A. R., and Chanock, R. M. (1971). *J. Immunol.* **106**, 907–916.
Brunner, H., James, W. D., Horswood, R. L., and Chanock, R. M. (1972). *J. Immunol.* **108**, 1491–1498.
Brunner, H., Greenberg, H. B., James, W. D., Horswood, R. L., Couch, R. B., and Chanock, R. M. (1973a). *Infect. Immun.* **8**, 612–620.
Brunner, H., James, W. D., Horswood, R. L., and Chanock, R. M. (1973b). *J. Infect. Dis.* **127**, 315–318.
Bryant, B. J., Adler, H. E., Cordy, D. R., Shifrine, M., and DaMassa, A. J. (1973). *Eur. J. Immunol.* **3**, 9–15.
Cantey, J. R., and Hand, W. L. (1974). *J. Clin. Invest.* **54**, 1125–1134.
Cassell, G. H., Lindsey, J. R., and Baker, H. J. (1974). *J. Immunol.* **112**, 124–136.

Clyde, W. A., Jr. (1971). *Infect. Immun.* **4,** 757–763.

Cole, B. C., and Ward, J. R. (1973). *Infect. Immun.* **7,** 691–699.

Cole, B. C., Golightly-Rowland, L., and Ward, J. R. (1975). *Infect. Immun.* **12,** 1083–1092.

Cole, B. C., Overall, J. C., Jr., Lombardi, P. S., and Glasgow, L. A. (1976). *Infect. Immun.* **14,** 88–94.

Cole, B. C., Aldridge, K. E., and Ward, J. R. (1977). *Infect. Immun.* **18,** 393–399.

Collier, A. M., and Clyde, W. A., Jr. (1974). *Am. Rev. Respir. Dis.* **110,** 765–773.

Cooper, M. D., Peterson, R. D. A., South, M. A., and Good, R. A. (1966). *J. Exp. Med.* **123,** 75–102.

Copperman, R., and Morton, H. E. (1966). *Proc. Soc. Exp. Biol. Med.* **123,** 790–795.

Costea, N., Yakulis, V. J., and Heller, P. (1971). *J. Immunol.* **106,** 598–604.

Costea, N., Yakulis, V. J., and Heller, P. (1972). *Proc. Soc. Exp. Biol. Med.* **139,** 476–479.

Couch, R. B., Cate, T. R., and Chanock, R. M. (1964). *J. Am. Med. Assoc.* **187,** 442–447.

Dajani, A. S., Clyde, W. A., Jr., and Denny, F. W. (1965). *J. Exp. Med.* **121,** 1071–1086.

Denny, F. W., Taylor-Robinson, D., and Allison, A. C. (1972). *J. Med. Microbiol.* **5,** 327–336.

Eckner, R. J., Han, T., and Kumar, V. (1974). *Fed. Proc., Fed. Am. Soc. Exp. Biol.* **33,** 769. (Abstr.)

Fernald, G. W. (1969a). *J. Infect. Dis.* **119,** 255–266.

Fernald, G. W. (1969b). *In* "The Secretory Immunologic System" (D. H. Dayton, P. A. Small, Jr., R. M. Chanock, H. E. Kaufman, and T. B. Tomasi, Jr., eds.), pp. 215–227. U.S. Govt. Print. Off., Washington, D.C.

Fernald, G. W. (1972). *Infect. Immun.* **5,** 552–558.

Fernald, G. W. (1973). *J. Infect. Dis.* **127,** Suppl., S55–S58.

Fernald, G. W., and Clyde, W. A., Jr. (1970). *Infect. Immun.* **1,** 559–565.

Fernald, G. W., and Clyde, W. A., Jr. (1974). *In* "Les Mycoplasmes de l'Homme, des Animaux, des Vegetaux et des Insectes" (J. M. Bové and J. F. Duplan, eds.), Colloques INSERM, No. 33, pp. 421–427. INSERM, Paris.

Fernald, G. W., and Clyde, W. A., Jr. (1976). *In* "Immunologic and Infectious Reactions in the Lung" (C. H. Kirkpatrick and H. Y. Reynolds, eds.), pp. 101–129. Dekker, New York.

Fernald, G. W., and Metzgar, R. S. (1971). *J. Immunol.* **107,** 456–463.

Fernald, G. W., Clyde, W. A., Jr., and Denny, F. W. (1967). *J. Immunol.* **98,** 1028–1038.

Fernald, G. W., Clyde, W. A., Jr., and Bienenstock, J. (1972). *J. Immunol.* **108,** 1400–1408.

Fernald, G. W., Collier, A. M., and Clyde, W. A., Jr. (1975). *Pediatrics* **55,** 327–335.

Fernald, G. W., Glyde, W. A., Jr., and Denny, F. W. (1979). *In* "Immunology of Human Infections" (R. Good, ed.). Plenum, New York. (In press.)

Foy, H. M., Nuget, C. G., Kenny, G. E., McMahan, R., and Grayston, J. T. (1971). *J. Am. Med. Assoc.* **216,** 671–672.

Foy, H. M., Ochs, H., Davis, S. D., Kenny, G. E., and Luce, R. R. (1973). *J. Infect. Dis.* **127,** 388–393.

Gabridge, M. G., and Schneider, P. R. (1975). *Infect. Immun.* **11,** 460–465.

Gale, J. L., and Kenny, G. E. (1970). *J. Immunol.* **104,** 1175–1183.

Ginsburg, H., and Nicolet, J. (1973). *Nature (London), New Biol.* **246,** 143–146.

Goiš, M., Kuksa, F., and Franz, J. (1974). *Zentralbl. Veterinaermed.* **21,** 176–187.

Goodwin, R. F. W., Hodgson, R. G., Whittlestone, P., and Woodhams, R. L. (1969). *J. Hyg.* **67,** 193–208.

Gourlay, R. N. (1975). *Dev. Biol. Stand.* **28,** 586–589.

Gourlay, R. N., and Shifrine, M. (1966). *Bull. Epizoot. Dis. Afr.* **14,** 369–372.

Heremans, J. F. (1969). *In* "The Secretory Immunologic System" (D. H. Dayton, P. A.

Small, Jr., R. M. Chanock, H. E. Kaufman, and T. B. Tomasi, Jr., eds.), pp. 309–324. U.S. Gov. Print. Off., Washington, D.C.

Hollingdale, M. R., and Lemcke, R. M. (1969). *J. Hyg.* **67,** 585–602.

Holmgren, N. (1974). *Zentralbl. Veterinaermed.* **21,** 188–201.

Howard, C. J., Taylor, G., Collins, J., and Gourlay, R. N. (1976). *Infect. Immun.* **14,** 11–17.

Howard, C. J., Gourlay, R. N., and Taylor, G. (1977). *Vet. Microb.* **2,** 29–37.

Hu, P. C., Collier, A. M., and Baseman, J. B. (1977). *J. Exp. Med.* **145,** 1328–1343.

Jones, T. C., and Hirsch, J. G. (1971). *J. Exp. Med.* **133,** 231–259.

Jones, T. C., and Yang, L. (1977). *Am. J. Pathol.* **87,** 331–346.

Kahane, I., and Brunner, H. (1977). *Infect. Immun.* **18,** 273–277.

Kaklamanis, E., and Pavlatos, M. (1972). *Immunology* **22,** 695–702.

Kaltreider, H. B. (1976). *Am. Rev. Respir. Dis.* **113,** 347–379.

Kenny, G. E., and Grayston, J. T. (1965). *J. Immunol.* **95,** 19–25.

Kenny, G. E., and Newton, R. M. (1973). *Ann. N.Y. Acad. Sci.* **225,** 54–61.

Lam, K. M., and Switzer, W. P. (1971). *Am. J. Vet. Res.* **32,** 1737–1741.

Leventhal, B. G., Smith, C. B., Carbone, P. P., and Hersh, E. M. (1969). *Proc. Leucocyte Cult. Conf., 3rd,* pp. 519–529.

Lindsey, J. R., Baker, H. J., Overcash, R. G., Cassell, G. H., and Hunt, C. E. (1971). *Am. J. Pathol.* **64,** 675–716.

Martinez-Tello, F. J., Braun, D. G., and Blanc, W. A. (1968). *J. Immunol.* **101,** 989–1003.

Masiga, W. N., and Windsor, R. S. (1975). *Vet. Rec.* **97,** 350–351.

Mizutani, H., and Mizutani, H. (1975a). *Jpn. J. Microbiol.* **19,** 157–162.

Mizutani, H., and Mizutani, H. (1975b). *Am. Rev. Respir. Dis.* **111,** 566–569.

Mizutani, H., Mizutani, H., Kitayama, T., Hayakawa, A., Nagayama, E., Kato, J., Nakamura, K., Tamura, E., and Izuchi, T. (1971). *Lancet* **1,** 186–187.

Mogabgab, W. J. (1973). *Am. Rev. Respir. Dis.* **108,** 899–908.

Mogensen, H. H., Andersen, V., and Lind, K. (1976). *Infection* **4,** Suppl., S21–S24.

Naot, Y., Tully, J. G., and Ginsburg, H. (1977). *Infect. Immun.* **18,** 310–317.

Newhouse, M., Sanchis, J., and Bienenstock, J. (1976). *N. Engl. J. Med.* **295,** 990–998, 1045–1052.

Powell, D. A., and Clyde, W. A., Jr. (1975). *Infect. Immun.* **11,** 540–550.

Powell, D. A., Hu, P. C., Wilson, M., Collier, A. M., and Baseman, J. B. (1976). *Infect. Immun.* **13,** 959–966.

Reynolds, H. Y., Thompson, R. E., and Devlin, H. B. (1974). *J. Clin. Invest.* **53,** 1351–1358.

Roberts, D. H. (1972). *Br. Vet. J.* **128,** 585–590.

Roberts, D. H. (1973). *Br. Vet. J.* **129,** 427–438.

Roberts, D. H., Windsor, R. S., Masiga, W. N., and Kariavu, C. G. (1973). *Infect. Immun.* **8,** 349–354.

Rouse, B. T., and Warner, N. L. (1972). *Nature (London), New Biol.* **236,** 79–80.

Schiefer, H. G., Gerhardt, U., Brunner, H., and Krupe, M. (1974). *J. Bacteriol.* **120,** 81–88.

Sethi, K. K. (1973). *Infection* **1,** 236–240.

Simberkoff, M. S., and Elsbach, P. (1971). *J. Exp. Med.* **134,** 1417–1430.

Simberkoff, M. S., Thorbecke, G. J., and Thomas, L. (1969). *J. Exp. Med.* **129,** 1163–1181.

Singer, S. H., Ford, M., and Kirschstein, R. L. (1972). *Infect. Immun.* **5,** 953–956.

Singer, S. J., and Nicolson, G. L. (1972). *Science* **175,** 720–731.

Smith, C. B., Chanock, R. M., Friedewald, W. T., and Alford, R. H. (1967). *Ann. N.Y. Acad. Sci.* **143,** 471–483.

Smith, P. F., Langworthy, T. A., and Mayberry, W. R. (1973). *Ann. N.Y. Acad. Sci.* **255,** 22–27.

Sobeslavsky, O., Prescott, B., James, W. D., and Chanock, R. M. (1966). *J. Bacteriol.* **91,** 2126–2138.

Sobeslavsky, O., Prescott, B., James, W. D., and Chanock, R. M. (1967). *Ann. N.Y. Acad. Sci.* **143,** 682–690.

Stanbridge, E. (1971). *Bacteriol. Rev.* **35,** 206–227.

Suzuki, M., Hayashi, Y., Arai, S., and Kumagai, K. (1976). *Jpn. J. Microbiol.* **20,** 191–196.

Taylor, G., and Taylor-Robinson, D. (1975). *Dev. Biol. Stand.* **28,** 195–210.

Taylor, G., and Taylor-Robinson, D. (1976). *Immunology* **30,** 611–618.

Taylor, G., Taylor-Robinson, D., and Fernald, G. W. (1974). *J. Med. Microbiol.* **7,** 343–347.

Taylor, G., Howard, C. J., and Gourlay, R. N. (1977). *Infect. Immun.* **16,** 422–431.

Vardaman, T. H., Landreth, K., Whatley, S., Dreesen, L. J., and Glick, B. (1973). *Infect. Immun.* **8,** 674–676.

Waldman, R. H., and Henny, C. S. (1971). *J. Exp. Med.* **134,** 482–494.

Waldman, R. H., Spencer, C. S., and Johnson, J. E., III (1972). *Cell. Immunol.* **3,** 294–300.

Whittlestone, P. (1972). *Ciba Found. Symp. Pathogen. Mycoplasmas* pp. 263–283.

Whittlestone, P. (1976). *Adv. Vet. Sci. Comp. Med.* **20,** 277–307.

Williams, R. C., and Gibbons, R. J. (1972). *Science* **177,** 697–699.

13 / MYCOPLASMA–TISSUE CELL INTERACTIONS

Michael F. Barile

I. INTRODUCTION

The ability to produce disease is the result of interactions between the membrane surface components of a pathogen and of the infected host cell. Pathogenicity and virulence are measures of tissue damage and disease resulting from such interactions. To produce disease, the pathogen must gain entrance, multiply, and resist the defense measures of the host (see Smith, 1977). The first encounter occurs at the portal of entry, where the pathogen must contend with the mucosal surfaces of respiratory tissues. Mycoplasmas initiate infection by attaching to ciliated bronchial tissues; this is followed by cell damage. The small mycoplasma cells can be seen attached to and nestled in crypts of bronchial epithelium surrounded by and hidden under multiple strands of microvilli, appearing inaccessible to and protected from the host defense mechanisms (Bredt, 1976a,b). At-

THE MYCOPLASMAS, VOL. II

tachment by the small membrane-bound mycoplasma parasites can pose special problems to the host. Because of attachment, the immune response must take place in close proximity to the infected cell membrane, with the possibility that the combatant interactions might cause damage to host tissues (Bredt, 1976a,b). Because mycoplasmas bind to sialic acid containing determinants, they may inhibit the normal, physiological function of these receptor sites, resulting in cellular dysfunction (Lloyd, 1975). Attachment and firm adherence anchor the agent and permit it to resist the mechanical flushing action of the moving lumen. Attachment also permits the mycoplasma to release harmful substances, such as hemolysins, and potent proteolytic enzymes, nucleases, and other toxic metabolites in close proximity to the infected cell, thereby disrupting the integrity of the membrane and causing cells to release essential components or interfering with essential functions. The liberation of toxins at the point of attachment is probably responsible for antigenic alterations in red blood cells, resulting in the loss of their antigen-I determinant. Attachment is also responsible for the development of cold (anti-I) agglutinins and plays an important role in the development of agglutinins to lung, brain, and smooth muscle tissues in patients infected with *M. pneumoniae*. In fact, if the cause of primary atypical pneumonia had not been shown to be due to *M. pneumoniae* (Chanock *et al.*, 1962), it would probably be regarded as an autoimmune disease (Thomas, 1969).

Most mycoplasma pathogens are not highly invasive, confine themselves to epithelial surfaces, and produce mild localized infections without penetrating the deeper tissues or disseminating to other organs. In fact, many of the respiratory pathogens can persist for months at the site of infection, even after cessation of clinical disease, without causing any great discomfort to the patient. Another example of quiet coexistence is illustrated by mycoplasma contamination of cell cultures (Barile, 1973a, see also Section III,B,2,a). At times, gross contamination can go unnoticed because some mycoplasma contaminants produce very little effect on the contaminated cell culture. In such cases, contamination can continue undetected for months, even though there may be hundreds more mycoplasmas than tissue cells in culture. In animals, certain potential pathogens, such as *Mycoplasma neurolyticum*, can readily be recovered from apparently healthy mice, and infection is initiated only after the animal has been provoked or stressed by either physical or biological means. In patients, *Mycoplasma pneumoniae* can be isolated from asymptomatic young children or from children with mild or inapparent disease (Brunner *et al.*, 1977; Brunner, 1976; Fernald *et al.*, 1975; see also Clyde, this volume, Chapter 9). Disease occurs in older children and young adults, and occasionally a patient may acquire repeated infection.

These findings suggest that mycoplasmas survive and persist for extended periods of time because they do not provoke the host to produce an intense immunological response. These observations also suggest that repeated exposure is necessary to produce severe mycoplasma disease, supporting the concept that hypersensitivity may play a role in the pathogenesis of primary atypical pneumonia (Biberfeld, 1974, Băizhomartov *et al.*, 1975; see also Fernald, this volume, Chapter 12). Because mycoplasmas usually produce localized diseases of mucosal surfaces with minimal systemic involvement, the humoral antibody titers are frequently low and unremarkable.

Several reports have shown that medium protein components can adsorb to mycoplasma cells during growth (Bradbury and Jordan, 1972; DeVay and Adler, 1976). Wise *et al.* (1978) reported that the interaction between *Mycoplasma hyorhinis* and an infected murine T-lymphoblastoid cell line resulted in the selective acquisition of host cell membrane alloantigen (e.g., Thy-1.1) on the mycoplasma cell. During disease, host cellular components could also adsorb onto mycoplasma cells. A host protein coat could protect the pathogen from host defenses and would also provide a mechanism to explain the development of autoantibodies during mycoplasma disease. Moreover, there is good evidence to suggest that the immune response may play an important role in the pathogenesis of *M. pneumoniae* disease. For example, human volunteers have a more severe disease following immunization with formalin-inactivated vaccine (Smith *et al.*, 1967); and experimentally infected hamsters produce a more severe cellular response, resembling a hypersensitivity reaction, following repeated reinfection with *M. pneumoniae* (Brunner *et al.*, 1976). In addition, Fernald and Clyde (1974) and Taylor *et al.* (1974) showed that the cellular response can be prevented by prior treatment of hamsters with anti-thymocyte antiserum, findings that support active participation of the immune response in the pathogenesis of *M. pneumoniae* infections.

In summation, pathogenicity, virulence, and ability to produce disease are dependent on the outcome of interactions between the mycoplasma pathogen and host tissue cells. A number of *in vitro* procedures are available to examine these mycoplasma–cell interactions and, in fact, most of our information regarding pathogenicity and virulence of *M. pneumoniae* has been derived from the use of cell tissue and organ culture systems (Taylor-Robinson, 1976). Because the target cell for mycoplasmal infection is the ciliated epithelium, tracheal organ culture procedures have been used effectively to examine (1) the course of a localized mucosal infection and the resulting cellular damage; (2) the ability of mycoplasmas to bind to receptor sites on mucosal tissues; (3) the chemical nature of the mycoplasma binding site and the tissue cell receptor site moieties; (4) the relative virulence of mycoplasma strains; (5) the role and function of virulence factors, such as mycoplasma hemolysins (i.e., peroxides) and other enzymatic metabolites in producing ciliary damage, and the effect of mycoplasmas on the metabolism and function of infected tracheal epithelial tissues (see Collier, this volume, Chapter 14). However, while *in vitro* models can provide much information on the course of a localized mucosal infection, one must resort to well controlled *in vivo* animal models to obtain an understanding of the localized, humoral, and cellular immune responses of the host to infectious disease (Brunner, 1976).

II. MYCOPLASMA–TISSUE CELL INTERACTIONS

A. Erythrocytes

1. Hemadsorption

Using a modification (Chanock *et al.*, 1958) of a viral hemagglutination procedure developed initially by Vogel and Shelokov (1957), Berg and Frothingham (1961) first reported the adsorption of guinea pig erythrocytes to monkey kidney cell cultures infected with *Mycoplasma pulmonis*, the causative agent of chronic respiratory disease (CRD) of mice. Hemadsorption was found useful for the serodiagnosis of CRD, and the technique was proposed for the characterization and classification of mycoplasma species. Del Giudice and Pavia (1964) reported that erythrocytes adsorbed to colonies of *M. pneumoniae* but not to the colonies of other human oral mycoplasma species. Convalescent sera of patients with *M. pneumoniae* disease inhibited hemadsorption. They proposed that the procedure be used for the identification of *M. pneumoniae* and for the serodiagnosis of human mycoplasmal disease. Because the hemadsorption inhibition antibody titers produced are generally low, this procedure has not been widely used. However, Grebe (1977) found the hemadsorption inhibition procedure useful as a rapid, specific, suitable field procedure for serodiagnosis of *Mycoplasma gallisepticum* disease.

In an extensive study, Manchee and Taylor-Robinson (1968) reported that a variety of animal erythrocytes adsorbed to colonies of various mycoplasma species, including *Mycoplasma gallisepticum*, *M. gallinarum*, *M. iners*, *M. pulmonis*, *M. canis*, *M. spumans*, *M. agalactiae*, *M. bovis*, and *M. bovigenitalium*, as well as *M. pneumoniae*. Not all strains of a given species hemadsorbed, nor did all strains of hemadsorbing species produce positive reactions with all animal host erythrocytes examined. Hemadsorption has also been used for the characterization of bovine (Jurmanova and Mensik, 1971; Ernø and Stipkovits, 1973), canine (Rosendal, 1973), equine (Kirchhoff *et al.*, 1973), and avian (Sato *et al.*, 1965) mycoplasma species. Whereas simian serotypes of *Ureaplasma* produced positive reactions (Shepard, 1967; see also Volume I, Chapter 17), only one of eight serotypes of human *Ureaplasma urealyticum* hemadsorbed weakly to guinea pig cells (Black, 1973, 1974). Data summarizing the ability of the established *Mycoplasma, Ureaplasma,* and *Acholeplasma* species to hemadsorb were reported recently by Tully and Razin (1977).

Manchee and Taylor-Robinson (1968) reported a lack of correlation between hemadsorption and hemagglutination. Some of the strains and species examined hemadsorbed; others hemagglutinated; some did both, and others did neither. These observations indicate that the mechanisms responsible for hemadsorption and hemagglutination may be different.

The ability to hemadsorb and hemagglutinate has been associated with virulence and pathogenicity, because many pathogenic mycoplasma have these properties, including *M. pneumoniae, M. gallisepticum, M. pulmonis,* and *M. agalactiae* (i.e., particularly the respiratory agents). The evidence obtained thus far indicates that adsorption may be important in initiating disease but that other factors are required to perpetuate the infection. Nonetheless, hemadsorption cannot be considered important in all mycoplasma diseases, because some highly pathogenic mycoplasmas (e.g., *Mycoplasma mycoides* subsp. *mycoides*) do not hemadsorb. In this case, pathogenicity is associated with the ability of *M. mycoides* subsp. *mycoides* to induce a hypersensitivity disease (Gourlay and Shifrine, 1966).

2. Hemagglutination

Van Herick and Eaton (1945) first reported hemagglutination by a strain of mycoplasma isolated from an infected developing chick embryo during passage of the "viral agent" of primary atypical pneumonia. Sera from chickens maintained at the hatchery from which the fertile eggs were obtained inhibited hemagglutination, indicating that the strain was probably an avian mycoplasma contaminant, and consequently they ruled out any relationship with the causative agent of primary atypical pneumonia. Later, Chanock *et al.* (1962) showed that the causative agent was in fact a human species of *Mycoplasma.* The hemagglutination inhibition test has been used extensively for the serodiagnosis of avian mycoplasma diseases, especially *M. gallisepticum* disease (Moore *et al.*, 1960; Adler, 1964), but avian diseases caused by *Mycoplasma synoviae* (Windsor *et al.*, 1975) and *M. meleagridis* (Thornton *et al.*, 1975) have also been diagnosed by this method. Hemagglutination inhibition has not been found useful for the serodiagnosis of bovine pleuropneumonia or of human primary atypical pneumonia. The active hemagglutinating component was closely associated with the mycoplasma cell membrane and was not present in culture supernates following sonication (Manchee and Taylor-Robinson, 1968). Optimal conditions for hemagglutination include a pH of 6.5–7.0, 37°C, and the use of guinea pig cells. The accumulative hemagglutination technique, which requires a combination of two agents (e.g., *M. pneumoniae* with either parainfluenza or measles virus), has been used to increase the titers and sensitivity of the hemagglutination and hemagglutination inhibition procedures (Jacob *et al.*, 1966).

3. Hemolysis

Warren (1942) first reported that some species of mycoplasma hemolyze horse and rabbit erythrocytes, whereas other species do not. Subsequently, hemolysis was used extensively for the characterization of mycoplasmas (Edward, 1950, 1954; Edward and Freundt, 1956), as well as for the presumptive identification of *M. pneumoniae* (Somerson *et al.*, 1963; Clyde, 1963a) and *M. gallisepticum* (Edward and Kanarak, 1959). The hemolysin of *M. pneumoniae* was identified as hydrogen peroxide (Somerson *et al.*, 1965a,b), and its role in the pathogenesis of mycoplasma disease was investigated by several investigators (Cohen and Somerson, 1967; Cole *et al.*, 1968; Cherry and Taylor-Robinson, 1970a,b,c; Manchee and Taylor-Robinson, 1970). Evidence that the hemolysin of *M. pneumoniae* is a peroxide is based on the inhibition of hemolytic activity by catalase or peroxidase and reversal of the enzyme inhibitory effect by the potent catalase inhibitor, 3-amino-1,2,4-triazole (Somerson *et al.*, 1965a,b). The peroxide hemolysins appear to be unique for mycoplasmas, since most of the bacterial hemolysins studied have been shown to be either proteins or lipids. Chanock *et al.* (1963) suggested that the development of cold agglutinins may be due to the host immune response to human erythrocytes which had been antigenically altered by the action of *M. pneumoniae* hemolysin. It is of interest that some of the established respiratory pathogens (i.e., *M. pneumoniae*, *M. mycoides* subsp. *capri*, *M. pulmonis*, and *M. gallisepticum*) produce the largest quantities of peroxide (Cole *et al.*, 1968). It is possible that some mycoplasma (*M. neurolyticum* and *M. bovigenitalium*) hemolysins are not peroxides, because even high concentrations of catalase do not completely suppress hemolytic activity. These nonperoxide hemolysins have not been characterized, however. Using chicken embryo tracheal explants, Cherry and Taylor-Robinson (1970a,b,c) observed that the hemolysin of *M. mycoides* subsp. *capri* inhibited ciliary activity, that catalase protected the cilia from damage, and that catalase inhibitors partially reversed the protective effect of the enzyme. Hydrogen peroxide added without mycoplasmas produced similar ciliary damage, indicating that the peroxide hemolysin plays an important role in the pathogenesis of infected tracheal organ cultures and suggesting that the liberation of hemolysin may also be important in the pathogenesis of natural mycoplasma disease. Whereas the liberation of peroxide is an important virulence factor in *M. mycoides* subsp. *capri* infection, catalase had no effect on ciliary damage produced by *M. gallisepticum,* indicating that a different mechanism is responsible for ciliary damage caused by this agent. Data on the hemolytic activity of the established *Mycoplasma* species have been summarized by Aluotto *et al.* (1970).

Shepard (1967) reported that certain serotypes of human *U. urealyticum* produced a soluble beta-hemolysin, but only small zones of hemolysis were produced. Cherry and Taylor-Robinson (1970c) found that these hemolysins were generally weak, were frequently of the alpha-prime type, and did not lyse human erythrocytes. Catalase inhibited the reaction, suggesting that the hemolysin of *U. urealyticum* was peroxide. With the use of a more sensitive procedure, Black (1974) found that each of the eight human serotypes of *U. urealyticum* examined produced clear, beta-type hemolysis against guinea pig and rabbit cells but not against human erythrocytes. He was unable to confirm earlier findings that the ureaplasma hemolysin was a peroxide, because catalase had no effect on hemolytic activity in his test procedure. Thus further studies are required to establish the nature of the ureaplasma hemolysin (see Shepard and Masover, Volume I, Chapter 17).

Several investigators have observed inhibition of hemolysis of red blood cells surrounding colonies in densely populated cultures of *M. pulmonis* (Fallon and Jackson, 1967), of *Mycoplasma salivarium* (Cole *et al.,* 1968), of *M. pneumoniae* (Lipman and Clyde, 1969), and of certain ureaplasmas (Manchee and Taylor-Robinson, 1970). Cohen and Somerson (1967) reported that *M. pneumoniae* liberates a peroxidase-like enzyme which prevents lysis of the erythrocytes bordering the colonies of *M. pneumoniae.* Wiebull and Hammarberg (1962) failed to detect catalase activity in several mycoplasmas tested.

B. Spermadsorption and Spermagglutination

Mycoplasmas and ureaplasmas can adsorb to and agglutinate human and animal spermatozoa (Taylor-Robinson and Manchee, 1967a; Gnarpe and Friberg, 1973a; Grossgebauer *et al.,* 1977). The ability to adsorb to sperm is dependent on the strain and species of mycoplasma, the age of the culture, the reaction temperature, and on the motility, viability, and animal source of the spermatozoa. There is generally good correlation between spermadsorption and hemadsorption (Taylor-Robinson and Manchee, 1967a). For example, bovine and human sperm adsorb readily to colonies of pathogenic, hemadsorbing species such as *Mycoplasma pneumoniae, M. gallisepticum,* and *M. pulmonis,* but not to the non-pathogenic, nonhemadsorbing species tested, e.g., *M. hominis* and *M. fermentans.* Bovine sperm adsorbed only to the bovine species, *M. bovigenitalium,* and neither human nor bovine sperm adsorbed to *M. agalactiae.* Mycoplasmas have been seen attached to the tails and embedded in the neck and head of sperm. Sperm appeared to be autolyzed at the contact surface interface of mycoplasma colonies. Mycoplasma-induced sperm damage was also reported by Grossgebauer *et al.* (1977). Specific antisera to *M. pneumoniae* and *M. gallisepticum* were shown to inhibit spermadsorption and spermagglutination (Taylor-Robinson and Manchee, 1967a). Busolo *et al.* (1975) used immunofluorescence procedures to demonstrate that *M. hominis* was attached to sperm in specimens of human semen. The presence of mycoplasmas in bull semen has been associated with impaired motility and reduced sperm counts (Jurmanova and Sterbova, 1977).

Some investigators believe that spermadsorption may be associated with the pathogenesis of infertility (Kundsin *et al.,* 1967; Gnarpe and Friberg, 1973a,b; Fowlkes *et al.,* 1975; Grossgebauer *et al.,* 1977). However, Taylor-Robinson *et al.* (1969) showed that ureaplasma-positive bull semen had very high fertilizing capacity and concluded that the ability to spermadsorb, taken alone, was not sufficient evidence to suggest a causative role in infertility. The role of ureaplasma in the pathogenesis of infertility is controversial, and additional data are required before it can be properly resolved.

Another consequence of spermadsorption and mycoplasma colonization of urogenital tissues may be their effects on embryonic development. Klein *et al.* (1969) demonstrated a direct correlation between the colonization of mothers with ureaplasmas and the delivery of babies with low birth weights. Fetal wastage disease was produced in newborn animals by experimentally infecting pregnant mice with *M. pulmonis* (Taylor-Robinson *et al.,* 1974, 1975). Subsequently, Fraser and Taylor-Robinson (1977) reported the effect of *M. pulmonis* on fertilization and preimplantation development in mice using an *in vitro* procedure developed earlier (Fraser and Drury, 1975). They showed that preincubation of mouse sperm with *M. pulmonis* markedly inhibited fertilization, implantation, and embryonic development. The reduced rate of fertilization was probably due to the effect of mycoplasma on the sperm, because the egg is generally considered the passive gamete at this stage. Live suspensions of *M. pulmonis* are required, because nonviable, sonicated, disrupted cells had no deleterious effects. Disintegration of the cell membrane of the embryo was a distinctive feature in the mycoplasma-treated group which also failed to form blastocytes.

C. Phagocytes

Interactions between human peripheral blood leukocytes and *M. pneumoniae, M. gallisepticum,* and *M. neurolyticum* were first reported by Zucker-Franklin *et al.* (1966a,b) using electron microscopy. They showed that an intimate relationship developed between the membrane of the attached mycoplasma and the mammalian cell. Mycoplasmas adhered to and were avidly phagocytosed by neutrophils and eosinophils. Mycoplasmas also adhered to mononuclear leukocytes and to a small percentage of "lymphocytes," findings which may have pathological, as well as immunological, implications. Organick and Lutsky (1968) showed that *M. pneumoniae* was phagocytosed by the alveolar pneumocytes of experimentally infected mice. Jones and Hirsch (1971) reported that *M. pulmonis* cells also attached to the surface of the leukocytes and were phagocytosed and digested within the lysosome vacuoles of the phagocytes. Specific antisera had a marked opsonic effect, suggesting that opsonic antisera probably play an important role in host resistance to mycoplasma disease. *Mycoplasma pulmonis* attachment to host leukocytes could not be blocked by low temperatures, hypertonicity, divalent cations, normal serum, or treating the mycoplasma or macrophages with trypsin, chymotrypsin, neuraminidase, or lysozyme. These findings indicate that attachment does not involve sialic acid receptors or calcium or magnesium -ion bridging (Jones *et al.*, 1972). Phagocytosis was increased by killing the mycoplasmas, by exposing them to proteolytic enzymes, and by adding antimycoplasma IgG, suggesting that *M. pulmonis* may produce a surface protein which blocks ingestion by mouse peritoneal macrophages. However, antiphagocytic proteins do not block attachment to the macrophage surface, conditions which might be comparable to the action of the M protein of *Streptococcus* (Lancefield, 1943) and its role in resisting phagocytosis (Jones and Hirsch, 1971). Howard *et al.* (1976) reported that *Mycoplasma dispar* and *M. bovis* (*M. agalactiae* subsp. *bovis*) were phagocytosed and digested by bovine macrophages in the presence of specific antisera, and that specific antiserum was an absolute requirement for destruction of the mycoplasmas. Jones and colleagues (1977; Jones and Yang, 1977) found that attachment, ingestion, and destruction of *M. pulmonis* by mouse peritoneal macrophages required specific antisera but no complement. Mycoplasma attachment to leukocyte membranes did not increase glucose metabolism via the hexose monophosphate shunt. In summation, mycoplasmas attach to and are ingested and destroyed by macrophages in the presence of specific antisera. Opsonic antisera are important for the destruction of mycoplasmas *in vitro* and are probably important factors in host resistance to mycoplasma disease (see Fernald, this volume, Chapter 12).

D. Adherence to Bacteria

Colonies of *M. hominis* and *U. urealyticum* were observed growing among or developing within colonies of *Neisseria gonorrhoeae* on primary isolation plates inoculated with urogenital specimens (Faur *et al.*, 1975). Electron microscope studies revealed nipplelike projections on the gonococcal cell wall to which the mycoplasmas appeared to be attached. Adherence was firm, because the mycoplasmas were not removed by repeated washings. The significance of these findings remains to be determined.

E. Adherence to Glass and Plastic Surfaces

Mycoplasma pneumoniae was shown to attach to and grow on the surface of glass and plastic containers, producing confluent colony growth (Somerson *et al.*, 1967). Subsequently, many strains (but not all) of various species have been successfully grown on glass and plastic surfaces; these include eight *Mycoplasma* species of human origin (Purcell *et al.*, 1971), as well as *M. gallisepticum, M. pulmonis,* and others. Colony growth is rapid, high yields are produced, and colonies can be washed repeatedly to remove medium components and metabolic by-products without detaching them from the surface. Colonies are removed by scraping the surface with a rubber policeman, treating with trypsin, or shaking with glass beads. Glass-grown colonies have been used to determine the ability of mycoplasmas to hemadsorb, spermadsorb, and cytoadsorb to HeLa cell cultures. There was no correlation between the ability to adsorb to red cells and to adhere to glass (Taylor-Robinson and Manchee, 1967a,b,c). Glass-grown colonies of *M. pneumoniae* have been used to prepare complement fixation antigens, to analyze membrane proteins by acrylamide gel electrophoresis, and to produce vaccines for human use (Somerson *et al.*, 1973; Wenzel *et al.*, 1976).

F. Attachment

1. Terminal Structures

Mycoplasmas have specialized terminal structures which may be responsible for attachment and/or motility. Indeed, three of the respiratory mycoplasma pathogens (i.e., *M. gallisepticum, M. pneumoniae,* and *M. pulmonis*) have been shown to have well-organized terminal structures. *Mycoplasma gallisepticum* has a terminal bleb structure connected by an infrableb region (Maniloff *et al.*, 1965; Maniloff, 1972). Because the terminal bleb of *M. gallisepticum* is generally seen positioned adjacent to the membrane of mammalian macrophages during attachment, Zucker-Franklin *et al.* (1966a,b) suggested that this device may have some sort of binding site. Uppal and Chu (1977) also observed that the terminal bleb of *M. gallisepticum* was generally seen attached to the membranes of ciliated epithelial cells of infected chicken tracheal organ cultures.

Biberfeld and Biberfeld (1970) first noted the appearance of a knoblike structure at the end of *M. pneumoniae* filaments and suggested that this terminal tip structure may be responsible for mycoplasma motility (Bredt, 1968, 1973). Subsequently, Collier (1972) observed that the side or tip of the specialized terminal structure was always seen in close proximity to or attached to host cell membranes and suggested that the tip was important in the attachment of *M. pneumoniae* to the bronchial ciliated epithelium.

Organick *et al.* (1966) showed that *M. pulmonis* attached to the surface of bronchial epithelial cells of infected mice. Subsequently, Richter (1970) illustrated, using electron microscopy, that the terminal structure of *M. pulmonis* was usually seen positioned at the membrane of infected bronchial cells.

It should be noted that these three species (i.e., *M. gallisepticum, M. pneumoniae,* and *M. pulmonis*) have several properties in common. Each is a respiratory pathogen that initiates infection by attaching to ciliated epithelium, each has a specialized terminal structure generally seen in close proximity to or attached to infected cells, and each is motile (Bredt, 1973). Since these mycoplasma species can also cause agglutination of erythrocytes, sperm, and HeLa cells, it is possible that these agents have more than one attachment site. These organisms move forward with the tip end out front. If the terminal tip is the motility apparatus which drives the agent, it could direct and move the pathogen tip-first through the maze of microvilli. Thus the terminal apparatus would be seen attached to membranes of host cells, because it would be the first point of contact between the pathogen and ciliated epithelium.

2. Host Cell Receptor Site

Gesner and Thomas (1966) reported that hemagglutination of turkey erythrocytes by *M. gallisepticum* was inhibited by mucoproteins containing sialic acid (e.g., egg white, ovomucoid, or gastric mucin) and by treatment of erythrocytes with neuraminidase. Treatment of these mucoproteins with neuraminidase reduced or abolished their inhibitory activity. Hemagglutination was inhibited by sialic acid (N-acetylneuraminic acid), was slightly inhibited by L-fucose, N-acetyl-D-galactosamine, and N-acetyl-D-mannosamine, but was not inhibited by simple sugars, D-glucose, D-galactose, D-mannose, or N-acetyl-D-glucosamine. Thus N-acetylneuraminic acid or an amino sugar closely related to sialic acid provides the binding site for M. gallisepticum. Because neuraminic acid receptors are also involved in the attachment of type-3 reoviruses (Gomatos and Tamm, 1962), myxoviruses (Gottschalk, 1958), and polyoma virus (Eddy et al., 1958), the binding site for mycoplasmas appears to be similar to that of viruses. Neuraminic acid has been shown to provide the attachment sites for influenza and parainfluenza viruses (Burnet, 1951). The differences in the cytadsorbability of M. gallisepticum strains indicate the probable existence of a binding gradient, which might reflect possible differences in the pathogenesis of M. gallisepticum strains for birds, analogous to the binding gradient demonstrated for myxoviruses (Burnet et al., 1946; Burnet and Anderson, 1946). Mycoplasma avidity for neuraminic acid receptors could affect firmness of attachment (binding) and the severity of disease. Sobeslavsky et al. (1968) reported that M. pneumoniae attaches to the neuraminic acid receptors of various cells. Manchee and Taylor-Robinson (1969a,b) found at least two types of receptors on HeLa cell cultures involved in mycoplasma attachment; i.e., neuraminic acid was involved with attachment of M. pneumoniae and M. gallisepticum, but neuraminidase had no effect on the adsorption of M. hominis and M. salivarium, implying a site with specificity other than sialic acid. Neuraminic acid has been shown to be present on membranes of HeLa cell cultures (Carubelli and Griffen, 1967).

3. Binding Moiety

Several workers have shown that neuraminic acid is probably involved in the attachment of M. gallisepticum and M. pneumoniae to host tissues, because neuraminidase treatment of the tissue cells inhibits mycoplasma adsorption (Gesner and Thomas, 1966; Manchee and Taylor-Robinson, 1969a,b). They also reported that a protein component of M. gallisepticum and M. pneumoniae membranes was involved in attachment because adsorption was reduced or abolished by treating mycoplasmas with proteolytic enzymes. Exposure of mycoplasma to neuraminidase had no effect. Moreover, treatment of these two mycoplasma species with mild buffered acid solutions at pH 3.8 abolished adsorption, a condition which would permit lipids and carbohydrates to remain unaffected but would produce protein denaturation. Protein participation in attachment was further supported by Powell et al. (1976), who reported that trypsin treatment inhibited M. pneumoniae attachment to ciliated tracheal cells.

Kahane and Brunner (1977) suggested that a glycoprotein in the membranes of *M. pneumoniae* may be involved because attachment to certain lectins was decreased following the proteolytic digestion of mycoplasma membranes. Similar results were obtained using *M. gallisepticum, M. neurolyticum,* and *Spiroplasma citri* (Kahane and Tully, 1976; Schiefer *et al.*, 1974, 1975, 1976). Membrane proteins have also been involved in the attachment of other mycoplasmas; e.g., the role of membrane proteins in the adsorption of *M. hominis* to animal cells was demonstrated by Hollingdale and Manchee (1972). Collier (1972) had shown earlier that virulent *M. pneumoniae* cells attached to the sialic acid receptors of respiratory ciliated epithelium by their tiplike organelle. Hu *et al.* (1977) reported that a protein membrane component of *M. pneumoniae* was responsible for the attachment. When *M. pneumoniae* was treated with proteases, attachment was inhibited and a major protein band in gel electrophoresis was markedly diminished. In summation, it appears that several mycoplasma species, but not all, attach or bind to sialic acid-containing receptor sites and that the attachment moiety is probably a protein.

G. Autoantibodies

1. Heterogenic Antibodies

Patients with primary atypical pneumonia frequently develop a variety of heterogenic antibodies during disease, including cold (anti-I) agglutinins and agglutinins to lung and brain tissues, to *Streptococcus* MG and to Wasserman cardiolipins (see Biberfeld, 1971a). In fact, the presence of cold agglutinins and agglutinins to *Streptococcus* MG was used for the serodiagnosis of primary atypical pneumonia long before the causative agent of this disease was established. The development of agglutinins to lung and brain tissues and to *Streptococcus* MG is due to serological cross-reacting glycolipids present in membranes of *M. pneumoniae, Streptococcus* MG, and host tissue cells (Lemcke *et al.*, 1967; Marmion *et al.*, 1967; Lind, 1968; Lemcke, 1969). However, cold (anti-I) agglutinins are probably produced as a result of antigenic alterations in human erythrocytes, resulting from the interaction between mycoplasmas and host cells (Feizi *et al.*, 1969).

2. Cold (Anti-I) Agglutinins

The presence of cold agglutinins in patients with primary atypical pneumonia was first reported by Peterson *et al.* (1943) and confirmed by many others (Turner *et al.*, 1943; Finland *et al.*, 1945a,b; Mufson *et al.*, 1961; Couch *et al.*, 1964). Cold (anti-I) agglutinins are directed against the antigen-I determinant of erythrocytes (Dacie, 1962; Costea *et al.*, 1966;

Feizi and Taylor-Robinson, 1967). Adsorption of immune sera with patients' erythrocytes did not reduce the antibody titer of *M. pneumoniae,* and adsorption of sera with *M. pneumoniae* had no effect on the cold agglutinin titer (Liu *et al.,* 1959; Biberfeld, 1966; Feizi, 1967). Although there has been some differences in results (Costea *et al.,* 1966), convincing evidence has been obtained to indicate that cold agglutinins are probably not developed because of cross-reacting antigens between *M. pneumoniae* and human red blood cells. Rather, they are the result of antigenic changes in red cells caused by *M. pneumoniae.* However, further data is needed before this question can be resolved. Because *M. pneumoniae* adsorbs and agglutinates erythrocytes and produces a hemolysin, Chanock *et al.* (1963) were the first to postulate that the development of cold agglutinins was due to an antigenic alteration of human red cells by *M. pneumoniae,* producing an autoimmune response. Experimental data have supported this view; i.e., cold agglutinins were developed in rabbits inoculated with human red blood cells that were preincubated with viable *M. pneumoniae* but not with *M. pneumoniae* or red blood cells inoculated alone (Feizi *et al.,* 1969; Lind, 1971). Cold agglutinins can develop in patients with bacterial and also with viral diseases such as influenza and adenovirus infections (Marmion, 1967; Lind *et al.,* 1970).

Whereas normal subjects have antigen-I-positive red blood cells, patients with primary atypical pneumonia lose antigen-I reactivity during disease (Smith *et al.,* 1967). Preincubation of antigen-I-positive red blood cells with suspensions of viable *M. pneumoniae* cells *in vitro* caused a loss in antigen-I reactivity (Schmidt *et al.,* 1965). Barile (1965) postulated that the presence of cold agglutinins, anti-I agglutinins, and antigen-I-negative cells in the same patient could be explained as follows: The antigen-I determinant is enzymically cleaved or altered by *M. pneumoniae* or an agent with similar activity, resulting in I-negative red blood cells. The altered antigen I behaves as a foreign antigen and stimulates the production of anti-I agglutinins. The antigenically altered red blood cells stimulate the production of cold agglutinins.

Increased agglutinin titers to erythrocytes modified by Newcastle disease virus were found in patients with infectious mononucleosis (Burnet and Anderson, 1946) and also in patients with *M. pneumoniae* disease (Aho and Pyhälä, 1974; Pyhälä, 1976). It has been suggested that increased agglutinin titers to virus-modified red blood cells might be due to cross-reacting antibodies evoked by *M. pneumoniae* during disease.

3. Lung and Brain Agglutinins

The development of antibodies to lung tissue antigens in patients with primary atypical pneumonia was first reported by Thomas *et al.* (1943). Some of the sera also reacted with liver, heart, and kidney tissues

(Thomas, 1964). The development of antibodies to brain tissues during *M. pneumoniae* disease was first noted by Biberfeld (1971a,b). Convalescent sera reacted with brain tissue derived from humans, monkeys, rabbits, and mice. Most of the patients (75%) showed a fourfold rise in antibody titer to lung and liver tissue antigens, but the highest titers developed against brain tissue antigens. The tissue agglutinins examined were generally of the IgM class. Adsorption of sera with *M. pneumoniae* glycolipid antigen removed most of the agglutinin activity, indicating that the development of brain and lung agglutinins resulted from cross-reacting glycolipid antigens present in the membranes of *M. pneumoniae* and human tissues (Biberfeld, 1971a,b). Two types of tissue agglutinins developed, i.e., cross-reacting and non-cross-reacting antibodies. Whereas most of the brain agglutinins examined were due to cross-reacting antibodies, the adsorption of some sera with *M. pneumoniae* did not completely remove all the agglutinin activity. The cross-reacting antigens are glycolipids present in the membranes of *M. pneumoniae* and human tissues (Beckman and Kenny, 1968; Plackett *et al.*, 1969; Razin *et al.*, 1970). Agglutinins to brain tissues developed in patients with and without complicating central nervous system involvement (Biberfeld, 1971a,b). Although the function of tissue agglutinins in the pathogenesis of human *M. pneumoniae* disease remains to be determined, it appears that they do not play a major role (Biberfeld, 1971b). Development of agglutinins to human tissues has also been noted in patients with adenovirus pneumonia (Van der Veen and Heyen, 1966).

4. Antibody to Wassermann (Cardiolipin) Antigens

An occasional, transient, false-positive serological reaction for syphilis has been found in cases of cold agglutinin-positive and -negative pneumonias (Florman and Weiss, 1945; Rein and Elsberg, 1944) and in well-documented cases of *M. pneumoniae* disease (Marmion, 1967). The sera from a portion (about 25%) of patients lose antibody activity to cardiolipin following adsorption with *M. pneumoniae* antigens (Biberfeld, 1971b). Whereas brain agglutinins were generally of the IgM class, antibodies to cardiolipins were IgM and IgG.

5. Antibody to Smooth Muscle

Biberfeld and Sterner (1976a) reported that about one-half of the patients infected with *M. pneumoniae* had antibodies (IgM class) to smooth muscle; one-half of these produced rises in antibody titers during the course of disease. Smooth muscle antibodies of the IgG class also developed in one-fourth of the patients, but significant antibody rises were seen in only two cases. Adsorption of sera with *M. pneumoniae* had no effect on the activity of smooth muscle antibody. The development of antibody to smooth muscle tissue also occurs in patients with active chronic hepatitis (Johnson *et al.*, 1965), infectious mononucleosis (Holborow *et al.*, 1973), and cytomegalovirus infections (Ajdukiewicz *et al.*, 1972). Adsorption studies have shown that the smooth muscle antibody (IgG class) occurring in cases of active chronic hepatitis is directed against actin (Gabbiani *et al.*, 1973; Lidman *et al.*, 1976). It is of interest to note that Neimark (1977) reported the presence of an actinlike component in *M. pneumoniae*.

III. MYCOPLASMA–CELL CULTURE INTERACTIONS

A. Effects on Lymphocyte Blast Formation

1. Specific Mitogenic Activity

Nowell (1960) first reported that phytohemagglutinin (PHA) was a nonspecific mitogen that stimulated mitosis and blast formation in lymphocyte cultures *in vitro*. Subsequently, it was shown that specific microbial antigens could also stimulate lymphocyte blast formation, and this procedure has received wide application in the study of lymphocytes from individuals sensitized to specific microbial antigens. Leventhal *et al.* (1968) first demonstrated that *M. pneumoniae* stimulated transformation (blast formation) and mitosis in lymphocyte cultures of patients with primary atypical pneumonia, and these findings were confirmed by others (Biberfeld *et al.*, 1974; Biberfeld and Sterner, 1976b; Morgensen *et al.*, 1976; see also Fernald, this volume, Chapter 12). Exposure of lymphocytes to *M. pneumoniae* and PHA given together stimulated erythrophagocytosis, but PHA or mycoplasmas given alone did not (Leventhal *et al.*, 1968). The mechanism of erythrophagocytosis is not well understood, but it could play an important role in the pathogenesis of mycoplasma disease. We have noted earlier that hemadsorption of *M. pneumoniae* may alter the antigenic surface of the red blood cell, so that it is recognized as a foreign antigen and is ingested. *In vitro* lymphocyte stimulation procedures appear to be sensitive methods for demonstrating cell-mediated immunity to *M. pneumoniae* and may help to provide useful information in establishing the role of cellular immunity in resistance to mycoplasma disease (see Fernald, this volume, Chapter 12).

2. Nonspecific Mitogenic Activity

In vitro lymphocyte blast formation can be stimulated by several nonspecific mitogens such as plant lectins (i.e., PHAs), streptolysin S, lipopolysaccharides, and other substances (Oppenheim, 1968). The non-specific mitogenic activity of various *Mycoplasma* and *Acholeplasma* species was first observed by Ginsburg and Nicolet (1973), Ginsburg (1974), and Naot *et al.* (1977), and confirmed by others (Kirchner *et al.*, 1977; Cole *et al.*, 1977). Murine mycoplasma species (*Mycoplasma pulmonis, M. neurolyticum*, and *M. arthritidis*) were strong mitogens for rat lymphocytes, and the mitogenic activity was strain-dependent. For example, strain Negroni was a potent mitogen, but other strains of *M. pulmonis* had no effect. Moreover, mouse strains (of *M. pulmonis*) activated human lymphocytes (Naot *et al.*, 1977), and mouse lymphocytes were stimulated by mycoplasma species not associated with mice, such as *S. citri, M. synoviae, M. gallisepticum, M. pneumoniae, M. fermentans*, and *Acholeplasma laidlawii*. There was no evidence of antibody activity against these mycoplasma mitogens in the sera of donor mice, indicating the absence of a proven sensitized lymphocyte subpopulation (Cole *et al.*, 1977). The mycoplasma mitogenic component was heat-stable. Biberfeld and Gronowicz (1976) also reported that a human species (*M. pneumoniae*) activated a polyclonal population of mouse B lymphocytes and that the mitogenic component was heat-stable. Because the mitogenic activity of many mycoplasmas is heat-stable, the active component might be an endotoxin-like substance. Some mycoplasmas have lipopolysaccharides which have endotoxin-like activity (Smith *et al.*, 1976). Thus mycoplasmas can induce lymphocytes to produce interferon (Cole *et al.*, 1978) and undergo nonspecific blast formation (Aldridge *et al.*, 1977a,b). Several mycoplasma species were also able to induce cytotoxic responses in normal mouse lymphocytes against allogeneic and syngeneic target cells. The mitogenic activity against normal lymphocytes may provide an explanation for mycoplasma-induced lymphocytotoxicity (Cole *et al.*, 1977). Soluble cytotoxic factors (lymphotoxins) are liberated during blastogenesis of normal lymphocytes in response to mitogens, and mycoplasmas can be mitogenic for normal unsensitized lymphocytes. Thus mitogenicity may be a general property of some mycoplasmas, providing them with a potential mechanism for damaging tissue cells (Cole *et al.*, 1977).

3. Inhibition of Mitogenic Activity by Arginine Depletion

Copperman and Morton (1966) observed that PHA stimulation of lymphocyte cultures could be inhibited by viable and nonviable cultures of *M. hominis* and that the inhibitory effect was reversible. These findings were confirmed by others using *M. arthritidis* (Spitler *et al.*, 1968; Cochrum *et al.*, 1969). Barile and Leventhal (1968) demonstrated that the inhibitory effect was due to depletion of arginine from the medium by the arginine-utilizing mycoplasmas. The lymphocytes were not killed, because changing the culture medium or replenishing it with additional arginine reversed the effect. The fermenting mycoplasmas examined had no effect or stimulated blast formation. Because certain *Mycoplasma* species utilize arginine for energy (Schimke and Barile, 1963a,b), they rapidly deplete and deprive cells of an essential amino acid, causing lymphocyte dysfunction. Simberkoff *et al.* (1969) reported that purified arginine-splitting enzyme (arginine deiminase) recovered from these mycoplasmas produced the same inhibitory effect and that the effect was reversed by enzyme-specific antisera. Because the antisera reversed the inhibitory effect of all arginine-utilizing mycoplasma species tested, they concluded that all arginine deiminase enzymes were closely related or identical. Subsequent studies have shown that there are at least three antigenically distinct arginine deiminase moieties (Weickmann and Fahrney, 1977). The purified enzyme also blocked the response of sensitized lymphocytes to tuberculin, to homograph antigens, and to secondary production of antibody to diphtheria toxoid *in vitro*. Mycoplasma contamination of membrane-associated measles antigens inhibited the ability to demonstrate *in vitro* lymphocyte responsiveness to measles (Ruckdeschel *et al.*, 1975). Mycoplasma infection can also immunosuppress the humoral antibody response of animals to various antigens (Kaklamanis and Pavlotos, 1972; Berquist *et al.*, 1974).

B. Effects on Cell Cultures

1. Mycoplasma Isolation and Propagation

Because primary atypical pneumonia was considered to be a viral disease, the "agent" was first grown in cell cultures and in developing chick embryos (Reimann, 1938; Dingle *et al.*, 1944; Chanock *et al.*, 1960). Using fluorescein-labeled antibody procedures, Liu (1957) first localized the agent on epithelial cells lining the bronchioles and air sacs of the developing chick embryo, and Clyde (1961) first observed the agent attached to the surface of monkey kidney cell cultures. Although Marmion and Goodburn (1961) and Clyde (1961) noted similarities between the agent of primary atypical pneumonia and known pleuropneumonia-like organisms, the causative agent was first grown on artificial medium producing typical mycoplasma colonies and identified as the cause of primary atypical pneumonia by Chanock *et al.* (1962). Cell culture procedures were also used initially to isolate the causative agents of chronic respiratory disease of mice (*M. pulmonis*) (Nelson, 1960) and enzootic pneumonia of swine (*Mycoplasma hyopneumoniae*) (Goodwin and Whittlestone, 1963). Growth of mycoplasmas in cell cultures can be detected by the type of cytopathic effect (CPE) produced (Section III,B,2), by subculture to agar culture medium (Section III,C,6), or by examining infected cell cultures using specific immunofluorescence or nonspecific histological or DNA-fluorochrome staining procedures (Section III,C,7).

2. Morphological Effects

a. Covert infection. Mycoplasma contamination of cell cultures may go unnoticed for several reasons; e.g., even large numbers of mycoplasmas do not produce overt turbid growth commonly associated with bacterial and fungal contamination. Also, cellular changes in some contaminated cultures can be minimal and inapparent, requiring careful microscopic examination, and the morphological changes caused by the depletion of amino acids, sugars, or nucleic acid precursors can be reversed by changing the medium or by replenishing it with fresh nutrients.

b. Cytopathic effects. Collier (1957) isolated a mycoplasma contaminant that produced CPE in a contaminated HeLa cell culture. The CPE was characterized by stunted, abnormal growth and by rounded, degenerated cells with a macroscopic "moth-eaten" appearance at the edge of the culture. O'Malley *et al.* (1961) isolated a cytolytic agent which was identified later as *M. gallisepticum* (O'Malley *et al.*, 1966) that produced a destructive CPE as well as plaque formation in primary rabbit kidney cell cultures. Subsequently, many species of mycoplasmas were shown to produce CPE. To a large extent, the biochemical activity of the mycoplasma contaminant predetermines the nature of the cytopathology (Barile, 1973a). Some mycoplasmas rapidly deplete arginine (Barile *et al.*, 1966b), depriving the cell culture of an essential amino acid (Morgan *et al.*, 1958), which may produce profound effects on cell morphology, cell function, nutrition, virus propagation, and chromosomal aberrations (Kenny and Pollock, 1963; Pollock *et al.*, 1963; Fogh *et al.*, 1971). Miller *et al.* (1971) reported that *Mycoplasma arginini* (Barile *et al.*, 1968) produces cellular lysis in some, but not all, human lymphoblastoid cell cultures and that the addition of arginine to the medium prevents the lytic activity, suggesting that the extent of the lytic activity produced was dependent on the arginine requirement of the contaminated cell cultures.

The most toxic cytolytic agents are mycoplasma fermenters which produce large amounts of acid metabolites from glycolysis, reducing the pH and causing destructive cellular damage. Some fermenters selectively colonize defined areas of the cell culture and produce microcolonies which develop microlesions and small foci of necrosis (e.g., *M. pulmonis*) or form plaques (e.g., *M. gallisepticum*) in an agar overlay system (O'Malley *et al.*, 1966). Microcolonization indicates that specific receptors may be concentrated in defined areas of some cell cultures. However, other fermenting mycoplasmas (e.g., *M. hyorhinis*) attach to every cell, producing a generalized CPE with destruction of the entire monolayer. Because large amounts of acids are produced, the fermenting contaminants (e.g., *Mycoplasma hyorhinis, M. pulmonis, M. capricolum,* and *A. laidlawii*) cause cells to detach from the glass, resulting in a V-shaped destructive CPE in cultures grown in test tubes (Sabin, 1967; Barile, 1973a). The mycoplasma fermenters known to produce CPE include (1) *M. pulmonis* (Nelson, 1960), (2) *M. hyorhinis* (Butler and Leach, 1964; Girardi *et al.,* 1965a; Sabin, 1967; Joncas *et al.,* 1969; Zgorniak-Nowosielska *et al.,* 1967; Hopps *et al.,* 1973), (3) *M. gallisepticum* (O'Malley *et al.,* 1966; Castrejon-Diez *et al.,* 1963; Grumbles *et al.,* 1964), (4) *M. bovigenitalium* (Afshar, 1967), and (5) *A. laidlawii* (Kagan *et al.,* 1969). *Mycoplasma pneumoniae* produces minimal morphological changes in infected cell cultures (Clyde, 1961, 1963b; Marmion and Goodburn, 1961; Chanock *et al.,* 1960), as do certain strains of *M. neurolyticum* and *M. fermentans* (M. F. Barile, unpublished observations).

c. Mistaken identity. Because some mycoplasmas grow readily in cell cultures, producing destructive CPE, some investigators have mistaken cytolytic mycoplasmas for viruses (e.g., Dingle *et al.,* 1944; Van Herick and Eaton, 1945; Grist and Fallon, 1964; O'Malley *et al.,* 1966; Cross *et al.,* 1970). Mycoplasmas share other properties with viruses, such as filterability, hemadsorption, hemagglutination, resistance to certain antibiotics, inhibition by antisera, induction of chromosomal aberrations, and sensitivity to detergents, ether, and chloroform. Consequently, the virologist must be cognizant of mycoplasmas and their properties in order to avoid misinterpretation of data.

3. Nutritional Effects

It has been well established that mycoplasmas can alter the metabolism and function of contaminated cell cultures by depleting the medium of essential nutrients. Attachment permits the mycoplasma to release enzymatic activity directly onto the host cell membrane. The effects of arginine depletion by the arginine-utilizing mycoplasma contaminants on cell cultures include alterations of protein synthesis, cell division and growth, lymphocyte blast formation (Section III,A), and virus propagation (Section III,B,5). Fermenting mycoplasmas rapidly degrade simple sugars to acid metabolites which produce severe CPE and alter cell functions. The specific nutritional requirements of mycoplasmas are discussed in Volume I (see Chapters 3–8). In brief, all mycoplasmas require nucleic acid precursors (free bases, nucleosides, or oligonucleotides) or nucleic acids, and an energy source (either arginine or dextrose, occasionally both). Several genera (e.g., the species of *Mycoplasma* and *Urea-*

plasma) require sterols (such as cholesterol), and others may require fatty acids or other lipids (see Razin, 1978). Because mycoplasmas have an absolute requirement for these substrates, contaminants can rapidly utilize and deplete the medium of these substances, depriving the infected cultures of essential nutrients and producing profound effects on cell metabolism and function. It has been well established that myco-plasmas can compete effectively for nucleic acid precursors and drasti-cally alter nucleic acid synthesis of contaminated cell cultures (Hakala *et al.*, 1963; Nardone *et al.*, 1965; Holland *et al.*, 1967; Levine *et al.*, 1968; Harley *et al.*, 1970; Perez *et al.*, 1972). As a consequence, the available pyrimidines are incorporated into mycoplasmal RNA rather than host cell RNA. Nuclease activity has been detected in broth cultures of myco-plasmas (Neimark, 1964; Pollack *et al.*, 1965; Huppert *et al.*, 1974), and mycoplasmal DNA polymerases have been purified, partially charac-terized (Mills *et al.*, 1977), and distinguished from cytomegalovirus-induced and tissue cell polymerases (Miller and Rapp, 1976). Mycoplasma contamination can also affect pyruvate dehydrogenase activity in cultured fibroblasts (Clark *et al.*, 1978).

4. Effects on Chromosomal Aberrations

The ability of mycoplasmas to interfere with normal cell division and cause chromosomal aberrations was reported independently by Paton *et al.* (1965) and Fogh and Fogh (1965) and confirmed by many others. Disturbances in chromosomal patterns have been observed (1) in human amnion cell cultures infected with an unspeciated mycoplasma (Fogh and Fogh, 1965), (2) in human diploid WI-38 cells infected with *Mycoplasma orale* (Paton *et al.*, 1965), with *M. hominis* (Paton *et al.*, 1967), and also with *A. laidlawii, M. hyorhinis,* and *M. pulmonis* (Stanbridge *et al.*, 1969), (3) in hamster fibroblasts infected with *M. salivarium* (MacPherson and Russell, 1966), (4) in human lymphocyte cultures infected with *M. salivarium, M. fermentans,* and *M. arthritidis* (*M. hominis* type 2) (Aula and Nichols, 1967) and with ureaplasmas (Kundsin *et al.*, 1971). The most common aberrations are chromosomal breakage, multiple translocation, reduction in chromosome number, and the appearance of new chromo-some varieties. Liao (1976) reported that infection with *M. hominis* caused a cell culture line (TT-1) to form two new additional chromo-somes. Because histones (the protein portion of nucleoproteins) are rich in arginine, Aula and Nichols (1967) postulated that chromosomal dis-turbances were due to inhibition of histone synthesis resulting from ar-ginine depletion. Freed and Schatz (1969) reported that mitosis was inhib-ited in arginine-deprived Chinese hamster cell cultures, supporting the concept that inhibition of histone synthesis may lead to disturbances in chromosomal replication. Because fermenting mycoplasmas and urea-plasmas (neither of which utilize arginine for energy) can also induce chromosomal aberrations, other mechanisms must be involved. Stan-bridge *et al.* (1969) reported that chromosomal damage could also be due to competition for nucleic acid precursors or to degradation of host cell DNA by mycoplasma nucleases (Paton and Allison, 1970; Stanbridge *et al.*, 1971). They showed that the addition of exogenously supplied DNAs increased chromosomal breaks in cultured cells. Mycoplasmas are known to have endonucleases (Neimark, 1964; Pollack *et al.*, 1965), and myco-plasma DNAs have been isolated from contaminated cell cultures by Stock and Gentry (1969). Thus both arginine-utilizing and fermenting myco-plasmas, ureaplasmas, and *A. laidlawii* have been shown to induce chromosomal aberrations *in vitro*. Although the implications of these findings remain to be determined, attempts to induce tumor formation with mycoplasmas have been universally unsuccessful using techniques involv-ing either newborn hamsters (Girardi *et al.*, 1965b) or the cheek pouch of cortisonized weanling hamsters (Fogh and Fogh, 1967). However, myco-plasmas can inhibit transformation of cell cultures by known onco-genic viruses. For example, *M. orale* can suppress multiplication of Rous sarcoma and Rous-associated viruses in chick embryo fibroblasts (Somerson and Cook, 1965) and can reduce the number of foci in simian SV40 and polyoma-infected cell cultures (Fogh, 1970; Fogh *et al.*, 1971). Arginine-utilizing mycoplasmas can also suppress growth of certain on-cogenic DNA viruses, e.g., adenoviruses (Section B,5).

5. Effects on Virus Propagation

While some mycoplasmas have no detectable effect, others can either increase or decrease virus yields *in vitro,* or they can alter the course of viral infections in animals. The effect produced depends on the strain and species of mycoplasma, the virus, and the cell culture substrate used. At least two mechanisms have been established for decreasing viral yields: (1) arginine-utilizing mycoplasmas decrease titers of arginine-requiring DNA viruses by depleting arginine from the medium, and (2) cytolytic mycoplasmas produce severe CPE, resulting in an unsuitable cell sub-strate for virus propagation. Mycoplasmas increase virus yields by inhibit-ing interferon induction and interferon activity (Barile, 1973a, 1977, 1978; Singer *et al.*, 1973).

a. Decreased virus yields. Rouse *et al.* (1963) reported decreased yields of adenovirus type 2 in human KB cell cultures contaminated with myco-plasmas. Changing the medium or replenishing it with additional arginine reversed the effect, and they concluded that decreased viral yields were due to arginine depletion by arginine-utilizing mycoplasmas. These findings were confirmed by Hargreaves and Leach (1970). Subsequently, mycoplasma contamination was shown to reduce titers of other arginine-requiring DNA viruses, such as *Herpes simplex* virus (Manischewitz *et al.*, 1975), vaccinia virus (Singer *et al.*, 1970), and simian SV40 virus (Fogh, 1970). Therefore it seems reasonable to conclude that arginine-utilizing mycoplasmas probably affect replication of other arginine-requiring viruses, i.e., adenovirus type 1 (Dubes *et al.*, 1969), adenovirus type 5 (Russell and Becker, 1968), polyoma virus (Winters and Consigli, 1971), and human and simian cytomegaloviruses (Minamishima and Benyesh-Melnick, 1969). Arginine was not required during the early stages of replication, including viral DNA synthesis, but was essential for the synthesis of late protein coat and the production of mature infectious adenovirus type-2 virion (viral progeny) (Rouse and Schlesinger, 1967). The arginine requirement for adenovirus type 5 was associated with the production of T protein, an antigen which is produced by oncogenic adenoviruses (Becker *et al.*, 1967; Russell and Becker, 1968). Control of the arginine level in virus infections may be important in determining whether the infection proceeds to (1) a lytic state (containing the arginine-rich late protein coat and the production of mature virus) or to (2) an abortive infection, either a latent viral infection or transformation and tumorigenesis, as seen with certain oncogenic adenoviruses. Although Tankersley (1964) first showed that arginine was essential for the replication of *H. simplex* virus, Becker *et al.* (1967) demonstrated that arginine was required for the synthesis of viral coat protein, i.e., similar to that described for adenoviruses. Goldblum *et al.* (1968) found that arginine was also required for the synthesis of coat protein for simian SV40 virus. Thus arginine-utilizing mycoplasmas can reduce titers of adenoviruses, herpesviruses, and papovaviruses by rapidly degrading and depleting arginine from the medium. Mycoplasma infection of cell cultures may provide a simple, useful procedure for establishing the arginine requirement of viruses (Barile, 1973a).

Butler and Leach (1964) reported decreased yields of measles virus in a human HEp-2 cell culture contaminated with a cytolytic, acid-producing mycoplasma identified later as *M. hyorhinis*. Decreased virus yields were due to the damaging CPE by the contaminant. Romano and Brancato (1970) reported reduced measles virus titers in cell cultures contaminated with the arginine-utilizing mycoplasma, *M. hominis*, and the restoration of virus growth by the addition of arginine. These findings demonstrate that measles virus titers can be reduced by more than one mechanism. The growth of Mengo encephalitis virus was also reduced in mycoplasma-infected mouse fibroblast cell cultures (Brownstein and

Graham, 1961). Kagan *et al.* (1967) reported that a variety of mycoplasma contaminants inhibited the growth of various RNA viruses, including eastern equine encephalitis virus, Venezuelan equine encephalitis
virus, and Newcastle disease virus.

b. Increased virus yields. Singer *et al.* (1969a,b) showed that *M. arginini*
and *M. hyorhinis* inhibited interferon production, interferon activity, and
cell resistance, resulting in increased yields of Semliki Forest virus.
Mycoplasmas inhibited interferon activity induced either by a virus (e.g.,
vesicular stomatitis virus) or by synthetic RNA copolymers (e.g.,
polyinosinic and polycytidylic acids). Mycoplasma contamination can
also render cell cultures less sensitive to exogenously supplied interferon,
and consequently contamination can affect the results of a standard interferon assay. To illustrate this activity, the mycoplasma–virus–cell
culture system must be properly standardized, because results can be
influenced by several factors. (1) Virus enhancement is only seen with low
virus input, which infects only a small number of cells, leaving most of the
cultured cells available to accept the interferon generated and to develop
cell resistance to viral infection. With high virus input, most of the cells
are infected initially, and consequently the inhibitory mycoplasma effect
can only be demonstrated by assay, i.e., by comparing the levels of
interferon produced. (2) The effect on virus titers cannot be demonstrated
in an agar overlay system, because interferon is not able to disseminate to
target cells as readily in an agar overlay. (3) The same number of cells
must be used in the mycoplasma-free and mycoplasma-infected cell cultures. (4) The same mycoplasma species may have several properties,
each of which may affect the cell culture in quite a different manner; e.g.,
M. hyorhinis can produce CPE and reduce virus yields, or it can inhibit
interferon and increase virus yields. Mycoplasma infection can conceivably be used to advantage; e.g., decreased interferon induction and activity
by mycoplasmas might be exploited to increase titers of latent viruses
(Barile, 1973a).

Mycoplasmas have been shown to alter the course of viral infections in
organ culture explants and in animals (see this volume, Chapter 1). Reed
(1971, 1972) reported that dual infection produced greater destruction of
the ciliated epithelium than either *M. hyorhinis* or swine influenza virus
given alone. *Mycoplasma gallisepticum* infection of pullets caused a dim-
inution of symptoms in Marek's disease (Katzen *et al.*, 1969) but increased the severity of Newcastle disease (Heishman *et al.*, 1969; Ranck
et al., 1970). Influenza A infections were enhanced in ducks infected with
Mycoplasma anatis (Roberts, 1964), in chickens infected with *M.
gallisepticum* (Berry, 1969), and in mice experimentally infected with *M.
pneumoniae* (Nakamura and Sakamoto, 1969). Swine adenovirus infection

was also enhanced in gnotobiotic pigs infected with *M. hyopneumoniae* (Kasza *et al.*, 1969).

6. Effect on Interferon

Mycoplasmas have been shown to depress, enhance, or have no effect on interferon induction and activity. The effect is dependent on the preparation of the mycoplasma (i.e., viable or nonviable cells) and whether an *in vitro* cell culture or animal assay system is used. Attempts to induce interferon in monolayer cell culture systems with a variety of mycoplasmas have been generally unsuccessful (Armstrong and Paucker, 1966; Yershov and Zhdanov, 1965; Singer *et al.*, 1969a,b). However, Smirnova and Kagan (1971) reported that preinfecting chick embryo fibroblast cultures with a variety of mycoplasmas 24 hr prior to virus infection increased interferon production fourfold, whereas interferon titers were markedly decreased in cell cultures chronically infected with mycoplasmas. This preinfection phenomenon resembles increased interferon activity following pretreatment of cell cultures with inactivated viruses before challenge with live virus, resulting in a synergistic effect (Mandy and Ho, 1964). Although attempts to produce interferon in monolayer cell cultures have failed, Rinaldo *et al.* (1973, 1974) reported that a variety of mycoplasmas induced interferon in ovine leukocyte cultures. Interferon activity can also be induced in animals inoculated with mycoplasmas. Fauconnier and Wroblewski (1974) reported that mice inoculated with a strain of *Acholeplasma* were protected against infection with Semliki Forest virus and that resistance to infection was mediated presumably by the induction of interferon. Most *Acholeplasma* species have been shown to have lipopolysaccharides with endotoxin-like activities (Smith *et al.*, 1976), which are known to induce interferon in mice. Some species (*M. arthritidis, M. pneumoniae,* and *A. laidlawii*) induced an earlier response in mice (6 hr after inoculation), while other species (*M. pulmonis* and an unspeciated species of *Acholeplasma*) produced a delayed response (Rinaldo *et al.*, 1974). Prior exposure of mice to viable and to nonviable, sonicated preparations of *M. arthritidis, M. pulmonis,* and *A. laidlawii* suppressed the interferon response to Newcastle disease virus, suggesting that prior experience with mycoplasmas can alter virus–host relationships in infected mice (Cole *et al.*, 1978).

Mycoplasmas can inhibit the induction of interferon produced by a virus (Semliki Forest virus) or synthetic RNA complexes (polyinosinic and polycyticylic acids) in monolayer cell culture systems. Mycoplasmas can also inhibit the activity of exogenously supplied interferon. Consequently, mycoplasma infections can drastically affect the results of a standard cell culture interferon assay (Singer *et al.*, 1969a,b, 1973).

C. Cell Culture Contamination

1. Incidence

Robinson *et al.* (1956) reported the first isolation of a mycoplasma from a contaminated HeLa cell culture. Subsequently, mycoplasmas have been established as common and bothersome contaminants capable of altering the activities and functions of cells and affecting the results of studies in laboratories throughout the world (Pollock *et al.*, 1960; Barile *et al.*, 1962; Herderscheê *et al.*, 1963; Rakovskaya and Neustroeva, 1967; MacPherson, 1966; Ogata and Koshimizu, 1967; Meloni *et al.*, 1969; Sethi, 1972; Kaluzewski and Jagielski, 1972). It has been well established that primary cell cultures are rarely contaminated (0–4%) and that continuous cell culture lines are frequently contaminated (50–95%). Original tissues used to prepare primary cell cultures are not a major source of contamination, and most contamination comes from outside sources (see Section III,C,3; see also Barile, 1968, 1973a, 1977; Fogh *et al.*, 1971; Ludovici and Holmgren, 1973). Because contamination comes from outside sources, the highest incidence is generally found in laboratories using large volumes of cell cultures and large numbers of containers, conditions which subject cells to greater risks. Cells in high passage are at greater risk and are more frequently contaminated (Barile *et al.*, 1962; Barile, 1973a). Because mycoplasmas colonize the oropharyngeal and urogenital tissues and are commonly recovered from neoplastic tissues of humans and animals (Barile, 1967), primary cell cultures prepared from colonized, infected, or neoplastic tissues have a greater risk and incidence of contamination. Cell cultures derived from all tissues, organs, and animals examined were found subject to contamination, including cultures derived from mammalian, avian, reptilian, fish, insect, and plant origin. All types of cell cultures are susceptible, including primary or continuous cultures, fibroblastic, epithelial, or lymphocytic cultures, diploid or heteroploid cells, and cultures grown in suspension or monolayer. Mycoplasma titers in contaminated cell cultures generally range from 10^4 to 10^9 colony-forming units (CFU)/ml of medium fluid. Some mycoplasma contaminants (e.g., *M. hyorhinis*, and *M. fermentans*) are avid cytadsorbing agents, and we have observed as many as 1000 mycoplasmal cells attached to 1 contaminated or infected cell in culture. Other contaminants are poor cytadsorbing agents and are found primarily in medium fluids. Consequently, procedures for establishing the mycoplasma titers of cytadsorbing agents are best estimated by examining infected cell cultures using specific immunofluorescence or nonspecific DNA-fluorochrome staining procedures (Section III,C,7). Populations of noncytadsorbing contaminants are best determined by dilution–colony count procedures.

2. Prevalence

Table I summarizes data collected primarily by Del Giudice in our collaborative efforts to establish the incidence and prevalence of mycoplasmas in contaminated cultures (Barile *et al.*, 1973, 1978; Del Giudice and Hopps, 1978). Approximately 2800 contaminants were isolated and identified from over 17,000 cell cultures examined during a 13-year study; 8% of the cultures had mixed contamination with two or more mycoplasma species. Several cell cultures were contaminated with three species, i.e., *M. arginini, M. orale,* and *M. hyorhinis.* Most of the contaminants (99%) were either bovine, human, or swine species of mycoplasmas.

The bovine mycoplasma species are the most frequent contaminants of cell cultures: 1262 bovine strains (45%) were isolated, representing at least 7 distinct bovine mycoplasma species, i.e., *M. arginini, M. bovis, M. bovoculi, Mycoplasma* sp. serogroup HRC 70-159, *Acholeplasma laidlawii, A. axanthum,* and 60 unspeciated strains of *Acholeplasma.* The major source of bovine mycoplasma contamination of cell cultures is contaminated commercial bovine sera (Barile and Kern, 1971) (Table II).

The second major group of contaminants consists of the human oral species of mycoplasmas; 929 strains (33%) were isolated and identified as *Mycoplasma orale, M. hominis, M. salivarium, M. fermentans,* or *M. buccale* (Table I). The most common mycoplasma species isolated throughout these studies was *M. orale*; a total of 832 (30%) strains were isolated from contaminated cell cultures.

The third major group of contaminants were the swine mycoplasmas; 590 strains (21%) of *M. hyorhinis* were isolated. Hopps *et al.* (1973) reported the isolation of a "noncultivable" strain of *M. hyorhinis* that failed to grow readily on standardized broth or agar medium and could only be identified by staining the contaminated cell cultures with specific fluorescein-conjugated antisera. Recently, Del Giudice and Hopps (1978) showed that the majority (70%) of the *M. hyorhinis* strains were noncultivable, i.e., did not grow on artificial medium, indicating that a cell culture procedure must be included in tests for detecting mycoplasma contaminants (Barile *et al.*, 1973, 1978). Failure to isolate mycoplasmas from contaminated cell cultures by the use of direct agar culture procedures has been reported by others (Zgorniak-Nowosielska *et al.*, 1967; House and Waddell, 1967; Stanbridge, 1971; Schneider and Stanbridge, 1975a,b).

Data summarizing mycoplasma contamination of primary cell cultures are presented in Table III (Barile *et al.*, 1973, 1978; Barile, 1973a, 1977; Del Giudice and Hopps, 1978). Of 3200 lots examined, 51 mycoplasmas, about 1%, were isolated from 42 contaminated primary cell culture lots.

TABLE I. Mycoplasma Contamination of Cell Cultures[a]

Source and species	Natural habitat	Number of isolations	Percent
Bovine			
M. arginini[b]	Oropharyngeal, urogenital	739	26.0
A. laidlawii[c]	Oropharyngeal, urogenital	240	8.5
Mycoplasma strain HRC 70-159	Cell cultures only	197	7.0
Acholeplasma sp. (unspeciated)	Presumably bovine	60	2.1
M. bovis	Oropharyngeal, joints, udder	23	0.8
A. axanthum[d]	Nasal, oropharyngeal	2	0.07
M. bovoculi	Conjunctival	1 1262	0.03 45.1
Human and primate			
M. orale	Oropharyngeal	832	29.5
M. hominis	Oropharyngeal	63	2.2
M. fermentans	Urogenital	28	1.0
M. salivarium	Oropharyngeal	4	0.14
M. buccale	Human oral (rare), monkey oral (common)	2 929	0.07 33.2
Swine			
M. hyorhinis	Nasal	590	21.0
A. oculi[e]	Conjunctival	1 591	0.03 21.1
Murine			
M. arthritidis	Rat tissues	5	0.36
M. pulmonis	Mouse and rat oropharyngeal	4 9	0.29 0.3
Avian (chickens and turkeys)			
M. gallisepticum	Oropharyngeal	3	0.21
M. gallinarum	Oropharyngeal	2 5	0.14 0.2

Canine				
M. canis		Oropharyngeal, genital	1	0.07
Mycoplasma sp. serogroup HRC 689		Urogenital	2	0.14
Total			$\dfrac{3}{2279}$	$\dfrac{0.1}{100}$

[a] From Barile et al. (1973a, 1978) and Barile (1973, 1977).
[b] Also isolated from sheep, goats, chamois, swine, and wild cats.
[c] Also isolated from avian, caprine, canine, equine, feline, murine, ovine, porcine, primates (including humans, rare) and plant tissues.
[d] Also from swine and equine tissues.
[e] Also from caprine and equine tissues.

454   Michael F. Barile

TABLE II. **Mycoplasma Contamination of Commercial Bovine Sera: Identification and Speciation**[a]

Species	Natural habitat	Number of isolations	Percent
M. arginini	Bovine: oropharyngeal, urogenital	65	33.7
M. alkalescens	Bovine: nasal	6	3.1
M. bovis	Bovine: oropharyngeal, joints, udder	5	2.6
M. bovoculi	Bovine: conjunctival	3	1.6
Mycoplasma sp. HRC 70-159[b]	Cell cultures only	3	1.6
M. hyorhinis	Swine: nasal	1	0.5
A. laidlawii	Bovine: oropharyngeal, urogenital	87	45.1
A. axanthum	Bovine: nasal, oropharyngeal	1	0.5
Acholeplasma sp.	Presumably bovine	22	11.4
Total		193	100.1

[a] From Barile and Kern (1971) and Barile and Del Giudice (1972).
[b] Distinct unspeciated serotypes unrelated to established species.

Mycoplasmas were isolated from cell culture lots prepared from (1) monkey kidney *(M. arginini, M. orale, M. hominis, M. buccale, A. laidlawii)*, (2) rabbit kidney *(M. orale, M. arthritidis, M. fermentans, M. hominis, A. laidlawii)*, (3) mouse embryo *(M. arginini, M. canis, Mycoplasma* sp. serogroup HRC689), (4) rat embryo *(M. pulmonis)*, and (5) chicken embryo cell cultures *(M. gallisepticum)*. Because the murine *(M. arthritidis, M. pulmonis)*, avian *(M. gallisepticum)*, canine *(M. canis, Mycoplasma* sp. strain HRC689), and monkey *(M. buccale)* contaminants were isolated only from primary cell culture lots derived from homologous murine, avian, canine, or monkey tissues, and because these same species are rarely found in contaminated continuous, heterologous cell culture lots, the probable source of these contaminants was the original organs used to prepare the primary cell culture.

3. Sources of Contamination

Barile and Kern (1971) reported that commercially prepared lots of bovine sera were frequently contaminated and that contaminated bovine serum was the major source of bovine mycoplasma contamination of cell cultures. Mycoplasma contaminants were isolated from 285 of 888 lots of either raw, unprocessed sera obtained from abattoir suppliers or from final lots of sera produced by the manufacturer for market. Successful isolations were made only with the large-specimen-volume broth culture medium procedure (Barile and Kern, 1971). The contaminants of bovine sera were similar or identical to the bovine mycoplasma species isolated

TABLE III. **Identification of Mycoplasmas Isolated from Contaminated Primary Cell Cultures**[a]

Primary cell culture	Number of lots contaminated[b]	Species identified[c]
Rabbit kidney	12[d]	M. orale (7), M. arthritidis (5), M. fermentans (2), A. laidlawii (2), M. hominis (1)
Monkey kidney	11[d]	M. arginini (5), M. orale (4), A. laidlawii (2), M. hominis (2), M. buccale (2)
Mouse embryo	9	M. hyorhinis (9)
Dog kidney	5	M. arginini (2), canine Mycoplasma serogroup HRC689 (2), M. canis (1)
Rat embryo	4	M. pulmonis (4)
Chick embryo	1	M. gallisepticum (1)
Total	42	51

[a] From Barile et al. (1973, 1978) and Barile (1973a, 1977).
[b] Approximately 3200 primary cell culture lots were examined.
[c] Number of strains isolated is given in parentheses.
[d] Five primary rabbit kidney and four primary monkey kidney cell cultures were contaminated with two mycoplasma species.

from contaminated cell cultures. At least eight distinct bovine mycoplasma species were isolated (Table II). In addition, one swine strain of *M. hyorhinis* was also isolated from one lot of contaminated serum, suggesting that bovine serum may also be a source of swine mycoplasma contamination of cell cultures. Final lots of sera from all commercial suppliers tested were found to be contaminated on one or more occasions. This high incidence of contamination was due primarily to the nonsterile, poor quality control conditions used for the collection of blood and the processing of serum at the abattoir. Blood obtained using sterile cardiac puncture and sera processed with good quality control procedures were found to be free of mycoplasmal contamination. Because the mucosal tissues of cattle are frequently colonized with mycoplasmas, the probable source of contamination is contaminated oropharyngeal, urogenital, and intestinal secretions which contaminate the blood and/or serum during harvest and manufacture. Commercially prepared serum is filter-sterilized using high-pressure filtration through filter packs containing a final filter of 220 nm. Filtration drastically reduces the amount of contamination but does not necessarily eliminate every mycoplasma cell. High-pressure filtration has been shown to force the pliable mycoplasma cell through a bacteria-retaining filter pack. Consequently, contaminated final lots of sera contain only very small numbers of mycoplasma contaminants. Because cell cultures are exquisitely sensitive for the growth of mycoplasmas, low orders of serum contaminants can reach high titers in cell cultures within a few days. Although the sterilization of sera poses difficult technical problems for the industry, it is relatively easy to filter-sterilize small (100-ml) volumes of sera for laboratory use, because high-pressure filtration can be avoided.

The original source of human oral mycoplasma contamination is laboratory personnel. However, the use of poor or inadequate quality control procedures is a major factor in the spread of human oral mycoplasma contamination; i.e., contaminated cells can cross-contaminate other cell cultures maintained in the same laboratory. Mouth pipetting is still a major vehicle of human oral mycoplasma contamination. Antibiotics present in medium destroy bacterial contaminants but permit mycoplasmas to grow unimpeded. Antibiotics tend to mask mycoplasma contamination and should be avoided.

Although the source of swine mycoplasma contamination is not established, trypsin and contaminated bovine serum have been incriminated as the possible culprits. Because swine and cattle are processed at the same abattoir, it is possible that bovine sera may become contaminated with swine mycoplasmas during collection and manufacture. However, attempts to grow mycoplasmas from commercial trypsin have failed, and only one strain of *M. hyorhinis* has been isolated from one lot of contaminated bovine serum.

The source of murine, avian, and canine mycoplasma contamination is probably contaminated organs used to establish primary cell culture lines (Barile *et al.*, 1973). In addition, contamination can be disseminated by using contaminated equipment, glassware, and other materials required in the preparation or maintenance of cell cultures. Virus suspensions have been found to be contaminated, and occasionally antiserum and other reagents used in cell culture studies have been contaminated [e.g., one lot of a commercially prepared, dry tissue culture powder medium (Low, 1974]. In sum, the initial sources of contamination (the original sin) are of human, bovine, and swine origin, but contamination can spread from cell to cell by contaminated cell cultures, virus pools, antisera, other reagents, and equipment commonly used in the preparation of cell cultures.

4. Prevention of Mycoplasma Contamination

The preventive measures used successfully are designed to control the sources and the spread of contamination (Coriell, 1962; Coriell and McGarrity, 1968; McGarrity, 1976; McGarrity *et al.*, 1978; Barile, 1973a,b, 1977, 1978). The major vehicles of spread are aerosols (O'Connell *et al.*, 1964), contaminated equipment and environment (McGarrity *et al.*, 1978), or contaminated reagents such as serum or antiserum (Barile and Kern, 1971). Several measures can be used effectively to reduce the risk and prevent the spread of contamination. Primary cell cultures should be used whenever feasible, since they are rarely contaminated. Mouth pipetting, which provides a vehicle for human oral mycoplasma contamination, should be avoided. Rigid sterile procedures must be employed. Commercial bovine serum should be treated to remove or inactivate potential contaminants by heating in small volumes (100 ml) at 56°C for 45 min, filtering twice through a 220-nm filter without the use of excess pressure, and/or adding the serum to medium and then filtering the complete medium twice through a 220-nm filter. The prepared working stock solution of trypsin should be filtered through a 100-nm filter twice, and whenever feasible a trypsin substitute should be used. Absolute Cambridge-type filters may be used to monitor and filter-sterilize the affluent and effluent air servicing the working area. Utilize laminar-flow hoods, decontaminate the working area daily and the room weekly with phenolic detergent-type disinfectants, and test the working cell culture passage weekly for mycoplasmal contamination. Discard contaminated cells immediately, because they can spread contamination rapidly to other cell cultures maintained in the same laboratory. Before initiating the study, prepare a large suspension of mycoplasma-free cell cultures in early passage and store frozen for future use in case the working cell culture passage becomes contaminated. Quarantine cell cultures until proven to be free of mycoplasmas. Keep records on mycoplasma tests performed; include dates and passage numbers for each substrate tested, and monitor working reagents for the presence of mycoplasmas (i. e., virus pools and antisera); treat contaminated reagents in a quarantined area. Mycoplasmas can be readily eliminated from virus pools by treating with 2:1 parts ether or chloroform to virus pool overnight in the cold, by adding detergents such as Triton-X, by filtering through a 100- or 220-nm filter twice, or by adding high concentrations of a pretested, effective antibiotic (e.g., 10,000 μg/ml kanamycin or tetracycline) or combinations of these varied approaches.

5. Elimination of Mycoplasmas from Contaminated Cell Cultures

Although many different procedures have been tried, there is no simple, rapid, universally effective method for eliminating mycoplasmas from cell cultures. Prevention is the most effective approach to quality control. Maintaining contaminated cell cultures poses risks in the spread of contamination to other cells maintained in the same laboratory and should not be done unless absolutely necessary. Nonetheless, the published procedures which have been used to eliminate mycoplasmas from contami-

TABLE IV. **Procedures Used to Eliminate Mycoplasmas from Contaminated Cell Cultures**

Procedure	Reference
Antibiotics	
Tetracyclines	Robinson *et al.* (1956); Hearn *et al.* (1959); Fogh and Hacker (1960); Carski and Shepard (1961); Perlman *et al.* (1967); Scriba (1968)
Kanamycin	Pollock *et al.* (1960)
Chloramphenicol and novobiocin	Balduzzi and Charbonneau (1964)
Tylosin	Friend *et al.* (1966)
Gentamicin	Casemore (1967)
Antibiotic in hypotonic solution	Gori and Lee (1964)
Aurothiomalate	Shedden and Cole (1966)
Tricine	Spendlove *et al.* (1971)
Triton-X	Reynolds and Hetrick (1969)
Sodium polyanethol sulfonate	Mårdh (1975)
Photodynamic inactivation	Grabowski *et al.* (1969)
Prolonged heat (41°C, 18 hr)	Hayflick (1960)
Specific, neutralizing antisera	Barile (1962, 1973a, 1977); Pollock and Kenny (1963); Herderscheê *et al.* (1963); Vogelzang and Compeer-Dekker (1969)
Antibiotic ard neutralizing antisera	Barile (1973a)

nated cell cultures are listed in Table IV. These include antibiotics such as tetracyclines, kanamycin, novobiocin, chloramphenicol [chloromycetin], tylosin, gentamicin, and treatment with antibiotics in hypotonic solution. The use of Tricine, Triton-X, aurothiomalate, and sodium polyanethol sulfonate have also been reported, as well as the use of prolonged heat, photodynamic inactivation, and treatment with specific antisera. Although some reports have generated widespread optimism, failures have been reported for each of these procedures. For example, the effectiveness of prolonged heat could not be confirmed by Herdersheê *et al.* (1963), Shedden and Cole (1966), Vogelzang and Comperr-Dekker (1969), or Barile (1973a). The treatment reagent must be removed and the cell cultures grown without reagent for several weeks before elimination of the contaminant can be established.

When a cell culture is irreplacable and the investigator is committed to spend the time and effort, the recommended treatment of choice is the combined use of high-titer specific neutralizing antisera and a pretested, effective antibiotic such as a tetracycline or kanamycin (100 μg/ml) (Barile, 1973b). The concentration of the antibiotic is predetermined as that which falls between the effective dose against the mycoplasma contaminant and the toxic dose for the cell culture. The cell culture is grown in medium containing the antibiotic and 5% noninactivated antiserum (which replaces the serum component of the medium) for at least 4 weeks with weekly subcultures or the equivalent, depending on the requirements of the cell substrate. Cell suspensions are examined weekly for the presence of mycoplasmas. In most cases, treatment causes a rapid drop in the mycoplasma titer, but low orders of mycoplasmas can persist for weeks or even months in the presence of antibiotics. Treatment must be continued, even though results appear to be negative. To establish an effective "cure," treatment is stopped, and the cell culture is grown without antibiotic and antiserum for 4 weeks and shown to be free of mycoplasmas by both the direct agar culture and cell culture procedures (Sections III,C,6 and C,7). If contamination persists, the contaminant must be identified and speciated, because mixed contamination with more than one mycoplasma occurs frequently. The treatment is then repeated with pretested antibiotic and high-titer specific antiserum.

Attempts have also been made to eliminate mycoplasmas from contaminated cell cultures by passage through animals. Van Diggelen *et al.* (1977) claimed that *M. hyorhinis* and *A. laidlawii* were eliminated by passing the contaminated cell culture in nude mice, but these findings have not been confirmed. Conversely, Schütze and Gericke (1969) failed in many attempts to eliminate an unspeciated mycoplasma from a contaminated lymphosarcoma cell line by passage through mice. Because animals have rich mycoplasmal flora and because mycoplasmas are frequently isolated from infected and neoplastic tissues, passage through animals could conceivably contaminate the cell culture.

Mycoplasma contaminants can readily develop resistance to antibiotics (Rahman *et al.*, 1967), and resistant strains have been isolated for each antibiotic tested. The effective concentration for each reagent varies widely among strains and species of mycoplasma, and each antibiotic, antiserum, or detergent must be pretested for effectiveness. Treatment is prolonged and can be toxic to cells because high concentrations of reagents are generally required. Moreover, treatment may induce the selection of a cell population which may not retain all the properties of the initial culture. Consequently, it is best to discard the contaminated culture immediately and to replace it with a mycoplasma-free cell culture.

6. Isolation of Mycoplasmas by Direct Agar Culture Procedures

Numerous media formulations and various culture procedures have been used by laboratories throughout the world for isolating mycoplasmas from contaminated cell cultures (see Barile, 1974). We have used four basic approaches (Barile *et al.*, 1958, 1973, 1978; Barile, 1973a, 1974, 1977, 1978): (1) a standardized culture procedure for routine specimens, i.e., cell cultures, biopsy tissues, throat cultures; (2) a semisolid broth culture procedure for screening cell cultures for bacterial, fungal, and mycoplasmal contamination; (3) a large-specimen-volume broth culture procedure for isolating small numbers of mycoplasmas from contaminated bovine sera; and (4) primary and continuous cell culture substrates for primary isolation, detection, and maintenance of fastidious mycoplasma pathogens and the cryptic noncultivable strains of *M. hyorhinis* (Hopps *et al.*, 1973).

a. **Standard culture procedure.** Our standardized medium (Barile, 1974) consists of the Edward–Hayflick formulation (rich basal medium, 20% pretested select horse serum, and 10% freshly prepared yeast extract), supplemented with either arginine (0.1%) or dextrose (0.5%) as energy sources, thymic DNA, vitamins and phenol red as an indicator. Penicillin (500 U/ml) and thallium acetate (1:4000) are added to medium used to examine specimens subject to bacterial contamination. Herderscheê *et al.* (1963) reported that the addition of 10% sucrose improved the growth-promoting properties of medium, and these findings were confirmed by Vogelzang and Van Klingeren (1974). In brief, 0.1 ml of the cell culture suspension is inoculated onto agar medium in duplicate and incubated in a 5% carbon dioxide–95% nitrogen atmosphere in humidified incubators or in the commercial Gaspak jars (Baltimore Biological Laboratories, Baltimore, Maryland) at $36 \pm 1°C$. Agar plates are observed weekly for at least 3 weeks before they are considered negative. Throat cultures are obtained by firmly scraping the infected area with a sterile cotton-tipped applicator and rubbing the specimen across the surface of the agar medium.

The preparation of the specimen can influence successful isolation and growth of mycoplasmas. Solid tissues and biopsied specimens should not be homogenized, because they may release mycoplasmacidal substances such as specific antibodies and complement (Tully and Rask-Nielsen, 1967). Accordingly, tissues were not homogenized in studies to establish the mycoplasma flora of dogs (Barile *et al.*, 1970) and monkeys (Del Giudice *et al.*, 1969; Barile, 1973c). Kaklamanis *et al.* (1969) reported that one of the mycoplasmacidal substances released was lysolecithin which developed during incubation of the culture. Mårdh and Taylor-Robinson (1973) found that cholesterol-requiring *Mycoplasma* species were four times more susceptible to lysolecithin than non-cholesterol-requiring *Acholeplasma* species.

Barile and colleagues (1958, 1962, 1966a, 1973; Barile and Schimke, 1963) first demonstrated that a 5% carbon dioxide–95% nitrogen atmosphere was superior to air for primary isolation and growth of mycoplasmas recovered from contaminated cell cultures and from normal and infected tissues of humans and animals, and these findings have been confirmed by many investigators.

The culture procedures must be standardized, and media must be pretested routinely to establish their ability to grow contaminants and fastidious mycoplasma pathogens. Because the quality of medium components varies from batch to batch, each component must be pretested for growth-promoting ability and for toxicity (see Barile, 1974). For example, whereas arginine (0.1%) stimulates the growth of many mycoplasma species, too much arginine (0.5%) can be toxic (Leach, 1976; Washburn and Somerson, 1977). Certain types of agar preparations can be very toxic to mycoplasmas, and only purified agar products should be used, such as Ionagar No. 2 (Oxoid), Noble agar (Difco), or an equivalent purified product. Growth-promoting properties should be established by comparing a new batch of medium with the existing medium, using a small, standardized inoculum (10^1–10^2 CFU) of frozen suspensions of selected fastidious mycoplasma strains, e.g., *M. hyorhinis, M. hyopneumoniae, M. pneumoniae*, and others.

b. Semisolid broth medium. To prepare this medium, a small amount of purified agar (0.05%) is added to broth medium dispersed in screw-cap tubes. The agar in broth permits mycoplasmas to produce turbid growth and microcolony formation. Arginine utilizers release ammonia, causing an alkaline shift, and the fermenters cause an acid shift, affecting the pH of the culture and changing the color of the indicator, which facilitates the detection of mycoplasma growth by visual examination. Semisolid broth medium is superior to broth for isolating and detecting small numbers of arginine-utilizing contaminants, whereas fermenters prefer broth to semisolid broth.

c. Large-specimen-volume broth culture procedure. Although many earlier attempts to isolate mycoplasmas from contaminated bovine sera had failed using standard agar culture procedures, successful isolations carried out by Barile and Kern (1971) by inoculating large volumes of commercial bovine serum into broth medium provided a more sensitive method for isolating small numbers of mycoplasma from contaminated sera. The serum specimen replaced the serum component of the broth medium (Barile and Del Giudice, 1972; Barile, 1973a,b). In brief, 25 or 100 ml of serum specimen is inoculated into 100 or 500 ml of broth medium and incubated aerobically at 36°C for 4 weeks with weekly subculture to agar medium. Agar plates are processed as above.

7. Staining and Biochemical Procedures for Detecting Noncultivable Mycoplasma Contamination

Because the noncultivable strains of *M. hyorhinis* cannot be grown readily on standardized agar culture medium, a cell culture procedure must be included in each test. Various cell culture procedures have been developed and are designed to detect one of several basic biological, biochemical, or antigenic properties of the mycoplasma contaminant. Many mycoplasma contaminants attach avidly to infected cell cultures and produce a characteristic pattern of infection. Because cytadsorption localizes the mycoplasmas onto the membranes of infected cell cultures and facilitates detection by ordinary microscopy, a variety of specific and nonspecific staining procedures have been developed and used successfully for the detection of mycoplasmas in contaminated cell cultures (Table V). These include hematoxylin and eosin, intensified Giemsa, May–Grünwald–Giemsa, and hypotonic orcein stains. Specific immunofluorescence procedures using fluorescein-conjugated and peroxidase-conjugated antisera have been used successfully, as well as nonspecific fluorescent stains such as acridine orange and DNA-binding fluorochromes, especially bisbenzimidazole (Hoechst No. 33258) and 4'-6-diamidino-2-phenylindole (DAPI). Occasionally, transmission and scanning electron microscopy studies have provided the initial evidence that a particular cell culture was contaminated with mycoplasmas (see Table V for references).

Other procedures used are based on the detection of an enzymatic activity present in mycoplasmas but not in mammalian cells, such as arginine deiminase activity or enzymatic activities utilizing nucleic acid precursors as substrates (Table V; see also Stanbridge, 1971; Schneider, 1975; Schneider and Stanbridge, 1975b; Levine and Becker, 1977). These latter procedures are designed to detect phosphorylation of thymidine, uridine, adenosine, or pyrimidine nucleoside, as well as to detect microbial hypoxanthine and uracil phosphoribosyltransferase activities. Some procedures are based on the isolation and identification of mycoplasmal RNA in contaminated cell cultures, and others on the comparative utilization of uridine versus uracil in contaminated and in mycoplasma-free cell cultures (Table V).

The bisbenzimidazole DNA-fluorochrome staining procedure is simple and inexpensive and has produced results comparable to those obtained with the direct agar and specific immunofluorescence procedures used for the study of cell culture specimens routinely submitted for examination (Del Giudice and Hopps, 1978). Comparable results were also obtained in detecting 22 established mycoplasma contaminants in experimentally infected Vero cell cultures using the DNA-fluorochrome staining procedure (Barile, 1978; Barile and Grabowski, 1978). Nonetheless, because not all mycoplasma contaminants are good cytadsorbing agents and because not all strains or species of mycoplasmas possess the enzymatic activity or certain cell cultures may have high levels of enzymatic activity under investigation, it is important to recognize that nonculture procedures have

TABLE V. **Staining and Biochemical Procedures for Detecting Mycoplasma Contamination of Cell Cultures**

Procedure	Reference
Histological staining	
Hematoxylin and eosin	Berg and Frothingham (1961)
Giemsa stain	Chanock et al. (1960); Clyde (1961)
May–Grünwald–Giemsa stain	Eaton et al. (1962)
Hypotonic orcein stain	Fogh and Fogh (1964)
Fluorescent staining	
Acridine orange	Jasper and Jain (1966); Ebke and Kuwert (1972)
DNA-binding fluorochrome stains	Russell et al. (1975)
DAPI[a]	
Bisbenzimidazole	Chen (1977); Barile (1977; 1978)
Specific fluorescein-conjugated antisera	Malizia et al. (1961); Carski and Shepard (1961); Barile et al. (1962); Barile and Del Giudice (1972)
Specific peroxidase-conjugated antisera	Hill (1978); Polak-Vogelzang et al. (1978)
Electron microscopy	Edwards and Fogh (1960); Anderson and Manaker (1966); Anderson (1969); Hummeler and Armstrong (1967); Dmochowski et al. (1967); Brown et al. (1974); Ho and Quinn (1967)
Autoradiography	Studzinski et al. (1973)
Biochemical assays	
Arginine deiminase	Barile and Schimke (1963)
Uridine/uracil ratio	Schneider et al. (1974)
Pyrimidine nucleoside phosphorylase	Hakala et al. (1963); Horoszewicz and Grace (1964); Nardone et al. (1965); Levine (1974); Schneider et al. (1973); Peden (1975)
Thymidine phosphorylase	Horoszewicz and Grace (1964); Perez et al. (1972); Van Roy and Fiers (1977)
Uridine phosphorylase	Perez et al. (1972); Levine (1974); Van Roy and Fiers (1977)
Adenosine phosphorylase	Hatanaka et al. (1975); Thomas et al. (1977)
Hypoxanthine phosphoribosyltransferase	Holland et al. (1967); Stanbridge et al. (1975); Van Diggelen et al. (1977)
Uracil phosphoribosyltransferase	Long et al. (1977)
Mycoplasmal RNA	Todaro et al. (1971); Reff and Stanbridge (1977)

[a] 4'-6-diamidino-2-phenylindole.

limitations. Therefore both a direct agar culture and an indirect cell culture procedure (we would recommend the DNA-fluorochrome staining procedure) must be included in each test for successful detection of all mycoplasma contaminants.

REFERENCES

Adler, H. E. (1964). *Am. J. Vet. Res.* **25**, 243–245.

Afshar, A. (1967). *J. Gen. Microbiol.* **47**, 103–110.

Aho, K., and Pyhälä, R. (1974). *Clin. Exp. Immunol.* **17**, 607–616.

Ajdukiewicz, A. B., Dudley, F. J., Fox, R. A., Doniach, D., and Sherlock, S. (1972). *Lancet* i, 803–805.

Aldridge, K. E., Cole, B. C., and Ward, J. R. (1977a). *Infect. Immun.* **18**, 377–385.

Aldridge, K. E., Cole, B. C., and Ward, J. R. (1977b). *Infect. Immun.* **18**, 386–392.

Aluotto, B. B., Wittler, R. G., Williams, C. O., and Faber, J. E. (1970). *Int. J. Syst. Bacteriol.* **20**, 35–58.

Anderson, D. R. (1969). *In* "The Mycoplasmatales and the L-Phase of Bacteria" (L. Hayflick, ed.), pp. 365–402. Appleton, New York.

Anderson, D. R., and Manaker, R. A. (1966). *J. Natl. Cancer Inst.* **36**, 139–154.

Armstrong, D., and Paucker, K. (1966). *J. Bacteriol.* **92**, 97–101.

Aula, P., and Nichols, W. W. (1967). *J. Cell. Physiol.* **70**, 281–289.

Băizhomartov, M. S., Prozorovskǐi, S. V., Irzhanov, S. D., and Tsǒi, I. G. (1975). *Zh. Mikrobiol. Epidemiol. Immunobiol.* **12**, 75–78.

Balduzzi, P., and Charbonneau, J. R. (1964). *Experientia* **20**, 651–652.

Barile, M. F. (1962). *Natl. Cancer Inst., Monogr.* **7**, 50–53.

Barile, M. F. (1965). *In* "Methodological Approaches to the Study of Leukemias" (V. Defendi, ed.), pp. 171–181. Wistar Inst. Press, Philadelphia, Pennsylvania.

Barile, M. F. (1967). *Ann. N.Y. Acad. Sci.* **143**, 557–572.

Barile, M. F. (1968). *Natl. Cancer Inst., Monogr.* **29**, 201–204.

Barile, M. F. (1973a). *In* "Contamination of Cell Cultures" (J. Fogh, ed.), pp. 131–172. Academic Press, New York.

Barile, M. F. (1973b). *In* "Tissue Culture, Methods and Applications" (P. F. Kruse and M. K. Patterson, eds.), pp. 729–735. Academic Press, New York.

Barile, M. F. (1973c). *J. Infect. Dis.* **127**, Suppl., 17–20.

Barile, M. F. (1974). *In* "Les Mycoplasmes de l'Homme, des Animaux, des Vegetaux et des Insectes" (J. M. Bové and F. Duplan, eds.), Colloques INSERM No. 33, pp. 135–142. INSERM, Paris.

Barile, M. F. (1977). *In* "Cell Culture and Its Application" (R. Action, ed.), pp. 291–334. Academic Press, New York.

Barile, M. F. (1978). *In* "Clinical Laboratory Sciences" (G. D. Hsiung and R. H. Green, eds.), CRC Handbook Series. CRC Press, Cleveland, Ohio. In press.

Barile, M. F., and Del Giudice, R. A. (1972). *Ciba Found. Symp. Pathogen. Mycoplasma* pp. 165–185.

Barile, M. F., and Grabowski, M. W. (1978). *In* "Mycoplasma Infection of Cell Cultures" (G. J. McGarrity, D. G. Murphy, and W. W. Nichols, eds.), pp. 135–150. Plenum, New York.

Barile, M. F., and Kern, J. (1971). *Proc. Soc. Exp. Biol. Med.* **138**, 432–437.

Barile, M. F., and Leventhal, B. G. (1968). *Nature (London)* **219**, 751–752.

Barile, M. F., and Schimke, R. T. (1963). *Proc. Soc. Exp. Biol. Med.* **114,** 676–679.

Barile, M. F., Yaguchi, R., and Eveland, W. C. (1958). *Am. J. Clin. Pathol.* **30,** 171–176.

Barile, M. F., Malizia, W. F., and Riggs, D. B. (1962). *J. Bacteriol.* **84,** 130–136.

Barile, M. F., Bodey, G. P., Snyder, J., Riggs, D. B., and Grabowski, M. W. (1966a). *J. Natl. Cancer Inst.* **36,** 155–159.

Barile, M. F., Schimke, R. T., and Riggs, D. B. (1966b). *J. Bacteriol.* **91,** 189–192.

Barile, M. F., Del Giudice, R. A., Carski, T. R., Gibbs, C. J., and Morris, J. A. (1968). *Proc. Soc. Exp. Biol. Med.* **129,** 489–494.

Barile, M. F., Del Giudice, R. A., Carski, T. R., Yamashiroya, H. M., and Verna, J. A. (1970). *Proc. Soc. Exp. Biol. Med.* **134,** 146–148.

Barile, M. F., Del Giudice, R. A., Hopps, H. E., Grabowski, M. W., and Riggs, D. B. (1973). *Ann. N.Y. Acad. Sci.* **225,** 251–264.

Barile, M. F., Hopps, H. E., and Grabowski, M. W. (1978). *In* "Mycoplasma Infection of Cell Cultures" (G. J. McGarrity, D. G. Murphy, and W. W. Nichols, eds.), pp. 35–45. Plenum, New York.

Becker, Y., Olshevsky, V., and Levitt, J. (1967). *J. Gen. Virol.* **1,** 471–478.

Beckman, B. L., and Kenny, G. E. (1968). *J. Bacteriol.* **96,** 1171–1180.

Berg, R. B., and Frothingham, T. E. (1961). *Proc. Soc. Exp. Biol. Med.* **108,** 616–618.

Berquist, L. M., Lau, H. S. B., and Winter, C. E. (1974). *Infect. Immun.* **9,** 410–415.

Berry, D. M. (1969). *Proc. R. Soc. Med.* **62,** 45–48.

Biberfeld, G. (1966). *Acta Pathol. Microbiol. Scand.* **66,** 284.

Biberfeld, G. (1971a). "Immunological, Epidemiological and Ultrastructural Studies of *Mycoplasma pneumoniae,*" Doctorate Dissertation, Karolinska Institutet, Stockholm, pp. 1–48. Tryckeri Balder AB, Stockholm, Sweden.

Biberfeld, G. (1971b). *Clin. Exp. Immunol.* **8,** 319–333.

Biberfeld, G. (1974). *Clin. Exp. Immunol.* **17,** 43–49.

Biberfeld, G., and Biberfeld, P. (1970). *J. Bacteriol.* **102,** 855–861.

Biberfeld, G., and Gronowicz, E. (1976). *Nature (London)* **261,** 238–239.

Biberfeld, G., and Sterner, G. (1976a). *Clin. Exp. Immunol.* **24,** 287–291.

Biberfeld, G., and Sterner, G. (1976b). *Infection* **4,** Suppl. 1, 17–20.

Biberfeld, G., Biberfeld, P., and Sterner, G. (1974). *Clin. Exp. Immunol.* **17,** 29–41.

Black, F. T. (1973). *Ann. N.Y. Acad. Sci.* **225,** 131–143.

Black, F. T. (1974). "Human T-Mycoplasma (*Ureaplasma urealyticum*)" Doctoral Dissertation, University of Aarhus, pp. 1–74. Bartholinbygningen, Universitetsparken, Aarhus, Denmark.

Bradbury, J., and Jordan, F. (1972). *J. Hyg.* **70,** 267–278.

Bredt, W. (1968). *Pathol. Microbiol.* **32,** 321–326.

Bredt, W. (1973). *Ann. N.Y. Acad. Sci.* **225,** 246–250.

Bredt, W. (1976a). *Infection* **4,** Suppl. 1, 9–12.

Bredt, W. (1976b). *Zentralbl. Bakteriol., Parasitenkd., Infektionskr.* **235,** 114–121.

Brown, S., Teplitz, M., and Revel, J. P. (1974). *Proc. Natl. Acad. Sci. U.S.A.* **71,** 464–468.

Brownstein, B., and Graham, A. F. (1961). *Virology* **14,** 303–311.

Brunner, H. (1976). *Zentralbl. Bakteriol., Parasitenkd., Infektionskr. Hyg. 1: Orig., Reihe A* **235,** 122–133.

Brunner, H., Brück, U., Lambert, D., Sziegoleit, D., and Schiefer, H. (1976). *Infection* **4,** Suppl. 1, 13–16.

Brunner, H., Prescott, B., Greenberg, H., James, W. D., Horswood, R. L., and Chanock, R. M. (1977). *J. Infect. Dis.* **135,** 524–530.

Burnet, F. M. (1951). *Physiol. Rev.* **31,** 131–150.

Burnet, F. M., and Anderson, S. G. (1946). *Br. J. Exp. Pathol.* **27,** 236–244.

Burnet, F. M., McCrea, J. F., and Stone, J. D. (1946). *Br. J. Exp. Pathol.* **27**, 228–236.

Busolo, F., Conventi, L., Bertoloni, B., and Meloni, G. A. (1975). *Atti Congr. Naz. Soc. Ital. Microbiol., 17th, Padua*, pp. 1111–1115.

Butler, M., and Leach, R. H. (1964). *J. Gen. Micribiol.* **34**, 285–294.

Carski, T. R., and Shepard, C. C. (1961). *J. Bacteriol.* **81**, 626–635.

Carubelli, R., and Griffen, M. J. (1967). *Science* **157**, 693–694.

Casemore, D. P. (1967). *J. Clin. Pathol.* **20**, 298–299.

Castrejon-Diez, J., Fisher, T. N., and Fisher, E., Jr. (1963). *Proc. Soc. Exp. Biol. Med.* **112**, 643–647.

Chanock, R. M., Parrott, R. H., Cook, K., Andrews, B. E., Bell, J. A., Reichelderfer, T., Kapikian, A. Z., Mastrota, F. M., and Huebner, R. J. (1958). *N. Engl. J. Med.* **258**, 207–213.

Chanock, R. M., Fox, H. H., James, W. D., Bloom, H. H., and Mufson, M. A. (1960). *Proc. Soc. Exp. Biol. Med.* **105**, 371–375.

Chanock, R. M., Hayflick, L., and Barile, M. F. (1962). *Proc. Natl. Acad. Sci. U.S.A.* **48**, 41–48.

Chanock, R. M., Mufson, M., Somerson, N. L., and Couch, R. B. (1963). *Am. Rev. Respir. Dis.* **88**, 218–231.

Chen, T. R. (1977). *Exp. Cell Res.* **104**, 255–262.

Cherry, J. D., and Taylor-Robinson, D. (1970a). *Appl. Microbiol.* **19**, 658–662.

Cherry, J. D., and Taylor-Robinson, D. (1970b). *Infect. Immun.* **2**, 431–438.

Cherry, J. D., and Taylor-Robinson, D. (1970c). *Nature (London)* **228**, 1099–1100.

Clark, A. F., Farrell, D. F., Burke, W., and Scott, C. R. (1978). *Clin. Chim. Acta* **82**, 119–124.

Clyde, W. A., Jr. (1961). *Proc. Soc. Exp. Biol. Med.* **107**, 715–718.

Clyde, W. A., Jr. (1963a). *Science* **139**, 55.

Clyde, W. A., Jr. (1963b). *Proc. Soc. Exp. Biol. Med.* **112**, 905–909.

Cochrum, K. C., Dykman, L., Najarian, J. S., and Fudenberg, H. H. (1969). *Proc. Leuco-cyte Cult. Conf., 3rd* pp. 169–176.

Cohen, G., and Somerson, N. L. (1967). *Ann. N.Y. Acad. Sci.* **143**, 85–87.

Cole, B. C., Ward, J. R., and Martin, C. H. (1968). *J. Bacteriol.* **95**, 2022–2030.

Cole, B. C., Aldridge, K. E., and Ward, J. R. (1977). *Infect. Immun.* **18**, 393–399.

Cole, B. C., Lombardi, P. S., Overall, J. C., Jr., and Glasgow, L. A. (1978). *Proc. Soc. Exp. Biol. Med.* **157**, 83–88.

Collier, A. M. (1972). *Ciba Found. Symp. Pathogen. Mycoplasma* pp. 307–320.

Collier, L. H. (1957). *Nature (London)* **180**, 757–758.

Copperman, R., and Morton, H. E. (1966). *Proc. Soc. Exp. Biol. Med.* **123**, 790–795.

Coriell, L. L. (1962). *Natl. Cancer Inst., Monogr.* **7**, 33–53.

Coriell, L. L., and McGarrity, G. J. (1968). *Appl. Microbiol.* **16**, 1895–1900.

Costea, N., Yakulis, V., and Heller, P. (1966). *Science* **152**, 1520–1521.

Couch, R. B., Cate, T. R., and Chanock, R. M. (1964). *J. Am. Med. Assoc.* **187**, 442–447.

Cross, G. F., Goodman, M. R., Chatterji, J., Beswick, T. S. L., and Chapman, J. A. (1970). *J. Gen. Virol.* **8**, 77–81.

Dacie, J. V. (1962). "The Haemolytic Anaemias," 2nd Ed., pp. 343, 530. Grune & Stratton, New York.

Del Giudice, R. A., and Hopps, H. E. (1978). *In* "Mycoplasma Infection of Cell Cultures" (G. J. McGarrity, D. G. Murphy, and W. W. Nichols, eds.), pp. 57–69. Plenum, New York.

Del Giudice, R. A., and Pavia, R. (1964). *Bacteriol. Proc.* p. 71.

Del Giudice, R. A., Carski, T. R., Barile, M. F., Yamashiroya, H. M., and Verna, J. E. (1969). *Nature (London)* **222**, 1088–1089.

DeVay, J. E., and Adler, H. E. (1976). *Annu. Rev. Microbiol.* **30,** 147–168.

Dingle, J. H., Abernethy, T. J., Badger, G. F., Buddingh, G. J., Feller, A. E., Langmuir, A. D., Ruegsegger, J. M., and Wood, W. B., Jr. (1944). *Am. J. Hyg.* **39,** 67–128, 197–268, 269–336.

Dmochowski, L., Dreyer, D. A., Grey, C. E., Hales, R., Langford, P. L., Pipes, F., Recher, L., Seman, G., Shively, J. A., Shullenberger, C. C., Sinkovics, J. G., Taylor, H. G., Tessmer, C. F., and Yumoto, T. (1967). *Ann. N.Y. Acad. Sci.* **143,** 578–607.

Dubes, G. R., Moyer, K. B., Halliburton, B. L., and Van deBogart, R. K. (1969). *Acta Virol. (Engl. Ed.)* **13,** 8–15.

Eaton, M. D., Farnham, A. E., Levinthal, J. D., and Scala, A. R. (1962). *J. Bacteriol.* **84,** 1330–1337.

Ebke, J., and Kuwert, E. (1972). *Zentralbl. Bakteriol., Parasitenkd., Infektionskr. Hyg., Abt. 1: Orig., Reihe A*: **221,** 87–93.

Eddy, B. E., Rowe, W. P., Hartley, J. W., Stewart, S. E., and Huebner, R. J. (1958). *Virology* **6,** 290–291.

Edward, D. G. ff. (1950). *J. Gen. Microbiol.* **4,** 311–329.

Edward, D. G. ff. (1954). *J. Gen. Microbiol.* **10,** 27–64.

Edward, D. G. ff., and Freundt, E. A. (1956). *J. Gen. Microbiol.* **14,** 197–207.

Edward, D. G. ff., and Kanarak, A. D. (1959). *Ann. N.Y. Acad. Sci.* **79,** 696–702.

Edwards, G. A., and Fogh, J. (1960). *J. Bacteriol.* **79,** 267–276.

Ernø, H., and Stipkovits, L. (1973). *Acta Vet. Scand.* **14,** 450–463.

Fallon, R. J., and Jackson, D. J. (1967). *Lab. Anim.* **1,** 55–64.

Fauconnier, B., and Wroblewski, H. (1974). *Ann. Microbiol. (Paris)* **125A,** 469–476.

Faur, Y. C., Weisburd, M. H., and Wilson, M. E. (1975). *Am. J. Clin. Pathol.* **63,** 106–116.

Feizi, T. (1967). *Ann. N.Y. Acad. Sci.* **143,** 801–812.

Feizi, T., and Taylor-Robinson, D. (1967). *Immunology* **13,** 405–409.

Feizi, T., Taylor-Robinson, D., Shields, M. D., and Carter, R. A. (1969). *Nature (London)* **222,** 1253–1256.

Fernald, G. W., and Clyde, W. A., Jr. (1974). In "Les Mycoplasmes de l'Homme, des Animaux, des Vegetux et des Insectes" (J. M. Bové and J. F. Duplan, eds.), Colloques INSERM, No. 33, pp. 421–428. INSERM, Paris.

Fernald, G. W., Collier, A. M., and Clyde, W. A., Jr. (1975). *Pediatrics* **55,** 327–335.

Finland, M., Peterson, O. L., Samper, H. E., and Barnes, M. W. (1945a). *J. Clin. Invest.* **24,** 454–473.

Finland, M., Samper, B. A., and Barnes, M. W. (1945b). *J. Clin. Invest.* **24,** 497–502.

Florman, A. L., and Weiss, A. B. (1945). *J. Lab. Clin. Med.* **30,** 902–910.

Fogh, J. (1970). *Proc. Soc. Exp. Biol. Med.* **134,** 217–224.

Fogh, J., and Fogh, H. (1964). *Proc. Soc. Exp. Biol. Med.* **117,** 899–901.

Fogh, J., and Fogh, H. (1965). *Proc. Soc. Exp. Biol. Med.* **119,** 233–238.

Fogh, J., and Fogh, H. (1967). *Proc. Soc. Exp. Biol. Med.* **126,** 67–74.

Fogh, J., and Hacker, C. (1960). *Exp. Cell Res.* **21,** 242–244.

Fogh, J., Holmgren, N. B., and Ludovici, P. P. (1971). *In Vitro* **7,** 26–41.

Fowlkes, D. M., Dooher, G. B., and O'Leary, W. M. (1975). *Fertil. Steril.* **26,** 1203–1211.

Fraser, L. R., and Drury, L. M. (1975). *Biol. Reprod.* **13,** 513.

Fraser, L. R., and Taylor-Robinson, D. (1977). *Fertil. Steril.* **28,** 488–498.

Freed, J. J., and Schatz, S. A. (1969). *Exp. Cell Res.* **55,** 393–409.

Friend, C., Patuleia, M. C., and Nelson, J. B. (1966). *Proc. Soc. Exp. Biol. Med.* **121,** 1009–1010.

Gabbiani, G., Ryan, G., Lamolin, J.-P., Vassali, P., Maino, G., Bouvier, C., Cruchaud, A., and Luscher, E. (1973). *Am. J. Pathol.* **72,** 473–488.

Gesner, B., and Thomas, L. (1966). *Science* **151,** 590–591.

Ginsburg, H. (1974). *Isr. J. Med. Sci.* **10,** 1165.

Ginsburg, H., and Nicolet, J. (1973). *Nature (London), New Biol.* **246,** 143–146.

Girardi, A. J., Hamparian, V. V., Somerson, N. L., and Hayflick, L. (1965a). *Proc. Soc. Exp. Biol. Med.* **120,** 760–771.

Girardi, A. J., Larson, V. M., and Hilleman, M. R. (1965b). *Proc. Soc. Exp. Biol. Med.* **118,** 173–179.

Gnarpe, H., and Friberg, J. (1973a). *Nature (London)* **245,** 97–98.

Gnarpe, H., and Friberg, J. (1973b). *Nature (London)* **242,** 120–121.

Goldblum, N., Ravid, Z., and Becker, Y. (1968). *J. Gen. Virol.* **3,** 143–146.

Gomatos, P. J., and Tamm, I. (1962). *Virology* **17,** 455–461.

Goodwin, R. F. W., and Whittlestone, P. (1963). *Br. J. Exp. Pathol.* **44,** 291–299.

Gori, G. B., and Lee, D. Y. (1964). *Proc. Soc. Exp. Biol. Med.* **117,** 918–921.

Gottschalk, A. (1958). *Nature (London)* **181,** 377–378.

Gourlay, R. N., and Shifrine, M. (1966). *J. Comp. Pathol. Ther.* **76,** 417–425.

Grabowski, M. W., Riggs, D. B., Moore, D. E., and Barile, M. F. (1969). *Bacteriol. Proc.* p. 33.

Grebe, H. H. (1977). *Zentralbl. Veterinaermed., Reihe B* **24,** 134–139.

Grist, N. R., and Fallon, R. J. (1964). *Br. Med. J.* **ii,** 1263.

Grossgebauer, K., Hennig, A., and Hartmann, D. (1977). *Hautarzt* **28,** 299–302.

Grumbles, L. C., Hall, C. F., and Cummings, G. (1964). *Avian Dis.* **8,** 274–280.

Hakala, M. T., Holland, J. F., and Horoszewicz, J. S. (1963). *Biochem. Biophys. Res. Commun.* **11,** 466–471.

Hargreaves, F. D., and Leach, R. H. (1970). *J. Med. Microbiol.* **3,** 259–265.

Harley, E. H., Rees, K. R., and Cohen, A. (1970). *Biochim, Biophys. Acta* **213,** 171–182.

Hatanaka, M., Del Giudice, R. A., and Long, C. W. (1975). *Proc. Natl. Acad. Sci. U.S.A.* **72,** 1401–1405.

Hayflick, L. (1960). *Nature (London)* **185,** 783–784.

Hearn, H. J., Officer, J. E., Elsner, V., and Brown, A. (1959). *J. Bacteriol.* **78,** 575–582.

Heishman, J. O., Olson, N. O., and Cunningham, C. J. (1969). *Avian Dis.* **13,** 1–6.

Herderscheê, D., Ruys, A. C., and van Rhijn, G. R. (1963). *Antonie van Leeuwenhoek: J. Microbiol. Serol.* **29,** 368–376.

Hill, A. C. (1978). *J. Infect. Dis.* **137,** 152–154.

Ho, T. Y., and Quinn, P. A. (1977). *Scanning Electron Microsc.* **2,** 291–300.

Holborow, E. J., Hemstad, E. H., and Mead, S. W. (1973). *Br. Med. J.* **iii,** 323–325.

Holland, J. F., Korn, R., O'Malley, J., Minnemeyer, H. J., and Ticklemann, H. (1967). *Cancer Res.* **27,** 1867–1873.

Hollingdale, M. R., and Manchee, R. J. (1972). *J. Gen. Microbiol.* **70,** 391–393.

Hopps, H. E., Meyer, B. C., Barile, M. F., and Del Giudice, R. A. (1973). *Ann. N.Y. Acad. Sci.* **225,** 265–276.

Horoszewicz, J. S., and Grace, J. T., Jr. (1964). *Bacteriol. Proc.* p. 131.

House, H., and Waddell, A. (1967). *J. Pathol. Bacteriol.* **93,** 125–132.

Howard, C. J., Taylor, G., Collins, J., and Gourlay, R. N. (1976). *Infect. Immun.* **14,** 11–17.

Hu, P. C., Collier, A. M., and Baseman, J. B. (1977). *J. Exp. Med.* **145,** 1328–1343.

Hummeler, K., and Armstrong, D. (1967). *Ann. N.Y. Acad. Sci.* **143,** 622–625.

Huppert, J., Delain, E., Fossar, N., and May, E. (1974). *Virology* **57,** 217–226.

Jacob, J. T., Stahl, M., and Fulginiti, V. (1966). *J. Bacteriol.* **92,** 1002–1004.

Jasper, D. E., and Jain, N. C. (1966). *Appl. Microbiol.* **14,** 720–723.

Johnson, G. D., Holborow, E. J., and Glynn, L. E. (1965). *Lancet* **ii,** 878–879.

Joncas, J., Chagnon, A., Lussier, G., and Pavilanis, V. (1969). *Can. J. Microbiol.* **15,** 451–454.

Jones, T. C., and Hirsch, J. G. (1971). *J. Exp. Med.* **133**, 231–259.

Jones, T. C., and Yang, L. (1977). *Am. J. Pathol.* **87**, 331–345.

Jones, T. C., Yeh, S., and Hirsch, J. G. (1972). *Proc. Soc. Exp. Biol. Med.* **139**, 464–470.

Jones, T. C., Minick, R., and Yang, L. (1977). *Am. J. Pathol.* **87**, 347–358.

Jurmanova, K., and Mensik, J. (1971). *Zentralbl. Veterinaermed., Reihe B* **18**, 457–464.

Jurmanova, K., and Sterbova, J. (1977). *Vet. Rec.* **100**, 157–158.

Kagan, G. Y., Ershov, F. I., Rakovskaya, I. V., Tsareva, A. T., and Zhdanov, V. M. (1967). *Vopr. Virusol.* **4**, 478–485.

Kagan, G. Y., Fleer, G. P., Rakovskaya, I. V., Smirnova, T. D., and Chumakov, M. P. (1969). *Zh. Microbiol., Epidemiol. Immunobiol.* **46**(3), 63–66.

Kahane, I., and Brunner, H. (1977). *Infect. Immun.* **18**, 273–277.

Kahane, I., and Tully, J. G. (1976). *J. Bacteriol.* **128**, 1–7.

Kaklamanis, E., and Pavlatos, M. (1972). *Immunology* **22**, 695–702.

Kaklamanis, E., Thomas, L., Stavropoulos, K., Borman, I., and Boshivitz, C. (1969). *Nature (London)* **221**, 860–862.

Kaluzewski, S., and Jagielski, M. (1972). *Exp. Med. Microbiol.* pp. 98–108.

Kasza, L., Hodges, R. T., Betts, A. O., and Trexler, P. C. (1969). *Vet. Rec.* **84**, 262–267.

Katzen, S., Matsuda, K., and Reid, B. L. (1969). *Poult. Sci.* **48**, 1504–1506.

Kenny, G. E., and Pollock, M. E. (1963). *J. Infect. Dis.* **112**, 7–16.

Kirchhoff, H., Basu, A., and Loh, M. (1973). *Zentralbl. Veterinaermed., Reihe B* **20**, 474–480.

Kirchner, H., Brunner, H., and Rühl, H. (1977). *Clin. Exp. Immunol.* **29**, 176–180.

Klein, J. O., Buckland, D., and Finland, M. (1969). *N. Engl. J. Med.* **280**, 1025–1030.

Kundsin, R. B., Driscoll, S. G., and Ming, P.-M. L. (1967). *Science* **157**, 1573–1574.

Kundsin, R. B., Ampola, M., Streeter, S., and Neurath, P. (1971). *J. Med. Genet.* **8**, 181–187.

Lancefield, R. C. (1943). *J. Exp. Med.* **78**, 465–476.

Leach, R. H. (1976). *J. Appl. Bacteriol.* **41**, 259–264.

Lemcke, R. M. (1969). *In* "The Mycoplasmatales and the L-Phase of Bacteria" (L. Hayflick, ed.), pp. 265–277. North-Holland Publ., Amsterdam.

Lemcke, R. M., Marmion, B. P., and Plackett, P. (1967). *Ann. N.Y. Acad. Sci.* **143**, 691–702.

Leventhal, B. G., Smith, C. B., Carbone, P. P., and Hersh, E. M. (1968). *Proc. Leucocyte Cult. Conf., 3rd* pp. 519–532.

Levine, E. M. (1974). *Methods Cell Biol.* **8**, 229–248.

Levine, E. M., and Becker, B. G. (1977). *In* "Mycoplasma Infections of Cell Cultures" (G. J. McGarrity, D. G. Murphy, and W. W. Nichols, eds.), pp. 87–104. Plenum, New York.

Levine, E. M., Thomas, L., McGregor, D., Hayflick, L., and Eagle, H. (1968). *Proc. Natl. Acad. Sci. U.S.A.* **60**, 583–589.

Liao, Y. L. (1976). *Chin. J. Microbiol.* **9**, 37–44.

Lidman, K., Biberfeld, G., Fagraeus, A., Norberg, R., Torstensson, R., Utter, G., Carlsson, L., Luca, J., and Lindberg, U. (1976). *Clin. Exp. Immunol.* **24**, 266–272.

Lind, K. (1968). *Acta Pathol. Microbiol. Scand.* **73**, 237–244.

Lind, K. (1971). *Acta Pathol. Microbiol. Scand., Sect. B* **79**, 239–247.

Lind, K., Ravn, T. J., and Moller, J. (1970). *Acta Pathol. Microbiol. Scand.* **78**, 6–14.

Lipman, R. P., and Clyde, W. A., Jr. (1969). *Proc. Soc. Exp. Biol. Med.* **134**, 1163–1167.

Liu, C. (1957). *J. Exp. Med.* **106**, 455–467.

Liu, C., Eaton, M. D., and Heyl, J. T. (1959). *J. Exp. Med.* **109**, 545–556.

Lloyd, C. W. (1975). *Biol. Rev. Cambridge Philos. Soc.* **50**, 325–350.

Long, C. W., Del Giudice, R., Gardella, R. S., Hatanaka, M. (1977). *In Vitro* **13,** 429–433.

Low, I. E. (1974). *Appl. Microbiol.* **27,** 1046–1052.

Ludovici, P. P., and Holmgren, N. B. (1973). *Methods Cell Biol.* **6,** 143–208.

MacPherson, I. (1966). *J. Cell Sci.* **1,** 145–167.

MacPherson, I., and Russell, W. (1966). *Nature (London)* **210,** 1343–1345.

McGarrity, G. J. (1976). *In Vitro* **12,** 643–648.

McGarrity, G. J., Vanaman, V., and Sarama, J. (1978). *In* "Mycoplasma Infections of Cell Cultures" (G. J. McGarrity, D. G. Murphy, and W. W. Nichols, eds.), pp. 213–241. Plenum, New York.

Malizia, W. F., Barile, M. F., and Riggs, D. B. (1961). *Nature (London)* **191,** 190–191.

Manchee, R. J., and Taylor-Robinson, D. (1968). *J. Gen. Microbiol.* **50,** 465–478.

Manchee, R. J., and Taylor-Robinson, D. (1969a). *J. Bacteriol.* **98,** 914–919.

Manchee, R. J., and Taylor-Robinson, D. (1969b). *Br. J. Exp. Pathol.* **50,** 66–75.

Manchee, R. J., and Taylor-Robinson, D. (1970). *J. Med. Microbiol.* **3,** 539–546.

Mandy, M. S., and Ho, M. (1964). *Proc. Soc. Exp. Biol. Med.* **116,** 174–177.

Maniloff, J. (1972). *Ciba Found. Symp. Pathogen. Mycoplasma* pp. 67–87.

Maniloff, J., Morowitz, H. J., and Barrnett, R. J. (1965). *J. Bacteriol.* **90,** 193—204.

Manischewitz, J. E., Young, B. G., and Barile, M. F. (1975). *Proc. Soc. Exp. Biol. Med.* **148,** 859–863.

Mårdh, P.-A. (1975). *Nature (London)* **254,** 515–516.

Mårdh, P.-A., and Taylor-Robinson, D. (1973). *Med. Microbiol. Immunol.* **158,** 219–226.

Marmion, B. P. (1967). *In* "Recent Advances in Medical Microbiology" (A. P. Waterson, ed.), pp. 170–250. Churchill, London.

Marmion, B. P., and Goodburn, G. M. (1961). *Nature (London)* **189,** 247–248.

Marmion, B. P., Plackett, P., and Lemcke, R. M. (1967). *Aust. J. Exp. Biol. Med. Sci.* **45,** 163–187.

Meloni, G. A., Rizzu, D., and Addis, S. (1969). *Boll. Ist. Sieroter. Milan* **48,** 23–38.

Miller, G., Emmons, J., and Stitt, D. (1971). *J. Infect. Dis.* **124,** 322–326.

Miller, R. L., and Rapp, F. (1976). *J. Virol.* **20,** 564–569.

Mills, L. B., Stanbridge, E. J., Sedwick, W. D., and Korn, D. (1977). *J. Bacteriol.* **132,** 641–649.

Minamishima, Y., and Benyesh-Melnick, M. (1969). *Bacteriol. Proc.* p. 170.

Moore, R. W., Grumbles, L. C., and Beasley, J. N. (1960). *Ann. N.Y. Acad. Sci.* **79,** 556–561.

Morgan, J. F., Morton, H. J., and Pasieka, A. E. (1958). *J. Biol. Chem.* **233,** 664–667.

Morgensen, H. H., Andersen, V., and Lind, K. (1976). *Infection* **4,** Suppl. 1, 21–24.

Mufson, M. A., Manko, M. A., Kingston, J. R., and Chanock, R. M. (1961). *J. Am. Med. Assoc.* **178,** 369–374.

Nakamura, M., and Sakamoto, H. (1969). *Proc. Soc. Exp. Biol. Med.* **131,** 343–348.

Naot, Y., Tully, J. G., and Ginsburg, H. (1977). *Infect. Immun.* **18,** 310–317.

Nardone, R. M., Todd, J., Gonzales, P., and Gaffney, E. V. (1965). *Science* **149,** 1100–1101.

Neimark, H. C. (1964). *Nature (London)* **203,** 549–550.

Neimark, H. C. (1977). *Proc. Natl. Acad. Sci. U.S.A.* **74,** 4041–4045.

Nelson, J. B. (1960). *Ann. N.Y. Acad. Sci.* **79,** 450–457.

Nowell, P. C. (1960). *Cancer Res.* **20,** 462–466.

O'Connell, R. C., Wittler, R. G., and Faber, J. E. (1964). *Appl. Microbiol.* **12,** 337–342.

Ogata, M., and Koshimizu, K. (1967). *Jpn. J. Microbiol.* **11,** 289–303.

O'Malley, J. P., Meyer, H. M., Jr., and Smadel, J. E. (1961). *Proc. Soc. Exp. Biol. Med.* **108,** 200–205.

O'Malley, J. P., McGee, Z. A., Barile, M. F., and Barker, L. F. (1966). *Proc. Natl. Acad. Sci. U.S.A.* **56,** 895–901.

Oppenheim, J. J. (1968). *Fed. Proc., Fed. Am. Soc. Exp. Biol.* **27,** 21–28.

Organick, A. B., and Lutsky, I. I. (1968). *J. Bacteriol.* **95,** 2310–2316.

Organick, A. B., Siegesmund, K. A., and Lutsky, I. I. (1966). *J. Bacteriol.* **92,** 1164–1176.

Paton, G. R., and Allison, A. C. (1970). *Nature (London)* **227,** 707–709.

Paton, G. R., Jacobs, J. P., and Perkins, F. T. (1965). *Nature (London)* **207,** 43–45.

Paton, G. R., Jacobs, J. P., and Perkins, F. T. (1967). *Ann. N.Y. Acad. Sci.* **143,** 626–627.

Peden, K. W. C. (1975). *Experientia* **3,** 1111–1112.

Perez, A. G., Kin, J. H., Gelbard, A. S., and Djordjevic, B. (1972). *Exp. Cell Res.* **70,** 301–310.

Perlman, D., Rahman, S. B., and Semar, J. B. (1967). *Appl. Microbiol.* **15,** 82–85.

Peterson, O. L., Ham, T. H., and Finland, M. (1943). *Science* **97,** 167–168.

Plackett, P., Marmion, B. P., Shaw, E. J., and Lemcke, R. M. (1969). *Aust. J. Exp. Biol. Med. Sci.* **47,** 171–195.

Polak-Vogelzang, A., Hagenaars, R., and Nagel, J. (1978). *J. Gen. Microbiol.* **106,** 241–249.

Pollack, J. D., Razin, S., and Cleverdon, R. C. (1965). *J. Bacteriol.* **90,** 617–622.

Pollock, M. E., and Kenny, G. (1963). *Proc. Soc. Exp. Biol. Med.* **112,** 176–181.

Pollock, M. E., Kenny, G. E., and Syverton, J. T. (1960). *Proc. Soc. Exp. Biol. Med.* **105,** 10–15.

Pollock, M. E., Treadwell, P. E., and Kenny, G. E. (1963). *Exp. Cell Res.* **31,** 321–328.

Powell, D. A., Hu, P. C., Wilson, M., Collier, A. M., and Baseman, J. B. (1976). *Infect. Immun.* **13,** 959–966.

Purcell, R. H., Valdesuso, J. R., Cline, W. L., James, W. D., and Chanock, R. M. (1971). *Appl. Microbiol.* **21,** 288–294.

Pyhälä, R. (1976). *Acta Pathol. Microbiol. Scand., Sect. B* **84,** 240–244.

Rahman, S. B., Semar, J. B., and Perlman, D. (1967). *Appl. Microbiol.* **15,** 970.

Rakovskaya, I. V., and Neustroeva, V. V. (1967). *J. Microbiol., Epidemiol. Immunobiol. (USSR)* **9,** 51–54.

Ranck, R. M., Grumbles, L. C., Hall, C. F., and Grimes, J. E. (1970). *Avian Dis.* **14,** 54–65.

Razin, S. (1978). *Microbiol. Rev.* **42,** 414–470.

Razin, S., Prescott, B., Caldes, G., James, W. D., and Chanock, R. M. (1970). *Infect. Immun.* **1,** 408–416.

Reed, S. E. (1971). *J. Infect. Dis.* **124,** 18–25.

Reed, S. E. (1972). *Ciba Found. Symp. Pathogen. Mycoplasmas* pp. 329–348.

Reff, M. E., and Stanbridge, E. (1977). *Int. J. Syst. Bacteriol.* **27,** 185.

Reimann, H. E. (1938). *J. Am. Med. Assoc.* **111,** 2377–2384.

Rein, C. R., and Elsberg, E. S. (1944). *Am. J. Clin. Pathol.* **14,** 461–469.

Reynolds, R. K., and Hetrick, F. M. (1969). *Appl. Microbiol.* **17,** 405–411.

Richter, C. B. (1970). *In* "Morphology of Experimental Respiratory Carcinogenesis" (P. Nellesheim, M. G. Hanna, Jr., and J. W. Deatherage, Jr., eds.), AEC Symposium Series, No. 21, pp. 365–382. USAEC, Washington, D.C.

Rinaldo, C. R., Jr., Overall, J. C., Jr., Cole, B. C., and Glasgow, L. A. (1973). *Infect. Immun.* **8,** 796–803.

Rinaldo, C. R., Jr., Cole, B. C., Overall, J. C., Jr., Ward, J. R., and Glasgow, L. A. (1974). *Proc. Soc. Exp. Biol. Med.* **146,** 613–618.

Roberts, D. H. (1964). *Vet. Rec.* **76,** 470–473.

Robinson, L. B., Wichelhausen, R. H., and Roizman, B. (1956). *Science* **124,** 1147–1148.

Romano, N., and Brancato, P. (1970). *Arch. Gesamte Virusforsch.* **29,** 39–43.

Rosendal, S. (1973). *Acta Pathol. Microbiol. Scand., Sect. B* **81**, 411–445.

Rouse, H. C., and Schlesinger, R. W. (1967). *Virology* **33**, 513–522.

Rouse, H. C., Bonifas, V. H., and Schlesinger, R. W. (1963). *Virology* **20**, 357–365.

Ruckdeschel, J. C., Kramarsky, B., and Mardinev, M. R., Jr. (1975). *Cell. Immunol.* **20**, 110–116.

Russell, W. C., and Becker, Y. (1968). *Virology* **35**, 18–27.

Russell, W. C., Newman, C., and Williamson, D. H. (1975). *Nature (London)* **253**, 461–462.

Sabin, A. B. (1967). *Ann. N.Y. Acad. Sci.* **143**, 628–634.

Sato, S., Matsui, K., and Yoshimitsu, Y. (1965). *Natl. Inst. Anim. Health Qt.* **5**, 45–46.

Schiefer, H.-G., Gerhardt, U., Brunner, H., and Krüpe, M. (1974). *J. Bacteriol.* **120**, 81–88.

Schiefer, H.-G., Krauss, H., Brunner, H., and Gerhardt, U. (1975). *J. Bacteriol.* **124**, 1598–1600.

Schiefer, H.-G., Krauss, H., Brunner, H., and Gerhardt, U. (1976). *J. Bacteriol.* **127**, 461–468.

Schimke, R. T., and Barile, M. F. (1963a). *Exp. Cell Res.* **30**, 593–596.

Schimke, R. T., and Barile, M. F. (1963b). *J. Bacteriol.* **86**, 195–206.

Schmidt, P. J., Barile, M. F., and McGinniss, M. H. (1965). *Nature (London)* **205**, 371–372.

Schneider, E. L. (1975). *Methods Cell Biol.* **10**, 261–275.

Schneider, E. L., and Stanbridge, E. J. (1975a). *Methods Cell Biol.* **10**, 277–290.

Schnieder, E. L., and Stanbridge, E. J. (1975b). *In Vitro* **11**, 20–34.

Schneider, E. L., Epstein, C. J., Epstein, W. L., Betlach, M., and Abbo Halsbasch, G. (1973). *Exp. Cell Res.* **79**, 343–349.

Schneider, E. L., Stanbridge, E. J., and Epstein, C. J. (1974). *Exp. Cell Res.* **84**, 311–318.

Schütze, E., and Gericke, D. (1969). *Zentralbl. Bakteriol., Parasitenkd., Infektionskr., Hyg., Abt. 1: Orig.* **209**, 536–544.

Scriba, M. (1968). *Z. Med. Mikrobiol. Immunol.* **154**, 267–276.

Sethi, K. K. (1972). *Zentralbl. Bakteriol., Parasitenkd., Infektionskr., Hyg., Abt. 1: Orig., Reihe A* **219**, 550–554.

Shedden, W. I. H., and Cole, B. C. (1966). *J. Pathol. Bacteriol.* **92**, 574–576.

Shepard, M. C. (1967). *Ann. N.Y. Acad. Sci.* **143**, 505–514.

Simberkoff, M. S., Thornbeck, J. G., and Thomas, L. (1969). *J. Exp. Med.* **129**, 1163–1181.

Singer, S. H., Kirschstein, R. L., and Barile, M. F. (1969a). *Nature (London)* **222**, 1087–1088.

Singer, S. H., Barile, M. F., and Kirschstein, R. L. (1969b). *Proc. Soc. Exp. Biol. Med.* **131**, 1129–1134.

Singer, S. H., Fitzgerald, E, A., Barile, M. F., and Kirschstein, R. L. (1970). *Proc. Soc. Exp. Biol. Med.* **133**, 1439–1442.

Singer, S. H., Barile, M. F., and Kirschstein, R. L. (1973). *Ann. N.Y. Acad. Sci.* **225**, 304–310.

Smirnova, T. D., and Kagan, G. Y. (1971). *Zh. Microbiol., Epidemiol. Immunobiol.* **48**, 54–58.

Smith, C. B., McGinniss, M. H., and Schmidt, P. (1967). *J. Immunol.* **99**, 333–339.

Smith, H. (1977). *Bacteriol. Rev.* **41**, 475–500.

Smith, P. F., Langworthy, A., and Mayberry, W. R. (1976). *J. Bacteriol.* **125**, 916–922.

Sobeslavsky, O., Prescott, B., and Chanock, R. M. (1968). *J. Bacteriol.* **96**, 695–705.

Somerson, N. L., and Cook, M. K. (1965). *J. Bacteriol.* **90**, 534–540.

Somerson, N. L., Taylor-Robinson, D., and Chanock, R, M. (1963). *Am. J. Hyg.* **77**, 122–128.

Somerson, N. L., Walls, B. E., and Chanock, R. M. (1965a). *Science* **150**, 226–228.

Somerson, N. L., Purcell, R. H., Taylor-Robinson, D., and Chanock, R. M. (1965b). *J. Bacteriol.* **89,** 813–818.

Somerson, N. L., James, W. D., Walls, B. E., and Chanock, R. M. (1967). *Ann. N.Y. Acad. Sci.* **143,** 384–389.

Somerson, N. L., Senterfit, L. B., and Hamparian, V. V. (1973). *Ann. N.Y. Acad. Sci.* **225,** 425–435.

Spendlove, R. S., Crosbie, R. B., Hayes, S. F., and Keeler, R. F. (1971). *Proc. Soc. Exp. Biol. Med.* **137,** 258–263.

Spitler, L., Cochrum, K., and Fudenberg, H. H. (1968). *Science* **161,** 1148–1149.

Stanbridge, E. J. (1971). *Bacteriol. Rev.* **35,** 206–227.

Stanbridge, E. J., Onen, M., Perkins, F. T., and Hayflick, L. (1969). *Exp. Cell Res.* **57,** 397–410.

Stanbridge, E. J., Hayflick, L., and Perkins, F. T. (1971). *Nature (London)* **232,** 242–244.

Stanbridge, E. J., Tischfield, J. A., and Schneider, E. L. (1975). *Nature (London)* **256,** 329–331.

Stock, D. A., and Gentry, G. A. (1969). *J. Virol.* **3,** 313–317.

Studzinski, G. P., Gierthy, J. F., and Cholon, J. J. (1973). *In Vitro* **8,** 466–472.

Tankersley, R. W. (1964). *J. Bacteriol.* **87,** 609–613.

Taylor, G., Taylor-Robinson, D., and Fernald, G. W. (1974). *J. Med. Microbiol.* **7,** 343–348.

Taylor-Robinson, D. (1976). *Infection* **4,** Suppl. 1, 4–8.

Taylor-Robinson, D., and Manchee, R. J. (1967a). *Nature (London)* **215,** 484–487.

Taylor-Robinson, D., and Manchee, R. J. (1967b). *Nature (London)* **216,** 1306–1307.

Taylor-Robinson, D., and Manchee, R. J. (1967c). *J. Bacteriol.* **94,** 1781–1782.

Taylor-Robinson, D., Thomas, M., and Dawson, P. L. (1969). *J. Med. Microbiol.* **2,** 527–533.

Taylor-Robinson, D., Rassner, C., Furr, P. M., Humber, D. P., and Barnes, R. D. (1974). *In* "Les Mycoplasmes de l'Homme, des Animaux, des Vegetaux et des Insectes" (J. M. Bové and J. F. Duplan, eds.), Colloques INSERM, No. 33, pp. 325–330. INSERM, Paris.

Taylor-Robinson, D., Rassner, C., Furr, P. M., Humber, D. P., and Barnes, R. D. (1975). *J. Reprod. Fertil.* **42,** 483–490.

Thomas, L. (1964). *N. Engl. J. Med.* **270,** 1157–1159.

Thomas, L. (1969). The *Harvey Lect.* **63,** 73–98.

Thomas, L., Curnen, E. C., Mirick, G. S., Ziegler, J. E., and Horsfall, F. L. (1943). *Proc. Soc. Exp. Biol. Med.* **52,** 121–125.

Thomas, M. A., Shipman, C., Jr., Sandberg, J. N., and Drach, J. C. (1977). *In Vitro* **13,** 502–509.

Thornton, G. A., Wise, D. R., and Fuller, M. K. (1975). *Vet. Rec.* **96,** 113–114.

Todaro, G. J., Aaronson, S. A., and Rands, E. (1971). *Exp. Cell Res.* **65,** 256–257.

Tully, J. G., and Rask-Nielson, R. (1967). *Ann. N.Y. Acad. Sci.* **143,** 345–352.

Tully, J. G., and Razin, S. (1977). *In* "Handbook of Microbiology" (A. I. Laskin and H. A. Lechevalier, eds.), 2nd ed., Vol. 1, pp. 405–459. Chem. Rubber Publ. Co., Cleveland, Ohio.

Turner, J. C., Nisnewitz, S., Jackson, E. B., and Berney, R. (1943). *Lancet* **i,** 765–769.

Uppal, P. K., and Chu, H. P. (1977). *Res. Vet. Sci.* **22,** 259–260.

Van der Veen, J., and Heyen, C. F. A. (1966). *Am. J. Epidemiol.* **84,** 396–404.

Van Diggelen, O. P., Shin, S. I., and Phillips, D. M. (1977). *Cancer Res.* **37,** 2680–2687.

Van Herick, W., and Eaton, M. D. (1945). *J. Bacteriol.* **50,** 47–55.

Van Roy, F., and Fiers, W. (1977). *In Vitro* **13,** 357–365.

Vogel, G., and Shelokov, A. (1957). *Science* **126,** 358–359.

Michael F. Barile

Vogelzang, A. A., and Compeer-Dekker, G. (1969). *Antonie van Leeuwenhoek; J. Microbiol. Serol.* **35**, 393–408.
Vogelzang, A. A., and Van Klingeren, B. (1974). *Antonie van Leeuwenhoek; J. Microbiol. Serol.* **40**, 316–317.
Warren, J. (1942). *J. Bacteriol.* **43**, 211–228.
Washburn, L. R., and Somerson, N. L. (1977). *J. Clin. Microbiol.* **5**, 378–380.
Weickmann, J. L., and Fahrney, D. E. (1977). *J. Biol. Chem.* **252**, 2615–2620.
Wenzel, R. P., Craven, R. B., Davies, J. A., Hendley, J. O., Hamory, B. H., and Gwaltney, J. M., Jr. (1976). *J. Infect. Dis.* **134**, 571–576.
Wiebull, C., and Hammarberg, K. (1962). *J. Bacteriol.* **84**, 520–525.
Windsor, G. D., Thompson, G. W., and Baker, N. W. (1975). *Res. Vet. Sci.* **18**, 59–63.
Winters, A. L., and Consigli, R. A. (1971). *J. Gen. Virol.* **10**, 53–63.
Wise, K. S., Cassell, G. H., and Acton, R. T. (1978). *Proc. Natl. Acad. Sci. U.S.A.* **75**, 4479–4483.
Yershov, F. I., and Zhdanov, V. M. (1965). *Virology* **27**, 451–453.
Zgorniak-Nowosielska, I., Sedwick, W. D., Hummeler, K., and Koprowski, H. (1967). *J. Virol.* **1**, 1227–1237.
Zucker-Franklin, D., Davidson, M., and Thomas, L. (1966a). *J. Exp. Med.* **124**, 521–532.
Zucker-Franklin, D., Davidson, M., and Thomas, L. (1966b). *J. Exp. Med.* **124**, 533–542.

14 / MYCOPLASMAS IN ORGAN CULTURE

Albert M. Collier

I. INTRODUCTION

The utilization of undifferentiated cell culture lines for the study of alterations produced by infecting microbial agents is well known. However, cell culture lines may or may not retain the characteristics of differentiated host cells. The use of organ culture to provide differentiated cells for examination of the microbial agent–host cell interaction has only recently been exploited. Organ culture permits the maintenance of complete rudiments or fragments of organs in a viable, differentiated,

THE MYCOPLASMAS, VOL. II
Copyright © 1979 by Academic Press, Inc.
All rights of reproduction in any form reserved.
ISBN 0-12-078401-7

functional condition in a nutrient medium *in vitro*. The technique of organ culture was first introduced in the late 1800s and has been instrumental in the advancement of knowledge in the areas of embryology, endocrinology, pharmacology, genetics, carcinogenesis, and infectious diseases (Hodges, 1976).

The employment of organ culture to study the effects of infectious agents on host tissue was begun in 1957 (Barski *et al.*, 1957). Hoorn (1966) used organ cultures to examine the effects of respiratory viruses on tracheal epithelium. Butler (1969) in England and Collier *et al.* (1969) in the United States first examined the effects of mycoplasmas on respiratory epithelium in tracheal organ culture. Since these first reports many mycoplasma species have been studied in organ cultures of many different host tissues. Tracheal organ cultures of various animal sources have proved particularly useful in studying the pathogenesis of respiratory mycoplasma infections.

Most mycoplasma species are extracellular pathogens that have as their target cells the epithelium lining mucosal surfaces. Organ cultures permit the maintenance of organized mucosal surfaces *in vitro* and thus allow direct observation of the interaction of mycoplasmas with these target cells and the injury produced. Organ culture studies have provided information that could not have been obtained from *in vivo* animal experiments; however, isolated tissue explants cannot provide any information on the systemic effect produced by the infectious agent.

For studies utilizing organ culture to be meaningful at least two criteria must be met. First, the cultured host tissue must be able to be maintained in a state of normal structure and functional activity throughout the duration of the experiment. Second, the response to the infectious agent of the cultured tissue *in vitro* must be substantially the same as the response of the target tissue in the natural disease *in vivo* (Fell, 1976).

II. METHODS OF ORGAN CULTURE PREPARATION AND MAINTENANCE

Organ cultures have been prepared from several organs for the study of mycoplasmas; however, trachea and fallopian tube tissue has been used most extensively. The tissues used have been obtained from humans and many different animal species. Several techniques have been described for establishing organ cultures, but the aim of all techniques is to transfer tissue from its *in vivo* location to the *in vitro* culture with the least trauma possible.

Rather than review all the different techniques that have been reported, we briefly describe the preparation of hamster tracheal organ cultures, a representative model which has been most extensively used for studying mycoplasma disease pathogenesis. This should at least give the reader who has had no experience with organ cultures an idea of what is involved in their preparation and maintenance. A more detailed description may be found in the Tissue Culture Association Manual (Collier, 1976).

Adult hamsters are anesthetized intraperitoneally with sodium pentobarbital, and enough blood removed from the heart to place the animal in shock. Under aseptic conditions the anterior neck is incised, and the trachea removed from just below the larynx down to the carina. The trachea is then placed in medium, and tracheal rings prepared by slicing between each cartilage ring. The rings are placed on small areas of crosshatch scratches on the bottom of a petri dish, and the medium to be used is added to a depth to just cover the tissue (Fig. 1). The dish is then placed in a 37°C incubator with a 5% carbon dioxide atmosphere.

The main variation in the above-described method for preparing tissue for organ culture has been to open the tubular trachea or fallopian tube longitudinally, exposing the inner ciliated surface. Small squares are then cut and placed in the bottom of a petri dish. The organ culture fragments can also be placed in closed tissue culture tubes. The tubes are then

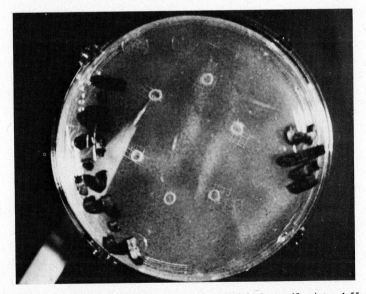

FIGURE 1.   Hamster tracheal organ culture system. Original magnification ×1.55. (From Collier and Baseman, 1973; reproduced by permission.)

incubated on a roller drum rotating at about 15 revolutions per hour (Reed, 1976).

For comparative studies the rings or fragments, consisting of tissue with the same genetic makeup, can be divided into separate dishes or tubes for control and infection. The culture of the particular mycoplasma species to be tested is then added to the culture vessels to be infected.

The types of media used in organ culture experiments have varied. The two main variations have been medium that supports growth of the mycoplasma species tested in the absence of the organ culture tissue, and medium that does not support growth of the mycoplasma species tested, requiring a nutrient or nutrients to be supplied by the organ culture tissue.

III. TECHNIQUES FOR MONITORING THE PHYSIOLOGICAL STATE OF MUCOSAL EPITHELIUM IN ORGAN CULTURE

A. Ciliary Activity

Both the trachea and the fallopian tube are lined with ciliated epithelium. The character and frequency of the ciliary beat of the ciliated epithelium in the culture vessel can be observed by microscopy at 100× magnification. When the rings of tissue are observed, the cilia can be seen by transmitted light; however, reflected light must be used for examination of ciliary activity in fragments of tissue. Ciliary activity has been shown to correlate with tissue viability and has been used as an indicator of injury. In studies with organ culture models ciliary activity has been quantitated as present or absent (Collier *et al.*, 1969), as the vigor of ciliary beating and the percentage of tissue surface with ciliary activity present (Cherry and Taylor-Robinson, 1970a), and as the frequency of ciliary activity measured by a stroboscope (Collier and Baseman, 1973).

B. Histology

1. Light Microscopy

The histopathological examination of fixed tissue from organ culture has been the most frequently used method to assess tissue injury. Tissue is removed from the culture vessel, fixed in an appropriate fixative, and embedded in paraffin, and sections cut. The sections are then stained and examined with the light microscope (Collier *et al.*, 1969). Most histopathological techniques available may be applied to organ culture material.

2. Immunofluorescence Microscopy

Immunofluorescence microscopy has been utilized to examine the relationship of mycoplasmal organisms to the tissue in organ culture. The tissue rings or fragments are removed from the culture vessel and quick-frozen in O.C.T. compound (Ames Company, Elkhart, Indiana), and 4-μm sections are prepared using a microtome cryostat. The sections are then exposed to rabbit antiserum against the mycoplasma species, followed by goat anti-rabbit globulin conjugated with fluorescein isothiocyanate. The sections are then examined using a fluorescence microscope (Collier *et al.*, 1971). The immunological specificity of this method provides precise localization of the organisms, which cannot be done with certainty using purely morphological methods.

3. Electron Microscopy

Because mycoplasmas are smaller than some of the larger viruses and are below the resolving limits of the light microscope, the electron microscope has been utilized to examine the relationship of individual organisms to the host tissue.

a. Transmission electron microscopy. Tissue to be examined by transmission electron microscopy is fixed with glutaraldehyde and osmium tetroxide, dehydrated in ethanol, and embedded in Epon 812. Thin sections are cut and stained with uranyl acetate and lead citrate, followed by examination in a transmission electron microscope (Wilson and Collier, 1976). Transmission electron microscopy of thin sections permits study of the internal ultrastructure of both organism and host cell but has the limitation of allowing only small areas of the sample to be thoroughly examined.

b. Scanning electron microscopy. Tissue for scanning electron microscope examination is fixed as above and then dehydrated through graded ethanol into Freon 113 and dried by the Freon 13 critical-point procedure. The dried specimens are then coated with gold in a sputter coater and examined in a scanning electron microscope (Muse *et al.*, 1976). This technique permits a large surface area to be examined but with less resolution than transmission electron microscopy. Scanning electron microscopy allows examination only of external surfaces.

C. Metabolic Activity

In order to gain information about the metabolic activity of the individual organized cells in tracheal ring organ cultures, Collier and Baseman (1973) examined hamster tracheal rings exposed to [^{3}H]amino acids and

[^{3}H]thymidine by radioautography. In studies utilizing radioisotopically labeled carbohydrate, protein, and nucleic acid precursors, Hu *et al.* (1975, 1976) examined alterations in hamster tracheal ring metabolism produced by *Mycoplasma pneumoniae* infection. The effects of *M. pneumoniae* infection on hamster tracheal rings have also been examined with respect to the kinetics of cellular respiration (Gabridge, 1975), gross oxygen uptake (Gabridge, 1976), dehydrogenase activity (Gabridge and Polisky, 1976), and ATP content (Gabridge and Polisky, 1977). The ability of erythromycin treatment of *M. pneumoniae*-infected hamster tracheal rings to prevent abnormalities in nucleic acid synthesis has also been studied (Hu *et al.*, 1975).

There is limited information on the metabolism of normal differentiated cells, and the organ culture model provides a tool that permits application of techniques that have been utilized for metabolic studies of cell culture systems with appropriate modifications. These metabolic techniques allow one to measure pathophysiological changes occurring at the molecular level of the host cells, and the organ culture system also permits correlation of metabolic changes with morphological changes.

IV. HUMAN ORGAN CULTURES INFECTED WITH MYCOPLASMAS

Tracheal tissue from human fetuses (16–24 weeks' gestation) has been infected with several mycoplasma species. This model was employed by Butler (1969) and Butler and Ellaway (1971) to examine the growth and cytopathogenicity of *Mycoplasma hominis, M. orale, M. salivarium, M. pneumoniae, Ureaplasma urealyticum, M. mycoides* subsp. *capri, M. mycoides* subsp. *mycoides, M. agalactiae, M. gallisepticum,* and *M. synoviae.* Growth of each mycoplasma species was demonstrated, except for *U. urealyticum* and *M. mycoides* subsp. *mycoides.* In these studies, Butler found that *M. mycoides* subsp. *capri* produced cessation of ciliary activity and epithelial cell damage. There were also changes in the cartilage cells. In one report by Butler (1969). *M. pneumoniae* inoculated at high titer ($10^{5.7}$ colony forming units/ml) produced damage similar to that induced by *M. mycoides* subsp. *capri*, but *M. pneumoniae* organisms could not be recovered from the culture at the end of the experiment. None of the other mycoplasma species tested produced cytopathology.

The interaction between mycoplasma species indigenous to humans (*Mycoplasma pneumoniae, M. hominis, M. fermentans, M. salivarium,* and *M. orale*) and human fetal trachea in organ culture has been studied by Collier and Clyde (1971) and Collier (1972). With *M. pneumoniae* infection there was impairment of cellular function reflected by ciliostasis and a sequence of cytopathological changes. There was epithelial cytoplasmic vacuolization and nuclear swelling with loss of cilia. By immunofluorescence and electron microscopy the *M. pneumoniae* organisms were found to be concentrated on the lumenal surface of the epithelium in an extracellular position. The organisms were filamentous in shape and attached to the epithelial cells by a specialized terminal structure which consisted of a fibrillar electron-dense central core surrounded by a lucent space enveloped by an extension of the unit membrane of the organism. There was intimate contact between the *M. pneumoniae* cell membrane and the membrane of the host cell, but no membrane fusion was seen (Fig. 2). An avirulent *M. pneumoniae* mutant that no longer retained the ability to attach to the epithelial cells produced no cytopathology, although it grew to high titers in the organ culture dish. No cytopathological changes were seen in human fetal tracheal organ cultures inoculated with *M. hominis, M. fermentans, M. salivarium,* or *M. orale*.

The effects of *M. mycoides* subsp. *capri* and *M. mycoides* subsp. *mycoides* on several human tissues in organ culture—trachea, nose, synovium, and oviduct—were examined by Cherry and Taylor-Robinson (1973). *Mycoplasma mycoides* subsp. *mycoides* was found to be more

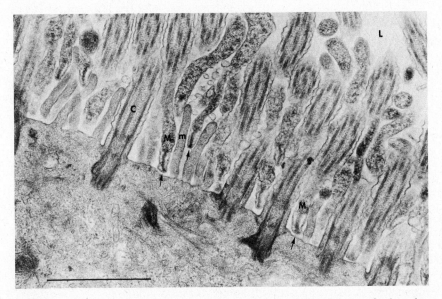

FIGURE 2.   Electron photomicrograph of *M. pneumoniae*-infected human fetal trachea after 48 hr in organ culture. M, Mycoplasma; C, cilia; m, microvilli; L, lumen; tip attachment structure (arrows). Original magnification ×43,000. Bar = 1 μm.

fastidious as far as growth in the organ cultures but was less damaging than *M. mycoides* subsp. *capri*. The effects of mycoplasmas on human fallopian tube organ cultures were studied by Taylor-Robinson and Carney (1974). *Mycoplasma orale,* a genital strain of *M. hominis,* oral and genital strains of ureaplasmas of human origin, ureaplasmas of simian and bovine origin, and *M. hyorhinis* of porcine origin were examined. None of these mycoplasma species produced ciliostasis or histopathological changes.

V. HAMSTER ORGAN CULTURES INFECTED WITH MYCOPLASMAS

Mycoplasmas were first studied in hamster tracheal organ culture by Collier *et al*. (1969). *Mycoplasma pneumoniae* produced cytopathology in this model system, consisting of ciliostasis and epithelial cell damage. The injury produced was dose-dependent, and a virulent *M. pneumoniae* strain produced tissue damage more effectively than an attenuated strain. Other human mycoplasma strains tested—*M. fermentans, M. hominis, M. orale,* and *M. salivarium*—did not produce ciliostasis or cytopathology in hamster tracheal organ culture.

The intimate association of *M. pneumoniae* and the lumenal aspect of the epithelium lining the trachea has been demonstrated by immunofluorescence and electron microscopy (Collier *et al.*, 1971). As in studies on human fetal tracheal organ culture, *M. pneumoniae* attached to the differentiated epithelial cells by the organism's specialized terminal structure. Attachment of the organisms to the ciliated cell was followed by a slowing of ciliary activity and eventual ciliostasis which could be measured by using a calibrated variable stroboscope (Fig. 3). The cytopathology following attachment of the infecting organisms consisted of ciliocytophthoria and eventual sloughing of the epithelial layer (Fig. 4). The attachment of *M. pneumoniae* to the epithelial cell could be blocked by prior treatment of the mammalian cells by neuraminidase (Collier and Baseman, 1973). At no time were *M. pneumoniae* organisms seen within cells.

Muse *et al*. (1976) examined the three-dimensional aspects of the surface parasitism of *M. pneumoniae* on the mucosal surface of hamster tracheal organ culture. These studies demonstrated the filamentous morphology of the *M. pneumoniae* organism and the attachment of numerous organisms to individual cells followed by cytopathology.

In order to examine the biochemical basis of alterations in epithelial host cells produced by *M. pneumoniae,* an assessment of carbohydrate,

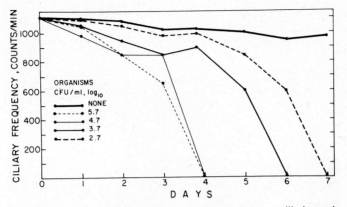

FIGURE 3. Effect of varying *M. pneumoniae* inocula on hamster cilia in tracheal organ culture. Ciliary beat frequency of tracheal rings was measured at intervals with a calibrated stroboscope. (From Collier and Baseman, 1973; reproduced by permission.)

protein, and nucleic acid metabolism was performed by Hu *et al.* (1975, 1976). In these studies precursors of carbohydrate (^{14}C-labeled galactose) and RNA (^{14}C-labeled orotic acid) synthesis which could be utilized by the mammalian cells but not by the mycoplasma were employed. Protein synthesis was examined by treating the infected rings after periods of infection with erythromycin to stop protein synthesis by the mycoplasma and then measuring the uptake and incorporation of ^{14}C-labeled amino acids by the mammalian cells. In these experiments a decline in protein and RNA synthesis was demonstrated within 24 hr after the initiation of *M. pneumoniae* infection of the tracheal rings, which preceded any histological change in the tissue. At that time the uptake of carbohydrate, protein, and nucleic acid precursors was similar to that of control rings and did not decrease until later in infection, paralleling the appearance of histological changes. From these studies these workers proposed that the primary effect of mycoplasma infection on tracheal organ cultures might be at a transcriptional or translational level.

Hu *et al.* (1975) presented evidence that *M. pneumoniae* organisms not only needed to attach to the epithelial cells to produce injury but that the organism must be metabolically active. The course of mycoplasma infection could be interrupted or reversed by erythromycin after the initial mycoplasma–host cell interaction. The addition of erythromycin 24 hr or earlier after infection prevented the onset of abnormal orotic acid uptake and subsequent cytopathology. However, 48 hr after infection, rescue of host cells by erythromycin did not occur, and pathological changes became evident.

Gabridge *et al.* (1974) reported that *M. pneumoniae* membranes inocu-

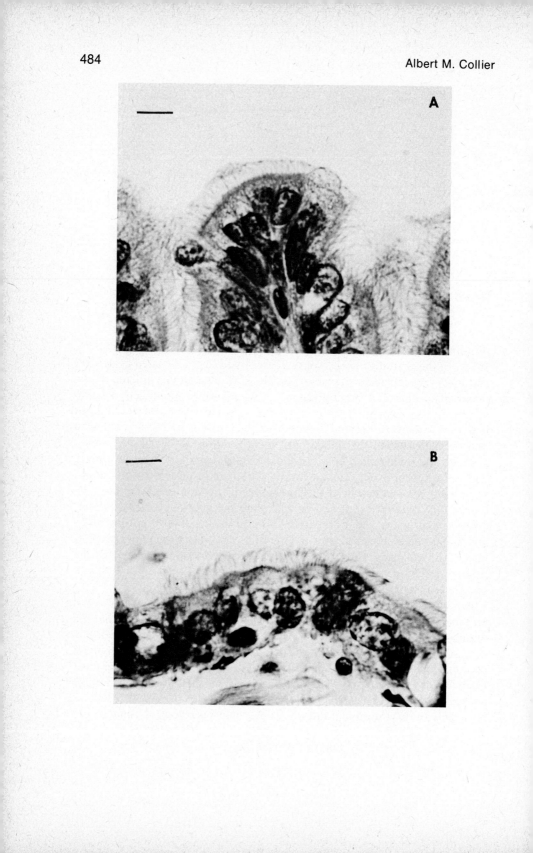

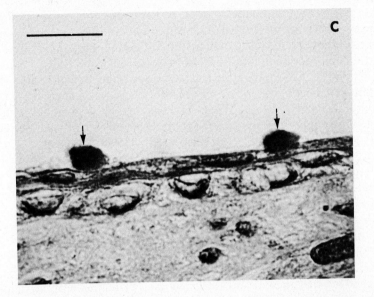

FIGURE 4. Organ culture of hamster trachea (hematoxylin and eosin). (A) Uninfected ciliated epithelium maintained in organ culture for 48 hr. Original magnification ×1000. Bar = 10 μm. (B) Trachea infected with *M. pneumoniae* for 48 hr. The epithelium shows nuclear swelling with chromatin margination, cytoplasmic vacuolization, and loss of cilia from some epithelial cells. Original magnification ×1000. Bar = 10 μm. (C) Trachea infected by *M. pneumoniae* for 96 hr in organ culture. The ciliated epithelium has been lost, and micro-colonies of mycoplasma (arrows) are seen on the remaining basal cells of the epithelial layer. Original magnification ×2100. Bar = 10 μm. (From Collier and Baseman, 1973; reproduced by permission.)

lated into hamster tracheal organ cultures produced ciliostasis and epithelial cell cytopathology. These findings lack confirmation by Hu *et al.* (1976). A more recent study by Gabridge *et al.* (1977a) reported that the mechanism of attachment of *M. pneumoniae* membranes was different from the sialic acid receptor site-mediated attachment of viable *M. pneumoniae* cells. This implies that the injury produced by the membrane preparation involved a mechanism different from that produced by the viable infecting organism in natural disease.

Gabridge (1975) demonstrated that hamster tracheas consumed measurable amounts of oxygen when incubated in a microchamber. In these studies *M. pneumoniae*-infected hamster tracheal rings utilized decreasing amounts of oxygen, which was dose-dependent with respect to the number of infecting organisms, in comparison to uninfected control rings. In 1976 Gabridge published studies showing that, when hamster tracheal organ cultures were infected with *M. pneumoniae,* there was significantly reduced ciliary activity, oxygen consumption, and tetrazolium reduction capacity; these studies also demonstrated that the three parameters were reduced in a coordinated fashion. In 1977 Gabridge and Polisky measured the amount of ATP in hamster tracheal rings. They demonstrated that in rings infected with virulent *M. pneumoniae* there was a decrease in ciliary activity and ATP content. When tracheal rings were infected with non-virulent mycoplasmas, the ciliary activity was only slightly decreased and ATP values rose slightly. Gabridge *et al.* (1977b) presented scanning electron microscope evidence that there were large patches of unciliated cells on the ventral surface of the trachea, especially in the middle third. The greatest attachment of tritium-labeled *M. pneumoniae* organisms was in these less ciliated areas.

The attachment of tritium-labeled *M. pneumoniae* organisms to ham-ster tracheal rings in organ culture has also been examined by Powell *et al.* (1976) using radioautography and liquid scintillation counting. With these techniques they demonstrated that virulent *M. pneumoniae* organisms attached but that an avirulent strain did not. Pretreatment of the rings with neuraminidase or sodium periodate decreased organism attachment.

The chemical nature of *M. pneumoniae* surfaces responsible for at-tachment has been unknown. However, Hu *et al.* (1977) utilized hamster tracheal organ cultures to demonstrate that virulent *M. pneumoniae* or-ganisms must possess a surface protein in order to attach to the respira-tory mucosa. This protein is trypsin-sensitive and, when the *M. pneumo-niae* organism is treated with a protease, attachment does not occur. After incubating the treated organisms in mycoplasma medium the protein is regenerated and the ability to attach returns.

The orientation of individual *M. pneumoniae* organisms when they attach to the epithelial surface of hamster tracheal organ cultures has been utilized by Wilson and Collier (1976) in ultrastructural chemical studies. Because *M. pneumoniae* attach by a specialized terminal structure, when thin sections of the lumenal border of infected tracheal rings are exam-ined, a large number of the attachment organelles can be visualized. By utilizing specialized electron microscope staining techniques the central core of the tip structure was shown to contain basic proteins. The *M. pneumoniae* organism was also shown to possess an extracellular muco-protein layer that was particularly concentrated in the area of the terminal structure.

Woodruff *et al.* (1973) examined the ultrastructural changes in hamster tracheal ring cultures infected with *M. pneumoniae.* They reported cytopathic mucosal changes and submucosal necrosis, along with the presence of submucosal macrophages that contained increased numbers of lysosomes and mycoplasma-like forms. No typical *M. pneumoniae* organisms as described above were demonstrated in this study.

VI. CHICKEN ORGAN CULTURES INFECTED WITH MYCOPLASMAS

A technique for the preparation and maintenance of chicken embryo tracheal organ cultures was first described by Cherry and Taylor-Robinson (1970a). The spectrum of growth and cilia-stopping effect of approximately 60 mycoplasma strains have now been studied in the chicken tracheal organ culture system (Cherry and Taylor-Robinson, 1970a,b,c, 1971, 1973; Taylor-Robinson and Cherry, 1972; Butler and Ellaway, 1971). In this model *Mycoplasma gallisepticum*, *M. mycoides* subsp. *capri*, *M. mycoides* subsp. *mycoides*, *M. pneumoniae*, *M. pulmonis*, *M. neurolyticum*, *M. hyorhinis*, *M. meleagridis*, and *M. agalactiae* adversely affected ciliary activity. However, *Mycoplasma gallinarum* possessed the ability to prolong the presence of ciliary activity in the chicken embryo tracheal organ culture compared to the uninfected control cultures.

In studies utilizing the chicken embryo tracheal organ culture system to delineate pathogenic factors of mycoplasma, Cherry and Taylor-Robinson (1970b,c) provided evidence suggesting that peroxide liberation but not cytoadsorption was an important virulence factor in *M. mycoides* subsp. *capri* infections. When *M. gallisepticum* was examined for virulence factors, neither cytoadsorption nor peroxide production appeared to play a role. However, a toxic substance other than peroxide was found in the medium of *M. gallisepticum*-infected organ cultures (Cherry and Taylor-Robinson, 1971). In the study of mixed mycoplasma infections in chicken embryo tracheal organ cultures, Taylor-Robinson and Cherry (1972) noted that the injury produced by *M. gallisepticum* could be prevented by prior infection of the organ culture with a nonpathogenic mycoplasma, *M. gallinarum*.

VII. BOVINE ORGAN CULTURES INFECTED WITH MYCOPLASMAS

The first studies involving mycoplasmas in bovine organ culture were made by Reed (1971). She examined the interaction of *M. hyorhinis* and swine influenza virus in bovine tracheal organ cultures. In this system the titers of virus were not altered by the presence of infection with *M.*

hyorhinis, nor was growth of the mycoplasma enhanced in bovine tracheal rings that had been infected with the virus. Reed also examined a bovine tracheal organ culture infected with a bovine ureaplasma and swine influenza virus. No evidence of interaction was seen. No cytopathology was produced by either *M. hyorhinis* or the ureaplasma in the bovine organ culture. Reed (1972a,b, 1976) also presented evidence that prior infection of bovine tracheal organ cultures with rhinovirus or parainfluenza virus—in contrast to swine influenza virus—enhanced the growth of *M. hyorhinis* by damaging the epithelium and releasing conditioning factors into the medium. *Mycoplasma hyorhinis* was found to associate more readily with the epithelium of rhinovirus-infected cultures than with normal cultures. Rhinovirus also enhanced the growth of *M. hominis* and *M. salivarium* in the bovine tracheal organ culture system.

Cherry and Taylor-Robinson (1973) examined the growth and cilia-stopping effect of *M. mycoides* subsp. *capri* and *M. mycoides* subsp. *mycoides* in bovine organ cultures. *Mycoplasma mycoides* subsp. *capri* grew in bovine embryo tracheal organ culture and produced ciliostasis. *Mycoplasma mycoides* subsp. *mycoides* grew in both bovine embryo tracheal and lung organ cultures but produced ciliostasis in only one out of five bovine tracheal organ cultures.

Thomas and Howard (1974) studied the effects of *Mycoplasma dispar, M. bovirhinis, Acholeplasma laidlawii,* and ureaplasmas on bovine tracheal organ cultures. Only *M. dispar* produced ciliostasis and epithelial destruction. Howard and Thomas (1974) presented evidence that the injury produced by *M. dispar* in bovine tracheal organ culture was dependent on the presence of serum in the organ culture medium.

Stalheim and Gallagher (1975) inoculated bovine uterine tube (oviduct) and fimbriae in organ culture with *M. bovis (M. agalactiae* subsp. *bovis), M. bovirhinis,* and *M. pneumoniae* strains FH and 1428. Of this group only *M. pneumoniae* strain 1428 inhibited ciliary activity. In a later study Stalheim *et al.* (1976) examined bovine uterine tube and fimbriae organ culture inoculated with ureaplasma strains P108, VMRI, 96, 5, 7139, and 7147. Each of the strains of ureaplasmas multiplied in the organ culture, stopped ciliary activity, and caused histological lesions. Ciliostasis was also produced by the addition of nonviable and disrupted ureaplasma cells to the organ cultures. The histological changes observed were collapse and sloughing of cilia with later epithelial disorganization, necrosis, and desquamation. Stalheim and Gallagher (1977) demonstrated the above pathophysiologic epithelial changes could be produced, without infection, by adding ammonia to the organ culture medium and by hydrolysis of urea in the medium with the addition of urease.

VIII. PORCINE ORGAN CULTURES INFECTED WITH MYCOPLASMAS

Studies of the effects of mycoplasma on porcine organ cultures were made by Reed (1971, 1972a,b, 1976). In these experiments *M. hyorhinis* produced minimal histopathological changes in the epithelium. She also reported that swine influenza virus infection of the porcine tracheal organ culture produced moderate epithelial damage. When a double infection of these agents, *M. hyorhinis* and swine influenza, was examined, there was increased destruction of the respiratory epithelium when compared to that of either agent separately. In the dual infection, the titer of virus remained the same, but growth of the mycoplasma was enhanced. The enhancement of *M. hyorhinis* growth was less prominent in porcine tracheal organ cultures infected with influenza A/WS strain virus.

Pijoan *et al*. (1972) assessed the pathogenicity of *Mycoplasma hyopneumoniae*, *M. hyorhinis*, *Acholeplasma granularum*, and *M. hyosynoviae* in porcine tracheal organ cultures. In these studies *M. hyorhinis* produced the most marked effect on ciliary activity and caused necrosis of the epithelium. *Acholeplasma granularum* and *M. hyosynoviae* produced a decrease in ciliary activity but no epithelial necrosis. Organ cultures infected with *M. hyopneumoniae* survived longer than the control cultures.

IX. MOUSE ORGAN CULTURES INFECTED WITH MYCOPLASMAS

Only a limited number of mycoplasmas have been studied in mouse tracheal organ culture. Westerberg *et al*. (1972) examined the effects of *M. pulmonis* in this system alone and in combination with influenza A/PR-8 virus. When *M. pulmonis*-infected mouse tracheal organ cultures were observed, there was inhibition of ciliary activity and histological epithelial damage. Influenza A/PR-8 replicated in the mouse tracheal organ culture and also produced inhibition of ciliary activity and tissue damage. When there was simultaneous infection by both *M. pulmonis* and influenza A/PR-8, there was more rapid inactivation of ciliary activity and greater tissue damage than that occurring with either agent alone. These investigators noted that the presence of the virus had no effect on growth of the mycoplasma; however, the mycoplasma produced a decrease in titer of the virus. Cherry and Taylor-Robinson (1973) infected mouse tracheal organ cultures with *M. mycoides* subsp. *capri* and observed ciliostasis.

X. CONCLUSIONS AND FUTURE OUTLOOK

From the preceding review of mycoplasma-infected organ cultures it is apparent that a wide range of studies has been made: These involve approximately 107 mycoplasma species or strains and 10 different tissues from 6 host species. The organ culture model system is now a well-established and accepted method for the study of mycoplasma disease pathogenesis. Because most mycoplasma species are extracellular parasites and attach to mucosal surfaces without entering the host cells, the ability to maintain organized, differentiated host cells *in vitro* to examine this interaction has proved exceedingly useful. Examples are:

1.   The organ culture model permits the use of tissue from the same animal, with identical genetic makeup, for control and test groups.

2.   The direct pathogenicity of the mycoplasma species for the host cell can be studied in the absence of the host immune and nonspecific host defense mechanisms.

3.   The tissue in the organ culture can be infected with a known number of a cloned mycoplasma species and maintained in a sterile environment, thus avoiding secondary invaders that are so common in animal experiments.

4.   By being able to infect small segments of mucosa with mycoplasma species, the interaction of the individual mycoplasmal organisms and host cells can be located using the electron microscope. This has permitted the investigator to see that the parasitic forms of certain mycoplasma species are not amorphous but have a recognizable shape and that some have attachment organelles.

5.   Organ culture studies provide evidence that certain mycoplasma species are able to injure specialized host cells by an extracellular attachment without evidence of the organisms entering the cell.

6.   The organ culture model permits sequential experiments utilizing isotopically labeled protein, carbohydrate, and nucleic acid precursors to delineate the level of metabolic injury in the host cell infected with mycoplasmas; this can be correlated with morphological and radioautographic changes in the organized tissue.

7.   The interrelationships of mycoplasmas and other microorganisms can be studied in organ cultures in order to gain information on synergism and antagonism between organism pairs.

As stated in Section I, for organ culture studies to be meaningful the cultured host tissue must be maintained in a state approximating normal structure and functional activity throughout the duration of the experiment. A large number of environmental factors must be evaluated carefully and controlled. Temperature, atmosphere, medium composition, and culture mode all may be critical for successful results with the particular tissue being used. There is no question that this may require more expertise than is needed to maintain an undifferentiated cell culture line. Therefore it is imperative for anyone wishing to become involved in organ culture work to take a basic course at a recognized center or to spend some time in an established organ culture laboratory.

During the past 10 years experiments with mycoplasmas in organ culture have demonstrated that this model system has a role to play in our understanding of mycoplasmal disease pathogenesis. As mentioned earlier, the response to the infectious agent of the cultured tissue in organ culture must be substantially the same as the response of the host tissue in the natural disease *in vivo*. In the case of *M. pneumoniae* in hamster and human tracheal organ culture, the close similarity between the interaction of this mycoplasma species with the host tissue *in vivo* and the host cell injury pattern has been demonstrated by Collier and Clyde (1974). In their studies on lungs from *M. pneumoniae*-infected hamsters and sputum from patients with natural *M. pneumoniae* disease, the parasite–host cell relationships were very similar.

In the future the ability to maintain differentiated, organized host target cells in organ culture will be further exploited to gain information on how mycoplasmas produce disease and the processes of tissue repair and protection. Because organ cultures have no blood supply and are devoid of the cells and products that the systemic circulation provide, this model should be ideal for reconstitution experiments in which the independent or combined roles of various host defense mediators (surface or humoral antibodies, immune cells, phagocytes) can be examined. Effects of hormones, pharmacological mediators, and antimicrobial agents are studied readily using the *in vitro* system provided by organ cultures. The organ culture model also should prove useful in assessing any portions of mycoplasmas or products of mycoplasmas isolated in the future. There is a particular need to develop methods which would permit one to free attached mycoplasma species from the host cell without injury, in order to establish by isotope studies whether or not attached extracellular mycoplasma species are truly parasites, competing with or depriving the more sophisticated host cells of needed metabolites with injurious consequences.

By combining the information obtained in the study of mycoplasma disease at the organ culture, experimental animal, and natural disease level, we should provide the best possible chance to gain the information needed to understand the mechanisms by which these most interesting prokaryotes produce disease.

REFERENCES

Barski, G., Nourilsky, R., and Cornefert, F. (1957). *Proc. Soc. Exp. Biol. Med.* **96,** 386–391.
Butler, M. (1969). *Nature (London)* **224,** 605–606.
Butler, M., and Ellaway, W. J. (1971). *J. Comp. Pathol* **31,** 359–364.
Cherry, J. D., and Taylor-Robinson, D. (1970a). *Appl. Microbiol.* **19,** 658–662.
Cherry, J. D., and Taylor-Robinson, D. (1970b). *Nature (London)* **228,** 1099–1100.
Cherry, J. D., and Taylor-Robinson, D. (1970c). *Infect. Immun.* **2,** 431–438.
Cherry, J. D., and Taylor-Robinson, D. (1971). *J. Med. Microbiol.* **4,** 441–449.
Cherry, J. D., and Taylor-Robinson, D. (1973). *Ann. N.Y. Acad. Sci.* **225,** 290–303.
Collier, A. M. (1972). *In* "Pathogenic Mycoplasmas. CIBA Foundation Symposium" (K. Elliot and J. Birch, eds.), pp. 307–327. Associated Scientific Publishers, Amsterdam.
Collier, A. M. (1976). *Tissue Cult. Assoc. Man.* **2,** 333–334.
Collier, A. M., and Baseman, J. B. (1973). *Ann. N.Y. Acad. Sci.* **225,** 277–289.
Collier, A. M., and Clyde, W. A. (1971). *Infect. Immun.* **3,** 694–701.
Collier, A. M., and Clyde, W. A. (1974). *Am. Rev. Respir. Dis.* **110,** 765–773.
Collier, A. M., Clyde, W. A., and Denny, F. W. (1969). *Proc. Soc. Exp. Biol. Med.* **132,** 1153–1158.
Collier, A. M., Clyde, W. A., and Denny, F. W. (1971). *Proc. Soc. Exp. Biol. Med.* **136,** 569–573.
Fell, H. B. (1976). *In* "Organ Culture in Biomedical Research" (M. Balls and M. Monnickendam, eds.), pp. 1–13, Cambridge Univ. Press, London and New York.
Gabridge, M. G. (1975). *Infect. Immun.* **12,** 544–549.
Gabridge, M. G. (1976). *J. Clin. Microbiol.* **3,** 560–565.
Gabridge, M. G., and Polisky, R. B. (1976). *Infect. Immun.* **13,** 84–91.
Gabridge, M. G., and Polisky, R. B. (1977). *In Vitro* **13,** 510–516.
Gabridge, M. G., Johnson, C. M., and Cameron, A. M. (1974). *Infect. Immun.* **10,** 1127–1134.
Gabridge, M. G., Barden-Stahl, J. D., Polisky, R. B., and Engelhardt, J. A. (1977a). *Infect. Immun.* **16,** 766–772.
Gabridge, M. G., Coe Agee, C., and Cameron, A. M. (1977b). *J. Infect. Dis.* **135,** 9–19.
Hodges, G. M. (1976). *In* "Organ Cultures in Biomedical Research" (M. Balls and M. Monnickendam, eds.), pp. 15–59. Cambridge Univ. Press, London and New York.
Hoorn, B. (1966). *Acta Pathol. Microbiol. Scand.,* Suppl. No. 183, 1–37.
Howard, C. J., and Thomas, L. H. (1974). *Infect. Immun.* **10,** 405–408.
Hu, P. C., Collier, A. M., and Baseman, J. B. (1975). *Infect. Immun.* **11,** 704–710.
Hu, P. C., Collier, A. M., and Baseman, J. B. (1976). *Infect. Immun.* **14,** 217–224.
Hu, P. C., Collier, A. M., and Baseman, J. B. (1977). *J. Exp. Med.* **145,** 1328–1343.
Muse, K. E., Powell, D. A., and Collier, A. M. (1976). *Infect. Immun.* **13,** 229–237.
Pijoan, C., Roberts, D. H., and Harding, J. D. J. (1972). *J. Appl. Bacteriol.* **35,** 361–365.
Powell, D. A., Hu, P. C., Wilson, M., Collier, A. M., and Baseman, J. B. (1976). *Infect. Immun.* **13,** 959–966.
Reed, S. E. (1971). *J. Infect. Dis.* **124,** 18–25.
Reed, S. E. (1972a). *In* "Pathogenic Mycoplasmas. CIBA Foundation Symposium" (K. Elliot and J. Birch, eds.), pp. 329–348. Associated Scientific Publishers, Amsterdam.
Reed, S. E. (1972b). *J. Comp. Pathol.* **82,** 267–278.
Reed, S. E. (1976). *In* "Organ Culture in Biomedical Research" (M. Balls and M. Monnickendam, Eds.), pp. 515–532. Cambridge Univ. Press, London and New York.
Stalheim, O. H. V., and Gallagher, J. E. (1975). *Am. J. Vet. Res.* **36,** 1077–1080.
Stalheim, O. H. V., and Gallagher, J. E. (1977). *Infect. Immun.* **15,** 995–996.

Stalheim, O. H. V., Proctor, S. J., and Gallagher, J. E. (1976). *Infect. Immun.* **13,** 915–925.

Taylor-Robinson, D., and Carney, F. E. (1974). *Br. J. Vener. Dis.* **50,** 212–216.

Taylor-Robinson, D., and Cherry, J. D. (1972). *J. Med. Microbiol.* **5,** 291–298.

Thomas, L. H., and Howard, C. J. (1974). *J. Comp. Pathol.* **84,** 193–201.

Westerberg, D. C., Smith, C. B., Wiley, B. B., and Jensen, C. (1972). *Infect. Immun.* **5,** 840–846.

Wilson, M. H., and Collier, A. M. (1976). *J. Bacteriol.* **125,** 332–339.

Woodruff, M. H., Schneider, E., Unger, L., and Coalson, J. J. (1973). *Am. J. Pathol.* **72,** 91–98.

SUBJECT INDEX